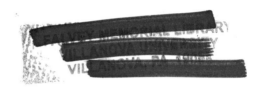

The
Psychoanalytic
Study
of the Child

VOLUME THIRTY-EIGHT

The Psychoanalytic Study of the Child

VOLUME THIRTY-EIGHT

New Haven
Yale University Press
1983

Designed by Sally Harris
and set in Baskerville type.
Printed in the United States of America by
Vail-Ballou Press, Inc., Binghamton, N.Y.

Library of Congress catalog card number: 45-11304
International standard book number: 0–300–03127–0
10   9   8   7   6   5   4   3   2   1

Anna Freud, one of the founding editors
of *The Psychoanalytic Study of the Child,*
died at her home in London on October 9, 1982.
A future volume will be dedicated to her.
The Editors

Contents

APPLICATIONS OF PSYCHOANALYSIS

In Memoriam
Marianne Kris

HENRY NUNBERG, M.D.

TWO YEARS HAVE PASSED SINCE THE DEATH OF MARIANNE Kris in London, at the home of Anna Freud, on November 23, 1980. Since then, we have had to learn to do without her unique talents of quiet leadership, sensitive understanding, and spirit of helpfulness. The passage of time has, if anything, made us all the more aware of her value to us. Her contributions to analysis, and in particular to the area of her own special interest, child analysis, were manifold, and endure in the scientific and educational legacy that she has left for us. Her legacy is a very special one: her meaning to our science was particularly hers, in that it depended so much on her personal qualities. She was a supreme teacher by example: her method and manner imparted not only knowledge to supervisees, students, and seekers of advice, but also an attitude and an approach to analysis that always took into account first of all the needs of patients. If ever she perceived that there was any chance that a conflict might arise between the aims of, for example, research and the interests of a patient, she would always choose the patient without a moment's hesitation—even if the chance of harm to the patient was remote. This attitude was a part of her view of psychoanalysis, and the requirements that she set for herself and imparted to all around her: as gentle and kind as she was, as tactful and patient with her students and others who consulted her, she always conveyed in a straightforward way her insistence on adherence to the basic principles of candor and

Read at the special Marianne Kris Memorial Meeting of the New York Society and Institute, November 9, 1982.

1

honesty both in self-examination and in dealing with others. An example was her Freud lecture which she would not publish even with disguises and modifications because of her concern that the patients might suffer. She insisted upon restricting the material for years to come. Although able to bring about compromises and resolve difficulties in practical situations, she was uncompromising in her adherence to these principles. Her adherence to principle included as well the need to meet the requirements of reality without resort to wishful or magical thinking.

She was not, however, a strict, superego-driven moralist. On the contrary: she had a mischievous streak, and a sense of humor about herself and others. She enjoyed life, and had the capacity to face hardships and difficulties with equanimity. She immersed herself to the full in all aspects of projects which interested her, in the same way that her attention was wholly focused upon the person with whom she was occupied—whether friend, relative, patient, supervisee, or colleague. She was a superb listener. She was as important to her relatives, as I can attest, as she was to her professional colleagues, for the good humor, equanimity, and sympathetic attention that went into her handling of the most difficult and delicate situations. She knew how to be a calm, unobtrusive presence, a talent which was appreciated especially by children. I recall her visits to my children when they were very young, and how immediately they were in comfortable communication with her. Children never felt that she was imposing her presence upon them. Her tolerance was such that she was inclined to persist where others would not, preferring to find a way to help a supervisee in difficulty, to improve a paper with drawbacks, and to treat a difficult patient. Her willingness to face difficulties in this way was based on her gentleness and regard for others. These were the characteristics which made her so avidly sought after as a supervisor, therapist, advisor, committee member and participant in seminars, projects and organizations. With all the demands on her time, it was a mark of her unique abilities that, in a field in which controversy and sharp disputes abound, she was loved and respected by so many.

Psychoanalysis was for Marianne Kris the encompassing expression of her interest in all aspects of life. She knew how to enjoy herself, whether at a dinner in her honor at the tenth anniversary celebration of the Association for Child Psychoanalysis, or taking photographs in family settings. It was an underlying cheerfulness, all the more striking in view of the depth and sincerity of her understanding and sympathy for the difficulties and pain of others. Perhaps this was in part because her capacity to understand was untainted by overidentification with others, again a quality which made her fit so perfectly into her profession. It seemed, indeed, as if she had been constitutionally endowed to become a psychoanalyst! With these perhaps innate qualifications, it was fortunate that she was born into the family of Dr. Oskar Rie, in 1900, just as Dr. Rie's close friend, Dr. Sigmund Freud, was developing the new science of psychoanalysis. The Rie and Freud families had close ties which lasted over more than one lifetime. Thus, the influence of psychoanalysis and its founder was of immense significance to the Rie family in many ways, an influence which was reflected in the personal ties of many members of the family to the circle of psychoanalysts.

Marianne knew from the age of 8 that she would become a physician. At 14, she thought about becoming a psychoanalyst, a decision which she crystallized at 19. She went to medical school, after having persuaded her at first reluctant father to allow her to prepare to become a doctor, and graduated in 1925. At that time, she went to Berlin and began analysis with Franz Alexander, at Freud's recommendation. Later, she was in analysis with Freud. Returning to Vienna, she married Ernst Kris in 1927.

In the Oral History interviews that she gave to the Institute, Marianne Kris recalled that her initial interest in medicine was to follow in her father's footsteps and become a pediatrician. When she later turned to psychoanalysis, she nevertheless retained her original interest in working with children. Through this interest, she was led into closer association with Anna Freud, who became her teacher and supervisor; it was from this connection that their firm adult friendship grew. Marianne's marriage to Ernst Kris was in itself an important event for the future of psychoanalysis, since it was through Marianne that

Ernst was introduced to Freud, and developed his serious interest in psychoanalysis. As was the rest of her life, Marianne's marriage was thus intertwined with psychoanalysis. The association of the Freud and Kris families continued through the disruptions brought about by the approach of war. Nearly simultaneously, the two families fled from Vienna to London in 1938. The Krises, with their two children, continued their journey two years later, arriving in New York in 1940, after a hazardous sea voyage during which they were constantly exposed to the danger of being torpedoed by Nazi submarines. Ernst began teaching at the New School for Social Research and established a psychoanalytic practice. Marianne, in addition to teaching and seeing some patients, took care of the children and prepared to take the examination required of immigrants to obtain a license to practice medicine. Thus, it was not until 1944 that she officially became a member of the New York Psychoanalytic Institute and Society, notwithstanding her membership in the Vienna Society from 1927 on, and her position as a training analyst in the British Psycho-Analytical Society from 1938 to 1940. The lack of official position did not, however, prevent her from playing an important role in the institute from the time of her arrival. She and Berta Bornstein, who was already established in New York by the time that Marianne Kris arrived, were the first teachers of child analysis in the New York Institute's program. Marianne Kris immediately began teaching a continuous case seminar in the technique of child analysis. She accepted as participants not only physicians, but also lay people with a professional interest in children who she felt were gifted as child analysts, with the proviso that they contributed to the seminar by presenting cases. She did not want passive observers. She felt that all analysts should, in the course of their training, become familiar with child analysis and learn about it, but she did not advocate that all candidates undertake the analysis of a child case. She was instrumental in introducing the child development sequence into the general curriculum. Most recently, she approved of the introduction of the current alternating continuous case seminar.

For Marianne Kris, there never was a sharp demarcation between the interests of her professional and personal life. Her understanding of life was imbued with the concepts and principles of psychoanalysis. This was clear in the context of her interest, along with Anna Freud, in the application of psychoanalytic understanding to extra-analytic situations, in particular to those involving children. Her work with educators and social workers at the Jewish Board of Guardians was an example of this outlook, as was her participation in the studies of children on kibbutzim, with Peter Neubauer and others. Her thinking was primarily oriented toward the practical and current. There was never the sense that she thought of psychoanalysis in terms of abstruse or difficult concepts which had meaning apart from their relationship to the stuff of life. Her research interests had the same quality, and reflected her interest in the clinical; she handled theoretical concepts as expressions of the reality of what she saw, heard, and felt. In the longitudinal studies at Yale, when a predicted outcome failed to occur, as in the cases that she described in her paper on prediction (1957), she sought explanations for the failure in the nature of the facts of the situation and the manifold nature of the variables involved. She did not concern herself particularly with more removed questions of metapsychology.

With the start of the association of Ernst with Milton Senn at the Yale Child Study Center, Marianne also began her long association with that project. From the beginning, her activities were clinical, concerned with the direct observation of children. In later years, when Marianne was asked to take over the chairmanship of the project, she took advantage of the opportunity presented by the fact that some members of a family were in analysis to study the analyses comparatively and thereby to gain an in-depth understanding of family interaction. At the time of Ernst's death, only some members of the family were in analysis. Marianne, responding to what she felt was important clinically, was instrumental in bringing the other members of the family into analysis. In a sense, it was the reverse of what had been the earlier procedure: she took advantage of an opportunity that presented itself as the basis for the study, rather than proceeding from a theoretical concern to a study design. In seminars and meetings, the same characteristics governed her: I remember particularly her ability to redirect and focus discussions in a seminar on reconstruction of the Psychoanalytic Research and Development Fund, in which the often highly developed reconstructive abilities of the participants tended at times to outstrip the data at hand. Marianne Kris gently but firmly reminded us that speculations were not, after all, data, and should not be mistaken as such!

Her tact and ability to compromise gave her a special place in the institutions and organizations of psychoanalysis. She did not like the limelight, so that her work was without fanfare, and thus more effective. In response to a perceived need, she was instrumental in organizing, in 1966, the Association for Child Analysis, an achievement of which she was justly proud. Sometimes, it seemed that she surprised herself by her achievements. Her feeling about the association was one of "I really did it!" As confident and energetic as she was in certain ways, she was genuinely modest and appraised herself and her abilities with a realistic eye, governing herself always according to the requirements of reality. She was able to see herself clearly, just as she had such a lucid and profound perception of her patients. That ability to perceive clearly was invaluable to me on those occasions when a knotty clinical problem required consultation.

In her long association with the New York Psychoanalytic Institute, these same qualities were invaluable to the contributions that she made in helping to shape and give a sense of direction to the child analytic program. In subsequent years, she was involved in child analytic programs in two other institutes in this city as well; each of them profited immensely from her association with them.

Of the many projects and activities in which she was involved, none was more important to Marianne Kris than her long association with Hampstead and Anna Freud, with whom she spent virtually every summer after the war, and in whose work she was intimately involved. It is sad that now we must mourn Anna Freud's death too, and reflect that, indeed, an era in psychoanalysis has passed. The close friendship of Marianne Kris with Anna Freud, which, as we have seen, had its origins far back in childhood, had professional as well as personal significance for both of them. From the early days of the "If I Were King" seminar in Vienna until the last day of Marianne Kris's life, their professional lives touched upon each other.

For many of us, I think that Marianne Kris represented the ideal of what a psychoanalyst should be: one who has a profound appreciation of unconscious life, together with a capacity for facing with honesty and courage the reality of life, self-aware and able to convey to others the importance of those qualities for the pursuit of psychoanalytic knowledge; who, withal, had a deep and abiding concern for human beings, with a desire to be helpful in the predicaments of their lives. In dedicating this volume to her, we celebrate these qualities, in the hope that in our own pursuit of psychoanalytic knowledge, each of us will try to be worthy of her memory.

On the Process of Mourning

JEANNE LAMPL-DE GROOT, M.D.

IN 1922, WHEN I CAME TO VIENNA TO BE TRAINED IN PSYCHO-
analysis, I met Marianne Rie, who then was still a medical student. We soon became friends. Marianne was a warm, lovely
young girl, perhaps a little shy. But so was I at that time. Later
on I moved to Berlin to gain more experience at the Berlin
institute, which was then the best and most flourishing psychoanalytic training center. I married Dr. Hans Lampl and, in
1933, when Hitler came to power, we again settled in Vienna,
Hans's birthplace. In the meantime the psychoanalytic scene
had changed. The Vienna psychoanalytic society and institute
had become prominent, with a number of young, bright, and
gifted analysts working there productively. Whereas in my
Berlin days Marianne and I had met only occasionally, we saw
much of each other in the '30s. Marianne, too, had married. As
a wife and mother, she had become a mature woman, as lovely
and likable as she had always been. Moreover, having completed her training, she became a valued colleague.

We were separated again in 1938 when Hitler overran Austria. Our friends emigrated mostly to England and the United
States, as did the Kris family. We went to Holland, my native
country. Good fortune allowed us to survive the German occupation. After the war, in 1946, Hans and I were invited by
our friends to the States, where we renewed our friendships
and saw a good deal of Marianne once more. We also continued
to meet at congresses and other analytic scientific meetings.

After both of us were widowed, Marianne in 1957 and I in
1958, the two of us became even closer. We always got together
whenever I went to New York or she came to England. In the
'70s we were together quite a few times with Anna Freud and

9

Dorothy Burlingham. The "four old ladies" had many a good time together.

ON THE MOURNING PROCESS IN CHILDREN

In 1976, I wrote a paper on "Mourning in a 6-Year-Old Girl" that originally was written in honor of Marianne on the occasion of her 75th birthday. Marianne wrote to me that she liked it very much, especially because she agreed with me that a child who has achieved some structuralization of the mind is capable of mourning the death of a beloved person in a way that is not much different from an adult's reaction, whereas many authors continue to deny a child's capacity to mourn.[1]

This is in sharp contrast to the overuse of the term "mourning" that has become prevalent in recent years. Some analysts describe the reaction to disappointments, frustrations, loss of love, the experience of powerlessness, feeling injured, etc., as mourning. For example, a younger colleague asked me how a postoedipal child copes with his "mourning." I think that this extended use of mourning blurs the precision of a valuable psychoanalytic concept. In analytic theory (Freud, 1917), mourning is a *process* that includes the gradual coping with the distress and pain caused by the *death* of a beloved one and the bereaved person's ability finally to invest another object with "libido" (as Freud called it originally, but later on widened to "drive energy").

In my 1976 paper I suggested the idea that an infant and preoedipal child lack the capacity to do just that. The very young child may feel bewilderment, pain, longing, distress, etc., but he or she is not able to cope with the finality of death and to shift libido to another object. The infant's reaction to death does not yet differ from his response to a parent's brief absence, or to being reprimanded by an angry mother, because the very young child has not yet acquired a cognitive notion of "future."

The postoedipal child, the adolescent, and the adult, however, *have* learned that absence of a love object does not mean

1. See Furman (1974) for a comprehensive review.

"forever," whereas death does. Thus, if the oedipal disappointment of the child is referred to as "mourning," the term is misused. The postoedipal child does not actually *lose* the parent whom he wants to be his sexual love object. A relationship continues to exist, though a much more ambivalent one, sometimes with more hostility and hate than sublimated love. In fact, individual reactions may differ very much; but one can observe that the actual death of a beloved one—parent, sibling, or grandparent—usually has a more traumatic impact than the estrangement caused by disappointments and frustrations due to lack of fulfillment of infantile sexual desires and fantasies.

Latency children, adolescents, and adults know intellectually that a dead person never returns; emotionally they all more or less deny this fact. In pathological cases, the denial cannot be corrected. If it overwhelms the personality, some circumscribed delusions may take hold of part of the personality and continue to exist in the unconscious. In extreme cases, a delusional psychosis may be the outcome. Various inner and outer factors determine whether a mourning process will lead to a "normal" or to a "disturbed" mental life. Among the many factors I draw attention to three: (1) a person's ability to master his unconscious guilt feelings and his need for punishment due to repressed infantile death wishes toward the deceased parent or sibling; (2) the overcoming of his unconscious triumph over the deceased: "You are dead, I am alive"—the survivor guilt; (3) the capability to sublimate destructive impulses into constructive activities.

MOURNING IN ADULT LIFE

In our middle years we encounter some age-specific life crises and losses, but I believe that here too we should not speak of mourning unless the event involves the death of a beloved person. Women in the menopause around age 50 may feel depressed, worthless, and weak. In my opinion, this is a neurotic reaction, as many women cope very well with the normal physiological process that ends the period of propagation and the ability to give birth to a child. Much depends upon their wish and capability to find other fields of activity.

With men one also speaks of "menopause." Some men feel distressed when their physical strength diminishes. They may become conscious of a fear of death and an anxiety about the prospect of their sexual potency diminishing. The latter, too, is a neurotic overanxiety. Sexual potency can be retained into old age. A depressive state of mind points to the reemergence of a neurotic disposition. Of course, if a life partner, a child, or another beloved relative dies, we expect a mourning process to start, but it may run the "normal" course already described.

Another typical distress that needs to be overcome during this phase of life is presented by the fact that children become independent adults and leave the parental home. But this belongs to the normal course of life as well. Much joy and satisfaction can be found in a grandparent's position, as well as in work and social activities, whether it is housework such as cooking and sewing and carpentry, or intellectual and artistic occupations, or a job performed outside the home.

As we grow older, other tasks confront us. One of the main ones concerns retirement from work. Most institutions in Western countries set a mandatory retirement age around 65 to 70 years. At present, however, there is a trend in many countries toward increasingly lowering the age of retirement—a trend that is dictated by economic and political factors rather than a person's ability to perform his job. From a psychological point of view, it is remarkable to observe the many differences in people's reaction to forced retirement. Some feel relieved, especially if their work was unsatisfactory or performed in an unpleasant environment. They may feel even "younger" and busy themselves with hobbies, ranging from painting and redecorating their house, gardening, taking trips, reading, studying, writing, to pursuing many forms of art. Others are distressed, desolate, angry, or depressed, and feel themselves to be real old-agers. They may even look many years older and become prone to hypochondriasis and fantasied physical illnesses or in fact undergo a rapidly accelerated aging process.

Old age—and I leave open the question when it starts—brings other important losses. The strength of the body declines; many organs fail to function well; mobility may be restricted; in some instances memory and other psychological functions may be diminished. All these contribute to a sense of loss of a self that cannot be regained. While I personally believe that the term mourning should be restricted to the actual loss of a love object, others might be inclined to include narcissistic considerations and extend the term mourning to parts of the self that have indeed been irretrievably lost, though here too interests may be channeled into new directions, comparable to a bereaved person's investment of new objects.

But old-agers not only have to confront the decline of their own capacities. They have usually lost, and continue to do so, very many persons dear to their hearts—parents and other relatives, marital partners, possibly children or grandchildren, and usually very many, more or less intimate friends. How can one cope with so many bereavements? How can one master the pain and distress, the feelings of loneliness and abandonment? How can an old-ager shift not only his or her libido but also the need for warmth, closeness, sharing thoughts and interests, etc., to new objects?

Some people even in their 80s and 90s might find new outlets and interests and under favorable conditions actually do. The individual variations of the mourning process are great indeed. But with declining age the opportunities for finding new love objects actually decrease. Perhaps what old people cathect instead are the memories of their past positive and satisfying relations. Retaining fine and happy memories is a wonderful blessing. Marianne left me many of them, for which I am very thankful.

BIBLIOGRAPHY

FREUD, S. (1917), Mourning and melancholia. *S.E.*, 14:237–260.
FURMAN, E. (1974), *A Child's Parent Dies.* New Haven & London: Yale Univ. Press.
LAMPL-DE GROOT, J. (1976), Mourning in a 6-year-old girl. *Psychoanal. Study Child*, 31:273–281.

SCIENTIFIC ASPECTS
OF PSYCHOANALYSIS

Freud's Use of Metaphor

JONATHAN T. EDELSON

IN 1930, SIGMUND FREUD RECEIVED THE GOETHE PRIZE FOR literature. No doubt, his masterful use of metaphor was a consideration in the awarding of this prize. Though Freud was a superb writer, as a scientist he was writing not merely to entertain but to inform. Metaphor in Freud's work is not a mere decorative flourish. Metaphor is a necessary part of Freud's formulation and exposition of his scientific theories. Therefore, much can be learned about Freud's work by studying the diverse roles metaphors play in his writings.

First, the metaphors orient Freud's readers to his place in intellectual history. They place him at a point of convergence of various intellectual currents.

Second, in part, Freud established himself at this nexus by using metaphors subtly to gain and hold his readers' attention. Metaphors helped ease the way to acceptance of Freud's work.

More important than their rhetorical value, however, metaphors were cognitively essential in Freud's introduction of a new scientific theory. Most scientific theories cannot even be formulated let alone comprehended without the use of metaphor. Freud's theories are no exception. Freud (1900) found metaphors particularly useful in formulating and explicating his theory of dreams. Probably the unique relationship obtaining between dreams and metaphors had something to do with

Philosophy major at Yale University (B.A., 1981); currently, third-year student at the University of Chicago Pritzker School of Medicine.

George Mahl read an earlier version of a part of this paper and encouraged me to prepare it for publication. I have, of course, benefited from a lifetime of discussions with Marshall Edelson, who kindled my interest in both psychoanalysis and language.

this. However, even in *The Interpretation of Dreams,* Freud's use of metaphor can be understood best in the context of a general explanation of why all scientists find it necessary to use metaphor in introducing new scientific theories.

Finally, Freud used metaphors to unify. Metaphors helped him to create a coherent picture of the interrelationships between his clinical hypotheses and his topographic and structural theories. Metaphors lent continuity to Freud's transition from his topographic to his structural theory. Metaphors integrate the various domains to which Freud applied his theory of the mind.

In this essay, I shall largely confine myself to examining Freud's use of metaphor in *The Interpretation of Dreams,* which from the point of view of science is exemplary. Unless otherwise indicated, when I refer to Freud's use of metaphor, I refer to his use of metaphor in this book. Only in discussing Freud's use of metaphor as he moves from his topographic to his structural theory will I have cause to examine the use of metaphor in his other works.

METAPHORS AND A SENSE OF HISTORY

The reader of *The Interpretation of Dreams* is struck by the variety of metaphors, which indicate the intellectual streams that came together to form the river of Freud's thought. Kearney (1971) identifies three intellectual traditions that came together to form the scientific revolution during the Renaissance: the Aristotelian or organic current; the magical current; and the mechanistic current. Kearney examined the kind of language each scientist used to identify which scientists of this revolution were most influenced by which of these currents. Each tradition had its own special language, its own imagery or figures of speech. The imagery of each current acts like a radioactively tagged molecule introduced into a stream of water. Even after the stream has merged into a river, the course of the water molecules from it can be followed by following the movements of the tagged molecules. Examining the imagery Freud uses identifies the intellectual traditions that influenced him.

The mechanistic tradition came to dominate Western science

after the scientific revolution. Mechanistic language was used by most postrevolutionary scientists. This language consists of mathematics and the imagery of mechanics. Not surprisingly, Freud (1900) used it. He repeatedly described the mind as a "mental instrument" (pp. 511, 607). He writes that one should attempt to discover the "mechanics of the processes" of this mental instrument (p. 599). He describes the mental instrument in optical terms: "I propose simply to follow the suggestion that we should picture the instrument which carries out our mental functions as resembling a compound microscope or a photographic apparatus, or something of the kind" (p. 536). And again:

> Everything that can be an object of our internal perception is *virtual*, like the image produced in a telescope by the passage of light-rays. But we are justified in assuming the existence of the systems . . . like the lenses of the telescope, which cast the image. And, if we pursue this analogy, we may compare the censorship between two systems to the refraction which takes place when a ray of light passes into a new medium [p. 611].

The reader also finds mechanistic imagery from the field of electronics: "The new connections [found in analyzing a dream] are, as it were, loop-lines or short-circuits, made possible by the existence of other and deeper-lying connecting paths" (p. 280). Later in the work, Freud refers to the point where two associative paths connect as a "switch-point" (p. 410). Freud also refers to these switch-points as "nodal-points," an image borrowed from wave physics (pp. 283, 340).

Even stronger evidence of the influence of the mechanistic tradition is to be found in Freud's central postulate of psychic determinism. Sulloway (1979) notes that "Freud's entire life's work in science was characterized by an abiding faith in the notion that all vital phenomena, including psychical ones, are rigidly and lawfully determined by the principle of cause and effect" (p. 94). The postulate of psychic determinism is a relative of the Newtonian axiom of physical determinism.

Kearney (1971) points to Pythagoras as one of the founding fathers of the magical tradition. While, as time passes, traditions have a tendency to become more diluted in the mainstream of thought, as do tagged molecules of a stream in a river, they do not disappear. While I find no metaphors to suggest Freud was influenced by the magical tradition, I do not think it absurd to assert that he was. Sulloway (1979) has documented that Freud was heavily influenced by this tradition through Fliess, a Pythagorean firmly ensconced in the magical tradition. Further, Fliess was not the last scientist to be influenced by this tradition. It is common knowledge that the twentieth-century physicist Heisenberg was a self-professed Pythagorean, believing in the magical, mystical power of numbers.

There is no question that the Aristotelean or organic tradition strongly influenced Freud, probably through his study of biology. Biology has its roots in the work of Aristotle, the so-called father of biology. Freud's psychological model of the mind is based on a model of the nervous system that was prominent when he studied biology as a young man: the reflex arc. In chapter 7, Freud (1900) writes that "the psychical apparatus must be constructed like a reflex apparatus. Reflex processes remain the model of every psychical function" (p. 538).

The figurative language of the organic tradition is not mechanistic. This language is domestic, drawn from the familiar, referring to mundane organic and political objects. *The Interpretation of Dreams* is saturated with organic figurative language. Some examples are:

> Dreams give way before the impressions of the new day just as the brilliance of the stars yields to the light of the sun [p. 45].
>
> When in the course of a piece of scientific work we come upon a problem which is difficult to solve, it is often a good plan to take up a second problem along with the original one— just as it is easier to crack two nuts together than separately [p. 135f.].
>
> The apparently innocent dreams turn out to be quite the reverse when we take the trouble to analyze them. They are, if I may say so, wolves in sheep's clothing [p. 183].

While these are rather short and simple examples, longer and more elaborate ones can be found. Freud describes how, in the formulation of a dream, somatic sources of stimulation during sleep

... are treated like some cheap material always ready to hand, which is employed whenever it is needed, in contrast to a precious material which itself prescribes the way in which it shall be employed. If, to take a simile, a patron of the arts brings an artist some rare stone, such as a piece of onyx, and asks him to create a work of art from it, then the size of the stone, its colour and markings, help to decide what head or what scene shall be represented in it. Whereas in the case of a uniform and plentiful material such as marble or sandstone, the artist merely follows some idea that is present in his own mind. It is only in this way, so it seems to me, that we can explain the fact that dream-content provided by somatic stimuli of no unusual intensity fails to appear in every dream or every night [p. 237f.].

Perhaps Freud's most elaborate metaphor in the organic tradition is his "entrepreneur-capitalist" metaphor:

A daytime thought may very well play the part of *entrepreneur* for a dream; but the *entrepreneur*, who, as people say, has the idea and the initiative to carry it out, can do nothing without capital; he needs a *capitalist* who can afford the outlay, and the capitalist who provides the psychical outlay for the dream is invariably and indisputably, whatever may be the thoughts of the previous day, *a wish from the unconscious* [p. 561].

This example points not only to the fertility of Freud's imagination but also to an important characteristic of Freud's use of organic language. He has anthropomorphized his theoretical construction of the mind into a miniature society. Besides entrepreneurs and capitalists, Freud has peopled the mind with borrowers, compromisers, guardians and watchmen, fools, mathematicians, paralytics, and dentists (pp. 564, 580, 233, 567, 444, 451, 555, 563). The society of the mind comes complete with politics: politicians, the public, dissenting newspapers, and censors (pp. 142, 144, 471, 516, 529).

In some ways, this sort of language seems outdated. One would expect it from a fifteenth-century prescientific revolution poet, rather than from a twentieth-century scientist. Freud seems more an Elizabethan than a Victorian. In *The Elizabethan World Picture*, Tillyard (1944) writes of a world view in which the world is filled with "correspondences." One of these correspondences was between the body politic and the microcosm of the body:

> The best known instance of this correspondence is in *Julius Caesar,* when Brutus, greatly perplexed, says, "Between the acting of a dreadful thing/ And the first motion, all the interim is/ Like a phantasma or a hideous dream./ The genius and the mortal instruments/ Are then in council; and the state of man/ Like to a little kingdom, suffers then/ The nature of an insurrection." It is a wonderfully full comparison. The commotion in the mind of man, the debate within the highest faculties of understanding and will and the executive faculties such as speech and motion, are likened to a debate of king and council [p. 94].

That Freud used this typically Elizabethan imagery does not necessarily reflect poorly on the scientific status of his work. The imagery merely places Freud in a tradition which, as Tillyard notes, goes all the way back to Plato. In fact, Temkin (1977) says that this tradition goes back even further to the pre-Socratic philosopher Alcmaeon. Freud is in good company. For example, William Harvey used organic metaphors in dedicating his masterwork *De Motu* to Prince Charles:

> The heart of animals is . . . the sovereign of everything within them. . . . The king, in like manner, is . . . the heart of the republic. . . . What I have here written of the motions of the heart I am more emboldened to present to your Majesty, according to the custom of the present age, because almost all things are done after human examples, and many things in a king are after the pattern of the heart [p. 3].

The scientific status of Harvey's work is considered to be exemplary. For his discovery that the function of the heart is to circulate a constant quantity of blood, Harvey is generally recognized as the father of modern biology and medicine.

Like Aristotle, Freud too was a teleologist. The teleological argument was the hallmark of Aristotle's physics, biology, and metaphysics. The influence of Aristotle's teleology on Freud is well illustrated by the following comment Freud (1900) makes as he tries to construct criteria for reviewing theories of dreaming and its function: "It need not necessarily be possible to infer a *function* of dreaming (whether utilitarian or otherwise) from the theory. Nevertheless, since we have a habit of looking for teleological explanations, we shall be more ready to accept theories which are bound up with the attribution of a function to dreaming" (p. 75).

One should not attack the scientific status of Freud's work just because he is a teleologist unless one is prepared to indict the rest of modern biology as well. As Hull (1974) wrote, "one might object, evolutionary theory did away with teleology, and that is that. Yet, the biological phenomena that gave rise to the idea of teleology are still with us, and biologists still continue to talk teleologically" (p. 101).

Metaphors as a Rhetorical Device

The influence of the Aristotelian tradition on Freud was probably not the only reason Freud used so many organic metaphors. Whether Freud was conscious of it or not, the use of organic metaphors was a clever tactic in propagating his work. By including so many organic metaphors, Freud made his work more accessible to members of the lay public, who would have had difficulty understanding technical, mechanistic metaphors.[1]

The philosopher Feyerabend (1979) believed that Galileo prospered scientifically "because of his style and his clever techniques of persuasion, because he writes in Italian rather than in Latin, and because he appeals to people who are temperamentally opposed to the old ideas and the standard of learning

1. In particular, Freud's use of the organic macrocosm-microcosm metaphor, by which he describes the mind in terms of a miniature society, serves, in addition to its other functions, a special function in making his work accessible to the lay public. A phenomenon such as dreaming is more easily understood if it is seen in a wider context. Freud (1900) states that a theory of dreams should define "the position occupied by dreams in a wider sphere of phenomena" (p. 75). Macrocosm-microcosm metaphors help to locate the phenomenon of dreams in this wider sphere. Temkin (1977) writes that macrocosm-microcosm metaphors serve "to co-ordinate the interests of our human life and the science of life. When the picture of the world and the spheres of interest changed, the metaphors of human biology tend to change, too" (p. 282).

connected with them" (p. 141). Like Galileo, Freud was aiming his work toward a new audience, not necessarily just the established scientific community. Further evidence to support this contention comes from the fact that, unlike his predecessors and contemporaries, when Freud refers to sexuality, he mostly uses his native German, not the concealing scientific Latin.

There are sound reasons justifying a scientist in attempting to find a new audience for his work. A scientist who worked all his life using and seeing the world through one paradigm (Kuhn, 1970) or theoretical predicate (Stegmüller, 1976) is loathe to change to a new paradigm or theoretical predicate. The most likely converts to a new paradigm or theoretical predicate are either the young scientist not yet steeped in an old theory or those who have been educated by, but are not within, the orthodoxy of mainstream science. Kuhn (1970) presents historical evidence illustrating how difficult it is for a "revolutionary" scientist to find a supportive audience for his work.

> Copernicanism made few converts for almost a century after Copernicus' death. Newton's work was not generally accepted, particularly on the Continent, for more than half a century after the *Principia* appeared. Priestley never accepted the oxygen theory, nor Lord Kelvin the electromagnetic theory, and so on. The difficulties of conversion have often been noted by the scientists themselves. Darwin, in a particularly perceptive passage at the end of his *Origin of Species,* writes: "Although I am fully convinced of the truth of the views given in this volume . . . I by no means expect to convince experienced naturalists whose minds are stocked with a multitude of facts viewed, during a long course of years, from a point of view directly opposite to mine . . . but I look with confidence to the future,—to young and rising naturalists, who will be able to view both sides of the question with impartiality" [p. 151].

So it was that Freud, in using German instead of Latin, and in using a profusion of organic metaphors instead of just mechanistic ones, was attempting to win an audience different from those steeped in the scientifically orthodox, mechanistic, somatically ruled view of the mind. Wolf (1971) points out that while Freud did not consciously intend it, his artful use of metaphor not only failed to win over this orthodoxy but positively offended it. Wolf believes that the eloquence of Freud's metaphors led Krafft-Ebing to call Freud's work a "scientific fairy tale" (Jones, 1953, p. 263).

Stegmüller (1976) states that it is not rhetorical tricks or "tactical moves" that determine whether a new scientific theory will replace an old scientific theory: "The victor of this contest is—despite all the beguiling talk of Kuhn and Feyerabend—not he who concocts the best propaganda for the scientific mob, or any other, but he who accomplishes all that his predecessor did and then some" (p. 218). While Stegmüller is probably right that rhetoric is not necessary for victory, the cause of Freud or other scientists introducing new theories cannot be hurt and is in fact often aided by the effective use of rhetoric. The lubricant of rhetoric is not necessary for progressive movement in science, but it surely makes the going easier.

METAPHORS AND DREAMS

The importance of metaphors as rhetoric in Freud's work is minor in comparison with the cognitive value of Freud's use of metaphor. I begin with a consideration of the cognitive value of metaphor by examining the special relationship that obtains between metaphors and dreams.

The dreamwork characterizes the mechanisms by which the unconscious works. Included among these mechanisms is one which can essentially be seen as creating metaphors. Freud (1900) writes, "Parallels or instances of 'just as' inherent in the material of the dream-thoughts constitute the first foundations for the construction of a dream; and no inconsiderable part of the dream-work consists in creating fresh parallels where those which are already present cannot find their way into the dream owing to the censorship imposed by resistance" (p. 320). Employing Chomsky's linguistic theories, M. Edelson (1972) adds that "unusual transformations of syntactically acceptable deep structures are probably involved in generating a metaphor. The dreamwork might very well include such unusual transformations" (p. 218).

The dreamwork is capable of creating isomorphic structures by taking the structure of one sentence, thought, or scene, stripping the structure of its content, and then filling the bare structure with the new content of the dream that the analyst finally analyzes. Freud (1900) fashions the rhetorical question: "Were not the formal structure of these sentences [describing the dream] and their antithetical meaning precisely the same as in the dream-thoughts I had uncovered?" (p. 424). A metaphor creates the same sort of isomorphism between "the implicative complex" of "the primary subject" and "the implicative complex" of "the secondary subject" of the metaphor.

THE TECHNICAL ANALYSIS OF METAPHOR

What is a metaphor? What are the primary and secondary subjects of the metaphor? What is an implicative complex? A metaphor "expresses an analogy" (Leatherdale, 1974, p. 224). And an analogy is a "correspondence in some respects, especially in function or position, between things otherwise dissimilar" (*American Heritage Dictionary*, 1969, p. 47). The philosopher Black (1980) states that "every metaphor may be said to mediate an analogy or structural correspondence" (p. 31). A metaphorical statement has two parts, to be identified respectively as the "primary" and "secondary" subjects. Freud (1900) attributes the metaphor, "the madman is a waking dreamer" (p. 90), to Kant. The primary subject of this metaphor is the madman. The secondary subject is the waking dreamer.

The implicative complex of the primary subject is the structure of relations between objects and ideas evoked by the primary subject. Similarly, the implicative complex of the secondary subject is the structure of relations between objects and ideas evoked by the secondary subject. Basically, a metaphor works when the hearer understands or sees the primary subject in terms of the implicative complex of the secondary subject. (For the purposes of this essay, metaphors and similes will be considered to be essentially the same device.[2])

2. A simile will be considered "a mere stylistic variation upon the metaphorical form" (Black, 1980, p. 32). A simile can be viewed as a weak version of a metaphor. As Black writes, "In discursively comparing one subject *with* another, we sacrifice the distinctive power and effectiveness of a good metaphor. The literal comparison lacks the ambience and suggestiveness, and the imposed 'view' of the primary subject, upon which a metaphor's power to illuminate depends" (p. 32).

DREAMS AS METAPHOR

Condensation in the dream works like a metaphor. A single element in the manifest content of the dream becomes an emblem for an expanded number of thoughts or associations. In a metaphor, it is the same process; the primary and secondary subjects become emblems for their implicative complexes.

Freud presents numerous examples of dreams which express metaphorical thoughts. In one dream, Freud urinates on a toilet seat to clean it: "what at once occurred to me in the analysis were the Augean stables which were cleaned by Hercules. This Hercules was I" (p. 469). This dream creates a metaphor in which Freud is Hercules. Freud is the primary subject of the metaphor. Owing to the egotistical nature of most if not all dreams, most if not all dreams create metaphors in which the primary subject is the dreamer.

Maury's "guillotine" dream is another example of a dream expressing a metaphorical thought. Maury believes himself to be in France at the time of the bloody Reign of Terror. Maury dreams he is about to be guillotined. The apparent stimulus for the dream is the impact of a piece of wood on Maury's neck, while he was sleeping. Commenting on this dream, Freud envisions the dreamwork as creating a metaphor out of this physical stimulus: "If the piece of wood had struck the back of Maury's neck while he was awake, there would have been an opportunity for some such thought as: 'That's just like being guillotined.' But since it was in his sleep that he was struck by the board, the dream-work made use of the impinging stimulus in order rapidly to produce a wish-fulfilment" (p. 496).

The obvious similarities between creating dreams and metaphors and, more importantly, in understanding them, points to an explanation of why Freud not only used so many metaphors but also used them so deliberately. Freud forces the reader to learn to think in terms of metaphors. The psychoanalyst needs a good implicit understanding of the metaphorical process in order to perform dream analysis because dreams are constructed out of metaphors. One could view the extensive use of metaphors in *The Interpretation of Dreams* as an actual training for dream interpretation. In order to understand the concepts

Freud expounds, the reader must understand the metaphors by which Freud introduces the concepts.

Freud makes numerous explicit references to his use of metaphor, thereby demonstrating that not only was he conscious of it but he also wanted his readers to be conscious of it. For example, Freud writes, "If I may venture on a simile from the sphere of psychiatry, the first group of theories construct dreams on the model of paranoia, while the second group make them resemble mental deficiency or confusional states" (p. 76). Another example is to be found when Freud writes of Robert's view of dreams, which holds that dreams "are somatic processes occurring every night in the apparatus that is concerned with mental activity, and they have as their function the task of protecting that apparatus from excessive tension—or, to change the metaphor—of acting as scavengers of the mind" (p. 80). And another example: "I hope I may be forgiven for drawing my analogies from everyday life, but I am tempted to say that the position of a repressed idea resembles that of an American dentist in this country: he is not allowed to set up in practice unless he can make use of a legally qualified medical practitioner to serve as a stalking-horse and to act as a 'cover' in the eyes of the law" (p. 563).[3]

The passage which best represents the deliberate attitude Freud has toward his use of metaphor occurs when he comments on his compound microscope metaphor:

> I see no necessity to apologize for the imperfections of this or of any similar imagery. Analogies of this kind are only intended to assist us in our attempt to make the complications of mental functioning intelligible by dissecting the function and assigning its different constituents to different component parts of the apparatus. So far as I know, the experiment has not hitherto been made of using this method of dissection in order to investigate the way in which the mental instrument is put together, and I see no harm in it. We are justified, in my

3. In fact, the reader can find over a dozen more explicit conscious references to the use of metaphor (pp. 90, 141, 144, 284, 467, 471, 491, 528, 530, 561, 595, 599, 610, 615).

view, in giving free rein to our speculations so long as we retain the coolness of our judgment and do not mistake the scaffolding for the building. And since at our first approach to something unknown all that we need is the assistance of provisional ideas, I shall give preference in the first instance to hypotheses of the crudest and most concrete description" [p. 536].

[And on p. 610:] we must always be prepared to drop our conceptual scaffolding if we feel that we are in a position to replace it by something that approximates more closely to the unknown reality.

These passages illustrate what I choose to call the "static" and "dynamic" use of metaphor. The static use of metaphor, which I have just illustrated, calls attention to and helps the reader understand the static structure of the finished dream. The dynamic use of metaphor is Freud's repeated pattern of replacing bad metaphors with good metaphors and good metaphors with better metaphors; e.g., replacing one metaphor with another that "approximates more closely to the unknown reality." The dynamic use of metaphor aids the reader in understanding the dynamic process of dream analysis.

Dream analysis consists in discovering the hidden unconscious wish (or wishes) being fulfilled by the dream. The wishes are hidden by the many transformations of the dreamwork. The analysis of the dream involves plowing through and discarding layer upon layer of disguises hiding the dream-wish. The analyst starts with the manifest content as the initial disguise. Through free association (on the analysand's part) and dream interpretation (on the analyst's part), the analyst comes to an interpretation; a motive-wish of the dream is discovered. For example, in analyzing his own Irma dream, Freud discusses a number of wishes which motivated the construction of the dream: various forms of his desire for revenge and his desire to prove his professional conscientiousness. However, these motive-wishes are not necessarily the "true" motive-wishes behind the dream. By "true" motive-wish, I mean the unconscious infantile wish which, according to Freud, is a necessary condition for the construction of any dream. In analyzing the Irma

dream, Freud notes that for two reasons he has not attempted
to find this basic wish: the analysis would take too long; and it
could prove embarrassing.

For Freud, an inadequate metaphor is something that must
be immediately replaced by another, disposed of, or bypassed
like the manifest content of a dream. This is not to say that an
inadequate metaphor or the manifest content is in any way
unessential. The scientist creating a metaphor as well as the
analyst interpreting a dream must have a starting point. After
disposing of the manifest content or inadequate metaphor, one
reaches intermediate motive-wishes or temporarily adequate
scientific metaphors. However, the investigator cannot stop
here. He must strive for the hidden unconscious infantile wish
or the hidden reality. The intermediate motive-wishes as well as
the temporarily adequate scientific metaphors must be replaced by new and deeper motive-wishes and metaphors. Commenting on the metaphors he has used to describe the structure
of the mind, Freud writes, "Let us replace these metaphors by
something that seems to correspond better to the real state of
affairs" (p. 610).

The literary critic Hyman (1974) says of this statement by
Freud that "since this turns out to be only a better metaphor,
we realize that his metaphors *are* his vision of reality" (p. 334).
Hyman is correct if by his statement he means that Freud saw
the world through his metaphors. All scientists do likewise.
Everyone's vision of reality is theory-laden, as the philosopher
of science Hanson (1979) has pointed out. We see the world
around us through metaphor-tinted glasses. However, this
does not prevent us from realizing that what we see is not
reality itself but only our best approximation of it. We cannot
know reality directly, as the philosophical realists say. Theories
are the scientist's metaphors for reality. Freud too was a philosophical realist: he believed reality can only be "unknown" (p.
610). He tried to approximate reality with his metaphors, not to
give an absolute and definite description of it. Hyman is incorrect if he means to say that Freud believed his metaphors did
give this absolute description of reality.

The fact that the ultimate goal of science, the description of
reality, is, on the realist interpretation, unattainable destroys

the perfect parallelism between analyzing dreams in psycho-analysis and analyzing metaphors of reality in science. In analyzing dreams, it is possible to achieve at least the goal of discovering an ultimate motive-wish—the unconscious infantile wish. (As there are actually more than one of these wishes to be found, *at least one,* although not all, of these wishes may be discovered at the dream's origin, the mushroom's mycelium [p. 525].) It is intrinsically impossible, however, to reach the goal of any absolute description of reality.[4]

The process of dream interpretation has a termination point, whereas the process of metaphor change in science has no termination; but this fact is in a way irrelevant to a comparison of these two enterprises. Processes are by nature dynamic. When a process reaches a termination point, it stops, becomes static, and is no longer a process. When a dream is thoroughly interpreted, the process of interpretation ceases. Therefore, what is only relevant to the comparison are two *processes,* not the static end result of either.

METAPHOR IN MOTION

As Eadweard Muybridge serially photographed an animal in motion to illustrate the beauty of the beast not only as a static object but also as a piece of kinetic art, Freud's readers may picture three linear progressions of metaphor change found in *The Interpretation of Dreams.* The first progression concerns the metaphors which come to represent the form the dream takes and its relationship to intelligibility. Freud first tells his readers of Strümpell's metaphor: "Dreaming has often been compared with 'the ten fingers of a man who knows nothing of music wandering over the keys of a piano'" (p. 78). Then Freud declares this to be an inadequate metaphor, and gives his reasons for believing so:

> Dreams are not to be likened to the unregulated sounds that
> rise from a musical instrument struck by the blow of some

4. In fact, strictly speaking, there is no goal toward which science moves. As Kuhn (1970) suggests, science's theories, like the natural species, do not evolve toward anything. Both evolve only from what they are. To characterize this process otherwise can only lead to trouble.

external force instead of by a player's hand; they are not meaningless, they are not absurd; they do not imply that one portion
of our store of ideas is asleep while another portion is beginning to wake. On the contrary, they are psychical phenomena
of complete validity—fulfilments of wishes; they can be inserted into the chain of intelligible waking mental acts; they are
constructed by a highly complicated activity of the mind [p.
122].

At this point, Freud has discarded the only metaphor he has
to describe the form the dream takes and its relationship to
intelligibility. His next step is to create a metaphor that will, at
least temporarily, work adequately within the framework of his
theory: "The dream-thoughts and the dream-content are presented to us like two versions of the same subject-matter in two
different languages" (p. 277). This metaphor is also inadequate, as we see when Freud immediately goes on to write:

> Or, more properly, the dream-content seems like a transcript
> of the dream-thoughts into another mode of expression,
> whose characters and syntactic laws it is our business to dis-
> cover by comparing the original and the translation. The
> dream-thoughts are immediately comprehensible, as soon as
> we have learnt them. The dream-content, on the other hand, is
> expressed as if it were in a pictographic script, the characters
> of which have to be transposed individually into the language
> of the dream-thoughts. If we attempted to read these charac-
> ters according to their pictorial value instead of according to
> their symbolic relation, we should clearly be led into error.
> Suppose I have a picture-puzzle, a rebus, in front of
> me . . . obviously we can only form a proper judgement of the
> rebus if we put aside criticisms such as these of the whole
> composition and its parts and if, instead, we try to replace each
> separate element by a syllable or word that can be represented
> by that element in some way or other. The words which are put
> together in this way are no longer nonsensical but may form a
> poetical phrase of the greatest beauty and significance. A
> dream is a picture-puzzle of this sort and our predecessors in
> the field of dream-interpretation have made the mistake of
> treating the rebus as a pictorial composition; and as such it has
> seemed to them nonsensical and worthless" [p. 277f.].

In this brilliant passage Freud elaborates a new metaphor which describes the form of the dream and explains how it can be seen as intelligible. Further, he uses this same metaphor to illustrate the misconceptions of past investigators with a metaphor which is more apt than theirs. A meaningless set of pictures is a more accurate representation of the manifest content than a meaningless set of sounds because dreams are primarily visual not aural. The ineptness of Strümpell's metaphor gives us an indication of how representative of a scientist's thought the metaphors he chooses are. Strümpell's choice of metaphor indicates he was thinking "aurally" not "visually." Yet the visual element of dreams is central to their comprehension. Strümpell's theory fell before a theorist who could think both visually and aurally.

The process of replacing inadequate metaphors with less inadequate metaphors goes on continually in Freud's work:

> When we reflect that only a small minority of the dream-thoughts revealed are represented in the dream by one of their ideational elements, we might conclude that condensation is brought about by *omission:* that is, that the dream is not a faithful translation or a point-for-point projection of the dream-thoughts, but a highly incomplete and fragmentary version of them. This view, as we shall soon discover, is a most inadequate one. But we may take it as a provisional starting-point [p. 281].

The second example of the dynamics of metaphor change concerns how a dream is constructed. In this example, Freud does not dismiss an inadequate metaphor of another investigator. He creates his own faulty metaphor and then replaces it with an accurate one:

> . . . a dream is not constructed by each individual dream-thought, or group of dream-thoughts, finding (in abbreviated form) separate representation in the content of the dream—in the kind of way in which an electorate chooses parliamentary representatives; a dream is constructed, rather, by the whole mass of dream-thoughts being submitted to a sort of manipulative process in which those elements which have the most numerous and strongest supports acquire the right of entry into the dream-content—in a manner analogous to election by *scrutin de liste* [p. 284].

Describing what a thing is not is often as valuable as describing what a thing is: the negative description saves the reader from falling prey to misconceptions.

The third example of the dynamics of metaphor change, similar to the second example, is also a combination of denying the secondary subject of one metaphor only to accept a similar formulation of the "contrary" secondary subject. Freud writes that "all dreams are in a sense dreams of convenience: they serve the purpose of prolonging sleep instead of waking up. *Dreams are the* GUARDIANS *of sleep and not its disturbers*" (p. 233). Later Freud elaborates upon the metaphor: sometimes in attempting to fulfill an unconscious wish, the dreamwork fails to disguise the wish sufficiently, so the dream can pass the censorship of the preconscious.

> In that case the dream is immediately broken off and replaced by a state of complete waking. Here again it is not really the fault of the dream if it has now to appear in the role of a *disturber* of sleep instead of in its normal one of a *guardian* of sleep; and this fact need not prejudice us against its having a useful purpose. [Freud supports the use of the guardian-of-sleep metaphor with a cogent biological argument.] This is not the only instance in the organism of a contrivance which is normally useful becoming useless and disturbing as soon as the conditions that give rise to it are somewhat modified; and the disturbance at least serves the new purpose of drawing attention to the modification and of setting the organism's regulative machinery in motion against it [p. 580].[5]

5. It is reasonable to assume that Freud took this argument from Helmholtz, whose work profoundly influenced Freud. For example, Sulloway (1979) notes, "Fliess's Christmas present to Freud in 1898 was, appropriately, a two-volume set of Helmholtz's lectures" (p. 138). Temkin (1977) puts Helmholtz in the Cartesian school, stressing the limitations and defects in nature's biological creations (in contrast to the Galenist school, which held nature's works cannot be improved). In the set of lectures Freud received before he wrote *The Interpretation of Dreams*, "Helmholtz, in considering the eye as an optical instrument, found it so full of defects that he for one would have felt justified in returning it to the optician who had dared to sell it to him" (Temkin, 1977, p. 277). Freud clearly belongs to the Cartesian school of biology.

THE COGNITIVE USE OF METAPHOR IN SCIENCE

The three examples presented show linear progressions of metaphor change, with each metaphor becoming less inadequate descriptively than the one preceding it. Each series of metaphors is a "diachronic" process. The metaphors used at any one point in the work exclude or subsume all metaphors that involve the same primary subject occurring at any previous point in the work. This diachronic use of metaphors is complemented by a "synchronic" use; that is, different metaphors are used and held simultaneously through the work in order to describe one and the same primary subject.

The cognitive value of the synchronic use of metaphors in science is illuminated by the work of the philosopher of science Boyd (1980). In particular, Boyd's work clarifies how Freud was able to use metaphor to surmount a problem he faced introducing his theory of the mind. How would readers grasp the hypothetical or intangible entities about which he wrote? Freud, determined to develop a psychological theory of the mind, could not point to physical entities. In this respect, Freud's competitors, those peddling the mechanistic, somatically controlled view of the mind, had it easier. For Freud, seeking an alternative form of exposition allowing him to refer meaningfully to hypothetical or intangible entities, metaphors were to prove the key.

Boyd adopts a nondefinitional theory of reference he associates with two other philosophers, Kripke and Putnam. The definitional theory of reference, propounded by the logical positivists, held that we refer to an object by giving a description of it. A nondefinitional theory of reference states that we refer to something by "naming" (Putnam) or "dubbing" (Kripke) that object and from then on we know how to refer to that object; we use the name we have given it.

Boyd's theory of metaphor is predicated upon the notion that our ability to refer to an object is necessary for us to have "socially coordinated epistemic access" to that object (p. 358); that is, we cannot learn about an object or understand it unless we can refer to it. One has somehow to be able to point to what one wants to talk about before talking about it. Every statement must have a referent or else it is vacuous nonsense. For Boyd, science progresses by giving us better and better epistemic access to the world. Since this access is mediated by language, it is the business of science to accommodate our language to match the reality outside of us ("the causal structure of the world"). Boyd writes of the process as getting our linguistic categories to "cut the world at its joints" (p. 358).

According to Boyd, metaphors play an essential role in the introduction of a new theory with its new concepts and objects of study. If a body of metaphors, all having the same metaphorical theme, that is, used synchronically, proves to be fruitful to science, then it is likely that these metaphors refer and, in fact, have the same referent. A metaphor that fails to refer to a single "natural kind" and thus fails to "cut the world at its joints" is dropped from science. For example, the metaphor of "ether" was dropped from physics because it failed to refer.

Freud makes numerous synchronic uses of metaphor in order to refer to the "natural kinds" that are theoretical entities in his system. In using metaphors synchronically, Freud is giving his readers epistemic access to his hypothetical or intangible psychological entities. This use of metaphor is, as expected, especially prominent in chapter 7, the most "theoretical" part of *The Interpretation of Dreams*. Here, Freud introduces a rather abstract and difficult conception of the structure of the mind. His metaphors are necessary to make the abstract and quite difficult ideas intelligible by relating them to concrete objects to which the reader already has epistemic access.

Freud uses two different metaphors, which are also in some ways similar, in a simple example of the synchronic use of metaphor, to describe the function of dreams as an outlet of unconscious discharge. Dreams function both as a "safety-valve" and as a "sally-port" (pp. 579, 581). In describing the process of condensation, Freud uses three metaphors within one passage:

> In the process of condensation, . . . every psychical interconnection is transformed into an *intensification* of its ideational content. The case is the same as when, in preparing a book for the press, I have some word which is of special importance for understanding the text printed in spaced or heavy type; or in

speech I should pronounce the same word loudly and slowly and with special emphasis. . . . Art historians have drawn our attention to the fact that the earliest historical sculptures obey a similar principle: they express the rank of the persons represented by their size [p. 695f.].

The process of censorship receives even more metaphorical attention from Freud than that of condensation. Is the degree of metaphorical attention a concept receives related to the importance of the concept within the theory? Is it related to the novelty and/or difficulty of the concept? It is probably a combination of all three factors—importance, novelty, and difficulty—and most likely the three are related to one another.

There are four separate metaphors which refer to the process of censorship. Three of these are political analogies (pp. 142, 144, 529); the fourth is not (p. 515). Is censorship a more novel or difficult concept than condensation? It is hard to say. Censorship is a more important concept than condensation; the censorship is a necessary condition for condensation.

Freud's Use of Metaphor to Unify His Dream Psychology and the Topographic and Structural Theories

Both Freud's general conception of the structure of the mind (his topographic and structural theories) and his general conception of the structure of dreams (his dream psychology) receive the greatest degree of metaphorical attention of any conception in his work. This is not surprising given that the structure of dreams and the structure of the mind are the most important, novel, and difficult conceptions in his work.

Freud uses three general types of metaphor to describe the structure of dreams: language and textual (including poetry) metaphors, weaving or spinning metaphors, and path metaphors. Of these, he uses path metaphors especially for describing the structure of the mind. Not surprisingly, Freud views the structure of the dreams in the same metaphorical light as he views the structure of the mind. After all, the structure of the mind is a precondition for the structure of dreams.

It is perhaps surprising that Freud's vision of the structure of the mind and of dreams is not as fragmented as the existence of three separate metaphors for the structure of dreams indicates it might be. All three metaphors can be reduced to one central metaphor. I speculate that language and text (especially poetry) metaphors are tied to weaving metaphors, because one of the basic metaphorical uses of weaving is the weaving of words into a written work, text, or poem.[6] The path metaphors are also tied to the weaving metaphors; paths (as will be seen) are envisioned by Freud as a crisscross meshwork forming a woven web. By virtue of a common relation to the weaving metaphors, the text metaphor is essentially the same as that of the path metaphor. Freud has a unified metaphorical vision of the mind and the dreams it creates.

Freud treats dreams as a text to be interpreted. Every word of this text is important and, in fact, indispensable to understanding the whole of the text: "in short, we have treated as Holy Writ what previous writers have regarded as an arbitrary improvisation, hurriedly patched together in the embarrassment of the moment" (p. 514). Freud views the dream-thoughts and dream-contents as two different languages, and then as two different forms of expression, "whose characters and syntactic laws it is our business to discover" (p. 277). Condensation is a process of printing a word in "spaced or heavy type" (p. 595). Secondary revision is a sort of printed joke like "the enigmatic inscriptions with which *Fliegende Blätter* has for so long entertained its readers" (p. 500). Dream symbols "frequently have more than one or even several meanings, and, as with Chinese script, the correct interpretation can only be arrived at on each occasion from the context" (p. 353).

Freud views dreams not only as a sort of "Holy Writ" but also as poems constructed by the dreamwork. The words attached to manifest dream images, understood as the words of a dream-rebus, "are no longer nonsensical but may form a poetical phrase of the greatest beauty and significance" (p. 278). Given the considerations of representability, creating a dream is like composing a poem.

6. The etymological root of "text" is "that which is woven" (*Oxford English Dictionary*, 10:238, 1961).

Any one thought, whose form of expression may happen to be
fixed for other reasons, will operate in a determinant and selective manner on the possible forms of expression allotted to
the other thoughts, and it may do so, perhaps from the very
start—as is the case in writing a poem. If a poem is to be
written in rhymes, the second line of a couplet is limited by two
conditions: it must express an appropriate meaning, and the
expression of that meaning must rhyme with the first line. No
doubt the best poem will be one in which we fail to notice the
intention of finding a rhyme, and in which the two thoughts
have, by mutual influence, chosen from the very start a verbal
expression which will allow a rhyme to emerge with only slight
subsequent adjustment [p. 340].

For Freud, who described the censorship as being responsible for weaving a cloak (dream) to hide the motive-wish behind
the dream (p. 515), the mind is a dream-weaver. First, the
dream is woven. "The currently active sensation [somatic stim-
ulation] is woven into a dream *in order to rob it of reality*" (p. 234).
The unconscious weaves its connections. "The unconscious
prefers to weave its connections round preconscious impressions and ideas which are either indifferent and have thus had
no attention paid to them, or have been rejected and have thus
had attention promptly withdrawn from them" (p. 563).
Thoughts are spun out from the mnemic image "to the moment at which the perceptual identity is established by the external world—all this activity of thought merely constitutes a
roundabout path to wish-fulfilment which has been made necessary by experience" (p. 566f.). What are spun out in a woven
dream are paths to wish fulfillment.

Here, weaving and path metaphors are explicitly connected.
The path metaphor also joins the weaving metaphor when
Freud, describing the dreamwork, writes about how "trains of
thought" ("associative paths") are interconnected in a dream:

Here we find ourselves in a factory of thoughts where, as in the
'weaver's masterpiece',—
　　. . . a thousand threads one treadle throws,
　　Where fly the shuttles hither and thither,
　　Unseen the threads are knit together,
　　And an infinite combination grows.
　　　　　　　　　Goethe, *Faust*, Part I [p. 283].

Once the dream has been woven into a fabric, Freud discusses how it might be unraveled. *"In regression the fabric of the
dream-thoughts is resolved into its raw material"* (p. 543). The psychoanalyst also unravels the dreamwork when he does his
work, although there is a tangle of dream-thoughts which cannot be unraveled.

> There is often a passage in even the most thoroughly in-
> terpreted dream which has to be left obscure; this is because
> we become aware during the work of interpretation that at that
> point there is a tangle of dream-thoughts which cannot be
> unravelled and which moreover adds nothing to our knowl-
> edge of the content of the dream. This is the dream's navel, the
> spot where it reaches down into the unknown. The dream-
> thoughts to which we are led by interpretation cannot, from
> the nature of things, have any definite endings; they are
> bound to branch out in every direction into the intricate net-
> work of our world of thought. It is at some point where this
> meshwork is particularly close that the dream-wish grows up,
> like a mushroom out of its mycelium [p. 525].

The associative paths of thought radiating out from the
dream are part of the structure of the dream. Yet these paths
radiate out from the dream only because the mind is structured
in terms of paths. The process of psychoanalytic interpretation
carries us along these paths through the mind. It is no wonder
that Freud writes that his patients imagine the psychoanalytic
process as a journey in a motor-car (p. 410).[7]

> It is true that in carrying out the interpretation in the waking
> state we follow a path which leads back from the elements of
> the dream to the dream-thoughts and that the dream-work
> followed one in the contrary direction. But it is highly im-
> probable that these paths are passable both ways. It appears,
> rather, that in the daytime we drive shafts which follow along
> fresh chains of thoughts and that these shafts make contact
> with the intermediate thoughts and the dream-thoughts now
> at one point and now at another. We can see how in this man-

7. Similarly, Freud (1913) compares the psychoanalytic situation to two in a
railway carriage with the one (the analysand) describing the passing scenery
seen through the window to the other (the analyst). Lewin (1970) has percep-
tively studied the genesis of this particular metaphor in Freud's life and work.

ner fresh daytime material inserts itself into these interpretative chains. It is probable, too, that the increase in resistance
that has set in since the night makes new and more devious
detours necessary. The number and nature of the collaterals
that we spin in this way during the day is of no psychological
importance whatever, so long as they lead us to the dream-
thoughts of which we are in search [p. 532].

Here are a few examples of the path imagery Freud uses in
chapter 7 to represent the structure of the mind: unconscious
wishes "represent paths which can always be traversed, whenever a quantity of excitation makes use of them" (p. 577). A
train of thoughts that has been set going in the preconscious
implies "that the energy attached to the train of thought is
diffused along all the associative paths that radiate from it" (p.
594). Finally, the paths of the mind are pictured as roads in
order to illustrate how the censorship replaces deep associations with superficial ones in dreams: "We may picture, by way
of analogy, a mountain region, where some general interruption of traffic (owing to floods, for instance) has blocked the
main, major roads, but where communications are still maintained over inconvenient and steep footpaths normally used
only by the hunter" (p. 530).

Characteristically, Freud reinforces his path conceptions of
the mind by using path metaphors to describe the reader's
progress through his book—a stylistic and heuristic device, similar to his frequent and explicit use of metaphors to get the
reader accustomed to thinking in terms of metaphors so he can
understand how the dreamwork functions. In a letter to Fliess
(August 20, 1899), Freud wrote that *The Interpretation of Dreams*
"is planned on the model of an imaginary walk. First comes the
dark wood of the authorities (who cannot see the trees), where
there is no clear view and it is very easy to go astray. Then there
is a cavernous defile through which I lead my readers—my
specimen dream with all its peculiarities, its details, its indiscre-
tions, and its bad jokes—and then, all at once, the high ground
and the prospect, and the question: 'Which way do you want to
go?'" (1950, p. 290).

Hyman (1976), who also quoted the above letter, misses a
significant path image in his discussion and documentation of

the use of this stylistic device by Freud. In building up to one of his most famous aphorisms, Freud writes that "dreams show us one of the paths leading to an understanding of the normal structure of our mental instrument" (p. 607f.). A paragraph later, Freud writes: "*The interpretation of dreams is the royal road to a knowledge of the unconscious activities of the mind*" (p. 608).

METAPHOR UNIFIES TOPOGRAPHIC AND STRUCTURAL THEORIES

In *The Interpretation of Dreams,* Freud delivered a new conception of the structure of the mind. He explicated this structure, making heavy use of metaphors. These metaphors are essential to understanding his exposition.

In the course of his life's work, Freud decided that the topographic theory of 1900 was in some ways inadequate. In particular, the mind could not be understood simply in terms of the systems Unconscious (*Ucs.*), Preconscious (*Pcs.*), and Conscious (*Cs.*). Through a series of publications (his "metapsychological papers") culminating in *The Ego and the Id,* Freud moved to his new structural view, with its new entities: ego, id, and superego. Concurrently, his old metaphors were replaced by a new set of metaphors.

How did Freud coherently make the transition from the topographic to the structural view? The new view is significantly different from the old. How do Freud's readers know that the mind described by the first theory is the same mind described by the second theory? Part of the answer to this question is obvious. Both theories have the same referent because there can only be one mind associated with man's brain. If one can assume that the structure of man's mind is in some way essentially dependent on the structure of the brain, then the structure of the mind did not actually change over the course of Freud's work. While the referent of the two theories did not change, the theories themselves did change.

While the two theories are in some ways radically different, they share elements that remain constant throughout the transition. For example, while, in the light of the new view, the concepts unconscious, preconscious, and conscious are no longer sufficient, these concepts retain much of their original meaning, but in the context of the new view now functioning as attributes.

Freud makes the transition coherent in part by showing the logical, theoretical connections between the new theory and the old, but principally by changing the metaphors he uses to describe the structure of the mind. An abstract transition between two theories is much more difficult to comprehend than a transition between somewhat more tangible metaphors. Throughout the transition, some metaphors of the mind are rejected and replaced. Others remain in place. These constant metaphors provide continuity between the new and the old theories, and, operating at an almost subliminal level, give coherence to the transition.

What were the logical, scientific reasons which led Freud to make this transition in the first place? Freud found the topographic theory inadequate for three reasons. First, seduction (and other) fantasies defy categorization in its terms. They belong neither to the *Ucs.* nor to the *Pcs.*: "On the one hand, they are highly organized, free from self-contradiction, have made use of every acquisition of the system *Cs.* and would hardly be distinguished in our judgement from the formations of that system. On the other hand they are unconscious and are incapable of becoming conscious. Thus *qualitatively* they belong to the system *Pcs.*, but *factually* to the *Ucs.*" (1915c, p. 190f.). Freud attempts to make this problem intelligible by constructing a metaphor to describe it: "We may compare them [seduction fantasies] with individuals of a mixed race who, taken all round, resemble white men, but who betray their coloured descent by some striking feature or other, and on that account are excluded from society and enjoy none of the privileges of white people" (1915c, p. 191).

How does this metaphor help the reader to understand the problem created by the existence of seduction fantasies? In a much later work (1933), Freud writes that "analogies, it is true, decide nothing, but they can make one feel more at home" (p. 72). Freud was correct. Metaphors make alien and often abstract concepts more intelligible by relating them to familiar and concrete situations which the reader can more easily comprehend. However, his is a rather inexact statement of the role of metaphors in scientific work. Boyd's theory about their role is more sophisticated. Freud's metaphor in this case, as in others, gives us epistemic access to the entities to which he is referring.

Freud's first problem with the topographic theory is that it does not, as Boyd would say, "cut the world at its joints." The seduction fantasy straddles the "cuts" of the topographic theory. Stated alternatively in terms of Freud's own metaphor: "If we throw a crystal to the floor, it breaks; but not into haphazard pieces. It comes apart along its lines of cleavage into fragments whose boundaries, though they were invisible, were predetermined by the crystal's structure. Mental patients are split and broken structures of this same kind" (1933, p. 59). If we were to split the crystal of the mind along the lines of cleavage suggested by the topographic theory, seduction fantasies would not be neatly found in any one piece of the split stone because they do not clearly belong to any of these pieces.

How one understands the structure of the mind has empirical consequences. The jeweler, who attempts to split a diamond based on an incorrect understanding of the stone, may shatter the jewel. The psychoanalytic jeweler does not split the psyche, but takes other equally consequential actions based on his understanding of its structure. To misapprehend the structure can have disastrous results.

The second problem with the topographic theory has to do with the censorship. Originally Freud postulated the existence of only one censorship, operating between the systems *Pcs.* and *Ucs.* Then Freud (1915c) writes, "Now it becomes probable that there is a censorship between *Pcs.* and *Cs.*" (p. 191). He tries to dismiss this problem. "Nevertheless we shall do well not to regard this complication as a difficulty, but to assume that to every transition from one system to that immediately above it (that is, every advance to a higher stage of psychical organization) there corresponds a new censorship" (p. 191f.). As a scientist, Freud is still left with a problem. The multiplication of theoretical entities is always a danger. Ad hoc explanations weaken the explanatory potency of a scientific theory. Each censorship added is like the addition of another Ptolemaic epicycle.

The third and final problem with the topographic theory is the breakdown of a theoretical equivalence central to it. No longer can the repressed be equated with the system *Ucs.* and the ego with the systems *Pcs/Cs.*

> . . . the attribute of being conscious, which is the only charac-teristic of psychical processes that is directly presented to us, is in no way suited to serve as a criterion for the differentiation of systems. Apart from the fact that the conscious is not always conscious but also at times latent, observation has shown that much that shares the characteristics of the system *Pcs.* does not become conscious; and we learn . . . that the act of becoming conscious is dependent on the attention of the *Pcs.* being turned in certain directions. Hence consciousness stands in no simple relation either to the different systems or to repres-sions. The truth is that it is not only the psychically repressed that remains alien to consciousness, but also some of the impulses which dominate our ego—something, therefore, that forms the strongest functional antithesis to the repressed. The more we seek to win our way to a metapsychological view of mental life, the more we must learn to emancipate ourselves from the importance of the symptom of 'being conscious' [1915c, p. 192f.].

Here again we see Freud moving away from the use of linguistic categories, such as consciousness, that do not cut the world at its joints.

Having found these defects in the topographic theory, Freud was forced to devise a new theory. In making the transition to it, as will be shown, Freud has once again used metaphors diachronically and synchronically. In fact, the metaphorical movement from the beginning to the end of *The Interpretation of Dreams* is a model for the metaphorical movement occurring during this transition.

Freud's most impressive synchronic use of metaphor is his unified metaphorical vision of the mind and the dreams it creates. It is because Freud maintains this vision of woven fabrics, texts, and paths throughout the transition from one theory to the other that the transition is coherent. This metaphorical construction is a stable base over which Freud could make his voyage from the topographic to the structural view.

The path metaphor can be seen to stay constant through the

transition, as the following examples show. Sexual instincts follow "the paths that are indicated to them by the ego-instincts" (1915a, p. 126). There are paths in the mind through which affects are released; paths along which wishful impulses may be dealt with; and paths of regression on which excitations may enter (1915d, pp. 225, 226, 234); which the libido tries to follow (1916, p. 316); and paths through the systems *Ucs.*, *Pcs.*, and *Cs.* by which the neurosis tries to regain its lost objects (1915c, p. 204). In 1920, Freud writes of repressed instincts attempting to find satisfaction "by roundabout paths" (p. 11). Finally, in 1923, "There are two paths by which the contents of the id can penetrate into the ego" (p. 55).

Again, Freud reinforces his path conception of the mind by using path metaphors to describe the reader's progress through his work. In 1920, the path image arises as "well-trodden ground": "If we turn now to the question of what circumstances are able to prevent the pleasure principle from being carried into effect, we find ourselves once more on secure and well-trodden ground" (p. 10). In the same work, with regard to the similarities between the idea of life and death instincts and Weismann's theory of living substance divided into mortal and immortal parts, "What strikes us . . . is the unexpected analogy with our own view, which was arrived at along a different path" (p. 46). Freud again implies a (sea) path image when he writes about the similarities between his dual-instinct theory and Schopenhauer's philosophy: "We have unwittingly steered our course into the harbour of Schopenhauer's philosophy" (p. 49f.). In 1923, Freud defends psychoanalysis against the criticism that it ignores "the higher, moral, supra-personal side of human nature" (p. 35). There "has been a general refusal to recognize that psychoanalytic research could not, like a philosophical system, produce a complete and ready-made theoretical structure, but had to find its own way step by step along the path towards understanding the intricacies of the mind by making an analytic dissection of both normal and abnormal phenomena" (p. 35f.). In 1933, Freud defends psychoanalytic research as better than mystical practices. "It may be safely doubted, however, whether this road [of mystical practices] will lead us to the ultimate truths from which salvation is to be expected" (p. 80).

The unified metaphorical vision of the mind created in *The Interpretation of Dreams* is also maintained through the transition from topographic to structural theory by the continued use of the weaving metaphor; e.g., "the patient can go on spinning a thread of such [free] associations, till he is brought up against some thought, the relation of which to what is repressed becomes so obvious that he is compelled to repeat his attempt at repression" (1915b, p. 150). Writing about *Rosmersholm*, Freud (1916) says, "The practising psycho-analytic physician knows how frequently, or how invariably, a girl who enters a household as servant, companion or governess, will consciously or unconsciously weave a day-dream, which derives from the Oedipus complex, of the mistress of the house disappearing and the master taking the newcomer as his wife in her place" (p. 330f.). In "A Metapsychological Supplement," the mind is constructed of woven materials, undone like our outer clothes before sleep: "We may add that when they [humans] go to sleep they carry out an entirely analogous undressing of their minds and lay aside most of their psychical acquisitions" (1915d, p. 222). In 1923, the ego "tries to remain on good terms with the id; it clothes the id's *Ucs.* commands with its *Pcs.* rationalizations" (p. 56). This formulation appears again in 1933: "In its [the ego's] attempts to mediate between the id and reality, it is often obliged to cloak the *Ucs.* commands of the id with its own *Pcs.* rationalizations, to conceal the id's conflicts with reality, to profess, with diplomatic ingenuousness, to be taking notice of reality even when the id has remained rigid and unyielding" (p. 78).

In *The Interpretation of Dreams* the mind is a miniature society. Freud not only maintains but increases the population of this society in his subsequent works. Under the structural view, the politics of the mind prosper. In "the matter of action the ego's position is like that of a constitutional monarch, without whose sanction no law can be passed but who hesitates long before imposing his veto on any measure put forward by Parliament" (1923, p. 55). The monarch has "dethroned the pleasure principle which dominates the course of events in the id without any restriction and has replaced it by the reality principle, which promises more certainty and greater success" (1933, p. 76). Again, the ego is a politician worried about his public image.

"In its position midway between the id and reality, it only too often yields to the temptation to become sycophantic, opportunist and lying, like a politician who sees the truth but wants to keep his place in public favour" (1923, p. 56).

Other aspects of the society of the mind flourish through Freud's transition from topographic to structural theory. In "Repression," the difference between an idea that represents an instinct being repressed after once having been conscious is opposed to a similar idea being repressed before it has ever reached consciousness. This "amounts to much the same thing as the difference between my ordering an undesirable guest out of my drawing-room (or out of my front hall), and my refusing, after recognizing him, to let him across my threshold at all" (1915b, p. 153). In "The Unconscious," we have seen how Freud compares seduction fantasies to a mixed race. He also compares the *Ucs.* to "an aboriginal population of the mind" (1915c, p. 195). In *The Ego and the Id,* neurotic acts of revenge are taken against the wrong people. "Such behaviour on the part of the unconscious reminds one of the comic story of the three village tailors, one of whom had to be hanged because the only village blacksmith had committed a capital offence" (1923, p. 45).

While conflict was always central to psychoanalytic theory, in the 1923 revision, the denizens of the mind are at war with one another. "We know that as a rule the ego carries out repressions in the service and at the behest of its super-ego; but this [hysteria] is a case in which it has turned the same weapon against its harsh taskmaster" (p. 52). Freud writes again of a beleaguered ego. "Helpless in both directions, the ego defends itself vainly, alike against the instigations of the murderous id and against the reproaches of the punishing conscience" (p. 53). Not only the triumvirate of ego, id, and superego have their armed conflicts, but even within the id the instincts battle it out. "Eros and the death instinct struggle within it; we have seen with what weapons the one group of instincts defends itself against the other" (p. 59). The ego is not always rebellious. Sometimes it is in control (see below); at other times Freud pictures it as absolutely servile. The ego "is not only a helper to the id; it is also a submissive slave who courts his master's love"

(p. 56). Freud has the ego actually talk to the id. "When the ego assumes the features of the object [erotic object choice], it is forcing itself, so to speak, upon the id as a love-object and is trying to make good the id's loss by saying: 'Look, you can love me too—I am so like the object'" (p. 30).

These synchronic uses of metaphor are central to the coherence and stability of Freud's transition from the topographic to the structural theory. The diachronic use of metaphor is central in taking the steps necessary to make this transition. If one can accept the notion that Freud's topographic and structural views are metaphors for the mind (as all of science is a metaphor for reality), then the transition between them constitutes the grandest example of Freud's diachronic use of metaphor. Within this diachronic use of metaphor other diachronic uses of metaphor are nested; that is, Freud uses a progression of metaphors to achieve better and more precise approximations of his new structural view, itself a metaphor.

For example, Freud uses a diachronic progression of metaphors in an attempt to describe the relationship of the ego to the id and superego. First, Freud (1923) creates this metaphor: "In its relation to the id it [the ego] is like a man on horseback, who has to hold in check the superior strength of the horse" (p. 25). However, Freud begins to find this metaphor inadequate in that within it there exists what is called a "negative analogy," that part of the metaphor which does not "work" when the metaphor is extended. The negative analogy is created by "this difference, that the rider tries to do so with his own strength while the ego uses borrowed forces" (p. 25). However, Freud keeps the metaphor because in it he finds a strong "positive analogy," that part of the metaphor which does work when the metaphor is extended. "The analogy may be carried a little further. Often a rider, if he is not to be parted from his horse, is obliged to guide it where it wants to go; so in the same way the ego is in the habit of transforming the id's will into action as if it were its own" (p. 25). Sealing the fate of this metaphor, Freud complains that it is an inadequate description of his metapsychology because the metaphor does not describe the relation of the superego (or ego ideal) to the other two parts of the mind. "It would be in vain, however, to attempt to localize the ego ideal, even in the sense in which we have localized the ego, or to work it into any of the analogies with the help of which we have tried to picture the relation between the ego and the id" (p. 36f.). In 1933, Freud disposes of the "horse" metaphor for a less inadequate one.

> We are warned by a proverb against serving two masters at the same time. The poor ego has things even worse: it serves three severe masters and does what it can to bring their claims and demands into harmony with one another. These claims are always divergent and often seem incompatible. No wonder that the ego so often fails in its task. Its three tyrannical masters are the external world, the super-ego and the id. When we follow the ego's efforts to satisfy them simultaneously—or rather, to obey them simultaneously—we cannot feel any regret at having personified this ego and having set it up as a separate organism [p. 77].

This metaphor is less inadequate than the "horse" metaphor for several reasons. First, Freud finds no negative analogies in the "masters" metaphor. Second, there is a place, not found in the "horse" metaphor, for the superego. Finally, the "masters" metaphor incorporates the roles not only of id, ego, and superego, but also of the external world in his new picture of the mind, thus making it more complete than the "horse" metaphor.

Another example of Freud's diachronic use of metaphor within the structural theory occurs when he tries to give an overall picture of the mind and its parts. First, as seen above, he pictures the mind as a crystal, whose parts can be cleaved neatly apart from one another (1933, p. 59). However, this picture of a neatly organized mind is dispelled and replaced when Freud (1933) pictures the mind as a configuration of different landscapes; component parts are its inhabitants, with a different place for each type of landscape; and the characteristics of its parts are the activities (fishing, farming, etc.) distinct for each ethnic group. Freud notes that while, for pedagogical reasons, one might like to present a simple picture of such a society as totally segregated, and one would be mostly accurate in depicting it as such, the reality of the situation forces one to present certain deviations from the ideal model: the ethnic groups are not totally segregated; some members of each group partake in activities usually found only in other groups; etc.

Not all the metaphors used to describe the structural theory were used diachronically. The readers of Freud are also given epistemic access to the parts of his new theory through the synchronic use of metaphor. The ego is pictured simultaneously in a number of different ways. First, the ego is a surface developed from the "surface" of consciousness, which "must lie on the borderline between outside and inside; it must be turned towards the external world and must envelop the other psychical systems" (1920, p. 23). One should picture "a living organism in its more simplified form as an undifferentiated vesicle of a substance that is susceptible to stimulation. Then the surface turned towards the external world will from its very situation be differentiated and will serve as an organ for receiving stimuli" (p. 26). This image is elaborated when Freud writes that this surface also serves as a shield from too much inner or outer stimulation (pp. 27, 29ff.). The metaphorical relation of this surface to the sphere of the id is further developed in 1923, where the surface rests atop, but does not completely cover, the sphere of the id. The ego in this role is also described as a "frontier-creature" (p. 56). As previously pointed out, the ego is also simultaneously pictured as a constitutional monarch as well as a servant to three masters.

METAPHORS UNIFY THE DOMAINS STUDIED BY FREUD

Freud uses metaphors to extend the domain of application of his theory of the mind, that is, to extend the kinds of human phenomena (more precisely, the kind of symbolic phenomena) which he examines in light of his theory. In order to understand how Freud uses metaphor in this fashion, one must make oneself familiar with Black's "interaction theory of metaphor." One sees the primary subject through the implicative complex of the secondary subject. The kernel or crux of the interaction theory is that the metaphor in addition "incites" the hearer to work the metaphor the other way around. That is, the secondary subject is viewed through the implicative complex of the primary subject. The net result of the metaphor is to change the hearer's understanding of both the primary *and* the secondary subject (Black, 1980; Hesse, 1970).

The interaction theory is marvelously and explicitly illustrated in *The Interpretation of Dreams*. Freud constructs a metaphor between childhood and paradise and then views not only childhood in terms of paradise but also paradise in terms of childhood: "When we look back at this unashamed period of childhood it seems to us a Paradise; and Paradise itself is no more than a group phantasy of the childhood of the individual" (p. 245).

The metaphor about "madmen" and "waking dreamers" leads Freud to see madmen in terms of dreamers and to view the thinking of madmen (more exactly, those who are psychotic) as a special case of primary process thinking, which is at the root of constructing dreams. Furthermore, psychoneurotics are seen as daydreamers: "The study of the psychoneuroses leads to the surprising discovery that these phantasies or day-dreams are the immediate fore-runners of hysterical symptoms, or at least a whole number of them" (p. 491).

The above two metaphors explicitly illustrate the interaction of subjects of a metaphor. A less obvious example of such interaction follows. Freud (1900) attempts to demonstrate that the case of Oedipus is merely a particular instantiation of a general formula or hypothesis of his psychology. Seeking to explain the myth of Oedipus, Freud writes that the legend's "profound and universal power to move can only be understood if the hypothesis I have put forward in regard to the psychology of children has an equally universal validity" (p. 261). Freud implicitly sets up the metaphor "Oedipus is us," in that Oedipus is just like any of us in our infantile sexual wishes. Yet, through the process of interaction, Freud finishes explaining us through the myth of Oedipus: "Like Oedipus, we live in ignorance of these wishes, repugnant to morality, which have been forced upon us by Nature, and after their revelation we may all of us well seek to close our eyes to the scenes of our childhood" (p. 263). The metaphor becomes "We are Oedipus."

The interaction theory shows how metaphors work in science. The relationship between primary and secondary subject is made reciprocal. Each is conceived in terms of the other. If one subject in the metaphor is thought of in terms of a certain scientific theory, e.g., psychoanalytic theory, then the hearer of the metaphor is led to thinking of both subjects in terms of that theory. If the metaphor works, it seems plausible to think of both subjects in terms of psychoanalytic theory. The subjects might not be single objects but classes of objects. In that case, the subjects are called "domains." For example, in the metaphor "The madman is a waking dreamer," "the madman" represents the domain of psychoneurotics, as does "the waking dreamer" the domain of daydreamers.

When Freud realized the implications of this metaphor, he made a scientific discovery. He discovered that two different domains (best put: neurotic symptoms and dreams) could be characterized by one scientific theory. Dreams and neurotic symptoms are indistinguishable in the sense that both belong to the domain of entities characterized by psychoanalytic theory.

This indistinguishability between two domains is the characteristic of "homogeneity" (described by Stegmüller, 1976, p. 164) shared by domains of application of a single theory. (To be historically accurate, Freud developed his theory around neurotic symptoms first and then went on to apply it to dreams. On the other hand, in *The Interpretation of Dreams,* his theory receives its fullest exposition up to 1900. After 1900, Freud went back to consider neuroses again in light of this fuller theory. This back-and-forth movement is all in the spirit of interaction.)

Freud (1900) brings together the two domains of neurotic symptoms and dreams by arguing that neurotic symptoms and dreams are analogous: "However many changes may be made in our reading of the psychical censorship and of the rational and abnormal revisions made of the dream-content, it remains true that processes of this sort are at work in the formation of dreams and that they show the closest analogy in their essentials to the processes observable in the formation of hysterical symptoms" (p. 607). Neurotic symptoms and dreams are indistinguishable in several essential features. "If we submit the content of the dream to analysis, we find that the anxiety in the dream is no better justified by the dream's content than, let us say, the anxiety in a phobia is justified by the idea to which the phobia relates" (p. 161). And, again: "We might also point out in our defence that our procedure in interpreting dreams is identical with the procedure by which we resolve hysterical symptoms" (p. 528).

The metaphor between neurotic symptoms and dreams created by Freud is imperfect if it is examined in terms of Hesse's theory of metaphors. Hesse (1970) builds upon the interaction theory of metaphors with her own notion of how positive, negative, and neutral analogies are built into a metaphor.

The positive analogy in a metaphor isomorphically relates the primary and secondary systems. In a less formal relationship between less formal systems, the positive analogy is that part of the comparison between systems that works. For example, dreams are neurotic symptoms because both are susceptible to analysis by psychoanalytic procedures.

The neutral analogy is that part of the metaphorical relationship where it is not clear whether an isomorphism is present or whether the comparison works. For example, contrary to what is probably historically the case, suppose Freud constructed the metaphor "dreams are neurotic symptoms" before he tried to analyze dreams with the same procedure he used to analyze neurotic symptoms. This metaphor would be termed a neutral analogy with respect to the procedure, possibly leading the scientific researcher to investigate whether in fact he could analyze dreams and neurotic symptoms with the same procedure. The scientific metaphor's success depends upon whether or not neutral analogies pan out.

The negative analogy is the part of the metaphorical relationship that is not isomorphic or does not work out. Failed neutral analogies become negative analogies. Freud pointed out an important negative or failed neutral analogy in the metaphoric relation between neurotic symptoms and dreams. He had made the "general assertion that *a hysterical symptom develops only where the fulfilments of two opposing wishes, arising each from a different psychical system, are able to converge in a single expression*" (1900, p. 569). But, he noted, dreams are not like hysterical symptoms in this respect: "all that we so far know about dreams is that they express the fulfilment of a wish from the unconscious; it seems as though the dominant preconscious system acquiesces in this after insisting upon a certain number of distortions. Nor is it possible as a general rule to find a train of thought opposed to the dream-wish and like its counterpart, realized in the dream" (p. 570).

That a scientist may find one negative analogy within the metaphorical relationship bringing two domains together under the figurative roof of one theory is usually not sufficient cause to dispense with the metaphor. If in most respects the metaphor works by demonstrating a largely significant number of positive analogies and promising neutral analogies, the scientist will probably keep the metaphor.

As already seen, Freud further enlarges the applicative range of his theory through metaphorical construction by bringing together domains other than those of dreams and neurotic symptoms. Each time Freud creates another metaphor bringing together a domain previously characterized in terms of psychoanalytic theory and a new domain not so characterized, he makes a potential scientific discovery. To make the discovery actual, all he must realize (by a mechanism described by the interaction theory) is that this new domain can also be characterized by psychoanalytic theory.

In extending the range of application of his theory to fairy tales, in particular, and to literature in general, Freud (1900) constructs a metaphor relating Hans Christian Andersen's version of the *Emperor's New Clothes* and dreams. "The imposter is the dream and the Emperor is the dreamer himself" (p. 244). This fairy tale, Freud explains, has its own origin in a "typical" dream, in which the dreamer sees himself naked and embarrassed in front of indifferent onlookers. Freud constructs the following metaphor between the fairy tale of the *Little Tailor* and dreaming. It is not "easy to credit the skill shown by the dream-work in always hitting upon forms of expression that can bear several meanings—like the Little Tailor in the fairy story who hit seven flies at a blow" (p. 523). The interaction theory of metaphor invites one to see the fairy tale in terms of psychoanalytic theory.[8]

8. This is, in fact, what Bettelheim (1977) has done in his book.

Similarly, metaphors involving Oedipus invite one to apply psychoanalytic theory to plays and, by extension, the progress of civilization as seen through these plays: "Another of the great creations of tragic poetry, Shakespeare's *Hamlet,* has its roots in the soil of *Oedipus Rex.* But the changed treatment of the same material reveals the whole difference in the mental life of these two widely separated epochs of civilization: the secular advance of repression in the emotional life of mankind" (1900, p. 264). Expanding the argument based on the analysis of the artifacts of civilization, Freud in 1930 attempts to analyze the progress of civilization.

Freud also leads his readers (including himself, most importantly) to apply his psychoanalytic theory to the domain of jokes by constructing metaphors relating dreams and jokes. Each of the following examples of this metaphor has dreams described as jokes. About the chains of thought that occur in dreams, Freud (1900) writes, "It is easy enough to construct such chains, as is shown by the puns and riddles that people make every day for their entertainment. The realm of jokes knows no boundaries" (p. 176). Freud discusses whether dreams have a means of expressing the relation of contradiction. "Another class of contraries in the dream-thoughts, falling into a category which may be described as 'contrariwise" or 'just the reverse', find their way into dreams in the following remarkable fashion, which almost deserves to be described as a joke" (p. 326). Again in a discussion of secondary revision:

> If I look around for something with which to compare the final form assumed by a dream as it appears after normal thought has made its contribution, I can think of nothing better than the enigmatic inscriptions with which *Fliegende Blätter* has for so long entertained its readers. They are intended to make the reader believe that a certain sentence . . . is a Latin inscription. . . . If we are to avoid being taken in by the joke . . . [p. 500f.].

According to the interaction theory of metaphor, the reader is led in 1905 to think of jokes in terms of dreams, which have been characterized by psychoanalytic theory. The reader is thus led to apply psychoanalytic theory to the domain of jokes.

CONCLUSION

The scientist is a poor detective. He seeks to discover nature's face behind a disguise of chaos. In the end, he thins the make-up on the mask a little; makes the lines a little clearer, a little more appealing, and perhaps a little less frightening. Yet he never finds the face. Why does he fail?

A scientific theory is a metaphor for reality. On the realist interpretation of science, we can never directly know the object of the scientific theory (e.g., the mind, in the case of Freud's topographic and structural theories). We can only say that it is like so-and-so, the secondary subject of the metaphor. The metaphors of science constitute a disguise for reality in much the same way that dreams are a disguise for our unconscious wishes. This is a two-edged sword. On the one edge, metaphors and dreams prevent us from observing that which we want to see directly, but never can. On the other edge, an understanding of how metaphors and dreams work can bring us closer to that which we want to obtain. It is only through our study of dreams that we can find that which is unconscious within us. Similarly, it is only through our studies of the metaphors of science that we can come to find that which is real.

There are some who do not accept the realist interpretation of science, those who think metaphors are reality. They risk the same sort of folly that those who do not recognize the distinction between manifest and latent content fall into. To those who recognize only the manifest content, dreams seem an absurd unintelligible mess. They are still at the bottom of Plato's Cave, mistaking the shadows for reality. The same is true of those who believe metaphors are reality. What they call reality seems to them an absurd unintelligible mess when the metaphors do not "pan out" in all respects; unfathomable anomalies erupt. The science they learn as students is for them immutable truth. They cannot comprehend, let alone create, scientific revolutions, because for them science as reality cannot change. They are never led to explore further, because there seems no hope of finding anything radically better. They are left in the dark. However, Freud, a philosophical realist, knew the difference between the manifest and latent content in dreams as

58   *Jonathan T. Edelson*

well as the difference between his metaphors and reality. Freud stood in the light.

BETTELHEIM, B. (1977), *The Uses of Enchantment.* New York: Vintage Press.
BLACK, M. (1980), More about metaphor. In *Metaphor and Thought,* ed. A. Ortony. London: Cambridge Univ. Press, pp. 19–43.
BOYD, R. (1980), Metaphor and theory change. In *Metaphor and Thought,* ed. A. Ortony. London: Cambridge Univ. Press, pp. 356–408.
EDELSON, M. (1972), Language and dreams. *Psychoanal. Study Child,* 27:203–282.
FEYERABEND, P. (1979), *Against Method.* London: Verso.
FREUD, S. (1900), The interpretation of dreams. *S.E.,* 4 & 5.
——— (1905), Jokes and their relation to the unconscious. *S.E.,* 8.
——— (1913), On beginning treatment. *S.E.,* 12:123–144.
——— (1915a), Instincts and their vicissitudes. *S.E.,* 14:109–140.
——— (1915b), Repression. *S.E.,* 14:141–158.
——— (1915c), The unconscious. *S.E.,* 14:159–215.
——— (1915d), A metapsychological supplement to the theory of dreams. *S.E.,* 14:217–235.
——— (1916), Some character-types met with in psycho-analytic work. *S.E.,* 14:309–323.
——— (1920), Beyond the pleasure principle. *S.E.,* 18:3–64.
——— (1923), The ego and the id. *S.E.,* 19:3–66.
——— (1930), Civilization and its discontents. *S.E.,* 21:59–145.
——— (1933), New introductory lectures on psycho-analysis. *S.E.,* 22:3–182.
——— (1950), *The Origins of Psychoanalysis.* New York: Basic Books, 1954.
HANSON, N. (1977), *Patterns of Discovery.* London: Cambridge Univ. Press.
HARVEY, W. (1628), *Excercitatio Anatomica de Motu Cordis et Sanguinis in Animalibus,* tr. C. Leake. Springfield, Ill.: Thomas, 1978.
HESSE, M. (1970), *Models and Analogies in Science.* Notre Dame, Indiana: Univ. Notre Dame Press.
HULL, D. (1974), *Philosophy of Biological Science.* Englewood Cliffs, N.J.: Prentice-Hall.
HYMAN, S. (1974), *The Tangled Bank.* New York: Atheneum.
JONES, E. (1953), *The Life and Work of Sigmund Freud,* vol. 1. New York: Basic Books.
KEARNEY, H. (1971), *Science and Change 1500–1700.* New York: World Univ. Library.
KUHN, T. (1970), *The Structure of Scientific Revolutions.* Chicago: Univ. Chicago Press.
LEATHERDALE, W. (1974), *The Role of Analogy, Model and Metaphor in Science.* Amsterdam: North-Holland Publishing Co.
LEWIN, B. D. (1970), The train-ride. *Psychoanal. Q.,* 39:71–89.

STEGMÜLLER, W. (1976), *The Structure and Dynamics of Theories*. New York: Springer.

SULLOWAY, F. J. (1979), *Freud: Biologist of the Mind*. New York: Basic Books.

TEMKIN, O. (1977), *The Double-Face of Janus and Other Essays in the History of Medicine*. Baltimore: John Hopkins Univ. Press.

TILLYARD, E. (1944), *The Elizabethan World Picture*. New York: Vintage Books.

WOLF, E. S. (1971), *Saxa loquuntur. Psychoanal. Study Child*, 26:485–534.

Is Testing Psychoanalytic Hypotheses in the Psychoanalytic Situation Really Impossible?

MARSHALL EDELSON, M.D., Ph.D.

IS THERE EMPIRICAL EVIDENCE THAT PROVIDES SUPPORT FOR the claim that psychoanalysis as treatment is efficacious? Is there empirical evidence that justifies provisional acceptance of psychoanalytic hypotheses about neurotic symptoms, dreams, and parapraxes as true over rival hypotheses? In our society (a society threatened by endemic irrationality and swept by anti-intellectual currents), those who are especially concerned to preserve, to put forward, and indeed to insist upon adherence to cognitive scientific canons increasingly and ever more emphatically tend to answer these two questions "No." More seriously, that negative answer has come to include the assertion "and it is in principle impossible to obtain such evidence by psychoanalytic methods of investigation."

Psychoanalysts should not remain mute before such an answer to these questions; dismissively belittle those who make it; or evade it by redefining psychoanalysis as a hermeneutic discipline—a branch of the humanities rather than a science.

Psychoanalysis as a science, like any other science, must conform in its reasoning and methods to scientific canons. These

Professor of Psychiatry, Yale University School of Medicine; Western New England Institute for Psychoanalysis.
This paper is based on material from my book *Hypothesis and Evidence in Psychoanalysis* (1983); it appears here with the permission of the University of Chicago Press.

canons presuppose a search for general statements about the actual (and not merely some possible) world, which are objectively true of it, in the sense that what they assert corresponds to something in that actual world.[1] The canons define what standards must be met by a particular kind of reasoning—the reasoning which leads to a conclusion that provisional acceptance of the truth of an assertion about the actual world is or is not justified in the light of empirical evidence. These canons also define what methods for obtaining this evidence are required if such reasoning is to meet these standards. While accepting that such canons are applicable to psychoanalysis, I shall in this paper refute the assertion that psychoanalysis never does and indeed in principle cannot satisfy them.

I intend in this paper to present a logical argument about the status of psychoanalysis as a scientific discipline. Therefore, I have avoided the use of clinical vignettes; these are likely to distract the reader from focusing on an evaluation of the validity and cogency of each step in the argument. Those clinical cases to which I do refer (the case of Anna O., the case of the Rat Man, and Luborsky's case of Miss X) are included not to raise questions about the merits of clinical work or the meanings of clinical phenomena, but because they are necessary to my argument. As a practicing psychoanalyst, I also allude to, and make use of, my knowledge of the complexities of the psychoanalytic situation, but only insofar as I judge such allusions will clarify my argument.

Can Psychoanalytic Hypotheses Be Tested in the Psychoanalytic Situation?

The philosopher of science Grünbaum addresses this question in a series of important and provocative papers (1980, 1981, 1982a, 1982b),[2] and his answer to it (a mistaken one, I shall show) is "No."

1. "Objectively" does not imply that science excludes interest in subjective phenomena. It does imply that the actual world, manifested in both objective and subjective phenomena, is as it is independent of our theoretical attempts to approximate it and our descriptions or knowledge of it.
2. J. Edelson, as an undergraduate major in the philosophy of science at Yale University, first brought Grünbaum's work to my attention.

Grünbaum takes four major steps to argue that while psychoanalytic hypotheses may be falsifiable, they have not achieved scientific credibility from data obtained outside the psychoanalytic situation and cannot achieve such credibility from data obtained in the psychoanalytic situation. (1) He points to the current unavailability of, and lack of interest by psychoanalysts in, experimental evidence. (2) He shows that Freud and others depended upon the so-called tally argument for establishing the credibility of psychoanalytic hypotheses nonexperimentally. (A premise of the tally argument is that interpretations owe their efficacy to the fact that they *tally* with what is true.) (3) He claims that, because of the inability of psychoanalytic clinical investigators to meet the requirements of the canons of eliminative inductivism, Freud and others have gradually had to abandon the tally argument. (4) He examines the data (the analysand's reports) available in the psychoanalytic situation and concludes that these data are unavoidably corrupted by the psychoanalyst's (unwitting) suggestions and selection biases, the analysand's own prior knowledge and theoretical preconceptions, and the fallibility of the analysand's memory and his reasoning about his own experience, and therefore cannot be used independently of the tally argument to support psychoanalytic hypotheses according to the canons of eliminative inductivism.

THE CANONS OF ELIMINATIVE INDUCTIVISM

Since Grünbaum's argument presupposes the canons of eliminative inductivism (essentially, in my view, canons of scientific reasoning and method), I shall begin a presentation of his argument with my own version (enlarging on his) of a stringent formulation of these canons.

Eliminative inductivism answers the question, "What evidence shall count as *scientific support* for a hypothesis?" in a way that distinguishes it from the enumerative inductivism associated with logical positivism and from Popper's falsificationism (1959). In brief, enumerative inductivism holds that any positive instance of a hypothesis—any observation entailed by it or deducible from it—confirms it. Falsificationism holds that the survival by a hypothesis of a rigorous attempt empirically to falsify it contributes to the degree to which it is regarded as corroborated. Psychoanalytic hypotheses are confirmable and falsifiable, but, while this has some importance, too much should not be made of it by psychoanalysts and philosophers of science (Edelson, 1983; Grünbaum, 1977a, 1977b, 1978, 1979).

Evidence shall count as scientific support for a hypothesis only if—

1. the evidence is entailed by, is deducible from, or is a positive instance of, the hypothesis (that the evidence confirms the hypothesis is necessary, but not sufficient, for it to count as support for the hypothesis);

2. the evidence justifies preferring the hypothesis to some other rival hypothesis (that is, justifies believing the hypothesis rather than this rival);

3. the evidence has been obtained in a way that eliminates from consideration plausible alternative explanations, which otherwise might have been held to account for it.

I shall now outline a more complete and precise explication of the canons of eliminative inductivism (which may seem to the reader more "technical" and forbidding than any other formulation in this paper will seem). This formulation, especially the fourth canon, makes explicit the dependence of eliminative inductivism in general on a notion of comparative support. Support is a comparative not an absolute concept. The support which evidence provides a hypothesis is always relative to the support the same evidence provides another rival hypothesis or alternative hypotheses. Evidence supports a hypothesis if it not only confirms the hypothesis but refutes, fails to confirm, or gives much less support to rival or alternative hypotheses. Evidence which is capable of supporting a hypothesis is probative—that is, tests the hypothesis. Merely confirming instances of a hypothesis as such cannot be probative.

An observable outcome of an experiment, or of some process, setup, or arrangement in nature, counts as probative evidence in support of a hypothesis about a domain, if the following statements are true.

Canon 1. The outcome is deducible, or follows logically, from the hypothesis. If the hypothesis is true, then the outcome must occur (the occurrence of the outcome is a necessary—although not a sufficient—condition for the truth of the hypothesis); or, if the hypothesis is probabilistic, then the process, setup, or arrangement has a much greater propensity to produce the outcome than it would have if the hypothesis were false. In other words, the criterion of confirmability has been met by the hypothesis, but the outcome does *not* qualify as support for the hypothesis just because it confirms or is a positive instance of the hypothesis.

Canon 2. The outcome is predicted on the basis of knowledge of the hypothesis before it has actually been observed. On the basis of what is already known (background knowledge), and without knowledge of the hypothesis, the outcome's occurrence would not have been predicted, or its failure to occur would have been predicted; its occurrence is, therefore, unexpected.

Canon 3. The outcome occurs. It must be possible that the outcome might not have occurred, so that the hypothesis could and would have been falsified had the outcome failed to occur. But as it turns out, the hypothesis is not falsified. The criterion of falsifiability has been met by the hypothesis, but the outcome does *not* qualify as support for the hypothesis, just because the hypothesis is falsifiable (although not actually falsified).

Canon 4. The hypothesis—which here I shall call H_1—has at least one rival, a hypothesis H_2, which is also about the same domain. The outcome warrants provisional acceptance of the hypothesis H_1 as true of the domain *over the rival hypothesis H_2*, on at least *one* of the following grounds. (At least one of three possible relations between the hypotheses H_1 and H_2 holds.)

a. The outcome is incompatible with (falsifies) the rival hypothesis H_2. (That the outcome will not occur is deducible from the rival hypothesis H_2.)[3] Or:

b. Neither the occurrence of the outcome nor its failure to occur is deducible from the rival hypothesis H_2. (The rival hypothesis H_2 has nothing to say about the outcome.) Or:

---

3. The hypotheses H_1 and H_2 can of course involve the same set of variables, but their claims will differ then, for example, with respect to: (a) whether or not some variables are related at all; (b) the kind of relation that exists between or among the variables; or (c) how strong the relation between them is.

c. Given the truth of the rival hypothesis H_2, the occurrence of the outcome is not simply rarer or more unexpected but much much rarer, much much more unexpected, than if the hypothesis H_1 were true. This possible relation between rival hypotheses has been explicated by Hacking (1965), whose formulation of a premise of comparative support may be paraphrased as follows.

IF (1) an observation statement describes an actual outcome, which is one member of a set of possible outcomes; and (2) that observation statement is consistent with the truth of any one of a set of alternative hypotheses, although each one of these hypotheses assigns different probabilities to the possible outcomes (each hypothesis entails a different probability distribution for the set of possible outcomes); and (3) given the truth of one hypothesis, the actual outcome is assigned a much much greater probability than it would be assigned given the truth of some alternative hypothesis;

THEN provisional acceptance of this one hypothesis instead of the alternative hypothesis is justified (the one is not simply better but far far better supported by the evidence than the other).

Platt (1964) describes how a domain can be systematically investigated by formulating rival hypotheses in such a way that possibilities with regard to what is true of the domain are progressively eliminated. For example, the most general contrary or contradictory pair of hypotheses about a domain are clearly stated and one of these, by whatever means will do the trick, is falsified. Then, given the provisional acceptance of the surviving hypothesis as true, one of a pair of less general hypotheses should be true. Again, with the use of whatever method is available and appropriate, one of these two hypotheses is falsified. The process is repeated. (This way of proceeding resembles that employed by a clinician studying a single case who, using psychodiagnostic data and information from interviews, for example, rules out possibilities listed in a differential diagnosis. Is this a case of neurosis, psychosis, or "other"? Given evidence which supports the diagnosis neurosis, is it this particular neurosis or that particular neurosis?) Platt claims that, whenever rapid advance occurs in a discipline (e.g., molecular biology), the use of the strategy of strong inference (avoidance of overdependence on any particular method of investigation, and emphasis instead on orderly and efficient conceptualization and on the progressive elimination of rival hypotheses) is responsible.

Canon 5. The plan for observing or obtaining the outcome is such that a convincing argument for eliminating plausible alternative explanations (other than the truth of the hypothesis H_1) for the occurrence of the outcome can be made from examining the outcome and the way in which the outcome is obtained. Some of these alternative explanations may seem both possible and plausible in one study after another, and may be in any particular study more or less extraneous to the investigator's focal interests. Such alternative explanations propose what variables might have acted to bring about the occurrence of the outcome even though the hypothesis H_1 be false, had their influence not been excluded or controlled.

Canon 6. The plan for observing or obtaining the outcome is such that a convincing argument for eliminating plausible alternative explanations (other than the falsity of the hypothesis H_1) for the failure of the outcome to occur can be made from examining whatever other outcome does occur and the way in which that outcome is obtained. These alternative explanations (some of which may seem plausible in study after study, and may be in any particular study more or less extraneous to the investigator's focal interests) propose what variables might have acted to prevent the occurrence of the outcome even though the hypothesis H_1 be true, had their influence not been excluded or controlled.

It is clear from the statement of these six canons that hypotheses can only be provisionally accepted as true, relative to the time of their testing, and to whatever specific rival hypotheses and plausible alternative explanations are available and eliminated at the time of testing. For the set of rival hypotheses about a domain, and the set of the plausible alternative explanations for the occurrence, or failure to occur, of an outcome, are infinite; and future members of these sets, which come into being in part as the result of the acquisition of new knowledge, are unforeseeable.

EXPERIMENTAL EVIDENCE

Grünbaum's argument begins with the observation that experimental evidence, providing support according to the canons of eliminative inductivism for psychoanalytic theory, has not been forthcoming. Freud and other psychoanalysts have claimed they do not need support from this source, because of the clinical observations available to them.[4] Furthermore, psychoanalysts have tended to regard failure here as inevitable, because phenomena to which the psychoanalyst has access in the psychoanalytic situation are simply not available in experimental situations.

THE TALLY ARGUMENT

That Freud and other psychoanalysts feel they can give such weight to clinical observations depends ultimately, according to Grünbaum, upon the tally argument.[5]

I am not clear whether Grünbaum in his statement and discussion of the tally argument always distinguishes between interpretations (hypotheses which are more or less general statements about a specific analysand) and general theoretical psychoanalytic hypotheses—or, for that matter, between interpretations that attribute some property, state, or attitude to the analysand, and interpretations that purport to explain causally some state, attitude, production, symptom, or other aspect of the analysand. Frequently, he seems to refer to causal interpretations, but treats these as if they were identical with the general theoretical propositions of psychoanalysis. In order to avoid complicating the paraphrase of his argument and my

4. "I have examined your experimental studies for the verification of the psychoanalytic assertions with interest. I cannot put much value on these confirmations because the wealth of reliable observations on which these assertions rest make them independent of experimental verification" (Freud, quoted by Luborsky and Spence, 1978, p. 356f.).

5. "After all, his [the analysand's] conflicts will only be successfully solved and his resistances overcome if the anticipatory ideas [interpretations] he is given tally with what is real in him. Whatever in the doctor's conjectures is inaccurate drops out in the course of the analysis; it has to be withdrawn and replaced by something more correct" (Freud, 1916–17, p. 452).

response to this argument, I have not insisted upon these distinctions here.

In fact, I hold that a psychoanalytic interpretation, frequently, is a supposition about a state of affairs (subjective or situational) in which the analysand is a participant. Such an interpretation follows or is logically entailed by one or more nontheoretical facts (what the analysand reports, or that he reports what he reports) in conjunction with at least one psychoanalytic theoretical hypothesis. Support for an interpretation depends in part upon whether a chain of similar entailments, involving other facts and hypotheses, converge independently upon the same interpretation.

I do not mean to imply by this formulation that the psychoanalyst in the clinical situation is wittingly making logical deductions to arrive at an interpretation. The psychoanalyst may arrive at his interpretations in many ways (here he is in the context of discovery and not in the context of justification)—for example, through preconscious mental processes, which are influenced by empathic identification with or reciprocal signal-responses to the analysand's activity. Justifying provisional acceptance of a hypothesis, however, requires a formal statement of its relation to evidence. Still, according to Glymour (1980), the Rat Man case (which I shall consider later in this paper) shows Freud interpreting nontheoretical facts (for example, the analysand's reports of his states and attitudes) by making inferences from a conjunction of these reports and theoretical psychoanalytic hypotheses.

The tally argument has the following form (I have altered Grünbaum's presentation somewhat):

Premise 1. Psychoanalytic therapy is successful only if the analysand achieves veridical insight (not pseudoinsight but objectively true—that is, scientifically credible—knowledge of himself) and he achieves veridical insight only if the interpretations of the psychoanalyst tally with what is objectively true.

Premise 2. Psychoanalytic therapy is successful.

Conclusion. Therefore, the analysand achieves veridical insight—and so psychoanalytic interpretations not only *seem* true to the analysand (that is, such interpretations are not simply regarded by the analysand as plausible or—as those who regard psychoanalysis as hermeneutics would say—as meaningful), but psychoanalytic interpretations are objectively true as well. (And, therefore, I would add, the general theoretical hypotheses of psychoanalysis which yield these interpretations have survived a test which might have resulted in their refutation.)

Grünbaum does not make explicit what he implies in the first premise—that whether interpretations tally with what is true of the analysand will determine assessment of the truth-value of general theoretical hypotheses of psychoanalysis to which these interpretations are logically related. So, if an inference (interpretation) is false, then the general theoretical hypothesis or the report by the analysand of his states and attitudes (for example, what he consciously believes, wishes, or perceives), or both, from the conjunction of which the interpretation was inferred, must be false. The general theoretical hypothesis is tested by predicting from it in conjunction with one or more facts that an interpretation (a statement about the analysand) is true. It is, therefore, important to have some outcome—such as therapeutic effect—which logically follows from a true interpretation, in order to evaluate whether the interpretation (the hypothesis about the analysand) can be accepted as true.

ABANDONMENT OF THE TALLY ARGUMENT

However, Grünbaum points out, Freud eventually had to abandon the tally argument. Spence (1982, p. 289f.) traces Freud's move away from "reconstruction" (recapturing memories, which tally with interpretations) to "construction" (Freud, 1937); I believe he is mistaken in concluding, on these grounds, that the tally argument is a straw man. It is precisely the implications for psychoanalysis of its own abandonment of the tally argument as a basis for warranting belief in psychoanalytic hypotheses as scientifically credible that Grünbaum is exploring. So, for example, current interest in the proposal to regard psychoanalysis as hermeneutics (as purveying subjective or narrative "truth" rather than objective truth) seems to have arisen as confidence in the tally argument has increasingly been eroded in the absence of any sense of what evidence obtainable in the psychoanalytic situation might replace therapeutic outcome to justify provisional acceptance of psychoanalytic interpretations as objectively true.

Here is Grünbaum's account of the abandonment of the tally argument.

1. The tally argument had its most convincing exemplification in such cases as Anna O. (Breuer and Freud, 1895). That the "talking cure," leading to recovery of the memory of a traumatic event, seemed to be effective in removing symptoms was used to argue that the hypothesis is true that repression is a necessary condition for the development of—and, therefore, a specific etiology of—such symptoms. Evidence is needed, of course, to support that it is just this specific feature of the treatment—talking, which leads to recovery of a repressed memory—and not some other aspect of the treatment (the relationship with the physician, for example) which is responsible for the disappearance of the symptoms. Such evidence was apparently obtained; the treatment was able to cause the disappearance of each symptom separately, without influencing other symptoms. This result tends to support the hypothesis that it is the recovery of the repressed memory—rather than the hypothesis that it is some general or inadvertent agent—which is responsible for the outcome of treatment.

2. However, the treatment effect was unreliable. Symptoms did not remain in remission. Instead, they recurred, apparently depending, according to Freud, upon the vicissitudes of the patient-physician relationship. In order to be able to account for the unreliability of outcome and continue to claim that the specific etiology of such symptoms is repression, Freud moved the past event even further backward in time. It is not repression of a recent traumatic event but of a childhood memory which is the etiologic agent. This extrapolation, however, does not have a convincing exemplification, such as would have been provided by the *independent* mitigation of different symptoms in such cases as Anna O., had that mitigation proved reliable.

3. There is no evidence to support, according to the canons of eliminative inductivism, the first premise of the tally argument (that therapy is successful only if interpretations are true). Suppose we disregard the increasingly accepted fact that life events and maturation itself may have profound "therapeutic"

effects, and are rival explanations of any therapeutic outcome. Suppose we also accept that the outcome of psychoanalytic therapy is better than the outcome that would have resulted from those influences as might have affected the patient if he had had no therapy at all. There is still no evidence supporting the hypothesis that veridical insights, effected by veridical interpretations, are necessary to achieve a presumed successful outcome of psychoanalysis. There is no evidence eliminating the possibility that other aspects of psychoanalytic therapy are responsible for its outcome, and no evidence that such an outcome is not achieved as well by other rival therapies, which relying on other means make no use of such interpretations.

So, even if the outcome of psychoanalytic therapy is better than that which would be expected to occur "spontaneously," there is no evidence which, by ruling out other plausible causes of such an outcome, supports the hypothesis that veridical psychoanalytic interpretations are responsible for it. Other possible causes include: (a) unwitting suggestion by the psychoanalyst (in the form of nonveridical or pseudoexplanations); (b) the belief of psychoanalyst and analysand in the truth and efficacy of the psychoanalyst's interpretations (inadvertent placebo effect); or (c) aspects of the psychoanalytic situation other than veridical interpretations (for example, the analysand experiences a new kind of relationship with the psychoanalyst), which aspects may, in fact, be the intended rather than inadvertent agents of change in other therapies.[6]

Symptoms have been removed by other therapies, apparently permanently and without substitution of other symptoms. When psychoanalysts account for this by supposing that symptoms so affected by other therapies are "ghost" symptoms which have achieved autonomy (are no longer connected to an active conflict), they have, unwittingly perhaps, undercut the argument that remission of symptoms through undoing of repression is evidence for the hypothesis that an active uncon-

6. Grünbaum does not add that psychoanalysts have not provided evidence eliminating the possibility that other aspects of the psychoanalytic situation might enable the analysand to achieve veridical insight even in the absence of interpretations (strictly defined) made by the psychoanalyst.

scious conflict is a necessary condition for the presence of a symptom and, therefore, that a prior repression is etiologically necessary for its having developed in the first place.

4. There is no evidence to support, according to the canons of eliminative inductivism, even the second premise of the tally argument (that psychoanalytic therapy is successful). Given the unavailability of prior knowledge of the propensity of different neuroses to spontaneous remission, a comparison of the effects of "psychoanalytic therapy" and the effects of "no formal treatment" (that is, the effects of life events and maturation, for example) upon similar patients (especially similar with respect to suitability for psychoanalytic treatment), who have the same kind and severity of illness, is required but has not been forthcoming.

5. The evidence required is difficult-to-impossible to obtain. The effects of interpretations are irretrievably and inseparably confounded in the psychoanalytic situation with inadvertent placebo effect and suggestion.

6. Therefore, Grünbaum concludes, the tally argument cannot be used to claim that psychoanalytic hypotheses have been or can be tested in the psychoanalytic situation.

DATA OBTAINED IN THE PSYCHOANALYTIC SITUATION

Finally, Grünbaum goes on to ask: if the tally argument fails, what evidence other than therapeutic effect can the psychoanalyst obtain in the psychoanalytic situation that would justify provisional acceptance of any psychoanalytic hypothesis?

1. Some have taken the position that unexpected statistical associations can be predicted from psychoanalytic theory and then observed in the psychoanalytic situation. Others have been impressed by the convergence of conclusions derived from analysis of symptoms, dreams, and parapraxes. These means of testing psychoanalytic hypotheses in the psychoanalytic situation are unacceptable, according to Grünbaum, because there is no way to eliminate, given the nature of the method of free association, alternative plausible explanations of such statistical associations and convergences.

That conclusions arrived at from analysis of symptoms,

dreams, and parapraxes converge does not constitute evidential support for them, because the apparently different data are
not really independent; they are all obtained by the same method, free association. Statistical correlations are also based on
data obtained by the method of free association, but Grünbaum
claims that this method yields probatively defective, contaminated data. There is no way, in other words, of eliminating
extraneous influences or adulterants, which provide plausible
alternative explanations for a convergence or correlation.

2. Data yielded by free association are contaminated by the
following influences:

a. These data may result from the inadvertent influence exerted by the psychoanalyst. Unwittingly, he conveys nonverbal
or paraverbal cues; he chooses when in the course of free association to remain silent and when to interrupt, when to ask and
when not to ask for further associations.

b. The psychoanalyst's own selection biases may determine,
especially in the absence of any prior criteria, which associations he uses and weaves together, and which he ignores, in
arriving at an interpretation.

c. The analysand may be led, by his own prior knowledge of
psychoanalysis and by his own beliefs about what is expected by
the psychoanalyst, to produce these statistical relationships and
convergent conclusions.

3. Any response of the analysand's to interpretations (other
than therapeutic outcome)—for example, assent to an interpretation previously resisted, or recovery of a memory—is
also nonprobative (cannot be used to support psychoanalytic
hypotheses), because it is impossible to eliminate as explanatory
candidates the following possible causes of these responses:

a. They may be determined by the psychoanalyst's witting or
unwitting suggestions.

b. They may be determined by the analysand's own theoretical preconceptions (not necessarily independent of psychoanalytic theory) about his introspections.

c. They may be determined by the analysand's logically fal-
lacious inferences concerning the reasons and causes of his
states and attitudes. He may, for example, attribute causal relevance to contents, because one follows another, when no such
attribution is logically warranted. Introspection gives no direct,

privileged access to objectively true knowledge of reasons and causes.

d. Memorics, especially, are untrustworthy. Fictitious events are "remembered" as having occurred. Memories are constructions, not mere registrations.[7] Confabulations enter into what is remembered.

e. Both assent and rejection following an interpretation cannot be taken at face value, but can only be evaluated in the light of new associations, including new memories, or, for example, a report that a symptom is aggravated. These data, in turn, also suffer from the defects previously mentioned.

4. Finally, it is the presumption of the causal role of repression which apparently provides warrant for inferences from free association.

a. But that presumption, as previously noted by Grünbaum in connection with the collapse of the tally argument, itself lacks warrant. Since it does not hold up even for the neuroses, its extrapolation from neuroses to dreams and parapraxes is also unwarranted, making even clearer the dubious evidential value of the fact that conclusions derived from analysis of symptoms, dreams, and parapraxes converge.

b. That an analysand has an association to some content does not warrant the conclusion that the association is causally related to that content. Even if one could support from free associations the hypothesis that a particular childhood event did occur and was then repressed (and it seems unlikely one could), the existence of that event does not support the hypothesis that the repressed event is causally (etiologically) relevant to an adult neurosis. For there is no way to show from the free associations of any analysand that the symptom would have developed only in case the event occurred and was repressed, and that therefore if the event had not occurred and/or had not been repressed the symptom would not have developed.[8] For the support of such etiologic hypotheses, extraclinical evidence from

7. A good discussion of the constructive aspect of memory, and indeed of the role of recovered memories in psychoanalytic treatment, can be found in E. Kris (1956b).

8. One does not need to assume at this point in Grünbaum's argument that the event is an external or situational rather than an internal or subjective event.

prospective studies, where manipulation of the causative factor is possible, is clearly required.[9]

Although Grünbaum claims to confine himself in his formidable critique to Freud's writings, I shall certainly refer in my response to developments in psychoanalysis that are not present or focal in, but which follow upon, Freud's work. Grünbaum does not hesitate to quote other psychoanalysts to buttress his arguments. If he does in fact confine his critique to the way in which Freud only among psychoanalysts carried out and reported his work, he limits that critique more than I think he intends to do.

Here, I address in particular Grünbaum's assertion that it is *in principle* impossible to test hypotheses in the psychoanalytic situation. I take him to assert, in other words, that it is *impossible* to obtain evidence in that situation, according to the canons of eliminative inductivism, warranting provisional acceptance of a hypothesis over some rival hypothesis.

I assume the phrase "testing hypotheses in the psychoanalytic situation" implies the use of data obtained in the psychoanalytic situation, whether that involves, for example, the analysis of the content of transcripts of psychoanalytic sessions (e.g., Luborsky, 1967, 1973), or the kind of reasoning a psychoanalyst might use in the psychoanalytic session (exemplified, for example, in Glymour's [1974, 1980] explication of the Rat Man case).

I do not intend, by casting doubt on Grünbaum's assertion, to imply that psychoanalytic investigators actually obtain such truly probative evidence every time they claim to confirm empirically psychoanalytic hypotheses in the psychoanalytic situation. Nor do I expect, even if psychoanalytic investigators

9. An impressive—as of this writing, the best and most complete—statement of his position and this argument will be found in Grünbaum (1982b). It includes both an appreciation of Freud as a scientist and methodologist and a trenchant analysis of the problems involved in the claim that psychoanalytic hypotheses can be tested in the psychoanalytic situation.

should be persuaded it is possible to obtain such evidence, that they will find it easy—or will necessarily be inclined to make the effort—to do so. I also do not intend, by maintaining it is in principle possible to test psychoanalytic hypotheses in the psychoanalytic situation, to imply that extraclinical or experimental testing of psychoanalytic hypotheses is therefore dispensable. Nor do I now, in accepting the usefulness of extraclinical or experimental tests, intend to imply that clinical or nonexperimental testing of psychoanalytic hypotheses is therefore unnecessary.

Briefly, in what follows, I shall question Grünbaum's interpretation of the canons of eliminative inductivism; he seems to consider these canons to be identical with what is actually only one method for satisfying them—*experimental* research, in which a comparison between or among *groups of subjects* is made, in such a way that *all* known relevant variables are controlled. I shall question as well his belief that the data obtained in the psychoanalytic situation are irretrievably contaminated. I shall argue that it is possible to explicate more precisely than has been done the objectives of psychoanalytic treatment, and, although this will not be any easier for psychoanalytic therapy than for any other psychotherapy, that it is also possible to assess whether in a particular case such objectives have been achieved. Finally, in what I consider to be a decisive refutation of Grünbaum's assertion, I shall show that psychoanalytic hypotheses not only can be but in fact have been tested in the psychoanalytic situation.[10]

10. I do not take up here, but have examined in some detail elsewhere (1983), issues that demand attention in any attempt by psychoanalysis to meet the challenge of eliminative inductivism: (1) the nature of psychoanalytic theory itself, the domain(s) to which it is applicable, the facts of interest to it, the kinds of explanations it provides for these facts, the relation it bears to theories in other disciplines (e.g., neural science), and the precise content of hypotheses that are to be tested; (2) the use psychoanalysis can make of recent conceptual and methodological developments in single-subject research; and (3) the importance of formulating at least some psychoanalytic hypotheses probabilistically and of making use of statistical reasoning in arguing the relation between the evidence and selected psychoanalytic hypotheses.

DOES ADHERENCE TO SCIENTIFIC CANONS NECESSARILY
REQUIRE AN EXPERIMENTAL METHODOLOGY

Grünbaum is unreasonably stringent in suggesting that the canons of eliminative inductivism can be met only through *experimental* research, that such experimental research in turn must involve a comparison between or among *groups of subjects*, and that in every study *all* known relevant variables must be controlled.

First, although I agree with Grünbaum about the importance of causal hypotheses, it is also true that other kinds of hypotheses may be of importance to a scientist and, therefore, to a psychoanalytic investigator (Bunge, 1979, pp. 255–262). Such hypotheses might make statements about: a structure's properties; a stochastic system's intrinsic propensities to manifest states or events (an example is the postulated cyclicity of instinctual drives); taxonomic associations (that is, relations between or among properties); relations between dependent variables (e.g., between two different responses, performances, or productions of the same subject, such as a self representation and an ideal representation); or trends (e.g., changes in propensities to manifest states or events over time, changes in capacities over time, or developmental trends in general).

Second, *nonexperimental* research, and also nonexperimental or experimental *single-subject* research (Campbell and Stanley, 1963; Chassan, 1970, 1979; Hersen and Barlow, 1976; Kazdin, 1981, 1982; Kratochwill, 1978), can be used to test causal hypotheses. Grünbaum argues as if manipulation of an independent variable is essential to obtain data that have relevance to causal hypotheses; and, by manipulation, he means especially the use of different treatment groups, or treatment and control groups, to which subjects have been assigned (ideally, randomly), so that each group can be exposed by the investigator to a different treatment or condition, or to different levels of a treatment.[11]

11. "Treatment" does not necessarily refer to therapeutic intervention but may be any explanatory factor, influence, intervention, property, or condition under study.

a. However, typically, data obtained in the psychoanalytic situation are nonexperimental. Causality can be argued, according to the canons of eliminative inductivism, from nonexperimental data by using, for example, causal modeling and statistical controls (Asher, 1976; Blalock, 1961, 1969; Cook and Campbell, 1979; Watson and McGaw, 1980).

b. Causality can be argued, according to the canons of eliminative inductivism, from single-subject data, if, for example, multiple measurements under baseline (no treatment) and treatment conditions, or multiple measurements under different treatments or conditions, are obtained for comparison (Hersen and Barlow, 1976).

Grünbaum, when he refers to single-subject research, argues as if the only possibility is an "on-off" intervention-baseline-intervention-baseline kind of design. He then supposes that this design is irrelevant to evaluating the efficacy of psychoanalysis because the long duration of the intervention makes it very difficult to eliminate alternative explanatory candidates that might be supposed to account for any effect observed. Other designs are available, however, including the time-series design with a single intervention, which may have a lasting effect, and the equivalent-materials design (designs 7 and 9 described by Campbell and Stanley, 1963); as well as the multiple-baseline design (which Grünbaum clearly sees is the prototype for cases like Anna O., where it implicitly serves as the basis for the argument that one is justified in eliminating a general placebo effect as an alternative explanation of the effects of the "talking cure" on different symptoms, because these symptoms are affected separately or independently).

That a multiple-baseline design is not in principle inapposite to hypothesis testing in the psychoanalytic situation, despite changes in the theory since the case of Anna O. was written, is suggested by the following characteristics of psychoanalytic treatment, among others. For long periods anyway, a particular focal conflict may be the focus of analytic work (Luborsky and Mintz, 1974). Working through (roughly, interpreting the manifestations of the same conflict in one context after another) is an important aspect of psychoanalytic treatment.

There is every reason to believe that such designs as these can be used in single-subject research to test psychoanalytic hypotheses in the psychoanalytic situation, although not necessarily those hypotheses focused on etiology or therapeutic efficacy with which Grünbaum appears to be especially concerned. Even with respect to these hypotheses, it is possible that etiologic hypotheses can be tested indirectly, by testing hypotheses deduced from them. If, for example, variations in the intensity of an unconscious conflict result in variations in severity or frequency of a symptom, that could be argued to be indirect though incomplete evidence for the role of unconscious conflicts in the *genesis* of neurotic symptoms.

Must ALL Known Relevant Variables Be Controlled in Every Study?

It is not necessary for psychoanalysis to submit to what seems to be a counsel of perfection. Does Grünbaum imply that all known plausible alternative explanations of an outcome must be eliminated or controlled in every research? I cannot think so. Better for the psychoanalyst to adopt the strategy of seeking in every research to eliminate at least one plausible alternative explanation, the one he sees as a truly plausible alternative, whose challenge most concerns him, and which in a particular study he is able to eliminate. Works on quasi-experimental design are apposite here (Campbell and Stanley, 1963; Cook and Campbell, 1976, 1979), and so is the GAP report on controls (1959). Campbell and Stanley argue that if a number of independent and different kinds of studies are tests of a particular hypothesis, and each study eliminates different alternative explanations of the credibilifying outcome, then it is more parsimonious to assume that the truth of the hypothesis accounts for this outcome in each study than to assume instead that in each study a different alternative explanatory candidate accounts for it (p. 36f.).

Of course, the converging studies must be independent and different in some way (different investigators, methods, settings, subjects). If one adopts this strategy, one accepts that a psychoanalytic hypothesis cannot be tested in the psychoanalytic situation alone, and so one employs various kinds of studies, of children as well as adults, experimental as well as nonexperimental. In referring to the necessity of using a variety of approaches, it is well to call attention to Platt's (1964) injunction not to depend upon or become overattached to a particular method of investigation.

Turning to other kinds of studies does not imply that studies in the psychoanalytic situation are dispensable, however. Making inferences from direct observation of children's behavior to psychological processes, for example, contrary to the impression sometimes given, is subject to many of the same kinds of problems that making inferences about the mind of the analysand from his reports is. Experimental studies, just because of the control exerted to exclude extraneous influences, are often problematic with respect to generalization of findings. Furthermore, intervening in an experimental situation, for example, to exacerbate symptomatology in order to test a critical hypothesis, poses immense and perhaps unsolvable practical and ethical problems.

Alternative Hypotheses Are Not Necessarily Plausible

Not all alternative hypotheses suggesting explanations for an observed outcome other than the one offered by an investigator are necessarily plausible. A psychoanalytic investigator should not be deterred from arguing in a study that a particular alternative hypothesis is not plausible, or from attempting to rule out in "nondesign" ways alternative interpretations of data, when these alternatives are threats to validity—that is, threats to acceptance of the conclusion that the investigator's hypothesis accounts for the outcome he has obtained.

> It should not be forgotten that experimental design is only one way to rule out alternative interpretations [of data] and that sometimes threats [to validity] can be ruled out in nondesign ways. This is especially the case when particular threats seem implausible in light of accepted theory or common sense or when the threats are validly measured and it is shown in the statistical analysis that they are not operating [Cook and Campbell, 1979, p. 96].

According to Cook and Campbell (p. 96), three factors in case studies in the social and clinical sciences often serve the same role (eliminating alternative explanations of an outcome) that pretest measures and control groups serve in formal experimental designs:

1. Often many different variables are measured after a subject has been exposed nonexperimentally to a treatment or condition in order to assess the effect of that treatment or condition.[12]

2. "Contextual knowledge is already rich, even if impressionistic."

3. "Intelligent presumptions can be made" about what the subject would have been like without exposure to the treatment or condition.[13]

> However, one would often recommend with the case study that scholarly effort should be redistributed so as to provide explicit evidence about conditions prior to the presumed cause and about contemporary conditions in social settings without the treatment that are similar to the setting in which the case study is taking place. All inference is comparative, and it is usually optimal to have comparable sorts of evidence, comparable degrees of detail and precision, about conditions prior to the implementation of a treatment and about factors that occur simultaneously with the treatment [p. 96f.].

Support for causal inference in a case study may be provided by either of the following circumstances (p. 97f.):

1. A hypothesis entails that different outcome variables will have different levels, and they do.

2. An effect is observed, which is rare (information is available about the probability of its occurrence), and for which there are few if any known causes other than the presumed cause (well-established causal hypotheses exist to justify this conclusion); and spatiotemporal contiguity links the subject to that cause.

---

12. "It may even be that in hypothesis-testing case studies, the multiple implications of the thesis for the multiple observations available generate 'degrees of freedom' analogous to those coming from numbers of persons and replications in an experiment" (p. 96).

13. For Cook and Campbell, a single group, exposed to a treatment and measured on outcome variables posttreatment, is the subject here.

Obtaining Support for vs. Falsifying Hypotheses

Even if one were to accept the canons of eliminative inductivism as providing the best basis for arguing the relation between hypothesis and evidence, one might adopt a weaker goal than achieving support for, or what Grünbaum calls "scientific credibilification" of, a hypothesis.

A psychoanalyst, for example, might seek, rather than to obtain confirmations of or support for the hypotheses he believes to be true, at least to get rid of false hypotheses. Then he will proceed by deducing a consequence of a hypothesis to be tested. This consequence is likely on background knowledge or another plausible hypothesis (which also may be and in most cases will be a psychoanalytic hypothesis) to be false. If this expected consequence does in fact fail to be the case, he can confidently regard the tested hypothesis as false and congratulate himself on having rid the world of still another false idea. (He still faces in some cases at least the problem of obtaining his data in such a way that he can argue that the consequence failed to be the case because the tested hypothesis is false, and not because the operation of other factors brought about this outcome, though the tested hypothesis is true.)

Such an investigator carries out the task of weeding so that plants in a garden can grow. A small set of hypotheses will survive this process of weeding out the unfit; these hypotheses remain possibly true. Without satisfying the canons of eliminative inductivism, the investigator is not warranted in going so far as to claim that they are scientifically credible. Nevertheless, his achievement, though minimal with respect to obtaining evidential support for any hypothesis, is not minor.

Wisdom (1967) argues in this connection that two facts tend to give weight to suggestion as a plausible alternative explanation of the effects of therapeutic intervention in psychoanalysis. One fact is that different conclusions are reached by different "schools of therapy." A second fact is that each school gets associations that confirm its theories. Both these phenomena, he points out, result from following procedures that aim at obtaining or enumerating mere confirming instances (on the mistaken notion that these give evidential support) rather than seeking refutations or falsifications.

Is there any reason to believe that the strategy of obtaining falsifications is in principle impossible in the psychoanalytic situation? It would appear not. No one can doubt that a marked increase in the number of single-subject researches carried out by psychoanalytic investigators that decisively refute empirical claims following from at least some psychoanalytic hypotheses would greatly enhance the scientific status of psychoanalysis.

ARE THE DATA OBTAINED IN THE PSYCHOANALYTIC SITUATION REALLY IRRETRIEVABLY CORRUPT?

I question Grünbaum's claim that there is no way of separating contaminated from uncontaminated data in the psychoanalytic situation.

Data Are Necessarily Theory-Laden

In any research one must provisionally accept some data statements as true in order to test any hypotheses at all (Glymour, 1980; Popper, 1959). What the analysand infers as a cause does not have to be included among such data, nor even what he purports to remember—but certainly, unless there is some evidence the analysand intends consciously to deceive, his conscious feelings, thoughts, beliefs, and perceptions can be included among such data.

Of course, these data are theory-laden, but the theory with which they are laden is not psychoanalytic theory, and with respect to psychoanalytic theory such data are nontheoretical facts (Edelson, 1983). As in any science, one can for reason ultimately question the truth of the data statement itself, but that does not mean there are no data statements that can be accepted at all. As Glymour points out, if one wishes to be especially cautious here, one can use as relatively indisputable nontheoretical data, not what the analysand refers to in his statements, but that the analysand reports what he reports.

Suggestion

There can be no question of minimizing or dismissing the problem of suggestion in the psychoanalytic situation. Freud himself took the problem of suggestion very seriously, as Grünbaum (1980, p. 320f.; 1982b) points out. It might be possible, however, to reduce the adulteration of data by suggestion in the psychoanalytic situation—perhaps to a vanishingly small degree, or at least to a degree it ceases to be a *plausible* alternative explanatory candidate. Many features of the psychoanalytic situation, in contrast to those of other psychotherapies, are in fact designed to control extraneous external influences on the analysand's productions. The disciplined use of a psychoanalytic technique which focuses on interpreting defense, rather than providing the analysand with suggestions about what he is defending against, also might cast doubt on a claim that suggestion is a plausible alternative explanation for an outcome observed in a particular single-subject research.[14]

In general, while an analysand may achieve insight into the nature of an unconscious conflict and its effects, interventions by the psychoanalyst which enable the analysand to achieve such insight do not necessarily do so by stating for him what the unconscious conflict or its constituents are. Many "interpretations" merely infer the analysand is having difficulties saying what is on his mind, point to the contexts in which he has such difficulties, or call attention to what is to be explained—for example, stereotypy in the images the analysand conveys from session to session, or in the way he resolves ambiguities in the psychoanalytic situation. Ideally, the psychoanalyst's interventions make it possible for the analysand to make discoveries about unconscious conflicts and their effects by making it easier and easier for him to say more and more of what is—with ever-increasing clarity and freedom from distortion—experienced by him as already "on his mind."

This description is meant to dissipate the impression sometimes given in writings by philosophers of science that "interpretations" in psychoanalysis are something like "you have an oedipal complex/castration anxiety/unconscious homosexual impulses." It is in fact here, with respect to the details about what is actually said by the psychoanalyst, using exactly what data, and with what actual response by the analysand, that the

---

14. For such an account of psychoanalytic technique, see, for example, Searl (1936), which was brought to my attention by S. Ritvo.

literature of psychoanalysis is especially (although considering problems of confidentiality somewhat understandably) lacking, and the literature of the philosophy of science (again, considering problems of access to such information, somewhat understandably) most misleading. An intervention by the psychoanalyst is frequently of the sort, "You seem to have some difficulty here, and I notice you have not said anything about what happened (just now/in yesterday's session), although we know in the past you have had strong feelings about that kind of thing." And the response of the analysand is frequently something like, "Oh yes, I was thinking about that when I came in, but forgot it by the time I got to the couch."

An interpretation, properly speaking, is an inference or hypothesis about the analysand (not necessarily a psychoanalytic hypothesis) which follows logically or with some degree of probability from what the analysand has (or has not) said in conjunction with a general and perhaps probabilistic psychoanalytic hypothesis. Moreover, an interpretation usually is an inference or hypothesis which follows from more than one such conjunction. That is, one general psychoanalytic hypothesis in conjunction with what the analysand has said, and another general psychoanalytic hypothesis (independent of the first) in conjunction with other things the analysand has said, and so on, all entail a particular inference or hypothesis about the analysand—all entail the same interpretation. Glymour (1980) has explicated this kind of relation between hypothesis and evidence in science.

The psychoanalyst, for example, following a passing reference by the analysand to the relationship between psychoanalyst and analysand, may infer, by making use of general psychoanalytic hypotheses, that subsequent associations, although not manifestly about the relationship, are a disguised elaboration of this reference; or, following the occurrence of a significant event in the relationship, may infer, by making use of general psychoanalytic hypotheses, that subsequent associations, although not manifestly about the relationship, are a disguised account of how the analysand experienced this event (Gill and Hoffman, 1982). Such an inference does not necessarily or even most often involve "unconscious" contents, or contents which refer to long past events, but rather it may and ideally often does involve contents which have recently been in the analysand's awareness and are rather easily recalled by the analysand to awareness.

In addition to minimizing, by a disciplined use of psychoanalytic technique, suggesting to the analysand what to produce in his associations, which will then provide the basis for interpretations, the psychoanalyst must also be able to argue that suggestion does not determine the analysand's responses to an interpretation, especially if that response is to be taken at face value as both true and a "confirmation" of the psychoanalyst's inference. Such an inference or interpretation, to the extent it can be accepted as true, may be regarded in turn as providing evidential support for the set of different general psychoanalytic hypotheses from which, in conjunction with different reports of the analysand, it logically follows.

In some cases, it can be argued that there is no reason to suppose that what the analysand says is untrue, especially if it is a report about mental contents in the present or very recent past (and not an inference he is making from these contents or a possible unreliable memory of contents in a more distant past).

In other cases, further productions or reports of the analysand follow from, and are predicted on the basis of, the interpretation or inference (perhaps in conjunction with some other general psychoanalytic hypothesis than the one from which, in conjunction with the analysand's reports, the inference was deduced in the first place). And just as sets of other reports in conjunction with other general psychoanalytic hypotheses may have led to or converged upon one particular interpretation or inference in the first place, so what the analysand reports or produces in response to that interpretation, in conjunction with some general psychoanalytic hypothesis (different from and independent of any psychoanalytic hypotheses used to deduce the interpretation), may also entail this same interpretation to which the analysand responds. These possibilities illustrate in part what is meant by the recommendation to rely on the production of new material by the analysand, rather than a "yes" or "no" response, in deciding whether the psychoanalyst's inference about the analysand is true.

Wisdom (1967) points out that the power of an interpretation to evoke a response can and should be distinguished from its truth. The only way to do so, he suggests, is for the investigator to predict what the analysand's response should be, or will be with some degree of probability, if the interpretation is to be provisionally accepted as true. Here, the interpretation or inference about the analysand, in conjunction with a general psychoanalytic hypothesis (different from and independent of any psychoanalytic hypothesis used to arrive at the interpretation), entails a given response or member of a finite class of responses from the analysand. What the psychoanalyst predicts will be the response to an interpretation clearly should not be merely an aspect of what has been previously manifested by the analysand and interpreted. For example, he may predict not only that an inferred motive will be preserved (and presumably become more explicit) in the analysand's response to an interpretation, but also that a particular defense, neither previously manifested nor suggested, will be apparent in the response.[15]

In addition to such efforts to reduce suggestion, the phenomenon of suggestion itself may be studied, and the extent of its influence measured. I have proposed (1975) investigating the "causes" in the psychoanalytic situation of interpretation itself, by examining, for example, the linguistic features of the contexts (in Luborsky's sense) in which acts of interpretation occur. Similarly, such contexts may be examined to test hypotheses that the psychoanalyst responds to some contexts and ignores others when he speaks, is silent, or emits various kind of verbal and nonverbal cues. Data can also be obtained to test,

15. For other discussions relevant to a consideration of the question of using an analysand's response to an interpretation (aside from any therapeutic effect it may have) to decide whether it should be accepted as true, see the volume edited by Paul (1963) on psychoanalytic clinical interpretation, which includes especially relevant papers by Ezriel, Fenichel, Freud, Loewenstein, Paul, Strachey, and Wisdom. See also A. Kris (1982) and E. Kris (1956a, 1956b).

with respect to a particular phenomenon under investigation, just how plausible the hypothesis is that suggestion explains the productions of the analysand or his response to interpretations.

It also may be possible in seeking probative data in the psychoanalytic situation to try to select for observation relatively suggestion-resistant performances of the analysand. These performances may not involve or perhaps do not even permit focal awareness—for example, the analysand's choice of syntactic structures in his speech (Edelson, 1975). These performances, insofar as they are relatively immune to the psychoanalyst's influence and to the analysand's own preconceptions, may provide the psychoanalytic investigator with probative data. (Whether such data will measure variables of interest to the psychoanalyst is another question, but not one to be dismissively prejudged.)

Finally, it should be noted that philosophers of science tend to focus, for example, on the recovery of memories in psychoanalysis and the fallibility of such evidence, and to be unaware of or to ignore the kind of evidence obtained in the psychoanalytic situation as symptoms subside or disappear and are replaced by the transference neurosis. The essential characteristic of the transference neurosis—indeed what makes it possible for the analysand, assisted by the interpretations of the psychoanalyst, ultimately to achieve insight into its nature—is just precisely that neither its manifestations nor their intensity, neither the emerging wishes nor the fears of the analysand directed to the psychoanalyst, can be justified or explained merely or solely in terms of the ordinary conscious mental life of the analysand, the observable properties of the psychoanalyst, or the present objective reality of, or anything that actually occurs in, the psychoanalytic situation, however much features of that situation may serve as occasions for the emergence of such wishes or fears.

The Psychoanalyst's Selection Bias and the Analysand's Preconceptions

The putative selection bias of the psychoanalyst is also subject to empirical study. How in fact does a focal theme or focal

conflict (Luborsky and Mintz, 1974), dominating one session
after another, emerge from a period of apparently "chaotic"
associations? Is it really at the prompting of the psychoanalyst?

What Grünbaum suggests is certainly not true—that the psychoanalyst has no prior criteria for selecting among associations. He can distinguish between, and give different weight to
the contents associated with, different types of "free" association. He observes the degree to which "free" association is deliberately or unwittingly monitored and organized by the analysand, or instead flows relatively unimpeded by tendentious
selectiveness, censorial judgments, or conscious purposiveness.

Indeed, it should not be supposed that it is always necessary
for the psychoanalyst to *infer* the analysand's unconscious wishes, thoughts, or fantasies. These progressively emerge into consciousness, often with an astonishing explicitness and degree of
convincing mundane detail, as conscious purposiveness is temporarily abandoned or suspended in the psychoanalytic situation.[16] Here, in observing variations in the quality of free association itself, the psychoanalyst is able to separate data "contaminated" by one kind of influence (the patient's selectiveness)
from data relatively uncontaminated by that kind of
influence.[17]

Furthermore, I think Grünbaum may be incorrect when he
implies that the psychoanalyst justifies his inferences from free
association by appealing to the "causal role of repression" in
neurosis (on the model of the case of Anna O.), a role which, of
course, Grünbaum is at some pains to show has not been established. What appears to me to be presupposed instead by the

16. Grünbaum is correct, of course, in pointing out that the existence of
such wishes, thoughts, or fantasies is not by itself sufficient to justify conclusions about their causal role or relevance, however plausible or irresistible
such conclusions may seem. That, however, poses no impossible difficulty.
Deducing and demonstrating covariations are, of course, the minimal next
steps.

17. Interest in obtaining "free associations" to an item, in order to explain
that item, has given way to interest in what accounts for the vicissitudes of free
association itself, expecially interest in what kinds of difficulties the analysand
has in reporting what is on his mind and what accounts for these difficulties
(Searl, 1936; A. Kris, 1982).

method of free association (in the same sense that laws of physics are presupposed in the use of a microscope or telescope), as far as Freud was concerned, is that mental processes are purposive. I take it that this presupposition is equivalent to the assertions that (1) all mental processes are related or oriented to, serve, or are governed, caused, or produced by purposes; and (2) therefore, that one particular content follows another is itself directly or indirectly determined by the purpose(s) governing a stream of associations. Freud (1900) mentions two additional theorems, apparently presupposed as well, which he claims provide the rationale for his method. The two theorems, which he calls the "basic pillars" of psychoanalytic technique are: "that, when conscious purposive ideas are abandoned, concealed purposive ideas assume control of the current of ideas, and that superficial associations are only substitutes by displacement for suppressed deeper ones" (p. 531).

If I am correct in assuming that these theorems are presupposed by the method of free association, then that method cannot, of course, be used to provide evidential support for them. Freud frequently appealed to the existence of independent evidence for what the method presupposes to be true. The phenomena of hypnosis are important to him, perhaps for this reason. In a 1909 footnote he claims that the two theorems have "been experimentally employed and confirmed by Jung and his pupils in their studies in word-association" (p. 532). It perhaps goes without saying that psychoanalysts should make explicit—following careful logical analysis—what assumptions about the mind are presupposed by the method of free association, and should accept the responsibility to obtain evidential support for these assumptions independently of this method that presupposes their truth.

The psychoanalyst is also especially alert to the analysand's biases in perceiving and organizing experience. Wherever experience is ambiguous, the analysand interprets it in a particular way. For example, he attributes motives, thoughts, feelings to others, and highlights one aspect of a situation, while casting another aspect in shadow. It does not make sense (here "does not make sense" is equivalent to "is improbable") that all ambiguous experiences should be given the same "reading," en-

dowed with the same features—that is, that reality-accommo-
dated interpretations would resolve ambiguity over and over in
the same way. Since it does not make sense, it calls for psychoanalytic explanation.[18]

Ambiguity and stereotypy in the analysand's resolution of
ambiguity are important prior criteria for what the psychoanalyst selects to attend and respond to, on the hypothesis that
such stereotypy may be an outcome of unconscious conflict
and, specifically, of the analysand's greater propensity, in an
ambiguous situation, to perceive opportunities for gratification
of unconscious wishes, to ferret out obstacles to that gratification, and to resolve ambiguity in the direction of wish fulfillment. These criteria underlie the technical importance of attention to transference phenomena and of working through. It
should not be difficult to make other prior criteria of selection,
in Grünbaum's sense, explicit, and to examine to what extent in
a particular study the psychoanalyst is governed by or departs
from them.

In general, the psychoanalyst is a clinical instrument with
many unknown and some remarkable properties. His properties, capacities, and performances need to be investigated—for
example, the preconscious processes making it possible for him
to conjoin different psychoanalytic hypotheses he knows and
different data in the psychoanalytic situation to which he is
exposed and of which he wittingly or unwittingly takes note; to
arrive at inferences about the analysand from such conjunc-
tions; to match these inferences about the analysand with each
other and with subsequent inferences; and to decide when and
how to convey such inferences in interpretations to the analysand, where the "when" and "how" of an act of interpretation—and not only its content—determine whether or not it
will lead to the achievement of veridical insight by the analysand. The psychoanalyst's ability to detect, accept, and reflect
upon small signs or signals of his own internal and regulated

---

18. I have suggested (1983) that phenomena which do not make sense in
any one of a variety of ways are the facts to be explained by psychoanalytic
theory.

reciprocations of, or empathic identifications with, the analysand's more or less covert wishes and fears (which in the psychoanalytic situation have reawakened and intensified in the transference) is surely important here. Manifestations of this ability, of course, belong to the context of discovery (generating hypotheses) and not to the context of justification (testing hypotheses).

Finally, with regard to the influence of the analysand's preconceptions about himself (which are not necessarily independent of psychoanalytic theory), as well as the influence of the psychoanalyst's suggestions and selection bias, I should wonder about a factor neglected in most writing about psychoanalysis by philosophers of science. It is neither general explanations nor obvious positive instances of psychoanalytic hypotheses that appear to be especially important to either psychoanalyst or analysand. Rather, what is given special weight by both is the emergence of circumstantial detail, having an astonishing degree of specificity and idiosyncratic nuance, in reports of fantasies and interpretations of experience. Such details have not previously been remembered by the analysand (or at least have not been an object of his focal awareness or conscious reflection) and almost certainly have not previously been imagined or guessed in advance by the psychoanalyst. A psychoanalysis without surprises cannot properly be termed a psychoanalysis at all. One cannot regard as plausible that such data have been suggested in any ordinary sense of that word. It is these data that may in the end prove to be most relevant to the search in the psychoanalytic situation for probative evidence providing support for psychoanalytic hypotheses.

The Fallibility of Memory

In general, I believe that Grünbaum's justifiable emphasis on the fallibility of memory does tend to underestimate the autonomous functioning of memory—that aspect of memory which, in Piaget's sense, is accommodative—and the possibility of detecting which aspects of memory are the results of accommodation to reality as it is and which are the outcome of distortion or fictive construction, as a result of unconscious conflicts involv-

ing wish fulfillment and defense. Psychoanalysts often feel that
they can intuitively distinguish between effects of what "really
happened to the analysand"—when an outcome is an adjustment to a noxious reality—and effects of what the analysand
imagined, where "what happened" was merely used as material
in his imagining. It is possible that making explicit the criteria
by which one separates one aspect of a memory from another—
appealing no doubt to general knowledge of what is possible
and impossible, as well as to internal evidence converging on
one conclusion rather than others in the mass of associations—
would prove a fruitful avenue of investigation, both theoretically and methodologically.

Spence (1982) is especially and, I believe, unduly pessimistic
about solving this problem. Like Grünbaum, he too dwells
upon the corruption of the data in the psychoanalytic situation,
particularly by the fallibility of memory, and concludes that
psychoanalytic hypotheses, especially about the past, cannot be
tested in that situation. Previously (1978), Luborsky and
Spence, both gifted empirical investigators, had written a cautiously optimistic review of the status of quantitative research
on psychoanalytic therapy. Now, disturbingly enough, Spence's
pessimism leads him to despair over the possibility of, and to
abandon the quest for, general objective truth in the psychoanalytic situation. He writes in a vein suggesting he has joined
others (for example, those who classify psychoanalysis as a hermeneutic rather than a scientific discipline) in concluding that
objective truth even about a single patient may not be obtainable in psychoanalysis. Instead, what is effective in a particular
clinical instance of psychoanalytic therapy is narrative "truth"
(what is merely possible and acceptable on aesthetic or hedonic
grounds to psychoanalyst and analysand). But this narrative
"truth" does not necessarily correspond to the actual world as it
is; and it "fits" one set of data only (it is not general or gener-
alizable). I believe that it is premature to give up on Freud's
attempt to approximate the unknown reality (1900, p. 610)—
and to turn instead, as Spence has apparently done, to the
pursuit of a satisfying, coherent, and nongeneralizable hermeneutic "reading" of a singular case.

HOW MIGHT ACHIEVEMENT OF THE OBJECTIVES OF
PSYCHOANALYTIC TREATMENT BE ASSESSED?

Grünbaum's discussion of the tally argument deserves special attention. It would be easy to reply to him, cavalierly, that there is no simple relation between theoretical knowledge and practical achievements. The truth of scientific hypotheses does not necessarily entail as a consequence the success of technological enterprises (such as therapy) in which these hypotheses are applied. Grünbaum knows this (1977a, p. 220f.). The failure to demonstrate that psychoanalytic therapy is efficacious may have any number of explanations, which are consistent with the truth of psychoanalytic hypotheses. It is also conceivable that psychoanalytic therapy might be demonstrated to be efficacious, even though psychoanalytic hypotheses be false.

The Achievement of Veridical Insight

It is difficult to escape the conclusion, however, that what is distinctive about psychoanalysis as treatment must surely be the shared quest by psychoanalyst and analysand for what is true about the analysand, about the particulars of his psychic reality (his acts of imagination) and also the particulars of the actual world in which he lives and has lived, and about how he has acted upon this world, how he has been acted upon by it, and what use he has made of it as material in producing psychological entities and structures.

The operative word is truth. Psychoanalyst and analysand seek accounts which—whether plausible, meaningful, satisfying, coherent, or eccentric, meaningless, painful, chaotic—can provisionally be accepted as closer and closer approximations to what is *true* of the analysand. The account sought is an account that corresponds to what the analysand is (and "what he is" includes his mental life, his fantasies, his wishes, and his propensities to interpret ambiguous experience one way rather than another). The analysand and his subjectivity are part of the world as it is, the same world which in another aspect is outside him, upon which he acts and which acts upon him. It is this actual world in both its internal (subjective) and external aspects—and not any possible world at all, however gratifying, plausible, or meaningful that possible world might be—that the psychoanalyst and analysand seek to know.

A psychoanalysis that does not seek an increase in veridical knowledge of self, that might be considered successful although no change in the accuracy of representations of—and no corresponding change in attitudes toward—oneself and the world in which one lives are part of its outcome, is a contradiction in terms.

The psychoanalyst wishes to make use of psychoanalytic hypotheses that he has some justification for provisionally accepting as true (in the "corresponding-to-the-actual-world" sense of "true") and which he intends to put to the test every time he makes an interpretation. For his aim, in the spirit of Freud's commitment to truth, is to enable the analysand to acquire veridical insight. The claim of psychoanalysis to distinctiveness as a treatment, in my view, depends upon the claim that the acquisition of veridical insight by the analysand is a necessary condition, although probably not a sufficient condition, for the efficacy of this treatment.

The Objectives of Psychoanalysis as Treatment

When I say efficacy, I allude to outcomes sought by psychoanalysis. Veridical insight is necessary, even if not sufficient, to bring about just these outcomes. What are they?

The problems involved in investigating the outcomes of psychoanalysis as treatment are vexing, but I do not believe that comparing with methodological rigor different treatment modalities according to their ability to achieve goals sought by some and not by others is any solution to these problems. For example, mitigation of symptoms in and of itself by any means is not a primary or distinctive objective of psychoanalytic treatment, but that is not to say that psychoanalysts have been especially helpful in making explicit what its primary and distinctive objectives are.

The following outcomes surely cannot be included among the primary, distinctive objectives of psychoanalytic treatment: (1) temporary remission of symptoms, whether due to suggestion or favorable life circumstances; (2) a mere inadvertent strengthening of (pathogenic) defenses or substituting of one (pathogenic) defense for another; or even (3) long-lasting alleviation of illness, when such alleviation depends upon continued exposure of the analysand to life circumstances so favorable they preclude recurrence of what previously instigated pathological formations.

The following statements, however, do express what probably should be included among the primary, distinctive objectives of such treatment.

1. Psychoanalysis aims to bring about not only a mitigation of symptoms but a permanent decrease in the patient's propensity to respond with symptom formation to the *same* kinds and degrees of frustration and deprivation that before treatment resulted in regression and symptom formation. Given Freud's postulation of a complementary series, which requires always assessing the relative contribution of both experience and constitution, and his postulation of constitutional predispositions or propensities to fixation and conflict in the genesis of neurosis, psychoanalysis cannot claim that, following therapy, *no* circumstances, *no* kind or degree of frustration or deprivation, will ever result in symptom formation. Psychoanalytic therapy cannot claim to mitigate constitutional pathogenic dispositions, nor can it claim that the patient's improved capacity to manage frustration, deprivation, or conflict without resort to symptom formation is adequate to *any* degree of challenge, no matter how severe. However, should symptom formation occur following a successful outcome of psychoanalytic therapy, one might expect that the analysand will achieve veridical insight with or without help more rapidly than before, and that, whatever symptoms occur, they will be less severe and more shortlived than before.

Clearly, there is no guarantee that an analysand will end up pleased or happy with himself, others, or the world he lives in— only that his discontent and misery are now determined by intransigent obstacles in the world impinging upon him, and by the unavoidable chasm yawning between his wish and his power to gratify it—and not by unconscious fantasies or conflicts.

2. Psychoanalysis aims to bring about deautomatization of

automatisms—automatic reactions, where one might expect reflection and choice. Not the least of such automatisms is the propensity to interpret experience, to the extent it is ambiguous, according to unconscious fantasies. Externalizations and internalizations or identifications provide—in unconscious and distorted attempts at wish fulfillment—ways of interpreting experience so that it conforms or alludes in a disguised form to unconscious fantasies. Therefore, because these fantasies are unconscious and result in wish fulfillment not gratification, the analysand's interpretations of experience are peremptory, automatic, stereotypic, and repeated over and over; ambiguities are resolved in different contexts and on different occasions in the same way, regardless of the consequences.

Veridical insights both diminish, and result from diminishing, motivational impediments to accommodative aspects of perception and memory, especially when these motivational impediments involve distortive transformations. Veridical insights eventually lead to changes in the analysand's attitudes toward (interpretations and appraisals of) himself, significant figures in his life, and the vicissitudes of his life—as well as expand the range of interpretations and appraisals he brings to bear in responding to experience. However, if (and to the extent) changes are inspired by *false* "insights" or pseudoinsights, then maladaptive action, inappropriate appraisals, distorted or stereotyped interpretations of experience, and symptom formation are more likely to continue or recur than not.

Veridical insight both causes and follows relaxation of automatic constraints upon psychological functioning, and diminution of the extent to which—and the number of contexts in which—psychological functioning proceeds in an automatic way to a predetermined end. As such changes occur, the analysand's interest, and the pleasure he takes, in his own mental processes (imagining, thinking, feeling), regardless of their content, increase. This emphasis on the mitigation of automatic responses to experience does not, of course, call into question that some automatisms have adaptive value (Hartmann, 1939).

The content or direction of changes in the analysand's attitudes is not specified in stating objectives of psychoanalytic treatment, for surely this content depends in part at least on what the analysand's veridical insights are; the psychoanalyst can have no foreknowledge of what these insights will be. The analysand's application of veridical insights acquired in psycho-analysis to his life also is not automatically predetermined by therapy; it is up to him, a matter of reflection and choice. He has acquired tools, but no a priori prescription exists telling him whether, when, or how to use them. He is free to attend to or ignore such insights, to change or not this or that about himself on the basis of such insights, to change in one way rather than another. So long as he possesses adequate knowl-edge and is able to reflect, what choices the patient actually makes should not affect any judgment about the success or failure of treatment.

3. The analysand's decreased propensity to form symptoms, decreased sphere of automaticity, and altered and expanded set of interpretations and appraisals of himself and his world may contribute to an enhanced capacity *both* to love and to work, although here too whether and how the analysand chooses, reflecting on veridical insights, to manifest this en-hanced capacity in the varied circumstances in which he finds himself should not affect any judgment about the success or failure of treatment.

Some Tasks Facing Psychoanalysis

What is striking about these objectives is that they involve changes in the analysand's propensities or dispositions, and not necessarily changes in how these are displayed; they do not stipulate unequivocal and unique changes in his manifest be-havior. A methodological task facing psychoanalysis, then, is to devise means of detecting and demonstrating alterations in such propensities or dispositions.

My guess is that it is first of all in the psychoanalytic situation itself that the psychoanalyst may be able to identify the condi-tions or contexts in which such dispositions manifest them-selves, and to detect changes in these dispositions throughout the process of the psychoanalytic treatment itself. Clearly, he must find a way to measure these dispositions and changes in their strength, for example, by observing and measuring changes in the way in which the analysand attempts in this

situation to convey in free association without judgment or selection everything on his mind; changes in the way the analysand in this situation resolves ambiguities; and exacerbations
and mitigations of the analysand's symptoms.

An additional task facing psychoanalysis is to specify not only
what properties in addition to truth an interpretation must
have for veridical insight to result, but what in addition to the
acquisition of veridical insight is necessary for these desired
objectives to be achieved. Interpretation in and of itself, insight
in and of itself, even though veridical, even though necessary,
do not seem to be sufficient. Otherwise, psychoanalysis might
be better deemed, rather than therapy, a purely cognitive educational intervention, which achieves its effects through the
transmission by an "instructor" of knowledge to a "student."

One need neither underestimate the difficulties of carrying
out such tasks, nor on the other hand abandon them. In any
event, the goal of obtaining evidential support for the hypothesis that such objectives as these are more likely to be achieved
by means of psychoanalytic treatment than by means of no
treatment, or by means of any other treatment (if there be any
such treatment) purporting to achieve the *same* objectives without recourse to interpretation or the acquisition of veridical
insight by the patient, is not to be despised.

Grünbaum is not convincing when he argues that there is no
evidence to show that psychoanalytic interpretations are necessary to achieve a successful outcome of psychoanalytic therapy,
because (so he says) the *same* kind of outcome (this is the hook-
er) has been shown to result from life events and the interventions of rival therapies. I do agree with him, however, that it is
the responsibility of psychoanalysis, not of its challengers, to
obtain evidence that supports the claim that psychoanalytic
treatment is efficacious. I do not believe, however, that testing
psychoanalytic hypotheses in the psychoanalytic situation must
wait achievement of this goal.

PSYCHOANALYTIC HYPOTHESES CAN BE AND HAVE BEEN
TESTED IN THE PSYCHOANALYTIC SITUATION

The existence of at least two counterexamples refutes or at least
casts strong doubt upon Grünbaum's generalization that it is in

principle impossible to test psychoanalytic hypotheses in the psychoanalytic situation. One counterexample is supplied by Luborsky's (1967, 1973) invention of a symptom-context method for obtaining quantitative probative data in the psychoanalytic situation to test psychoanalytic hypotheses according to the canons of eliminative inductivism, and his use of this method in single-subject research (Luborsky and Mintz, 1974). Luborsky devised a matched-samples design to satisfy the requirement that a comparison between at least two conditions be included in describing an effect or outcome of interest—a requirement the importance of which Grünbaum so emphasizes and which he apparently regards as impossible to meet in the psychoanalytic situation.

The second counterexample is supplied by Glymour's (1974, 1980) explication of a so-called bootstrap strategy in testing scientific theories (viewed as sets of multiple, interrelated, but independent hypotheses), which he believes is characteristic of actual scientific practice—and as much exemplified by Freud's Rat Man case study as, for example, by Newton's way of testing the laws of particle mechanics.

The Case of Miss X

Luborsky and Mintz (1974) do not present their study clearly as a test of a psychoanalytic hypothesis, but they certainly could have chosen to do so, and I shall formulate the argument about hypothesis and evidence in the study as they might have formulated it, if they had chosen to present the study as that kind of test.

Here, then, is the argument about the relation between hypothesis and evidence in the study, stated in terms that will make clear how and to what extent the study satisfies the canons of eliminative inductivism.

1. Miss X manifests 13 instances of momentary forgetting in around 300 sessions of psychoanalysis. [Phenomena of interest—variations in presence and absence of momentary forgetting.]

2. An increase in the intensity of a focal conflict is necessary to cause the appearance of neurotic symptoms or parapraxes, or to cause an aggravation of their severity. [Hypothesis to be tested.]

3. An instance of momentary forgetting is an instance of a neurotic symptom or parapraxis. [Follows from a characterization of momentary forgetting as meeting definitional criteria for "neurotic symptom" or "parapraxis."]

4. If Miss X is emotionally involved with her psychoanalyst, a focal conflict is intensified. [Follows from psychoanalytic hypotheses about transference phenomena and the development of a transference neurosis in the psychoanalytic situation.]

5. Given that Miss X suffers an episode of momentary forgetting, her propensity on that occasion to be emotionally involved with her psychoanalyst is stronger than it is on some occasion when she suffers no such episode of momentary forgetting. In other words, the degree of emotional involvement of Miss X with her psychoanalyst is much greater in those contexts in which momentary forgetting occurs than it is in those contexts in which momentary forgetting does not occur. [This is the predicted outcome of the study, stated probabilistically. It follows from 2, 3, and 4.]

6. A context is a passage from a psychoanalytic session of a certain length preceding and following the occurrence of a symptom. A control context is a matched passage, of similar length and the same amount of time into the session, from a nearly contiguous session in which no symptom occurred. In an ideal execution of this research design, all contexts are scored blindly for emotional involvement with the psychoanalyst (not just any old kind of emotion) by judges who do not know in which contexts the symptom occurred; thus the possibility that the bias of judges is responsible for the outcome is excluded.

7. Each pair of contexts, different with respect to whether momentary forgetting has or has not occurred, has been matched (with respect to the temporal proximity of sessions and the temporal location of passages in the sessions), so that the contexts can otherwise in crucial respects be regarded as equivalent. Such matching is intended to exclude the possibility that some other difference between the contexts accounts for the fact that momentary forgetting occurs more frequently in association with one kind of context than the other. The contexts are matched by a method (using automatic criteria) which excludes the influence of a selection bias as accounting for the outcome.

8. The predicted outcome is observed. The null hypothesis that the outcome might be expected to occur by extraneous influences alone, acting randomly (not all in one direction), even in the absence of any relation between emotional involvement with the psychoanalyst (resulting in intensification of conflict) and momentary forgetting, is eliminated by statistical test. That is, the particular outcome observed would be much rarer if the null hypothesis were true than if the hypothesis being tested were true, and therefore the outcome tends to support the latter rather than the former.

It is important to note the rarity of the phenomenon (13 instances of momentary forgetting in something like 300 sessions), which in itself tends to eliminate unwitting suggestion by the psychoanalyst (arising from his interest in the phenomenon) as a cause of its appearance. It is even more difficult to see how suggestion, or the preconceptions or expectations of the analysand, could play a role in ensuring that instances of momentary forgetting occur more frequently in relation to certain contexts than others, and that, in the kind of contexts in which they do tend to occur, they do so not invariably but in fact relatively rarely. (This latter fact is, of course, consistent with the hypothesis that the intensification of conflict is, put nonprobabilistically, a necessary but not a sufficient condition for the occurrence of a symptom or parapraxis.)

It is true, of course, that the relation between intensification of conflict and momentary forgetting is a statistical association. No evidence has been obtained which supports the hypothesis that this relation is also causal. However, while it does not follow from the fact that a relation is a statistical association that it is also causal, the reverse is not the case. That a relation between two variables is causal does entail that there is a statistical relation between them. Therefore, the study tests the causal hypothesis. For, if the evidence did not support that a statistical relation holds between the variables, the hypothesis that a causal relation holds between them is falsified.

Therefore, in turn, the research hypothesis did in this study stand in risk of being falsified. The risk was considerable, since the investigator has no warrant from background knowledge or any other theory for believing that the phenomenon of momentary forgetting depends in any way or in this way upon the degree of Miss X's emotional involvement with her psycho-analyst (not just any increase in emotion).

I do not, of course, claim that the study is a perfect one, regarded, for example, from the point of view of the canons of eliminative inductivism. There are, no doubt, methodological problems here. However, there is no reason to dismiss it as an achievement that successfully casts considerable doubt on Grünbaum's conclusion.

The Case of the Rat Man

Glymour (1980) holds a theory to be a set of interrelated but independent hypotheses. He rejects the hypothetico-deductive model of testing a theory in toto by deducing an empirical consequence from it. Instead, he regards scientists such as Newton—also, Freud (1909) using the existence or nonexistence of states of affairs as data in the Rat Man case, and social scientists using nonexperimental data and the strategy of causal modeling—to be testing *subsets* of the interrelated but independent hypotheses of a theory through a kind of bootstrap strategy. This strategy makes it possible to reject and revise a subset of hypotheses without abandoning an entire theory. The bootstrap strategy, prototypically, matches a prediction made from the conjunction of at least one fact and one hypothesis with a prediction made from the conjunction of at least one other fact and the same or another hypothesis.

The form of relations between or among different variables in a theory is stated by each hypothesis that is part of the theory. Some of the variables of a theory are nontheoretical. Their values are obtained by making empirical observations, carrying out operations, or taking measurements. Some of the variables of a theory are theoretical. The value of a theoretical variable is obtained by calculating it, using a law or hypothesis and the value assigned to another variable (nontheoretical or theoretical) to which the theoretical variable is related by some function.

According to the bootstrap strategy, IF (1) the hypothesis in a set of hypotheses about a domain are interrelated (hypotheses have one or more than one variable in common), but independent (no one hypothesis is entailed by any other); and (2) one of the hypotheses, together with a set of observation statements, entails a statement; and (3) the statement that is entailed by this hypothesis and set of observation statements is also entailed by a second hypothesis in conjunction with another set of observation statements, or the statement entailed by this hypothesis and set of observation statements is also an instance of (entailed by) the second hypothesis; and (4) this result occurs repeatedly if one compares what is entailed by the same hypothesis and different sets of observation statements, or what is entailed by different hypotheses each with different sets of observation statements;

THEN it is justifiable to accept provisionally as true a *conjunction* of just those hypotheses so tested.

A competition between rival theories is decided by referring to a complicated set of criteria, including: the number of independent hypotheses in each which have survived such tests; the extent to which hypotheses in each have survived multiple tests; and the extent to which hypotheses in each which have survived such tests are central rather than peripheral.

In the Rat Man case, the variables are states of affairs, and their values are not quantities but the classificatory or categorical values "exists" and "does not exist."

The patient's report of conscious guilt over his father's death in conjunction with a psychoanalytic hypothesis stated by Freud entails the interpretation that there exists an unconscious thought for which guilt is appropriate. The patient's report of the fears he felt at the conscious thought of his father's death in conjunction with another independent psychoanalytic hypothesis stated by Freud entails the interpretation that the patient unconsciously wished for his father's death. But this conclusion in turn entails the *same* states of affairs entailed by the other fact and hypothesis—the existence of an unconscious thought for which guilt is appropriate.

In turn, the unconscious wish for the father's death in conjunction with another psychoanalytic hypothesis entails an infantile conscious wish for the father's death. This state of affairs in conjunction with another psychoanalytic hypothesis entails an infantile conflict with the father over sensual desires. This state of affairs in conjunction with another psychoanalytic hypothesis entails that such a conflict with the father occurred before the age of 6. This state of affairs in conjunction with another psychoanalytic hypothesis entails that, before the age of 6, the patient was punished by the father for masturbating.

According to Glymour, since this last prediction was disconfirmed, Freud chose to revise the set of hypotheses by rejecting the hypothesis that called for such an actual event. He added instead a hypothesis about the causal role of fantasy or psychic reality.

Grünbaum seems to accept the validity of Glymour's strategy; he certainly does not argue that it violates the canons of eliminative inductivism. At the same time, Grünbaum dismisses the particular application of the strategy to Freud's Rat Man case study. His argument that the data here are contaminated ignores Glymour's basis for regarding as reasonable the selection of the analysand's reports of certain conscious thoughts and feelings as nontheoretical facts, since these do not require knowledge of psychoanalytic hypotheses to obtain or to evaluate as true or false.

Grünbaum also chooses to regard the appeal in this case to extraclinical data (historical information)—required to confirm the particular set of hypotheses here being tested—as somehow inevitable in any use of the bootstrap strategy to test psychoanalytic hypotheses with data obtained in the psychoanalytic situation. Such tests, he concludes, will always be parasitic on extraclinically obtained data; Glymour's analysis of Freud's reasoning in this case, then, actually supports the conclusion that psychoanalytic hypotheses cannot be tested with data obtained *solely* in the psychoanalytic situation.

However, there is nothing in Glymour's explication of his strategy or analysis of its use in the Rat Man case to suggest that reliance on extraclinical data is necessarily required by this strategy or this kind of use of it. Surely, the need for extraclinical nontheoretical facts in any instance will depend on which particular hypotheses are tested (they need not, for example, be etiologic hypotheses or concerned with the genesis of a neurosis in the distant past), and whether what nontheoretical facts are needed in any instance are in fact available in the psychoanalytic situation itself.

Glymour provides psychoanalysis with one way of arguing

the relation between hypothesis and evidence in a single-case study—even though the study is both nonexperimental and nonquantitative. His strategy is an important contribution (whatever the imperfections in the argument or data in one or another study). Making use of it, instead of telling a "story" which mixes hypotheses and facts indiscriminately, is very likely to increase the cogency of scientific reasoning in psychoanalysis.

CONCLUSION

The demands upon psychoanalysis should it accept the challenge of attempting to satisfy the canons of eliminative inductivism will be great. A research program—a set of formidable theoretical, methodological, and substantive problems for psychoanalytic investigators to solve—is implied by the response to that challenge adumbrated in this paper. But eliminative inductivism is not some artificial prescription of logicians. It is another name for scientific reasoning, which found one expression in the writings of John Stuart Mill, and which has proved itself as a means for testing our beliefs about the world. Considering the implications of ignoring persistent, troublesome, and well-reasoned questions about the scientific status of psychoanalysis, I do not see any alternative for a new generation of psychoanalytic investigators except to bestir itself to carry out the needed work. That is just one of the responsibilities that goes with being a psychoanalyst.

BIBLIOGRAPHY

ASHER, H. (1976), *Causal Modeling*. Beverly Hills, Calif.: Sage Publications.
BLALOCK, H. (1961), *Causal Inferences in Nonexperimental Research*. New York: Norton, 1972.
———— (1969), *Theory Construction*. Englewood Cliffs, N.J.: Prentice-Hall.
BREUER, J. & FREUD, S. (1895), Studies on hysteria. *S.E.*, 2.
BUNGE, M. (1979), *Causality and Modern Science*, 3rd ed. New York: Dover.
CAMPBELL, D. & STANLEY, J. (1963), *Experimental and Quasi-Experimental Designs for Research*. Chicago: Rand McNally.
CHASSAN, J. (1970), On psychodynamics and clinical research methodology. *Psychiatry*, 33:94–101.

108   *Marshall Edelson*

_____ (1979), *Research Design in Clinical Psychology and Psychiatry*, 2nd ed. New York: Irvington.

COOK, T. & CAMPBELL, D. (1976), The design and conduct of quasi-experiments and true experiments in field settings. In *Handbook of Industrial and Organizational Psychology*, ed. M. Dunnette. Chicago: Rand McNally, pp. 223–326.

_____ _____ (1979), *Quasi-Experimentation*. Boston: Houghton, Mifflin.

EDELSON, M. (1975), *Language and Interpretation in Psychoanalysis*. New Haven & London: Yale Univ. Press.

_____ (1983), *Hypothesis and Evidence in Psychoanalysis*. Chicago: Univ. Chicago Press.

FREUD, S. (1900), The interpretation of dreams. *S.E.*, 4 & 5.

_____ (1909), Notes upon a case of obsessional neurosis. *S.E.*, 10:153–320.

_____ (1916–17), Introductory lectures on psycho-analysis. *S.E.*, 15 & 16.

_____ (1937), Constructions in analysis. *S.E.*, 23:257–269.

GILL, M. M. & HOFFMAN, I. (1982), A method for studying the analysis of aspects of the patient's experience of the relationship in psychoanalysis and psychotherapy. *J. Amer. Psychoanal. Assn.*, 30:137–167.

GLYMOUR, C. (1974), Freud, Kepler, and the clinical evidence. In *Freud*, ed. R. Wollheim. Garden City, N.Y.: Anchor, pp. 285–304.

_____ (1980), *Theory and Evidence*. Princeton, N.J.: Princeton Univ. Press.

GROUP FOR THE ADVANCEMENT OF PSYCHIATRY (1959), *Some Observations on Controls in Psychiatric Research*, rep. no. 42. New York: GAP Publications.

GRÜNBAUM, A. (1977a), How scientific is psychoanalysis? In *Science and Psychotherapy*, ed. R. Stern et al. New York: Haven, pp. 219–254.

_____ (1977b), Is psychoanalysis a pseudo-science? I. *Z. philos. Forsch.*, 31:333–353.

_____ (1978), Is psychoanalysis a pseudo-science? II. *Z. philos. Forsch.*, 32:49–69.

_____ (1979), Is Freudian psychoanalytic theory pseudo-scientific by Karl Popper's criterion of demarcation? *Amer. Philos. Q.*, 16:131–141.

_____ (1980), Epistemological liabilities of the clinical appraisal of psychoanalytic theory. *Nôus*, 14:307–385.

_____ (1981), The placebo concept. *Behav. Res. Ther.*, 19:157–167.

_____ (1982a), Logical foundations of psychoanalytic theory. In *Festschrift for Wolfgang Stegmüller*, ed. W. Essler & H. Putnam. Boston: D. Reidel (in press).

_____ (1982b), Can psychoanalytic theory be cogently tested "on the couch"? *Psychoanal. Contemp. Thought*, 5:155–255; 311–436.

HACKING, I. (1965), *Logic of Statistical Inference*. Cambridge: Cambridge Univ. Press.

HARTMANN, H. (1939), *Ego Psychology and the Problem of Adaptation*. New York: Int. Univ. Press, 1958.

HERSEN, M. & BARLOW, D. (1976), *Single-Case Experimental Designs*. New York: Pergamon Press.

KAZDIN, A. (1981), Drawing valid inferences from case studies. *J. Consult. Clin. Psychol.*, 49:183–192.

———— (1982), Single-case experimental designs. In *Handbook of Research Methods in Clinical Psychology*, ed. P. Kendall & J. Butcher. New York: Wiley, pp. 461–490.

KRATOCHWILL, T. (1978), *Single Subject Research*. New York: Academic Press.

KRIS, A. O. (1982), *Free Association*. New Haven & London: Yale Univ. Press.

KRIS, E. (1956a), On some vicissitudes of insight in psycho-analysis. *Int. J. Psychoanal.*, 37:445–455.

———— (1956b), The recovery of childhood memories in psychoanalysis. *Psychoanal. Study Child*, 11:54–88.

LUBORSKY, L. (1967), Momentary forgetting during psychotherapy and psychoanalysis. In *Motives and Thought*, ed. R. R. Holt. *Psychol. Issues*, monogr. 18/19. New York: Int. Univ. Press, pp. 177–217.

———— (1973), Forgetting and remembering (momentary forgetting) during psychotherapy. In *Psychoanalytic Research*, ed. M. Mayman. *Psychol. Issues*, monogr. 30. New York: Int. Univ. Press, pp. 29–55.

———— & MINTZ, J. (1974), What sets off momentary forgetting during a psychoanalysis? *Psychoanal. Contemp. Sci.*, 3:233–268.

———— & SPENCE, D. (1978), Quantitative research on psychoanalytic therapy. In *Handbook of Psychotherapy and Behavior Change*, ed. S. Garfield & A. Bergin. New York: Wiley, pp. 331–368.

PAUL, L., ed. (1963), *Psychoanalytic Clinical Interpretation*. New York: Free Press.

PLATT, J. (1964), Strong inference. *Science*, 146:347–353.

POPPER, K. (1959), *The Logic of Scientific Discovery*, rev. ed. New York: Harper & Row, 1968.

SEARL, M. (1936), Some queries on principles of technique. *Int. J. Psychoanal.*, 17:471–493.

SPENCE, D. (1982), *Narrative Truth and Historical Truth*. New York: Norton.

WATSON, G. & McGAW, D. (1980), *Statistical Inquiry*. New York: Wiley.

WISDOM, J. (1967), Testing an interpretation within a session. *Int. J. Psychoanal.*, 48:44–52.

PSYCHOANALYTIC
DEVELOPMENTAL THEORY

Development

SAMUEL ABRAMS, M.D.

IN PSYCHOANALYSIS THE WORD "DEVELOPMENT" IS A SOURCE of confusion and a center of controversy. It is confusing because it has both conventional meanings and special technical ones; because the special technical meanings express descriptive and conceptual usages; and because the conceptual usage encompasses various levels of abstraction. It is controversial because it has become a symbol of disagreements about technique and the treatment process. Both the confusion and the controversy have often clustered about the theories of psychological growth proposed by various researchers and clinicians, as each contributor stakes a legitimate claim to the word (Wolff, 1960; Thiel and Treurniet, 1976; Goodman, 1977; Peterfreund, 1978; Glenn, 1979; Krent, 1979; Levine, 1979).

In its broadest *conventional usage,* a development is an event, a happening, an *occurrence* of any sort. It may be expected or come as a surprise; it may be viewed with pleasure or with alarm, seen as desirable or untoward. Within the context of this customary meaning almost anything can develop in the course of an analysis. Fate can intrude, a somatic disorder may erupt, or something may happen to one of the participants. Such developments (i.e., occurrences) may facilitate or intrude upon the therapeutic process, depending upon what they are and how they are addressed.

In its more restricted *conventional usage,* a development is a specific happening, the *outcome* of a sequence of related events whose causal links may be tracked. Functioning as historians, analysts trace such developments retrospectively by establishing

Director, The Psychoanalytic Institute at The New York University Medical Center.

the logical connections in a set of antecedent events. This type
of development (i.e., outcome) may evoke surprise, be viewed
with satisfaction or dismay, be seen as desirable or disagreeable.
In an analysis a completely new symptom may appear, a lost
phobia from childhood may surface, or a patient may make
transference demands. Such developments are aspects of the
treatment and always require study. In fact, psychoanalytic
technique has been partly designed to facilitate the appearance
of certain specific outcomes, e.g., transference neuroses. Determining their dynamic and historical explanations is the commonplace labor of the psychoanalytic clinician.

A still more restricted yet frequent *conventional use* of the
term development implies *enhancement* or positive growth. So
defined, a development is a particularly favored outcome, a
consequence of a successful clinical experience. In the course of
analysis skills may develop (i.e., grow) with the lifting of inhibitions, social interactions may broaden, the range of interests
widen as defensive constrictions are resolved.

Used in the context of *occurrence, outcome,* or *enhancement,* the
term development produces only minimal confusion. However,
development also has a highly specialized meaning in psychoanalysis, conceptually more complex by far. Psychoanalysis is a
general psychology, and included within its frames of reference
are propositions of development. In this *conceptual context,* development defines a *process* of growth, i.e., an expectable progressive sequence. The sequence is observable while one studies
children longitudinally and can also be reconstructed in adults
in retrospect within the psychoanalytic situation. This process
meaning of the word is embedded in the phrases "developmental orientation" and "developmental point of view" and implied
when the substantive noun (developmental) is used.

Psychoanalytic developmental psychology is based on a view
of growth as a progressive differentiation and integration;
progressive—forward-moving; differentiation—increasing discrimination of the constituent elements; integration—a more
complex organizing of the discriminated constituents (Freud,
1913, p. 182ff.; Murphy, 1947; Hartmann, 1950; Rapaport,
1960a; Blanck and Blanck, 1972; Zetzel and Meissner, 1973;
Neubauer, 1976; Abrams, 1978). In psychoanalytic theory, a

developmental orientation or *approach* (see, e.g., Goodman, 1977) is often distinguished from a developmental *point of view*. Both encompass sets of hypotheses, but they operate at different levels of abstraction. A developmental orientation is closer to empirical data; it is "clinical theory" at a lower level of abstraction. Thus "oriented," researchers view and structure data as products of an evolving interaction between intrinsic and extrinsic factors. Psychoanalytic concepts of health and disease are partly rooted in such an orientation. Such a developmental orientation may be contrasted with approaches that see psychological growth as merely the enhancement of fundamental givens or as simply a mirroring of the environment.

A developmental *point of view* is at a higher level of theoretical abstraction, farther removed from clinical observation. It is conceptually analogous to the dynamic or structural points of view, each presumably of equivalent value for constructing highly abstract explanations. Thus, at this level, the developmental point of view is an expression of theoretical scaffolding. It is found as a component of the *genetic hypothesis,* one of the five recognized coordinates of psychoanalytic metapsychology (Rapaport and Gill, 1959). The genetic hypothesis contains propositions of both a developmental and historical point of view; this sometimes adds a further note of confusion since the former involves transformations of prior positions, while the latter involves continuous links to antecedents. I have made the suggestion that sharply differentiating the two components might reduce this source of confusion (Abrams, 1977).

The developmental component of the genetic hypothesis rests on several postulates:

1. Intrinsic maturational factors, constitutional givens, provide a program for growth and the impetus for its emergence (e.g., Freud, 1919b, p. 188; 1924, p. 174).

2. Stimuli arising from external sources help activate the constitutionally determined program.

3. Experiences, the concrete products of the maturational and environmental, become the nuclei for the realization of the program's potential (Van der Waals, 1952; Escalona, 1968).

4. The potential is fully realized in the form of a sequence of stable, hierarchically ordered phase organizations. These orga-

nizations are composed of structures that mediate psychological functions. The effect is a continuity of function and a discontinuity of the organized phases with their inherent mediating structures. Consequentially, steps in growth are neither simply linear nor mere enhancements; they involve transformations of earlier achievements and modes of being. For example, contrasting the components of later and earlier psychological organizations, the defense of repression supersedes disavowal, the cognitive structures underlying secondary process thought are substantively more complex than those underlying primary process thinking, and the postoedipal organization of the psychic apparatus is of an entirely new and more advanced order than the preoedipal ones. The word "discontinuity" describes, and the word "transformations" conceptualizes, this sequential passage into the novel.

Phases are labeled in a variety of ways. This is yet another source of confusion (Piaget, 1956). They can be named in accordance with hypothetical coordinates (Freud's original approach), clinically observable characteristics (quite common), primary achievements (also common), the disequilibrating transitions (crises) that bring the stability of an earlier phase to a close while introducing a new one (somewhat less common); the inherent structural makeup of the stabilized organizations (the rarest); and finally, by combinations of many of these (the most frequent).

5. The overall progression is usually uneven; arrests may appear, or a labored effort past a particular junction may mark a point of fixation. Regressions occur. Since psychological growth is determined by such staggered to-and-fro movements, the developmental process is subject to variations. For example, sequential organizations may coexist, overlap, or remain sharply distinct, and the ease of shifts from one to the other may vary considerably.

History of Development as Process

When the term development is used to define a process of progressive growth based on a set of postulates, this highly specialized use gives rise to ambiguity and quarrel. This is partly a consequence of history. The developmental point of view has been treated with indifference in some periods while raised to superordinate status during others. Sometimes its postulates have been especially emphasized and at other times neglected altogether. There have also been occasions when particular components of personality have been studied developmentally without attempts being made to incorporate the new knowledge into earlier discoveries. Often such studies have led to recommendations for innovations in technique, presumably as a consequence of new "developmental" insights. Such recommendations have provided a focus for controversy, since the innovations have often challenged accepted tenets of the theory of the therapeutic process.

FREUD

Freud assumed a developmental orientation quite early in his career. The probable ingredients that influenced his readiness to do so were the scientific Zeitgeist of Darwinism, Hughling Jackson's theory of hierarchies of neurological functioning (Rapaport, 1960b), and his own research background in embryology (Spitz, 1959). In his treatise on sexuality (1905), Freud outlined underlying phases of organization mediating the sexual function. In doing so, he not only linked sexual behavior to psychological structures, but he also delineated the postulates of psychoanalytic developmental metatheory with considerable precision.

The usefulness of a developmental framework for understanding the origins of psychological functioning and for conceptualizing a theory of the therapeutic process seemed immediately apparent to Freud; however, he was more uncertain about its applicability to systematizing the technique of analysis, a technique which seemed more propitiously derived from other orienting perspectives.

Normal adult sexuality, Freud assumed, is the expression of a specific "firm" psychological organization that emerges for the first time during puberty; the new organization reintegrates the components of its infantile precursors, effecting a progressive transformation of antecedent aims, goals, and objects. According to Freud (1905), those precursors also constitute a "sexual régime of a sort . . . [involving] phases of sexual organization . . . normally passed through smoothly, without giving more than a hint of their existence" (p. 198). The phases and smooth passage are codetermined by the constitution and the environment. The constitutional encompasses at least two features: the existence of an intrinsic factor (the instinctual drives fueled by libido) and a blueprint of the sequential evolvement of the set of expected organizations. The environment, assuming it is what Hartmann later (1939) labeled "average expectable," supplies the opportunity for stimuli necessary to transform drives into mental representations and thereby converts the maturationally determined blueprint into the actuality of the structured, stable developmental phases.

Freud hypothesizes the existence of zones—oral, anal, and phallic—the experiential junction where the constitution meets the environment, and called the libidinal phases in accordance with these hypothetical coordinates. The zones are envisioned as natural regions for the nuclear experiential libidinal products because they coincide with anatomical locales that are rich crossroads of environmental interplay. Thus, the fate of the developing sexual function and of the phases of libidinal (or psychosexual) organization emerging to structure stimuli and implement sexuality rests upon the drives, the surrounds, the experiential products of the two at the zones of interactions, and the intrinsic program of to-and-fro movements (see also Freud, 1916–17). Psychopathology can be traced to some adverse influences upon the formations of such organizations destined to threaten the anticipated transformations and new integration of puberty. Freud (1905) offered what became a model conceptualization of the etiological relationship between the extrinsic and intrinsic:

> It should . . . on no account be forgotten that the relation between the two [constitution and the accidental] is a co-operative and not a mutually exclusive one. . . . The constitutional factor must await experiences before it can make itself felt; the accidental factor must have a constitutional basis in order to come into operation. To cover the majority of cases we can picture what has been described as a complementary series, in

which the diminishing intensity of one factor is balanced by the increasing intensity of the other; there is, however, no reason to deny the existence of extreme cases at the two ends of the series [p. 239f.].

Summarizing neurosogenesis from the vantage point of his theory of libidinal phase organizations, Freud (1937) implicated as causal agents excesses of stimulation that could disrupt sequences, "temporal" factors affecting phase progression, and libidinal pertinacity or adhesiveness. Psychoanalytic treatment is to be regarded as effective if the excluded components of infantile sexuality can be brought into the later organization. Technically, it requires the exploration of the origin and course of neurotic disorders. Freud was skeptical of suggestions that the analyst could promote the integration by specific activities, probably because he feared that any attempt to do so would compromise basic procedures. He compressed his argument into the following:

> In actual fact, indeed, the neurotic patient presents us with a torn mind, divided by resistances. As we analyse it and remove the resistances, it grows together; the great unity which we call his ego fits into itself all the instinctual impulses which before had been split off and held apart from it. The psycho-synthesis is thus achieved during analytic treatment without our intervention, *automatically and inevitably*. We have created the conditions for it by breaking up the symptoms into their elements and by removing the resistances. It is not true that something in the patient has been divided into its components and is now quietly waiting for us to put it somehow together again [1919a, p. 161; my italics].

Despite the clarity of his developmental presentation, the concepts were not entirely devoid of ambiguities—even initially. Freud's *postulate* of the sequential emergence of phases was easily confused with his empirically observable *discovery* of the infantile sexual function. While phases and functions influence one another, each is substantively a different phenomenon. The blurring between the two that became a feature in psychoanalysis was partly a result of the zonal labeling and partly a consequence of Freud's early attempt to organize all of mental life around his theory of instinctual drives. Initially, his psychoanalytic psychology was almost exclusively drive-derived. The libidinal phases were expected to encompass much more than sexuality alone. Object choice and goals were seen as expressions of zonal interests, anxiety as a consequence of repressed libido, and restraints such as reaction formation as merely vicissitudes of instincts. For more than a decade Freud tried to make the psychosexual phases serve as general phases of psychological development with libidinal energy at the core.

New discoveries strained his efforts. As aggression became implicated in neurosogenesis, its ontogenetic sequence was hypothetically tracked as well. In addition, the recognition of the importance of self-feelings forced Freud to push his outline of phase sequences to an even earlier period than orality. By adding a second instinct and extending the timetable backward to autoerotism, he could hold the drive-based phases in place for a short while. The outlined sequence that was to be the heritage of the period of drive-derived psychoanalytic psychology proved to be quite a conceptual mix. There was a narcissistic phase, primary and secondary (albeit no zone of self); oral, anal, and phallic zones, each subdivided and comprised of libidinal and aggressive components (ambitiously used by Abraham [1924] to classify mental disorders); an oedipal phase, sometimes included as a feature of the phallic, but sometimes separated from it (labeled in accordance with the characteristic object interplay); a phase of latency—subsequently, early, middle, and late—featuring a reduction of the sexual along with an enhancement of other functions (without a zone); and, finally, adolescence (similarly fated for multiple subdivisions), a new organization comprising zone, objects, and diverse activities.

By the '20s additional clinical data led Freud from his relatively exclusive interest in the instinctual drives to a consideration of the restraining and adaptive functions of the psychic apparatus. During this period, his drive-derived general psychology became more of a conflict-derived one. Freud (1923) hypothesized a structural point of view, demarcating the contenders in that struggle. He revived the "ego," a substructure of the personality that he had defined, decades earlier in 1895, as a coherent organization "with a constant cathexis" characterized by a group of functions. The drive-restraining aspects, heretofore seen as vicissitudes of instincts, were now designated defenses, originating and strategically deployed by the psychological system, ego. Anxiety, no longer merely repressed libido, became one of the ego's functions, a phylogenetically guaranteed signal of danger. Furthermore, situations of danger which evoked conflict and promoted adaptive strategies were seen as evolving in their own expectable sequence (Freud, 1926). Logic dictated that the system ego as well as the psychic apparatus as a whole must also proceed in phase sequences. Freud was presented with a new theoretical task: it would be necessary to outline an ontogeny of the ego and the psychic apparatus. He willed this task to succeeding generations; but he also willed several dilemmas. One was the heritage of his earlier definitions. Freud had used the term "ego" sometimes to mean a psychic organization, sometimes to imply a phenomenon akin to the "self," and occasionally in an ambiguous fashion bridging system and self. A second dilemma arose because Freud had offered no hypothetical nodal point analogous to the erotogenic zones around which ego phases could be centered. Several were to be suggested, yet none was destined to be as parsimonious as the zones. Consequently competing centers of the ego evolved, since any ego function that attracted an investigator's attention might be construed as its core feature. And the final dilemma: as far as the development of the psychic apparatus was concerned, Freud clearly defined only the tripartite structure that emerged at the end of the oedipal period, the harmonious coexistence of the systems id, ego, superego, each differentiated along functional lines. He suggested that this organization derived from an initial undifferentiated state dominated by a different regulatory principle; however, he proposed no outline of the steps in progressive hierarchies that might be expected to exist between these positions. For these reasons, ego phases and the phases of psychic organization never approached the earlier conceptual elegance or the illusion of clarity possessed by the libidinal phases. This may account for the continuing preference of psychoanalytic clinicians to use libidinal phase terminology as a professional shorthand.

Freud's ambiguous definitions of the term ego fostered two

somewhat divergent paths of inquiry into its development. His suggestion that it is a repository of abandoned past relationships opened one pathway that led to the examination of the interplay with the environment; his suggestion that the ego is derived from an undifferentiated state led to a second—the investigation of its constitutional determinants.

GLOVER

Glover chose the first path. He viewed ego development as a result of the instincts intersecting with the "world of objects" (1932, p. 167; 1943). The forward-propelling impetus, therefore, is drive-derived. For him, an autonomously arising ego seemed too close to the propositions of Melanie Klein (Glover, 1932) or of Jung (Glover, 1966). Later, he also used his theories as arguments against Jacobson's propositions of the self and object world and Erikson's of ego identity. Glover designates the ego as an organ of adaptation, places it between instinct and environment, and defines it as an organized system of psychic impressions. It emerges from conflict; its function is to effect a compromise between the demands of instinct and the amount of gratification possible in the external world (1932, p. 167). The ego develops gradually, evolving as a composite of antecedent ego nuclei. The disparate nuclei, initially diffuse, gradually integrate and organize, and become a coherent ego during a time that parallels the anal libidinal phase. Glover suggested no new labels for his hypothesized sequence. He applied his conceptualization to clinical psychiatry, by suggesting a classification of mental disorders based upon fixations to stages in ego development, analogous to Abraham's libidinal phases.

HOFFER

Hoffer (1950), in an approach akin to Glover's, suggests that a "mouth ego" emerges at ages 12 to 16 weeks, followed by a "body ego" beginning in the latter half of the first year. These structures facilitate the growth of self-feelings and the differentiation of self from nonself. Hoffer speaks of ego structure and self-feelings in a manner that blurred the distinction of ego and self rather than facilitating the establishment of clear differences. By retaining such an ambiguity as well as one between the constitutionally versus the environmentally determined origins of each, Hoffer's hypothetical constructs could be cited by those who chose the first road of investigation of ego development as readily as by those who came to choose the second.

ANNA FREUD

Anna Freud (1936) took a constitutionally determined path. Beginning with a suggestion of Freud's that defenses might be traced ontogenetically, she underscored the new view of the defenses as ego functions, implied a sequence in their development, and emphasized their active deployment toward affects and reality as well as to instincts. In addition, she made at least two conceptual contributions to the question of the development of structures. She labeled the earliest period of life the "undifferentiated phase" and described characteristic defensive operations during adolescence, implying a new organizational consolidation in that period. In selecting the defensive functions, her attention was naturally drawn to the conflict-derived sources of structure formation. However, she did not feel it was possible to name the steps in ego development after characteristically evolving defenses, i.e., the disavowal ego, the isolation and reaction-formation ego, the repression or sublimation ego. The parallel with the erotogenic zones was simply not there.

HARTMANN

At about the same time, Hartmann (1939) took a similar constitutional road, but tracked a different byway. Like Glover, he promoted the adaptive and synthesizing aspects of the ego; and like Anna Freud, he underscored the significance of the relatively recently conceived structural hypothesis. However, unlike either, his attention was drawn to features that went beyond conflict.

Hartmann views ego development as a progressive differentiation in its regulatory mechanism (p. 49) along with an increasingly available maturation of the inborn apparatuses.[1] A nonconflictual sphere emerges, coordinating with the conflictual. This ego that serves adaptation and synthesis has expected steps in development. Hartmann stipulates three: the first, at age 3 months, is marked by the appearance of intentionality; the second, occurring in the latter half of the first year, features "object comprehension," by which Hartmann meant the capacity to recognize and distinguish things; and a third, at about age 6, is characterized by the formation of the superego, the emergence of new regulatory mechanisms. He implied that additional steps existed between object comprehension and superego formation and that additional consolidations followed the oedipal period. As Freud had done with sexuality, Hartmann tilted his treatise in the direction of the constitutional guarantees, the biological timetable. His theory of ego development was designed to promote psychoanalysis as a general psychology. It was not intended to provide the foundation for a new concept of the therapeutic process, nor did it lend itself to any radical revisions of technique. The naming of the hypothesized ego phases—"intentionality," "object comprehension," and "superego formation"—never became popular, despite the fact that there were recognizable empirical correlates for each of the labeled steps and a sophisticated rationale in basing phases of ego growth on the emergence of higher-order regulatory principles.

ERIKSON

By the end of the '30s and for the next several decades, psychoanalysis was confronted with an increasing demand that it bring environmental issues into its fundamental hypotheses. Erikson's developmental theory was one of several responses to this demand. Erikson proposed the use of the term *epigenesis* to characterize his conceptualizations. The term was borrowed from nineteenth-century biological research. During that period two camps arose within the circle of embryologists, the first

---

1. Years later Weil (1978) pointed out how variations in the maturation and functioning of the ego apparatuses might influence psychic structure and conflicts.

dedicated to the principle of "preformism," the second to "epigenesis." The preformists held that all structures existed in the earliest germinating cells, but the structures were too small to be seen. Growth was simply the enhancement of those existing preformed elements. The epigeneticists held that only the potential for the emergence of structures existed, a potential that required the proper surround conditions for realization (Dobshansky, 1962, p. 245). An explicitly critical feature of epigenesis is the temporal one. Structures emerge at specifically anticipated time periods. If an impairment arises because of an inadequate milieu at a particular point in time, the resulting defect can be expected to be carried along into subsequent hierarchies. To Erikson, the analogy was plain: environmental requirements for human growth are highly time-related; they cannot be adequately compensated for once the critical moments have lapsed. Normal sequence contains proper rate and specific timetable and both are ingredients in a healthy outcome.

Within this theoretical atmosphere, Erikson (1940) focused on the milieu. He proposed three "organizations" that impact on human behavior: man as mammalian organization whose physical and mental equipment is epigenetically determined; societies as socioeconomic organizations varying in their provisions, demands, ideals, and evils; and ego organizations, the composite of each individual's unique experiences, a product of the first two. The individual's ego organization was hypothesized as proceeding through eight stages, each labeled in accordance with an expectable "psychosocial crisis" to be met and resolved. Societies are obliged to safeguard this series of discontinuous yet culturally and psychologically consistent steps leading to transformations and to expansion of life tasks.

Ego identity is the comprehensive gain that appears at the end of adolescence, and the struggle to achieve it the psychosocial crises of the phase. Defined as a persistent selfsameness and sharing of some kind of essential character with others (Erikson, 1956), identity formation is noted as neither beginning nor ending in adolescence. A sequence of selves evolves through life, each falling prey "to the discontinuities of psychosocial development." Ego identity grows as a result of the transformations of earlier achievements of unipolarity, bipolarity, play identification, and work identification; after adolescence, it further transforms into a sense of solidarity. So much of ego as self. But what of the *system* ego in Erikson's schemata? The ego's function is to integrate the psychosexual and psychosocial aspects at each level of development and harmonize them with those already in existence.

Erikson's theory was a developmental one; it encompassed differentiation and integration, while discontinuities and transformations abounded on several fronts. However, it was more of a psychoanalytic sociology than a psychoanalytic psychology. Furthermore, neither the psychosocial crises nor the ontogeny of identity formation proved to be substantive contributions to the phases of development of the *system* ego.

HARTMANN, KRIS, AND LOEWENSTEIN

Erikson's work broadened the scope of psychoanalytic interest; however, for many, it seemed somewhat outside the immediate concerns of the psychoanalytic clinician. A more focused study on child development might fill the gap, by sharpening reconstructions, for example. The schematic outline which encompassed those child studies was provided by Hartmann, Kris, and Loewenstein in 1946. Their contribution may be said to have been—among other things—the definitive attempt to outline the developmental phases of structural organization.

The 1946 paper proved to be rich in definitions and conceptual proposals. It defines the three psychic substructures or systems of the personality, underscores the centrality of conflict, specifically distinguishes maturation from development, clarifies the concept of phases, and explains the impact of phase-specific processing on stimuli. Hartmann, Kris, and Loewenstein enunciate what became a psychoanalytic dictum: "the essential elements in the structure of personality exist in children of our civilization at the age of five or six" so that developmental processes occurring after that age "can be described as modifications, as enrichments, or, in pathological cases, as restriction of the then existing structure. Developmental processes before that age can be described in terms of formation of this structure" (p. 19). They then propose a sequence of the formation of that structure and suggest this timetable:

1. In the newborn they hypothesize an undifferentiated phase in which ego and id are not yet separable.

2. Steps suggesting ego formation slowly become apparent. The "first and most fundamental" (p. 20) early pre-ego phase (first half year of life) is the infant's distinguishing his self and the world around him. This differentiation leans on several determinants: expectable experiences of gratification and frustration; the maturation of the apparatus governing motility, perception, and cognition; the distribution of psychic energy and characteristic instinctual modes of incorporation and ejection. In the view of Hartmann et al., the most important facilitating feature in the environment is the mother. The mother-infant tie contains a libidinal and a cognitive component—the libidinal, determined by instinctual drives; the cognitive, by communication. The early identification of the child with his mother gradually develops into what they call object relations (p. 22).[2]

3. A later pre-ego phase appears in the second half of the first year of life. Further maturational changes influence the child's relationship to his own body and the world of inanimate objects. The beginning shift from the pleasure to the reality principle becomes discernible.

4. An ego-id differentiation phase emerges. It coincides with a more definitive distinction between the self and the environment and appears in the second year of life. Hartmann et al. state that ambivalence plays a central role in this phase of development, and they suggest the various determinants that can influence the degree and nature of the ambivalent tendencies. Three specific ones are outlined: first, the maturation of the instinctual drives, expressed in anal erotism; second, the maturation of the ego, expressed through control over its apparatus, the capacity to appraise danger, and the ability actively to deploy defenses; and the third, an object-relations determinant,

2. Regrettably, the term is regularly confused with object representations, i.e., the "internalized objects." For a study indicating the impact on development of variations of parental attitudes, see Coleman et al. (1953).

i.e., the present and prior relations to the real adults who provided attitudes, modes of functioning, expression of feelings, with a resultant facilitating or inhibiting influence on the entire interaction.

5. The phase of ego-superego differentiation. A final step in the formation of the psychic organization occurs when the third psychic substructure, the superego, appears. The superego is less dependent upon, albeit not totally devoid of, maturational factors. The new formation is a result of social influences, and the process of identification with parental values; however, it is especially a consequence of the resolution of the oedipal conflict. This last phase is marked by the appearance of guilt.

Although Hartmann, Kris, and Loewenstein felt that the psychic organization was concluded at this point, they allowed for the possibility of important modifications in later years, especially of the ego ideal during adolescence. Jacobson (1964) and Blos (1979) among others actively exploited this idea.

This 1946 contribution was a milestone for psychoanalytic developmental theory. It defined and illustrated the psychoanalytic concept of development, attempted a preliminary schematization of the sequence of growth of the psychic apparatus as a whole, and outlined three crucial influences affecting growth: drives, ego, and object relations, acting separately and interdependently (see also Hartmann, 1952). The phases were not labeled in a consistent or precise fashion, and characteristic empirical features were described for only the latter two. Their paper was not meant to conceptualize psychopathology in a new way, to modify the theory of technique, or to refashion the concept of therapeutic action. However, it became the theoretical starting point for many subsequent developmental studies and for changes in the way analyses were conducted (Hartmann, 1951; Kris, 1951; Loewenstein, 1951a, 1951b).

SPITZ

One of the pioneer child observational researchers was Spitz. On the basis of his work (1957, 1959, 1965), he hypothesized a sequence of the earliest phases of structural development. In an initial "nondifferentiated phase," the newborn's responses to stimuli are random and reflexive. Within the first 2 or 3 months, a higher-level organization evolves—recognizable by the smiling response. Reactions are no longer merely reflexive; they now entail reciprocal communication. A "rudimentary body ego" has formed. The next great change takes place somewhere between 6 and 10 months of life; the indicator and organizer of this change are marked by the appearance of "8-month anxiety." Spitz hypothesized the emergence of a "libidinal object proper" during this phase; i.e., a particular figure in the outside world becomes specifically distinguishable from all others. While maturational determinants previously influenced ego development, developmental (i.e., those containing a greater environmental component) now become more influential. There also occurs a fusion of libidinal and aggressive drive energies, energies that had heretofore been unfused. The last of Spitz's earliest phases appears sometime between 10 and 18 months. It organizes around a particular turn in speech development, the emergence of the symbolic "No." The ego, interacting with the manifestations of the anal stage, can now initiate defense mechanisms, and the self becomes differentiated from the world of objects.

Spitz saw his observations and theories as helpful for preventing deficiency disorders and ameliorating developmental imbalances during childhood. He also proposed a modification of the accepted Freudian view of the adult therapeutic process. He felt that it was possible for a facet of development, bypassed in the childhood years, to appear for the first time in analysis as a result of its liberating influences. Initially (1957), he cautioned against any innovations in basic technique intended actively to foster such structural growth, holding that such innovations might disturb the natural developmentally unfolding process and thereby impede the healing action. Later (1965), he somewhat altered his view. Narcissistic patients, he suggested, had to be treated with technical modifications. "What has been lacking in the patient's object relations should be provided by the therapist" (p. 295).

JACOBSON

While Spitz narrowed his field of inquiry to the development of a portion of the psychic apparatus at a very early period, Jacobson attempted to reconstruct a wider variety of sequences over a longer time span. In *The Self and the Object World* (1964), she took as her starting point Hartmann's distinction between the ego and the self and set out to trace the growth of the system, ego, and its substructure, self. At the same time, she outlined sequences in the development of the id, the superego, and what she called the representational world of objects. While she acknowledged that both constitution and environment determine the fate of the psychic apparatus, much of her attention focused on the influences arising from the child's immediate caretaking.

Jacobson saw her work as valuable in accounting for a broad spectrum of psychological disorders. Aspects of her treatise were used (by Kernberg, for example) as a theoretical foundation for altering analytic procedures so as to be able to treat a wider scope of patients. Jacobson (1971) herself felt that "severely depressed" patients require specific modifications, sometimes in frequency of visits and often in respect to alterations in customary stance (p. 281ff.).

Like Hartmann, Anna Freud, and Spitz, Jacobson (1964) assumed the existence of an initial undifferentiated phase. However, the undifferentiated elements harbor much more than ego and id. For Jacobson, the mental apparatus begins as a "primal psychophysiological self." It is structurally undifferentiated and contains a composite of energies still not distinguishable as libido or aggressiveness. Hence, it is also economically undifferentiated. It is further undifferentiated in respect to drive distribution and the direction of discharge. While the proportion of drive *distribution* might have many determinants, Jacobson theorizes that a pathological tilt toward aggressivity probably originates in poor maternal care. There are mitigating possibilities later on. The two drives inevitably undergo fusion, thus reducing the aggressive-drive potential, and the expected sequential change in drive quality from a fully instinctualized to a neutralized state further reduces the perils of an initial excessive aggressiveness. The proportion of the *direction* of drive discharge also is subject to variations. The direction might be more inside or more outside: inside, toward the soma; outside, along the motor pathways of activity. These distinctions are important for Jacobson since they allow her to hypothesize an early source of psychosomatic disorders, i.e., enhanced aggressive energies excessively discharged inwardly (compare Schur, 1955). The inside discharges also are viewed as precursors of the self, and the outside as forerunners of object representations. Consequently, the initial proportion of tilt in distribution and direction inevitably shapes all future growth, normal and abnormal. Stable self and object representations slowly emerge from the undifferentiated primal psychophysiological state and its early tilts. Jacobson saw the simultaneously evolving phases of psychosexual and ego development and the emerging object relationships as additional influences on the nature and quality of the representations.

In this context, identifications also drew her attention. Many evolving ego attitudes, interests, and functions are viewed as reflections of parental prototypes. The pattern or modes of identification also undergo a sequential development from an earlier magical illusory form to a later more reality-bound type. For Jacobson, progressive structuralization is closely tied to both the modes of identifications and the actualities of the prototype persons available in the milieu setting. All of this transpires within an autonomous ground plan of stages in the progressive differentiation of the self and object world: initial self-object fusion, subsequent distinctions between self and others, and ultimate self and object constancy.

Finally, writing of the core development of the superego, Jacobson describes yet another sequence—steps in an inevitably evolving value system. Values initially concretize about polarities of pleasure versus unpleasure, move to issues of strength versus weakness, progress to phallic strength as contrasted with the castrated state, and finally, following oedipal resolution, transform into a system of moral values—good and bad. Jacobson notes that idealization undergoes additional changes during adolescence.

All of these developmental processes, assuring energic and

structural progressive differentiation, are intimately cross-linked with one another, and each is highly responsive to the environmental setting within which the patterning evolved. It is evident that Jacobson viewed the parent-child relationship as the "most influential" determinant in that setting. She asserted, "Parental love is the best guarantee for the development of object and self constancy, of healthy social and love relations, and of lasting identifications, and hence for a normal ego and superego formation" (p. 55).

MAHLER

Mahler's developmental research may be seen as a highly focused sector of Jacobson's constructs. It is centered on a specific feature in the first 3 years of life, the process of establishing separateness and individuality. Mahler underscored her view of the significance of this process for the formation of the psychic structure by designating it "psychological birth." She paid close attention to a feature of one of the three basic determinants of psychic structure hypothesized by Hartmann et al.—the object-relations determinant. Freud initially viewed structural growth as a response to libidinal phases; in effect, he studied the development of the ego in the presence of average expectable object relations and an average expectable autonomous ego. Hartmann and Spitz concentrated on the autonomous aspects of early ego development, in effect in the presence of average expectable object relations and instincts. Mahler's study complemented the others in examining ego development under circumstances of an average expectable id and average expectable autonomous ego factors.

Mahler et al. (1975) delineate an anticipated sequence of discontinuous steps unfolding in a forward direction and culminating in two complementary outcomes, the intrapsychic awareness of separateness and the acquisition of a distinct and unique individuality (p. 292). Viewing the sequence as codetermined by intrinsic maturational factors and specific environmental responses, Mahler et al. propose that "a major organization of intrapsychic and behavioral life develops around issues of separation and individuation" (p. 4); consequently they regard that period of psychic growth as a separation-individuation phase. Four steps are seen as nuclei or four subphases. The ultimate achievements include the consolidation of representations of self and objects (crucial prerequisites for the sense of identity), structuralization of the ego, and the emergence of basic moods. The separation-individuation phase is pictured as antecedent to and an important influence upon the oedipal phase that shortly follows it. Acknowledging that issues of separation and individuation may occur throughout different periods of life, Mahler et al. emphasize that their study concentrates only on the original occurrences, the core of all such future activities. Mahler (1974) regards her work as particularly useful for clinicians since it permits a more precise reconstruction of the preverbal period. Many patients, otherwise inaccessible to analysis, can be helped as a result of these insights into the origin of structural deficiencies. In addition, idiosyncratic features of the oedipal phase might be traced to defects in the antecedent separation-individuation phases, and thereby also enhance the work of analysis (see, e.g., McDevitt, 1971; Kramer, 1979). Mahler did not recommend any fundamental modifications in technique, nor did she call for a change in the theory of the therapeutic process. Some clinicians, however, have seen implications in her research that have moved them to do one or the other (see, e.g., Fleming, 1975; Settlage, 1977).

ANNA FREUD

Anna Freud (1965) attempted to broaden developmental theory so that it might prove useful in a wider array of clinical situations. She extended the concept to include not simply selected systems or functions or facets influencing substructures but observational correlates—"historical realities" (p. 64)—involving the total personality. "What we are looking for are the basic interactions between id and ego and their various developmental levels, and also age-related sequences . . . comparable to the maturational sequence of libidinal stages or the gradual unfolding of the ego functions" (p. 63). She conceptualized this schema as "developmental lines" and suggested several that could be clinically useful in working with children and adults.[3] The prototype line was the movement from dependency to emotional self-reliance and adult object relationships, a prototype that attempted to organize the development of self and objects in steps from infancy to adulthood. The labeling of the steps proved less felicitous than the concept promised, since the terms were drawn from various theoretical perspectives and levels of abstraction. For example, the prototype line begins in infancy as a biological unity encompassing narcissistic features, is further divided in terms of Mahler's subphases, proceeds to the step of Melanie Klein's part object, then to the stage of object constancy (a hypothetical construct), to the ambivalence reflecting the anal-sadistic stage, to the object-centered phallic-oedipal, to a latency period (where the features become more descriptive than hypothetical), to a preadolescent "prelude," and finally to the genital supremacy of adolescence. By adding clinical descriptions to each labeled step, Anna Freud was able to utilize her schema of developmental lines for constructing psychoanalytic profiles to assess normality, classify types and degrees of disorders, determine analyzability, and evaluate the effectiveness of therapeutic efforts. The concept was not conceived as a basis for changes in basic technique or revisions in the concept of the therapeutic process.

KOHUT

Kohut's developmental concepts (1979), on the other hand, have evoked many controversies, chiefly because of the changes in technique and the revisions in the concept of the analytic process explicitly emerging from them. Designed to be particularly useful for understanding the causes of a specific group of patients diagnosed as having "narcissistic personalities" or "disorders of the self," the concepts have also been thought to be applicable to the understanding of psychological growth in general. Kohut saw the self as the core of personality, derived

3. For a similar ambitious attempt utilizing libidinal phases to outline sequences, see Flapan and Neubauer (1979).

from both inherited and environmental determinants. It is a composite of constituents acquired in the interplay with those persons in the earliest environment described as self-objects, i.e., persons in the surrounds experienced as part of the self. A "firm" self, the result of optimal interactions between the child and his self-objects, is seen to emerge from three sources: a polar component striving for power and success, a second pole harboring idealized goals, and "an intermediate area of basic talents and skills that are activated by the tension arc that establishes itself between ambitions and ideals" (Kohut and Wolf, 1978, p. 414). Once the self crystallizes, it aims toward the realization of "its own specific program of action," a program determined and created by the patterns of the constituents.[4]

The seqeunce of the development of the integrated self can be tracked in terms of the degree of cohesiveness that is achieved. Specific requirements of parenting during different periods are suggested as necessary to promote the sequence. A classification of disorders linked to stumbling on the steps of self-development is described. Kohut's developmental theory seems based on the traditional psychoanalytic postulates. However, his nosology, technique, and conceptualization of the psychoanalytic process are not customary psychoanalytic positions. To some analysts, the changes are of such an order as to seriously compromise the expected treatment process. The word developmental has become the harassed hostage during disputes about such applications (see, e.g., Levine, 1979).

Conclusion

Many psychoanalytic developmental theories have been proposed over time, some concordant, some in conflict. One common aim has been to account for the growth of the psychic apparatus; another, to help create a psychoanalytically useful classification of health and disease. The theories differ in a variety of respects. They differ in the degree of focus on constitutional as contrasted with environmental determinants (more the former in the initial decades of psychoanalysis, more

4. Compare Lichtenberg's (1975) three sources of self.

the latter in recent years). They differ in their scope (Hartmann et al., Jacobson, and Anna Freud the broadest; Kohut, Mahler, Hoffer, and Spitz more narrow). They differ in localizing impairments in development and hence assigning causative factors in diseases, although all share the position that the earlier the area of weakness, the more serious the disorder. They differ in the degree to which the theories have posed a threat to the fundamental technique of psychoanalysis or the concept of the therapeutic process (less challenging in the initial years, somewhat increasingly so in the last decade or two). They differ in origins, some having been derived exclusively from reconstructions in adult clinical work, while others are largely products of direct observational studies of children. They differ in the approach of labeling the developmental sequences, some using abstract concepts, others concrete observable phenomena, a few both. And finally they differ in the ways they view what is fundamental for phase evolvement: drives, inherent structural potential, object relations.

BIBLIOGRAPHY

ABRAHAM, K. (1924), A short study of the development of the libido, viewed in the light of mental disorders. *Selected Papers on Psycho-Analysis.* London: Hogarth Press, 1949, pp. 418–479.

ABRAMS, S. (1977), The genetic point of view. *J. Amer. Psychoanal. Assn.,* 25:417–425.

――― (1978), The teaching and learning of psychoanalytic developmental psychology. *J. Amer. Psychoanal. Assn.,* 26:387–406.

BLANCK, G. & BLANCK, R. (1972), Toward a psychoanalytic developmental psychology. *J. Amer. Psychoanal. Assn.,* 20:668–710.

BLOS, P. (1979), *The Adolescent Passage.* New York: Int. Univ. Press.

COLEMAN, R. W., KRIS, E., & PROVENCE, S. (1953), The study of variations of early parental attitudes. *Psychoanal. Study Child,* 8:20–47.

DOBSHANSKY, T. (1962), *Mankind Evolving.* New Haven & London: Yale Univ. Press.

ERIKSON, E. H. (1940), Problems of infancy and early childhood. In *Outline of Abnormal Psychology,* ed. G. Murphy & A. Bachrach. New York: Modern Library, 1954, pp. 3–36.

――― (1956), The problem of ego identity. *J. Amer. Psychoanal. Assn.,* 4:56–121.

ESCALONA, S. K. (1968), *The Roots of Individuality.* Chicago: Aldine.

FLAPAN, D. & NEUBAUER, P. B. (1979), *The Assessment of Early Child Development*. New York: Aronson.

FLEMING, J. (1975), Some observations on object constancy in the psychoanalysis of adults. *J. Amer. Psychoanal. Assn.*, 23:743–760.

FREUD, A. (1936), The ego and the mechanisms of defense. *W.*, 2.

—— (1965), The concept of developmental lines. *W.*, 6:62–92.

FREUD, S. (1905), Three essays on the theory of sexuality. *S.E.*, 7:125–245.

—— (1913), The claims of psycho-analysis to scientific interest. *S.E.*, 13:165–190.

—— (1916–17), Some thoughts on development and regression—aetiology. *S.E.*, 16:339–357.

—— (1919a), Lines of advance in psycho-analytic therapy. *S.E.*, 17:159–168.

—— (1919b), 'A child is being beaten.' *S.E.*, 17:175–204.

—— (1923), The ego and the id. *S.E.*, 19:3–66.

—— (1924), The dissolution of the oedipus complex. *S.E.*, 19:173–179.

—— (1926), Inhibitions, symptoms and anxiety. *S.E.*, 20:77–174.

—— (1937), Analysis terminable and interminable. *S.E.*, 23:216–253.

—— (1950 [1895]), Project for a scientific psychology. *S.E.*, 1:283–397.

GLENN, J. (1979), The developmental point of view in adult analysis. *J. Phila. Assn. Psychoanal.*, 6:21–38.

GLOVER, E. (1932), A psycho-analytical approach to the classification of mental disorders. In *On the Early Development of Mind*. New York: Int. Univ. Press, 1956, pp. 161–186.

—— (1943), The concept of dissociation. In *On the Early Development of Mind*. New York: Int. Univ. Press, 1956, pp. 307–323.

—— (1966), Metapsychology or metaphysics. *Psychoanal. Q.*, 35:173–190.

GOODMAN, S. (1977), Child analysis. In *Psychoanalytic Education and Research*, ed. S. Goodman. New York: Int. Univ. Press, pp. 49–102.

HARTMANN, H. (1939), *Ego Psychology and the Problem of Adaptation*. New York: Int. Univ. Press, 1958.

—— (1950), Psychoanalysis and developmental psychology. *Psychoanal. Study Child*, 5:7–17.

—— (1951), Technical implications of ego psychology. *Psychoanal. Q.*, 20:31–43.

—— (1952), The mutual influences in the development of ego and id. *Psychoanal. Study Child*, 7:9–30.

—— KRIS, E., & LOEWENSTEIN, R. M. (1946), Comments on the formation of psychic structure. *Psychoanal. Study Child*, 2:11–38.

HOFFER, W. (1950), Development of the body ego. *Psychoanal. Study Child*, 5:18–23.

JACOBSON, E. (1964), *The Self and the Object World*. New York: Int. Univ. Press.

—— (1971), *Depression*. New York: Int. Univ. Press.

KOHUT, H. (1979), The two analyses of Mr. Z. *Int. J. Psychoanal.*, 60:3–27.

—— & WOLF, E. S. (1978), The disorders of the self and their treatment. *Int. J. Psychoanal.*, 59:413–425.

KRAMER, S. (1979), The technical significance and application of Mahler's separation-individuation theory. *J. Amer. Psychoanal. Assn.*, 27 (Suppl.): 241–262.

KRENT, J. (1979), Some thoughts about the impact of psychoanalytic developmental psychology upon adult psychoanalysis. *J. Phila. Assn. Psychoanal.*, 6:73–82.

KRIS, E. (1951), Ego psychology and interpretation in psychoanalytic therapy. *Psychoanal. Q.*, 20:15–30.

LEVINE, F. J. (1979), On the clinical application of Heinz Kohut's psychology of self. *J. Phila. Assn. Psychoanal.*, 6:1–20.

LICHTENBERG, J. D. (1975), The development of the sense of self. *J. Amer. Psychoanal. Assn.*, 23:453–484.

LOEWENSTEIN, R. M. (1951a), The problem of interpretation. *Psychoanal. Q.*, 20:1–14.

———— (1951b), Ego development and psychoanalytic technique. *Amer. J. Psychiat.*, 107:617–622.

McDEVITT, J. B. (1971), Preoedipal determinants of an infantile neurosis. In *Separation-Individuation*, ed. J. B. McDevitt & C. F. Settlage. New York: Int. Univ. Press, pp. 201–226.

MAHLER, M. S. (1974), Symbiosis and individuation. *Psychoanal. Study Child*, 29:89–106.

———— PINE, F., & BERGMAN, A. (1975), *The Psychological Birth of the Human Infant*. New York: Basic Books.

MURPHY, G. (1947), *Personality*. New York: Harper, p. 619.

NEUBAUER, P. B. (1976), *The Process of Child Development*. New York & Scarborough, Ontario: New American Library.

PETERFREUND, E. (1978), Some critical comments on psychoanalytic conceptualizations of infancy. *Int. J. Psychoanal.*, 59:427–441.

PIAGET, J. (1956), The general problems of the psychological development of the child. In *Discussion in Child Development*, ed. J. M. Tanner & B. Inhelder. New York: Int. Univ. Press, 4:3–27.

RAPAPORT, D. (1960a), Psychoanalysis as a developmental psychology. In *The Collected Papers of David Rapaport*, ed. M. M. Gill. New York: Basic Books, 1967, pp. 820–852.

———— (1960b), *The Structure of Psychoanalytic Theory. Psychol. Issues*, monogr. 6. New York: Int. Univ. Press.

———— & GILL, M. M. (1959), The points of view and assumptions of metapsychology. *Int. J. Psychoanal.*, 40:153–162.

SCHUR, M. (1955), Comments on the metapsychology of somatization. *Psychoanal. Study Child*, 10:119–168.

SETTLAGE, C. F. (1977), The psychoanalytic understanding of narcissistic and borderline personality disorders. *J. Amer. Psychoanal. Assn.*, 25:805–834.

SPITZ, R. A. (1957), *No and Yes*. New York: Int. Univ. Press.

———— (1959), *A Genetic Field Theory of Ego Formation*. New York: Int. Univ. Press.

———— (1965), *The First Year of Life*. New York: Int. Univ. Press.

THIEL, J. H. & TREURNIET, N. (1976), Panel on 'The implications of recent advances in the knowledge of child development for the treatment of adults.' *Int. J. Psychoanal.*, 57:429–439.

VAN DER WAALS, H. G. (1952), The mutual influences in the development of ego and id. *Psychoanal. Study Child*, 7:66–68.

WEIL, A. P. (1978), Maturational variations and genetic-dynamic issues. *J. Amer. Psychoanal. Assn.*, 26:461–481.

WOLFF, P. H. (1960), *The Development Psychologies of Jean Piaget and Psychoanalysis. Psychol. Issues,* monogr. 5. New York: Int. Univ. Press.

ZETZEL, E. R. & MEISSNER, W. W. (1973), *Basic Concepts of Psychoanalytic Psychiatry.* New York: Basic Books.

Adoptive Parents

Generative Conflict and Generational Continuity

HAROLD P. BLUM, M.D.

> So God created man in his own image, in the image of
> God he created him; male and female he created
> them. And God blessed them, and God said to them,
> "Be fruitful and multiply" (Genesis 1:27–28).

ANALYTIC STUDIES OF ADOPTION HAVE HIGHLIGHTED MANY
of the problems encountered by adoptive parents and their
adopted children. These problems are not necessarily different
from those encountered in other patients, and no special syndrome or disturbance has been associated with adoption. All
parents and children have conflicts and problems; all parents
and children are ambivalent toward each other; and parenting
may be added to the list of the impossible professions. However, the reality of adoption does color the family situation of
the adoptive parents and their adopted child; influences the
activation, magnitude, and solution of various psychological
conflicts; and has an impact on the personality development of
the adoptive child (Panel, 1967; Schechter, 1970; Wieder,
1978; Brinich, 1980). This paper deals especially with problems
which have received insufficient attention in the psychoanalytic

Editor, *Journal of the American Psychoanalytic Association;* Clinical Professor of
Psychiatry, New York University.

This paper is respectfully dedicated to and written in honor of the late Dr.
Marianne Kris who was so extraordinarily attuned to parent-child relationships and the nuances of human development.

literature and which are related to the special reality of adoption and to the type of adoption which is consequent to infertility.

The reality of adoption influences the parent-child relationship, the fantasy systems of parent and child, their unconscious communications, and the nature of the unconscious intrafamilial identifications, defenses, and attitudes. The motives, circumstances, facts, and feelings regarding adoption are part of the reality and ambiance of the entire family. It is a reality to which the adopted child responds, which he alters with his own reactions, and which is mediated and communicated to the child through the relationship with his adopted parents.

Earlier psychoanalytic contributions have highlighted the complex influences on and the special problems in personality development encountered by adopted children. Analyses of adopted children have, in addition, been especially geared to an understanding of the fantasy system of the adopted child, those fantasies which have been intensified and seemingly validated in reality by the actual circumstances of adoption. While much has been written about the fantasied natural parents who may still be alive and who may be found or who may choose to find and even reclaim their own natural child, little has been said about the influence of the other set of natural parents, namely, the natural parents of the adoptive parents, the grandparents. (Biological parents' real attributes are important if known to the adoptive parents and adopted child.) The conflicts of the generations are highlighted and intensified in the adoptive family situation, and the reaction of the adoptive parents to their own parents has to be understood alongside their reactions to adoption and their fantasies about the natural parents of their adopted child. Becoming a parent activates old parent-child conflicts in the adoptive parents and their natural parents. Where there are living grandparents, there may be many current interactions and communications which influence the entire adoptive family situation.

There are many motives for adoption, but infertility of one or both marital partners is a frequent one. Before the decision to adopt is reached, the infertile spouse had to cope with his or her infertility as well as the partner's reactions to it—the challenge, conflicts, and marital crisis which may lead to progressive resolution and/or to regressive adaptations and personality disturbance. Most infants adopted within days of their birth arrive in a setting in which the adoptive parents are still engaged in the active, ongoing, and often long-standing struggle to come to terms with their infertility and feelings of castration; their narcissistic injuries; their bitter frustration, disappointment, threats of divorce, and often recrimination due to their inability to be natural parents. The adoption has gratifying, defensive, and developmental implications for the adoptive family which thus impinge upon the infant from the day of adoption.

This conflict-rife situation may be one of the factors in adoptees' seemingly greater vulnerability for psychiatric disorders (McWhinnie, 1969; Bohman, 1970), although it must be noted that the adoptive population may be overrepresented in the statistics. The intensive scrutiny to which adoptive parents are subjected, the requirement that they prove themselves to be desirable parents before they are given a child and then allowed to keep the baby, and their own need to be superior parents to compensate for feelings of parental inadequacy may be factors in the higher incidence of adoptees in clinic populations. The problems of adoption may also serve as a developmental challenge and may lead to various creative solutions (Blum, 1969; Glenn, 1974). Adopted children can be just as much loved and lovable as natural children; and in families where there are both adopted and natural children, it is not necessarily the natural child who is favored. Parental love can certainly be gratified in the rearing of an adopted or a natural child, and this love as well as the mature qualities that all parents can bring to their parenting mean that adoptive parents can be the full equivalent of natural parents (Deutsch, 1945). The reciprocal object love and relatedness will be just as important in the adopted family as in any other family. Child abuse, neglect, and other deviant pathological forms of child rearing occur with natural as with adopted children, and the reality of adoption by no means implies inevitable developmental disturbance. However, "blood is thicker than water," and for many grandparents and some adoptive parents, the fact that the child has come from another person's "seed" or is born of another woman's body and is not of the bloodline, may lead to particular problems in the attachment and relationship to the adopted child.

The reality of adoption does tend to be associated with unresolved conflicts in the parents which tilt the parent-child relationship in various ways, and promote certain shared fantasies and collusive denials. For example, the adopted child who is told he was chosen by his adoptive parents has to deal with the underlying reality that he is not a child of choice, that he was abandoned rather than chosen by his natural parents, and that his adoptive parents may have had no other choice of raising a child. The parents, in turn, might continue to harbor hopes that the misfortune of their barrenness will change and that they might yet have a natural child. The deprivation of a "natural parenthood" is denied when the adopted child is told he was "chosen." And so is the fact that agencies sometimes exert subtle pressures, and that the adopted child has often actually been bartered for money or favors. Moreover, the infertility which is the cause of the adoption is sometimes cured by it, leading subsequently to natural parenthood which is preferred.

Studies of adoptive parents and children have led to the delineation of characteristic fantasies and defenses as well as adaptive reaction. The nature of the parents' relationship to each other and to their parents as well as to the adopted child are of fundamental importance in understanding a child's fantasies and attitudes. The infertile parent's need to adopt and the child's having been abandoned by his or her natural parents are intrinsic elements in the adoptee's fantasy system and are responsible for both intensifying and modifying their family romance fantasies in specific ways (Wieder, 1977; Brinich, 1980). In the typical family romance of natural children, the biological parents are denigrated while the wished-for ("adoptive") parents are idealized. In contrast, the adoptive child denigrates both the adoptive parents and the (unknown) biological parents. In addition, the adoptee may also show self-denigration and self-blame as a "rejected" child of the natural parents and as an artificial child of the "pretend" parents. He is also the biological and genealogical survivor of parents whom, in his fantasies, he "killed" or alienated and with whom he seeks reunion. The denigration of himself and both sets of parents will be further influenced by the real attitudes and reciprocal fantasies of the adoptive parents. Adoption themes come to life not only in the psychology of the adopted child (Wieder, 1977) but also in the inner life of the adoptive parents. In addition to the fantasy and reality of abandonment, there is the child's fantasy and realty of rescue by the adoptive parents; the fantasy system surrounding the sterility such as castration and punishment; the parents' fantasies of having stolen a child from someone else or the child's of having been kidnapped; the child's fantasies of return to and reunion with the biological parents as well as the parents' fears of the biological parents reclaiming or kidnapping the child; loyalty conflicts between adoptive and biological parents; incestuous temptation between adoptive parents and child who are not biologically related; turning to the adopted child for proof of potency or fertility of which one parent feels deprived by the infertile spouse, etc. The boundaries between who is the real parent and who is the real child, between reality and fantasy, may be blurred where reality has been validated or anchored in fantasies and where familial secrecy surrounds adoption (Blum, 1969). The child's sense and testing of reality may have been hampered by conspiracies of silence, misrepresentation of facts by the parents, parental ambivalence and conflict, and unresolved parental injury, guilt, and shame over the adoption.

To this confusion may be added the parental uncertainties regarding infertility which may not be considered absolute by themselves or their medical consultants; the waiting period with its uncertain screening procedures probing the prospective parents' motivation and the fear of being found wanting; the secrecy of motive and procedure; the fragmented communications of extended family and friends; the mixed and confused messages that may actually be given, consciously and unconsciously, not only to the child but to the adoptive parents; the admixture of facts and fantasy concerning the natural parents and their reasons for placing the child for adoption; the different attitude of the adoptive parents toward adoption; and their inability to deal fully with their attitudes toward each other and the desire to abandon the partner for a new one. Guilt, recrimination, and fantasied affairs in adoptive parents are legion, and extramarital affairs with hopes of impregnation are not uncommon in individuals with problems of infertility.[1]

The problems of the infertile couple who have no natural children and choose to adopt a neonate are particularly poignant and pertinent at this time because of the increasing number of out-of-wedlock babies, the availability of abortion, and the paradoxically relatively decreasing number of babies available for adoption since 90 percent of single mothers keep their babies (Menning, 1977). Infertility is on the rise in the United States with the rising frequency of venereal disease and its consequences, the rising age of marriage and parenthood, the decreasing fertility in women past 30, the postponement of parenthood because of career pressures and ambitions, and frequent moves which interfere with nesting and social support for parenthood. It is also possible that medical advances in correcting infertility have led to longer waiting periods and more protracted procedures before infertile couples achieve even a limited resigned acceptance of their infertility and reach the decision to adopt.

This means that adopting parents and their parents are likely to be older than biological parents and grandparents, likely to have been married longer, and probably more likely to have siblings who have become parents and who have presented the grandparents with natural grandchildren. There are great individual variations in the altered life situation of parenthood through adoption, and much depends on the parents' attitude toward each other as well as on the conflicts engendered, and the support received from grandparents, relatives, and friends. Further studies are needed on the motives for adoption, and on those childless couples who choose not to adopt, as well as those who have a natural child before or after adopting a child (Neubauer in Panel, 1967).

1. Donor insemination is growing in popularity in the United States, but this is a different type of reality than the adoption without pregnancy referred to in this paper. The status of children born of donor insemination is legally dubious; while the pregnancy is an open fact, the artificial insemination is usually concealed.

Considering the transmission of communications about adoption, one has to take three generations into account. For it proceeds not only from adoptive parent to child but also among the three generations, with complementary and shared fantasies and circular interactions. The attitudes of their own parents toward the adoption is central among the communications, conscious and unconscious, verbal and nonverbal, which may encourage the adopting parents, support their sense of being effective and competent in their parenthood, or undermine and denigrate their infertility and lack of biological reproduction. The idea that the adopted child might be legally returned as damaged goods within a year of the adoption—the probationary period required by most states—finds its counterpart in the adoptive parents' sense of themselves as damaged which may also reflect the attitudes of their own parents toward them and their adopted child. Legal strictures testify to intergenerational ambivalence toward adoption and fear and stigma concerning the identity and motives of the biological parents.

Adoptive parents are more likely to be subject to various generational strains and conflicts with their own parents. The psychological meaning of the adoption, conscious and unconscious, is highly variable and associated with phase-specific developmental conflicts in the adoptive parents and child. Solnit, noting that such meanings could be focused and magnified, pointed to the continuum of "Who am I?" "Who was I?" "Who shall I become?" representing a reciprocating search by parents and child (Panel, 1967). The identity conflicts of the adopted child and the parental identity of the adoptive parent are also influenced by the attitude and communication of the grandparents. Past and present identifications with their parents, the quality and content of parental ideals and the superego, and the nature of the parental relationships shaped during the adoptive parents' own familial and social development influence the reactions of the adoptive parent to the child. The grandparents may convey warm acceptance or cold indifference in their attitudes toward adoption as well as in their continuing interaction with the adoptive family. Deutsch (1945) noted that the motherliness of the adoptive mother can be enriched by the same joys and sorrows that fall to natural motherhood; what transpires in the adoptive situation is closely related to the mother's relationship to her own mother. These remarks can be amplified to include fathers and mothers and the grand-parents on both sides of the family.

The adoptive mother needs to work through her narcissistic injuries, lest there be too ready a tendency to blame the adopted child for not providing narcissistic compensation and satisfaction and to communicate her disappointments to the child. The mother and her family are exonerated, and the sense of blame and defect is shifted to the adopted child. This may be rationalized in terms of the child's inadequate genetic endowment. Because of injured family narcissism, the adoptive parent or relatives may tend to reject the child as not being of the bloodline. If the grandparent does not regard the adopted child as a true grandchild, this will have an impact upon parent and child. Grandparent and parent may regard the child both as an exception and an "outsider" and unconsciously condemn and reject the child as born in sin and out-of-wedlock, viewing the child as the product of the "wild seed" of a delinquent or prostitute mother. The adopted child, assuming his abandonment by his natural parents, may feel that he is the bad seed of "bad parents," but this fantasy may also be shared and mediated in unconscious communications from parents and grand-parents. The adopted child of different blood and denigrated descent will then feel the familial disappointment in the most diverse communications, extending far beyond those involving when and how the child is informed of being adopted. Some adoptive parents prefer to adopt girls which could be related to the fact that a daughter is not expected to continue the family name. The frustrated narcissistic expectations of the parents may be more readily disguised along with their fear that an adopted child might prefer his natural parents, changing his identity and loyalty if he finds his natural parents. The adoptive parents' fear of being rejected is often a projection of their own and their parent's original preference for a natural child. Fantasies of abandonment and rejection are related to identifications with the attitudes of their own natural parents, the natural parents of the abandoned-adopted child, the attitude of the natural father toward the presumed out-of-wedlock natural mother, and the threat of divorce between infertile spouses.

Familial narcissism, with its group idealization and quest for immortality, may be an obstacle to acceptance of adoption. The importance of narcissistic injuries in the adoptive situation cannot be underestimated, because the narcissistic fantasies of the three generations have reciprocal influences. Freud (1914) observed a fundamental narcissistic motivational theme in parenthood and delineated parental narcissistic goals and satisfactions.

> . . . he shall once more really be the centre and core of creation—'His Majesty the Baby', as we once fancied ourselves. The child shall fulfil those wishful dreams of the parents which they never carried out—the boy shall become a great man and a hero in his father's place, and the girl shall marry a prince as a tardy compensation for her mother. At the most touchy point in the narcissistic system, the immortality of the ego, which is so hard pressed by reality, security is achieved by taking refuge in the child. Parental love, which is so moving and at bottom so childish, is nothing but the parents' narcissism born again, which, transformed into object-love, unmistakably reveals its former nature [p. 91].

The parent wishes for physical and psychological immortality and hopes to see his idealized self in the child, who also represents idealized objects. Parents may tend to idealize their own childhood and, from the point of view of narcissism, will yearn for the fulfillment, through the child, of all their narcissistic ambitions and expectations and the undoing of all their disappointments and injuries. It is, of course, necessary for optimal development that the parental narcissistic demands and expectations shall have been tamed and that narcissistic injuries shall have been worked through by the mature ego. But this is complicated by the fresh narcissistic injuries associated with the adoptive situation.

The need for a generational continuity and the concern about the bloodline and the child being of true blood is ubiquitous in the world literature. Commenting on this theme, Freud (1911) notes its significance in Schreber, who was childless and quite concerned about the familial line of descent. Schreber had fantasies of being impregnated by God the Father and creating a new race of men. By "behaving as though he were himself a descendant of the sun and were submitting his children to a test of their ancestry," and by boasting "that he can look into the sun unscathed and undazzled, he has re-discovered the mythological method of expressing his filial relation to the sun" (p. 81). Schreber's preoccupations with parents, parenthood, and progeny are of universal import. The universal myths of descent and of the birth of the hero demonstrate the continuity of the generations, the identification of descendants and ancestors with each other, and the familial narcissism of aggrandized parents, idealized children, and parental perpetuation with immortality.

It is important not to overlook the intergenerational conflicts that may ensue. The adoptive mother has the same hopes and fears as the natural mother, but the adoptive parent may feel guilt toward the natural parents for not having fulfilled their narcissistic goals and for not having lived up to the expectations of the internal parents, that is, their own ego ideal of natural parenthood. Adoptive parents may not complete their identification with their own natural parents, remaining immature and unfulfilled and not feeling the equal of their parents.

The approval and encouragement of the natural parent normally are embodied in the parental ego ideal and in the actual reactions of the living grandparent (Blum, 1981). The resolution of the oedipus complex contributes to the definition, separation, and identifications of the generations, and assures the succession and continuity (and preservation rather than hostile destruction) of generations. Perpetual familial descent in the Bible is established through the tracing of genealogy and generations. The line of the fathers establishes true paternity when there might have been suspicion or confusion, but also represents parental eternity. In the Bible and other literature, a fantasied solution to potential female sterility lies in miraculous impregnation, e.g., Sarah and the Virgin Mary. That the adopted child is mythically born of an immaculate conception magically reverses "original sin" and the stigma of unmarried or otherwise degraded parenthood. The child's feeling of having been a gift to his adoptive parents and rescued by them counterbalances the seemingly inevitable fantasies of abandonment and rejection that occur when the child is informed that he has been adopted. The narcissistic injury for all the generations is intertwined with the oedipal disappointment of parents and grandparents.

To present a natural grandchild to one's parents symbolically renews their procreation, perpetuation, and phallic-oedipal gratification. The child identifies with the biological-sexual parents of the primal scene and with the parental care and attitudes of psychologically invested parenthood. He wants to have and rear children and unconsciously also wishes to reproduce himself and his own parents. The intergenerational, intrafamilial, and bisexual identifications are essential to familial and social empathy and cohesion. In this context, Freud's (1910) remarks are very relevant to the psychology of adoption: "His mother gave him a life—his own life—and in exchange he gives her another life, that of a child which has the greatest resemblance to himself. The son shows his gratitude by wishing to have by his mother a son who is like himself" (p. 173). Freud's observations are directly pertinent to the issue of familial resemblance. How often children are told they look just like one or the other parent and that siblings resemble each other as a parental blend. Resemblance is an important issue in adoption. There is often concealment of nonbiological issue and an attempt to give adoption the appearance of natural kinship. The narcissism of self-perpetuation is injured for many parents if the offspring bears no resemblance, and this reaction may be intensified if the parents of adoptive parents also suffer narcissistic disappointment. The child was to be created in the image of the parent who was commanded "to be fruitful and multiply." The inability to fulfill the superego injunction and narcissistic ideal is a blow to the self-esteem of the adoptive parent.

Both the resolution of revived oedipal conflicts associated with parenthood and the confidence in parenting may be impaired in the adoptive situation. The years of waiting and hoping for pregnancy; anxiety with pregnancy because of repeated miscarriage; the heightened concern in connection with the menstrual cycle; the probability that many irregular periods were mini miscarriages, and that a missed period became a missed opportunity; menstrual depression; the anxious questioning of family and friends; the medical procedures, tests, and treatments—all heighten the adoptive parents' ambivalence and feelings of frustration and inadequacy. The pleasure and spontaneity of sexual relations may be lost in command performance and repeated failure to conceive. Unresolved oedipal and sibling rivalries may assume new intensities. The infertility itself may be experienced as a punishment for rivalrous oedipal fantasies or past misdeeds. If infertility follows abortions or venereal disease, it will tend to validate fantasied punishment for sexual "transgression."

Case 1. The following material derives from the analyses of an infertile couple, Mr. and Mrs. A., who both were in analysis with different analysts.[2] After 6 childless years of marriage, a 28-year-old Catholic man entered analysis under pressure from his wife, then in her sixth year of analysis. Basically, he wished the analyst could restore his fertility, allay his castration anxiety, and spare him the further narcissistic injury of adoption at the insistence of his wife. He unconsciously feared his wife would desert him, as his mother had left his father for alcoholism. He was guilty about his unconscious complicity and gratification in driving his father out, feeling he had injured his mother at birth, and was now injuring his wife by depriving her of "birth." The slip of paper with his abnormal sperm count and function became a "pink slip" of dismissal by his wife, his analyst, and his employer.

Regarding his parents as withholding love, money, and concern, he also was unconsciously gratified by withholding their posterity from them. He readily joined his wife in mutual withholding and provocative behavior. She was a silent patient in her analysis, and what was not verbalized was sexually enacted at home. She was angry, demanding, and then excited by sadomasochistic sex, requesting her husband to spank her and obtaining her orgasm after he inserted his finger in her rectum. She demanded intercourse and impregnation and then insisted upon adoption and getting a baby through an alternate route. He would have preferred rectal intercourse at times since it assuaged his castration anxiety and helped him maintain his

2. I wish to thank Dr. Warren Goodman for sharing his analytic data and ideas with me.

denial of the fertility test data. While he could minimize his wife's rageful demands and their frequent quarrels, he simultaneously felt like punching the doctor who informed him of his infertility.

His penis was represented in dream imagery as a defective "split frankfurter," and his testes were equated with his abnormal kidney stones and abnormal sperm. He was identified with his father who had a malignant bladder disease and with his mother who was afflicted with a potentially fatal, chronic kidney disease. His parents had been an older couple when he was born after years of childless marriage. Thus, he saw his infertility as an inherited biological disorder. He was faced with real and threatened loss. He withheld from the analyst by silences and missed sessions. In conjunction with "command sexual performances" coordinated with his wife's fertile period, he became phobic of sexual relations. His wife referred to his analyst as Dr. Goodballs, implying her husband was "badballs." Indeed, she once pinched his scrotum in rage, prompting more castration anxiety and retaliatory withholding. Surgical repair of a varicocele only increased his castration anxiety but not his sperm count. He was demeaned, and she really had fantasies of leaving him, having affairs, and marrying a fertile husband.

He also fantasied having affairs in revenge and to reassure himself of his manhood and virility. The infertility and fantasied affairs were associated with fantasies of cheating and being cheated. His father had "cheated" on his mother. He was cheating his wife of a child, his parents of a grandchild; and he wept at the thought that since he was an only child, there were and would be no children of his to present to his parents. He would not be a father like his father, and he stressed the importance of biological fatherhood and natural progeny which would please his parents and continue the family. Adoption itself was cheating and fraudulent, and the stealing of the penis-child from others involved danger. In the transference he wanted to cheat the analyst and feared the analyst might cheat him. He fantasied that doctors at the hospital stole his father's organs after his death, reflecting his wish to steal the analyst's and his father's genitals to impregnate his wife. Simultaneously, he unconsciously identified with his fertile mother and was homosexually excited by fantasies of his wife being artificially inseminated by her gynecologist. He wanted the analyst to penetrate and impregnate him, behind which were also fantasies of his wife's analyst impregnating her. His analyst became not only "Dr. Goodballs" but "Dr. Bigbucks" by an equation of potency, fertility, and wealth. The analyst was also identified with the urologist who analyzed his semen after ordered masturbation and prescribed testosterone. He fantasied being both fertile and fertilized through this magic potion which in reality did not prove to be beneficial. Jealous of and competitive with his own father, he was now identified with the drunken, defective, castrated father. After his father died, he received no consolation from his dying mother. Nor did she support the couple's plans to adopt a child.

After a "site visit" by the adoption agency, he was impotent. He then dreamed of disarming two intruders and shooting one of them. The intruders were the agency personnel, the biological parents, and the adopted child. He was afraid of his aggression and of his wish to shoot live semen, like his father impregnating his mother in the primal scene where he was the original intruder. He wanted to blame his wife for not compensating for his deficiency by being especially fertile (doctors often suggested a bilateral couple contribution to infertility). A natural child would be a far more welcome intruder, replacing his lost parents and carrying on the bloodline.

As the day of adoption inevitably approached, he became apprehensive about his low bank balance, attempted to build a reservoir of semen through pornographic stimulation without ejaculation, and withheld payment of the analytic fees. When he was forced to accept adoption (or divorce) at the insistence of his wife, he abruptly terminated his analysis. His peremptory interruption of analysis was sudden, merciless, and irreversible, like his defect and his wife's decision to adopt. At the time of adoption, these potential parents were feeling defective, different, depressed, disappointed in themselves and each other. Unconsciously they believed they also were disappointments to their parents and so felt unloved and singled out for special punishment. His "castration" was a supreme narcissistic injury which also meant death. He could not replace his dead father and dying mother with a natural child who would establish generational continuity with fantasied perpetuity.

The setting in which an adopted child arrives is frequently one of mourning rather than celebration, with the collusive denial concealing the unresolved conflicts over infertility. It is not surprising that many adopted children feel rejection and estrangement. They have been "rejected" by their biological parents, and their adoptive parents and grandparents may have difficulties in attachment to the new baby. The real attitude of the grandparents and their unconscious fantasies influence the adoptive situation, as the following case shows.

Case 2. Mrs. B. was extremely competitive with her young, pretty, vivacious, and sexually active married daughter, who for several years had been trying to get pregnant without success except for one brief pregnancy which culminated in miscarriage. Mrs. B. was consciously supportive of her daughter's desires for pregnancy, although it became clear that she was unconsciously gratified when her daughter's period recurred. There were frequent subtle messages between mother and daughter—to keep trying, the next menstrual cycle will be successful—and attempts to comfort yet provoke the distressed and increasingly depressed daughter after each new disappointment. Mrs. B. was much more concerned about this daughter than about a younger son who had just become a father and whose life seemed to be progressing more favorably. It was clear that, although Mrs. B. was ambivalent about her daughter becoming pregnant and achieving motherhood, she was even more ambivalent about the possibility of adoption. It seemed she neither wanted the daughter to become pregnant nor to have a child by adoption. The daughter had hinted at adoption by mentioning other adoptive parents, but Mrs. B. did not pursue this line of thought. She tended to denigrate her son-in-law, consciously attributing her daughter's infertility to her son-in-law's putative sexual inadequacy. Since he was not a natural father and could not impregnate her daughter, he was not a "real man," and she would not be his child's grandmother. She thought she could probably love a child, after more and more contact, whether or not the child was adopted, but then a grandmother has after all less contact and less re-

sponsibility for a grandchild than her own child. She really was
not the least bit enthusiastic about adoption, and this could be
recognized in the very expression on her face and in her tone
of voice. She would try, but not always succeed, in avoiding
references to her daughter being childless, and not directly
discuss adoption when her daughter raised the issue. On the
other hand, she thought it might be a good idea for the couple
to adopt, because they might have a baby after they stopped
worrying so much about becoming pregnant. However, while
this would be good for the daughter and son-in-law, Mr. B.
indicated that he would not be able to bring the same affection
and interest to an adopted child as he did to the natural grandchild his son had fathered. Furthermore, one could not be sure
of the inheritance, it might be a bad seed, and if it wasn't from
his own seed, their own blood, why should he become overinvolved and overinvested? He joked to his wife, "What do we
need a little bastard in the family for, anyway?" Actually Mrs. B.
shared her husband's attitudes about adoption (but was also
ambivalent about her daughter becoming pregnant). He doubted that they should invest the same funds for an adopted child
as for a "real" grandchild.

   This mother displayed a reactive overconcern about her
daughter's physical state and menstrual cycle as well as inconsistent, ambivalent communications concerning the possibility of
her daughter adopting or remaining childless. Unfortunately,
it was not possible to follow the further course of this genera-
tive and generational conflict since the patient terminated analysis before her daughter had either become pregnant or
adopted a child. At the time Mrs. B. terminated analysis, the
daughter was still enlisting her support for adoption while trying to invoke the mother's blessing for a magical pregnancy
that would solve the problem. Mrs. B. surmised that her daughter had seriously considered divorce, and she took seriously her
daughter's occasional jokes about extramarital affairs. In view
of the need for planned and command sexual performances as
opposed to more spontaneous sex in a couple where infertility
and impregnation are not problems, this mother knew when
her daughter was ovulating and when she had intercourse. The
knowledge of the daughter's sexual activity increased Mrs. B.'s

primal scene curiosity and excitement. All the anxiety and guilt engendered by the primal scene appeared to be bilaterally reactivated as the daughter conveyed aspects of her sexual activity to her parents. The reciprocal, incestuous excitement heightened the oedipal guilt for the mother and presumably also for her daughter. Mrs. B.'s oedipal rivalry with her daughter was particularly dangerous because of the daughter's infertility. The daughter rebelled against her mother's gifts of nightgowns and underclothes, but at the same time bought these clothes for herself on her mother's charge card. We can see elements here of very deep affection, antagonism, and identification between mother and daughter, and how a miscarriage may validate an abortion fantasy in the potential grandmother. Though reactively disguised, Mrs. B.'s anxiety and guilt were communicated to her daughter, doubtless feeding the latter's anxiety and guilt. The grandparents' real attitudes as well as the internalized ones may assume the role of a benevolent auxiliary superego at the point of adoptive parenthood or interfere with parental acceptance, attachment, and authority. The punitive or persecutory superego may prohibit parenthood and adoption.[3]

The activated primal scene fantasy in my patient was also connected with the familial secrecy surrounding her daughter's infertility, the secrecy surrounding the possible adoption and where the adopted baby might come from, and the revived thoughts of castration and genital damage. Women could be damaged in sexual relations, and her daughter might have been further damaged in utero because of Mrs. B.'s omnipotent fantasies of envy and enmity. One cannot help but be reminded here of the fairy tales in which the little girl's feminine sexuality and future motherhood are threatened by the wicked witch. The interpretation should include both the daughter's and the mother's oedipal fantasies and the recipro-

3. Guilt and punishment may follow abortion but may also be one of the motives for abortion. Sometimes when a pregnancy is carried to term after repeated induced abortions, the infant rather than the fetus may be subject to the mother's acting out of infanticidal, abusive fantasies and be given away for adoption as both an expression of and a protection against the mother's aggressive attitudes toward her baby and a punishment for her own aggression toward her mother.

cal effects of daughter and mother on each other during development.

Mrs. B. profited from the analytic work and the ensuing insight into her conflicts with her daughter and earlier with her own mother and siblings. Although an adoption had not yet occurred, it was clear that the potential grandmother was developing a much more benign attitude toward adoption.

The adoptive parents do not have either the benefit or the rigors of going through the physical and psychological changes of pregnancy. The adoptive mother does not have the experience of pregnancy, delivery, and lactation. Neither the child nor the child's milk is from her own body-self, and she may need more contact with and care and response of her adopted child to elicit her full motherliness. Similar reactions may be postulated for the adoptive father before he feels fully responsible and identifies with being a father and fatherhood. To some extent, then, adoptive parents may be in greater need of their parents' support and approval than natural parents. Coping with their own conflictual feelings, they are particularly sensitive and vulnerable to their parents' attitudes. They quickly sense whether the grandparents are as excited by the adopted baby as they were by the birth of natural grandchildren, and as eager to lend a hand, e.g., with baby care or baby-sitting. It soon becomes apparent whether grandparents were more concerned about the strains and stresses, the joys and sorrows of their children who became natural parents or are just as much concerned about their children who adopted a child. Long before the adoption is completed, their feelings about their child's infertility, their attitude toward adoption, and their empathy, sympathy, and support, or direct and nonverbal expression of disappointment and regret are communicated to their child. This may be empathic with the child's bitter disappointment, or may express disappointment in their child (the adoptive parent), and in the prospect of adoption. The grandparents may not consider themselves true grandparents or an adopted child a true grandchild.

The grandparents will have reacted earlier to their child's denial or acknowledgment of infertility. The inevitable grief, the mourning for a loss of reproductive function, the regressive turning to parents or parent surrogates for comfort will all have involved the grandparents or the imagined reactions of absent grandparents. For adults, the real grandparents are usually far less important than internalized fantasies and images. However, old tendencies toward shared fantasies, shared denial, secret collusion may be reactivated and repeated in a new mode. Secrecy surrounding adoption and knowledge of the biological parents may be shared with grandparents. Awareness of disappointment may be well-defended with silent collusion of the two generations and with a feeling that complaint might complicate efforts to adopt. An adoption agency might convey that the infertile couple are lucky to get a baby and have no right to disappointment.

I shall briefly report some additional clinical material as further illustrations of grandparental reactions and variations on the theme of disappointment and conflict between the generations.

Case 3.[4] Mr. and Mrs. C. decided to adopt on being told that Mrs. C. had almost no chance of conceiving after an entire ovary and three-quarters of the other had to be removed. Mrs. C.'s parents were Conservative Jews with a strong interest in family and lineage. They were overbearing and intimidated both Mr. and Mrs. C. who did not tell them that they were considering adoption until a private obstetrician they had contacted called to tell them that he had a baby girl for them. The grandparents, upset because they had been excluded from the decision-making, questioned the C.s about the biological parents of the child and were not satisfied with the few identifying data provided by the obstetrician.

The dark-haired, olive-skinned couple were presented with a blue-eyed baby girl whose hair was so light at birth as to be almost white. The grandparents were open in their double disappointment—that their son and daughter-in-law could not have a biological child, and that the child appeared to be of Scandinavian origin. (Of course they blamed their daughter-in-law for the infertility.)

---

4. I am indebted to Dr. Selma Kramer for sharing her clinical material and analytic observations.

The grandfather said, while looking at the lithe, active, quite beautiful blond-haired child, "This baby is *no* C. [common Jewish name]." Later he said, "It's just as well it's not a boy. I wouldn't want someone looking like that to carry on the family name."

Young Mrs. C. became pregnant within 6 months and gave birth to a dark-skinned, dark-haired little girl. The grandparents were ecstatic, for they now had a sense of family continuity which was so important to them. It is noteworthy that they repetitively forgot birthday gifts for the adopted child, while never failing to remember all occasions involving the second child. Such denigrating behavior by the grandparents is not uncommon and has psychological meaning for the adoptive parents and their adopted child. The grandparents urged the young C.s to have additional children, probably in the hope that they would have a grandson. However, the pain and inability to accept the adoption were considerably ameliorated by the birth of their first "real" grandchild.

Case 4. A reactive overenthusiasm for adoption was shown by a woman, Mrs. D., who was in psychotherapy. She was a Quaker from a family that traced their origin to early settlers. Just as in the case of the C.s—in fact, even more so—"family" meant a great deal to her, including lineage and descent.

When her only daughter could not become pregnant, Mrs. D. introduced the idea of adoption, although the idea caused much inner turmoil in her. She could accept and handle the adoption because she could focus on how fine a home the adopted child would be given. She used many defenses, especially denial, and also used the Quaker philosophy she had been raised with. These defenses helped her to deal with the blow of "not having my own flesh and blood grandchild," as she once admitted.

Her Quaker beliefs then allowed her to suggest that her daughter and son-in-law were such good people to have adopted a poor homeless child that they should consider adopting the unadoptables—children with birth defects, mental retardation, etc.—which certainly revealed what she thought of the adoption of any child at all. For her, biology was bedrock, and an adopted child was incurably defective, just as sterility was a severe biological defect.

CONCLUSION

The clinical material and theoretical inferences indicate that adoption involves a reality of several sets of parents, and that the real parents of the adoptive parents are important, overlooked grandparents. They are usually natural parents who are known to the adopted child and his parents. The network of relationships, identifications, and communications between the generations has complex effects upon all the related persons. The real reactions and fantasies of the grandparents are part of the wider adoptive situation. Unconscious fantasies, especially the oedipal constellations of the family romance, the primal scene, and the castration complex are linked to issues of generational difference, continuity, and discontinuity. If adoption provokes negative counterreactions in the grandparents, this will have an adverse influence on the adoptive situation. The love, support, sanction, and facilitating attitudes of grandparents are needed by new parents. Such support may be especially needed and yet not forthcoming for deeply distressed adoptive parents. Their parental identity may not be confirmed by their own parents, which may later contribute to the adopted child's identity confusion, "bad seed" fantasies, and fears of rejection. The "bad seed" may refer to the "sinful" biological parents, the abnormal sperm or eggs of the adoptive parents, and the narcissistic injury of all sets of parents and the "exceptional" child. The adopted child's fantasies may contain more than a grain of truth of the shared attitudes and fantasies of his adoptive parents and grandparents. The adopted child may be the "blacksheep" of the family (but, of course, may be favored in specific situations). Moreover, identifications with fertile biological parents are often modeled on the actual grandparents as well as on the mythical or fragmentary knowledge of the biological parents. The child will identify with the extended family and lineage, with his parents' childhood and origins. The need to establish full identity and generational continuity, to synthesize a childhood in terms of the real and ideal childhood of parents and grandparents, and to become a parent like one's own, within one's own lineage, may be a major factor in the adopted adolescent's search for the biological parent, as it is in other adolescents disengaging from their own caretaking parents.

SUMMARY

The adoptive situation is intergenerational; it involves the adopted child, the adoptive and natural parents of the child, and the grandparents, namely, the parents of the adoptive parents and sometimes the parents of the biological parents. Adoptive parents and grandparents and the adopted child form a communal network of interaction, identification, conscious and unconscious conflict, fantasy, and communication which influence the entire adoptive situation. The conflicts of the generations will have a positive or negative impact upon the adoptive parents' attainment of parental identity, attachment, and confidence in their rearing of the child. The reciprocal reactions of the adoptive parents and their own parents coexist with their fantasies concerning the biological parents of the adopted child. The natural parents of the adoptive parents may be more important in the adoptive situation than the physically (but not psychologically) absent biological parents of the adopted child. Becoming a parent reactivates old parent-child conflicts. Adoption may intensify universal oedipal and intergenerational conflicts and may leave the adoptive parent feeling unfulfilled as a person and as a parent. Unless the intrapsychic conflicts surrounding adoption are resolved, adoptive parents may feel disappointed in themselves and a real or fantasied disappointment to their own parents. Along with underlying feelings of castration and narcissistic injury, extrafamilial adoption associated with infertility may challenge the continuity and perpetuity of the generations. The identifications among the generations, the tracing of ancestry and descendants, the child's need to identify not only with the parents but with their life history and childhood—all are powerful factors which may contribute to the conflicts activated in the adoptive situation. The adoptive parent may not have fulfilled the wishes of the actual grandparent or of the unconscious superego to procreate in the image of the idealized parent and to insure generational, genealogical, and personal continuity. The wish for concrete flesh and blood immortality can also be understood in relation to both parental and infantile narcissism as well as protection against intrafamilial aggression and death wishes.

BIBLIOGRAPHY

BLUM, H. P. (1969), A psychoanalytic view of *Who's Afraid of Virginia Woolf. J. Amer. Psychoanal. Assn.*, 17:888–903.

———— (1981), The maternal ego ideal and the regulation of maternal qualities. In *The Course of Life*. Washington: N.I.M.H., 3:91–114.

BOHMAN, M. (1970), *Adopted Children and Their Families*. Stockholm, Sweden: Proprius.

BRINICH, P. M. (1980), Some potential effects of adoption on self and object representations. *Psychoanal. Study Child*, 35:107–133.

DEUTSCH, H. (1945), *Psychology of Women*, vol. 2. New York: Grune & Stratton.

FREUD, S. (1910), A special type of choice of object made by men. *S.E.*, 11:163–175.

———— (1911), Psycho-analytic notes on an autobiographical account of a case of paranoia. *S.E.*, 12:3–82.

———— (1914), On narcissism. *S.E.*, 14:67–102.

GLENN, J. (1974), The adoption theme in Edward Albee's *Tiny Alice* and *The American Dream*. *Psychoanal. Study Child*, 29:413–429.

MCWHINNIE, A. (1969), The adopted child in adolescence. In *Adolescence*, ed. G. Caplan & S. Lebovici. New York: Basic Books, pp. 133–142.

MENNING, B. (1977), *Infertility*. Englewood, N.J.: Prentice-Hall.

PANEL (1967), Psychoanalytic theory as it relates to adoption. M. Schechter, reporter. *J. Amer. Psychoanal. Assn.*, 15:695–708.

SCHECHTER, M. (1970), About adoptive parents. In *Parenthood*, ed. E. J. Anthony & T. Benedek. Boston: Little, Brown, pp. 353–371.

WIEDER, H. (1977), The family romance fantasies of adopted children. *Psychoanal. Q.*, 46:185–200.

———— (1978), On when and whether to disclose about adoption. *J. Amer. Psychoanal. Assn.*, 26:793–812.

The Prerepresentational Self and Its Affective Core

ROBERT N. EMDE, M.D.

A "PREREPRESENTATIONAL SELF" MAY SEEM A CONTRADIC-
tion in terms. How can there be a self before the development
of a mental capacity for representation? Still, I hope this contradictory phrase serves a purpose in introducing this essay,
one which sets up a questioning frame of mind for thinking
about self as process rather than as fixed attainment. Other
contradictions of this sort will follow.

This essay will enumerate several fundamental principles for
a theory of self-development. These principles emerge from
recent research in developmental psychology and from a psy-
choanalytic-biological systems perspective. Following a review
of this research, I shall propose an "affective core" of the self, a
notion previously hinted at by Rangell (1976) and Izard (1977).
My conclusion will then press the following thesis: because of its
biological organization, *our affective core guarantees our continuity
of experience across development in spite of the many ways we change;* it
also guarantees that we can understand others who are human.

Professor of Psychiatry, University of Colorado School of Medicine,
Denver.

This paper is dedicated to the memory of Marianne Kris. Understanding
individuality and adaptive patterns of early development were topics she
considered central in research and in clinical work (e.g., Kris, 1957). A modified version of this paper was presented at the Los Angeles Psychoanalytic
Society in February 1982 and at the Chicago Institute for Psychoanalysis in
June 1982; I am grateful for the discussions of many colleagues in both
places.

Support for this research comes from Public Health Service Grants MH
22803 and MH 35808 from the National Institute of Mental Health.

SELF AS PROCESS

Most developmentalists would agree that organized self-experience, as we usually know it, requires the capacity for "reflection," and that awareness of self in this sense emerges in a convincing way during the infant's second year. This emergence occurs along with the beginnings of representational intelligence. It is then that there are increasing cognitive capacities for going beyond the immediate action-world of experience. It is then that the infant is able to evoke the image of an object or of an event which is not present and reflect upon these evoked representations; thus, the infant can regard his own image and the organization of his own acts as separate from the acts themselves. Since this may seem fairly abstract Piagetian theory, I shall move to some recent research which gets at a vivid aspect of this.

The onset of *self-recognition* has now been studied experimentally, and the convergence of findings is quite dramatic. Three different laboratories have found similar results with infants observed in front of a mirror. A typical experiment goes like this. Before exposing the infant to the mirror, a mother wipes her infant's face with a washcloth and covertly marks a region (for example, the nose) with a rouge spot. The infant is then allowed to look at the mirror, as mother moves aside. Mark-directed recognition behavior is determined by the infant's looking at his image in the mirror, noticing the spot, and then touching his own face in the marked region, or directing a gesture toward it. Such recognition began at the same age in all studies. It was not found before 15 months; it occurred in some infants between 15 to 18 months; and it occurred in most infants between 18 and 20 months (Amsterdam, 1972; Schulman and Kaplowitz, 1977; Lewis and Brooks-Gunn, 1979). Lewis and Brooks-Gunn, who have done the most extensive work in self-recognition development, also studied infant responses to videotaped images of themselves and to others and to such images presented in photographs. The findings paralleled the mirror studies. For all modes of representation, the majority of infants experienced self-recognition between 18 and 21 months of age. Further, personal pronouns began to be used at the end of this age period when infants looked at their own pictures.

What does this mean? At the very least, these recognition studies indicate that, beginning at 15 months and certainly by 20 months, the infant has a concept of self which involves a sense of continuity over time and space. Whether in the mirror, the videotape, or the picture image, the capacity to identify one's own image and respond differentially to it shows that there is some kind of preexisting identity on the part of the 1½-year-old making such an inference (see discussion in Gallup, 1979).

Other studies (Kagan, 1981) used a variety of cognitively oriented tasks instead of self-recognition tasks. A similar conclusion was reached: that self-awareness emerges during the last 6 months of the second year. Observations which led to this conclusion included the emergence of self-descriptive utterances, gestural directives to adults which indicated a desire to have the adult behave in a specific manner, distress when the child could not imitate a complex adult behavior, and mastery smiling upon successfully accomplishing a goal.

These recent experimental studies seem to anchor what psychoanalytic observers have documented so richly, namely, that this is an age when there are corresponding developments concerning "willfulness" (Freud, 1905), autonomy (Erikson, 1950), the semantic no (Spitz, 1957), the beginnings of the representational world of self and objects (Sandler and Rosenblatt, 1962), and, most poignantly, the awareness of separateness which inaugurates the subphase of rapprochement for separation-individuation (Mahler et al., 1975).

I cannot resist citing one further vivid observation concerning the development of self-awareness. Freud (1920) recorded observations of his 1½-year-old grandson who allowed his mother to go away without protesting, but, when she was away, repeated a disappearance-and-mastery game using a wooden reel with an attached piece of string. Freud interpreted the child's accompanying utterances (*o-o-o-o* and *da*) as showing an awareness of "gone" (the German *fort* upon throwing the reel) and "there" (the German *da* upon retrieving it). He then alluded to a further observation presumably at the same age. During another maternal absence, the child made himself disappear and reappear again in front of a full-length mirror with the accompanying words, "Baby o-o-o-o!" In a footnote added to *The Interpretation of Dreams* (1900) in 1919, Freud recorded an observation of his grandson's first dream at 20 months. Since the child's words which were called out from sleep dealt with separation, Freud alluded to the fact that for several months before this time, his grandson had played at "gone" with his toys (p. 461). Clearly, Freud documented self-awareness at 1½.[1]

These convergent observations are extraordinary. Still, I believe we must avoid getting caught up in the idea of a sharply focused age period in which the self emerges. Such a way of thinking tends to reify the self as a developmental acquisition and implies that it is something like walking, learning to ride a bicycle, or beginning speech. Nothing could be further from the truth. I believe we must remind ourselves that the self is a *process,* and refers to a vital set of synthetic functions which increase in complexity and depth as development proceeds throughout the life-span. In order to emphasize this point, I wish to allude to some important later developments. *Gender identity* becomes consolidated in the second and third years, as observations from several different disciplines now indicate (Galenson and Roiphe, 1971; Money and Ehrhardt, 1972; Jacklin and Maccoby, 1978; Galenson, 1982); and *emotional object constancy* also becomes established during this time (Mahler et al., 1975). During the fourth through the sixth years, there is the consolidation of *oedipal identifications leading to the superego and the ego ideal,* a process which has now been commented on by nearly four generations of analytic observers.

The special maturation of the *sense of self in adolescence* has been richly documented, most notably by Erikson (1959, 1968). The importance of a new integration of *self-experience in mid-life* has been a focus of theorizing by Jung (1939), who described age 40 as "the noon of life" for full individuation. Jung's thinking about self-consolidation in mid-life proved particularly useful in interpreting the results of the recent much-publicized

1. W. Ernest Freud, the grandson who was the subject of these observations, is now a supervising and training analyst at the Hampstead Child-Therapy Clinic. He participated in the discussion of this paper as a member of the guest faculty of the Los Angeles Psychoanalytic Institute and UCLA Extension Division, February 1982.

adulthood study of Levinson (1978). Finally, it is noteworthy that two major psychoanalytic theorists of the self, Erikson and Kohut, each give special importance to the new level of *integrative self-experience in later life.* Erikson (1959) writes of "ego integrity" (as opposed to "despair") for his eighth stage of man. Kohut (1977) writes of late middle age as a "crucially significant . . . point in the life curve of the self," a time when we "ask ourselves whether we have been true to our innermost design" (p. 241).

Thus, the self is not usefully regarded as a psychic structure which is simply acquired at age 1½. It is better thought of as a process, as a descriptor of an expanding, individualized, and creative aspect of the personality. This process view of the self was recognized by Kohut as a continuing coherent "center of initiative," by Erikson as "identity," and by Jung as "individuation."

Once we accept the self as a *process concept,* its developmental aspects *fall into place.*[2] Self-awareness begins in the second year and successively evolves to higher levels of organization; it becomes heightened at later times of developmental change and in certain contexts. Further, this perspective invites us to consider an aspect of self process earlier than 15 months, namely, the prerepresentational self. I submit that when we do this, we find principles which are absolutely fundamental for any theory of self. These are systems principles. In some ways, they seem obvious, but, in other ways, novel. Ineluctably, they lead us to our affective core.

THREE BIOLOGICAL PRINCIPLES

Self-regulation is the first principle. Modern biology has taught us that self-regulation is basic for all living systems. At the level of physiology, it is built into cardiorespiratory and metabolic systems; were it otherwise, life would not be possible. But beyond this there is regulation for behavioral systems, not only in

2. It is noteworthy that two recent reviews in developmental psychology arrive at a strong process-oriented view of the self (Damon and Hart, 1982; Kopp, 1982); it would seem this is a topic of increasing interest for developmentalists as well as clinicians.

the short-term sense for arousal, attentiveness, and sleep-wakefulness cycles, but in the longer term sense for growth and vital developmental functions. The developing individual maintains an integrity during major environmental changes and during developmental transformations. From a biological point of view, development is goal-oriented and, for species-important developmental functions, there are multiple ways of reaching developmental goals, something Bertalanffy (1968) referred to as "equifinality" in development. Examples of this are provided by children who are congenitally blind (Fraiberg, 1977), or congenitally deaf (Freedman et al., 1971), or who are without limbs (Decarié, 1969), or who have cerebral palsy (Sameroff, 1981). All go through infancy and have different sensorimotor experiences, but all typically develop object permanence, representational intelligence, and self-awareness in early childhood.

A related aspect concerns *self-righting tendencies* in development. For important functions, there is a strong tendency to get back on a developmental pathway after deficit or perturbation (Waddington, 1962; Sameroff and Chandler, 1976; Sacket et al., 1981). Recent observations of developmental *resiliency*—i.e., severe infant retardation due to deprivation which is corrected by later environmental change—are illustrations of this aspect of self-regulation (see examples in Clarke and Clarke, 1976).

Self-regulation is perhaps the most fundamental biological principle of self. Although it is a general life principle, it takes on the specific properties of the life-span trajectory for any given species. For man, this trajectory includes a variety of superimposed developmental changes in self-awareness. Curiously, the newer subfield of developmental psychology, known as social-cognition, treats self-regulation in a quite limited sense. There, self-regulation refers to the child's awareness of socially approved behaviors; in other words, it is a developmental outcome of early cognitive development and socialization process (see the review of Kopp, 1982).

Social fittedness is the second biological principle underlying the prerepresentational self. More and more we have come to appreciate that the human infant comes to the world pre-adapted for participating in human interactions. Our biology ensures organized capacities for initiating, maintaining, and terminating such interactions with others. Some of these capacities are present at birth and include: a propensity for participating in eye-to-eye contact; a state responsivity for being activated and soothed by human holding, touching, and rocking; and a propensity for showing prolonged alert attentiveness to the stimulus features contained in the human voice and face (see reviews by Ainsworth et al., 1974; Emde and Robinson, 1979; Papousek and Papousek, 1981). Indeed, the integrative capacities of the young infant (for processing sequential information, for generating complex patterns of motor activity, for cross-modal perception, and for orienting) can be thought of as magnificent preadaptations for the complex dynamic circumstances of human interaction (Papousek and Papousek, 1981).

The biological principle of social fittedness can also be discussed from the parents' side. A variety of parenting behaviors with young infants are done automatically, beyond awareness, and, in fact, are apt to be disrupted if they are pointed out. Since they appear to be species-wide, and do not seem to be the product of individual experience, the Papouseks (1979), who are currently describing the full repertoire of these behaviors, believe they are biologically based and refer to them as "intuitive parenting behaviors." These include a variety of parental behaviors which minimize transitory states (such as drowsiness or REM states) and maximize either wakefulness or quiet sleep. These authors also include parental behaviors supporting visual contact, such as a positioning of the infant so that eye-to-eye distance meets the newborn's accommodative abilities (20–25 cm) and not the parents' own optimal reading distance. (Interestingly, even parents who believe that newborns cannot see do this.) The Papouseks also include exaggerated greeting responses, parental imitation of the newborn's facial and vocal expressions, and parental use of simple repetitive structure for interactional episodes in a way which nearly matches the infant's ideal requirements for learning. Intuitive parenting is especially clear in the universal parental tendency for "baby talk." In this, speech, gestures, and facial expressions are directed to the infant with slow, simple, repetitive patterns. In addition, there is an exaggeration of the musical features of speech with a pitch that is higher and more variable than that for adult-directed speech, and with the talker frequently enlivening things with "mock surprise" expressions (see also Snow, 1971; Stern, 1977). The biological basis of baby talk is indicated not only by its universality in adults who speak to babies this way, but also by its consistent use in children who speak to babies this way beginning at about 3 and 4 years of age (Slobin, 1968).

This leads to current research in which *behavioral synchrony* is being examined. Behavioral synchrony implies the biological predisposition of parent and infant to mesh their behaviors in a timed mutual interchange during social interaction. This has been examined from the point of view of behavioral state (Sander, 1975), the microanalyses of looking and arousal (Stern, 1977; Als et al., 1979; Brazelton and Als, 1979), and the microanalysis of voice and movement (Condon and Sander, 1974). Butterworth (1979; Butterworth and Jarret, 1980) replicated earlier observations (Scaife and Bruner, 1975) of 6-month-old infants, seated opposite mother, looking in the direction mother looks. Since this occurs regularly without the infant following mother's eye tracking or head movement, it is presumed to represent a capacity for joint visual referencing and an inborn potential for a "shared visual reality" between mother and infant. In this way of thinking, Butterworth comes close to the state of early biological communicative connectedness which Trevarthen (1979) describes as "primary intersubjectivity."

Affective monitoring is the third biological principle. The first two principles indicated that the self-regulating human is from the start actively social, and that psychological functions related to self-experience will necessarily emerge from a social matrix. The principle of affective monitoring indicates that this self-regulating, social being monitors experience according to what is pleasurable and unpleasurable (Emde, 1981). In other words, there is a preadapted organized basis in the central nervous system for guiding behavior. The extent of the organization for affective monitoring will be detailed later when I discuss the affective self. For now, I would merely like to point out that in *early* infancy, such monitoring is preeminently social in terms of its adaptive functioning. That is, infant affective expressions are used to guide caregiving. The mother hears a cry and acts to relieve the presumed cause of distress. She sees a smile and hears cooing and cannot resist maintaining a playful interaction. *Later,* the infant makes use of the affective monitoring system for guiding his own behavior, whether mother intervenes or not.

By now it probably has become apparent that affective monitoring serves self-regulatory processes. Our central nervous system is constructed in such a way that all experience is affective; this helps us avoid what is too little or too much; and it provides incentives for developmental goals (Emde, 1980a; 1980b). I also wish to emphasize that these three biological principles of self are inseparable. Together they guide adaptive functions beginning at birth and throughout the life-span so that there is organized coherence to an individual's activity.

DEVELOPMENTAL PRINCIPLES

The following developmental principles illustrate today's scientific appreciation of the fundamental activity of the infant who moves toward increasing psychological complexity. This is quite different from our previous ways of thinking in terms of a fixed reality to which the infant must adapt, and in terms of drive reductionism and reflexology. To highlight this newer way of thinking, I briefly present these developmental principles in the form of paradoxes. Paradoxes are apparent contradictions which, from my point of view, serve to illustrate two themes. First, they illustrate, by contrast, how far we have come from our earlier static view of reality in which the world was a "given" rather than something actively constructed by the infant. Second, they serve to illustrate that human experience is organized according to polar opposites which must be continually integrated by individualized experience. The theme of opposites and their integration is implicit in Freud (1905, 1915), but has been made explicit by such psychoanalytic thinkers as Erikson (1950) and Sander (1962, 1964, 1980). Writing about developmental polarities, Sander (1980) commented that "the mystery in pathogenesis is less that of discovering where conflicts come from than of accounting for what holds us together in the face of them" (p. 1). Thus, in a general way, paradoxes illustrate the self-organizing aspect of psychobiological functioning. I shall enumerate four such paradoxes.

1. *The Development of Others and the Development of Self.*[3] That the infant must develop a notion of others confronts us with a paradox. How can the infant who is so "immature" and "inexperienced" fit into a social world of significant others when he himself must develop a notion of these others? How can he make use of others when he must construct them? Yet this happens. Following Piaget, whose work has so compellingly shown us how the infant constructs his inanimate world, we are now coming to learn how the infant does indeed construct his social world as he interacts with others (Lamb and Sherrod, 1981). He does this through self-regulating developmental processes of assimilation and accommodation, wherein knowledge is gained through successive increments of experiencing the novel against a background of the familiar.

But there is another angle to this paradox. The development of the self occurs as part of the development of the other; from a process point of view, they seem inseparable. The interconnectedness of the development of self-knowledge and knowledge of others was pointed out long ago by Cooley (1912) and Mead (1934) and has been reemphasized by later psychoanalytic theorists, including Erikson (1950, 1959), Jacobson (1964), and Mahler and her colleagues (1968, 1975). But perhaps the most explicit psychoanalytic theory along these lines was developed by Spitz, whose thinking I shall review in the light of recent research.

---

3. Since this essay was completed, the incisive statement of Stern (1982) has come to my attention. After his review of recent findings in developmental psychology, he concludes that much of a self-other distinction exists quite early in the infant's world as a consequence of predesigned discriminations. My view is that while many elements for a self-other distinction are, indeed, present soon after birth (see "social fittedness" principle), the distinction itself requires considerable development and "construction." Certainly I agree with Stern's point that there is no evidence for the infant experiencing an early self-other "confusion" or "anxiety" about a lack of self-other differentiation. The latter assumption makes no sense on either logical or empirical grounds.

Spitz inferred that the infant's basic sense of being separate from the world emerges around 3 months, at the time social smiling becomes prominent. After this, the infant, through recurrent social interactions, begins to work out an awareness of the "I" by means of actions performed in his relations with the "non-I." The idea is that as the infant perceives differences in the "non-I" (e.g., mother versus others), there will be a corresponding enrichment in the infant's sense of the "I." Interestingly, although Spitz thought that this development would require several months, recent research indicates that it occurs earlier. By 3 to 4 months of age, infants can distinguish between mother and unfamiliar people as measured by a variety of responses. (These include differential smiling [Emde et al., 1976]; differential vocalizing [Rebelsky, 1971; Turnure, 1971]; differential cardiac deceleration [Banks and Wolfson, 1967]; and other behaviors [Wahler, 1967; Bronson 1972]; see discussion in Lewis and Brooks-Gunn [1979].) Spitz was unequivocal in his view that the objectification of self goes hand in hand with the objectification of the other. This process culminates in a new level of organization at 15 months which, he felt, is marked by the acquisition of the semantic "no" and an emergent autonomy and self-awareness. Concerning the latter, he stated, "An unmistakable testimony of this self-awareness is provided around eighteen months, when the child begins to speak of himself in the third person" (1957, p. 130).

Thinking of the self-as-object again emphasizes the experiential interrelationship of self and other development. For Mead, the development of self required that the developing child anticipate the other's reactions, take the role of the other, perceive the self as other, and engage in an internal dialogue with a "generalized other." As Spitz and Lewis and Brooks-Gunn (1979) have pointed out, this could not take place before the representational self at 15 to 18 months. But the latter have also pointed out an earlier aspect of the self-as-object. If one assumes that knowledge about others is knowledge about the self, then this is so because infants before 12 months are able to distinguish others on the basis of familiarity, age, and gender. (For a review of studies, see Lewis and Brooks-Gunn, 1979.)

The self is, however, a body self as well as a social self. The body self has received primary emphasis in psychoanalysis (e.g., by Hoffer, 1949; Jacobson, 1964; Anna Freud, 1965) as well as in neuropsychiatry in general (Schilder, 1935); but if we think of its prerepresentational origins, our understanding of the self-other differentiation is enhanced. As the Papouseks (1979) point out, neurophysiological considerations make it obvious that touching something else is perceived differently than touching oneself or being touched. By the same token, one has afferent feedback from one's own movement which one also sees; this must be experienced quite differently from just seeing another's movement. The same is true for hearing and otherwise sensing one's own voice as compared to the voice of another. All of this must operate from early infancy to build up progressively more integrated schemas of body self as compared with other selves. Still, as Spitz (1957) so poignantly observes, this double origin of the self (which he referred to as the narcissistic and social) continues with us after infancy. In his view, all later self-awareness combines the awareness of one's own body and the awareness of "'other's' reactions to it" (p. 121).

2. *The Development of the Past and the Development of the Future: the Janus Principle.* That the past develops and the future develops both seem paradoxical if one thinks of it from our preconstructivist point of view. But the paradox runs deeper. I have come to realize that perhaps the basic psychological principle of development can be thought of as the Janus principle: *we must look back in order to look forward;* we must *use the past* in order *to anticipate.* In other words, just as the development of other and self go hand in hand, so do the development of past and future (anticipation).

For the development of the self, we know there is a development in early infancy from a world of immediate perception and action to a world involving increasing memory with a sense of the past and a use of the past. Memory is required for anticipations involved in the simplest kind of learning (for example, classical conditioning) as well as for the expectations involved in more complex learning (for example, coordinating sensorimotor schemas). A lot remains to be investigated about the development of memory in infancy, but several generalizations can be made. First, there is a major enhancement of learning which

takes place around 2 months; habituation, classical conditioning, and operant learning are difficult to demonstrate before
that time and easy to demonstrate afterward. (For a review, see
Sameroff, 1979; or Emde and Robinson, 1979.) Second, there
is another enhancement of memory at 7 to 9 months (for a
review, see Kagan et al., 1978).[4] Third, it has been a recurrent
observation that memory for social features in the infant's environment proceeds in advance of memory for nonsocial features. (Even this is awaiting thorough systematic study, but virtually all infancy researchers know it to be so. Piaget, for
example, commented that cognitive development around
mother probably would be enhanced due to her comings and
goings and being at the interface of so many sensorimotor schemas.) Finally, it is quite likely that memory is enhanced by affect. This is a topic of considerable interest to psychoanalysts
(for example, Spitz, 1972) and, although it has not been systematically investigated in infancy, it now seems about to gain attention in the midst of some exciting research concerning "re-
instatement learning." In this form of learning, as Rovee-
Collier and Fagan (1981) have shown, reinstating the original
context in which learning takes place enormously enhances the
infant's memory. As this research proceeds, I would expect that
the relevant context for memory enhancement will be shown to
be social and affective.

3. *The Development of Causality.* In this principle we are confronted with the paradox of the infant having to "construct" a
notion of causality as he is having to learn the specifics of what
leads to what. In a sense, he must teach himself about learning
in order to be taught. But this does occur, as Piaget's work so
richly documents (e.g., 1936, 1937). A knowledge of contingencies soon becomes of central importance to the infant.[5] Indeed,
it is possible to think of contingency awareness as one of the
earliest aspects of the prerepresentational self—an aspect in
which there is self-environment differentiation based on what

4. Some may note that these age points correspond with those of Spitz's
first two organizers. For a review of this aspect, see Emde et al. (1976).

5. A form of contingency awareness in mirror behavior has been shown at
5 months (Papousek and Papousek, 1979) and in the latter part of the first
year (Lewis and Brooks-Gunn, 1979).

the infant causes versus what the infant does not cause (Papousek, personal communication).

But the most salient aspect of this linkage between contingency awareness and the early development of self may come from *parental "mirroring"* of infant behavior. Psychoanalytic observers such as Mahler and Furer (1968), Kohut (1971), Call (1980), and Pines (1982) have alluded to the functional importance of this for self-development, but the Papouseks are now studying this in detail. For them, mirroring is an example of intuitive parenting, since parents across cultures engage in such behaviors automatically and do this beginning with the newborn. Parents show a strong tendency to imitate the baby's facial expressions and vocalizations, especially with newly developing patterns of behavior. Thus, from earliest infancy, parental mirroring seems to provide natural contingencies which offer the infant chances for controlling parental behavior.[6] In fact, because of parental mirroring, most contingencies that the infant can control are social, whereas most he cannot are nonsocial—an important aspect of self-development. Beginning at 2 to 3 months, "parental echoing" takes place. This is a form of mirroring in which the parent repeats the infant's sounds. Around 6 months, parents repeat babbling syllable sounds, usually amplifying such sounds with an explosion of pleasure and making a word. Thus, "ba ba" becomes "baby" with a rising intonation. Usually, words which mothers create from baby sounds relate to the self. Mothers make a game of this, and the Papouseks believe that through these games, an infant gradually comes to learn that he is labeled differently from mother, father, sister, or object. The infant becomes labeled as an individual.

As mirroring continues, there is apt to be a considerable amount of mutual pleasure in this process. Undoubtedly this contributes to the infant's incentive for learning from the face and voice and for modeling adult behavior in general.

4. *The Development of Language before Language.* A decade ago this would have sounded more paradoxical to us than it does today. By and large we now appreciate that there is an impor-

6. It may be that the newborn tongue-protruding and mouth-opening "imitative behaviors" described by Meltzoff and Moore (1979) are part of such a mirroring process.

tant communication system in infancy and one which can easily be observed in the reciprocal interactions between infant and caregiver (Brazelton et al., 1974; Stern, 1977; Call, 1980). Yet, even now, it is not sufficiently appreciated that this communication system is affective (Basch, 1976); that there is an *affective signaling* which is biologically based, highly organized, and undergoes development. The infant's signals of distress, smiling, interest, surprise, fear, anger, sadness, and disgust are used for caregiving and are exchanged between parent and infant. In early infancy, such signals predominantly flow from infant to parent, but in later infancy (beginning at 7 to 9 months), they increasingly flow from parent to infant. By the end of the first year, the infant and another person can communicate about a third event by means of affective signaling.

THE AFFECTIVE SELF

By way of introducing a discussion of the affective self, I briefly mention two more paradoxes. The first is a basic biological paradox. *Biologically based principles are species-general,* yet through their functioning *they seem to assure individuality.* Because of man's complexity and the fact that no two individuals are born the same, the general biological principles of self-regulation, social fittedness, and affective monitoring work toward the coherent uniqueness of each developing person. Thus, it seems a paradoxical truth of self that our heritage guarantees both our species-wide commonness and our individual uniqueness.

The final paradox of this presentation is one I consider to be the basic paradox of development. In developmental psychology, this is usually stated in terms of the continuity-discontinuity issue. From decades of prospective longitudinal observation, we have become aware that development is not simply continuous, and that there are times of major transformation. I like to think of this paradox from the point of view of personal experience: *how can we change so much, and yet we know we are the same?* This is obviously a profound paradox, and one central to the emergence of self. I think our understanding of it is helped immeasurably by a theory of the affective self.

An orienting thesis for such a theory is this: our *affective life gives continuity* to our experience in spite of the many ways we change. This is so because its central organization is biological and its vital relations are unchanging (Izard, 1977). Further, not only is the continuity of experience across development guaranteed, but what I call our "affective core" ensures that we are able to understand others who are human. Finally, because our affective core touches upon those aspects of experience which are most important to us as individuals, it also allows us to get in touch with the uniqueness of our own (and others') experience.

The following arguments support this thesis.

First is the *clinical-humanistic* argument. Both clinical practice and everyday experience illustrate how much we rely upon knowing other people by means of understanding their feelings. Once we are in touch with another's emotional life, we are in touch with his or her humanity; this kind of understanding then becomes a basis for going further and appreciating that individual as a unique human being. This aspect of our lives, this shared "affective core," enables us to appreciate a wide variety of characters in novels and plays. It enables us to travel in foreign countries and have a basis for communicating, even without fluency in a foreign language. (It is part of being human that I can have considerable rapport with another, even though our experiences are different; I can do that by being guided by my understanding of that person's feelings and by my own feelings occurring in response to them.)

The second argument for affective continuity concerns the *similar organization of emotional expression in infants, children, and adults.* In our infancy studies, we found a striking consistency concerning the organization of infant facial expression of emotions. We used a multidimensional scaling approach for analyzing adult judgments of photographed infant facial expressions which were sampled in a variety of ways. We sampled expressions at 2½, 3½, 4¼, and 12 months of age, and we carried out 8 different judgment studies using 25 judges in each study. At 2½ months, scaling solutions were two-dimensional with the first dimension easily characterized as hedonic tone and the second best characterized as "state." However, after 3 months, three-dimensional scaling solutions predominated. In these, hedonic tone carried the most variance, activation appeared as the second dimension, and an internally/externally oriented dimension was the third.[7]

These results show a striking continuity with studies of adult emotional expression. A history of similar conclusions goes back to the thinking of Spencer (1890), Wundt (1900), and Freud (1915) who, from a somewhat different vantage point, wrote that our instinctual impulses were influenced by *"the three great polarities that dominate mental life"* (p. 140). These included pleasure/unpleasure, active/passive, and subject (ego)/object (external world). But most impressive are the similar conclusions from a host of experimental investigations which include Woodworth and Schlosberg (1954), Abelson and Sermat (1962), Gladstone (1962), Frijda and Phillipszoon (1963), Osgood (1966), and Frijda (1970). As in our results, "pleasantness-unpleasantness" emerges as the major dimension, "activation" or "intensity" is the next most prominent dimension, and a third dimension is often suggested but is usually difficult to interpret. (The third dimension is sometimes called "acceptance-rejection," sometimes "control," and sometimes "expressed feeling versus inner feeling.")

Until recently, there was an age gap between infancy and adulthood in these scaling studies of emotion. Now that gap has been filled as Russell and Ridgeway (1982), in a series of studies of school children from grades 3 through 7, have reported a similar organization according to predominant dimensions of hedonic tone and arousal.

The third argument for affective continuity concerns *cross-cultural evidence for discrete emotions.* Although Darwin (1872) had long ago postulated the species-wide existence of discrete emotional expressions, and although Tomkins's theoretical work (1962–63) and empirical work (Tomkins and McCarter, 1964) had revived this proposition, it remained for more recent investigators to provide a systematic test of it. In the early 1970s

---

7. As in other dimensional scaling studies mentioned below, our third dimension accounted for relatively little variance and was sometimes difficult to interpret. I infer that this third dimension is not a central aspect of emotional organization and probably represents a related subsystem of mental functioning.

two separate teams of investigators (Izard, 1971; Ekman et al., 1972) reported on their programmatic cross-cultural research. Results were dramatic. Using still photographs of adults who posed peak expressions, both research programs found remarkable agreement about specific facial expression of emotion. Agreement was found among adults in non-Western as well as Western cultures and in nonliterate as well as literate cultures. Agreement was found for the emotions of joy, surprise, anger, fear, sadness, disgust, and to a lesser extent for interest. This agreement seemed to imply the universal basis not only for the expression of particular emotions but also for their recognition; furthermore, the specific facial movements involved in each of these patterns of emotion have now been specified (see Izard, 1971; Ekman and Friesen, 1975). Thus, an implication from this work is that such discrete emotional expressions are part of our biological heritage and that members of our species are born with a preadapted readiness to express and recognize these emotions. A natural question then arises: are discrete emotional expressions present in infancy?

The fourth argument concerns just that, the *presence of discrete patterns of emotional expression in infancy*. Although the story is far from complete, there are already consistent conclusions as a result of ongoing infancy research in several laboratories. Facial expressions of emotion can be judged reliably by those who know nothing about the eliciting circumstances to which a baby is exposed, and such expressions fit the patterning suggested by the theoretical and empirical analyses of adult discrete emotions (Izard, 1971; Tomkins, 1962–63; Ekman and Friesen, 1975; Plutchik, 1980). Thus far, the infancy discrete emotions for which this is true include happiness, fear, sadness, surprise, anger, disgust, and pain (Emde et al., 1978; Hiatt et al., 1979; Izard et al., 1980; Gaensbauer, 1982; Stenberg et al., 1982). Furthermore, other studies have shown that there is impressive agreement among groups of judges about context-free emotions expressed in still photographs of infants; such studies have been replicated both within and across laboratories (Emde et al., 1982).

Emotion is, of course, not expressed solely by the face. Everyday experience tells us that the voice is extremely important. Research on vocalic expressions of emotion, although relatively recent, is now becoming a lively area. Thus far, there appears to be clear evidence for discrete vocalic expressions of emotion in adults (Scherer, 1979). Work in infancy is also encouraging, but is just beginning.

EMOTIONAL AVAILABILITY AND SOCIAL REFERENCING

I hope the final argument for the continuity in our affective life, for its human patterning, and for its significance in self-development will be the most convincing. This argument concerns the importance of *emotional availability* and *emotional referencing* before and during the time of self-awareness. The importance of the emotional availability of the caregiver in infancy has been implicit in investigations of attachment (Bowlby, 1969; Matas et al., 1978) and has been explicit in the work of Mahler and her colleagues (1975). In a recent experimental study of 15-month-olds, we found striking effects of mother's emotional availability on infant exploration and play. The experimental effects in our playroom setting depended upon whether mother was reading a newspaper or not (Sorce and Emde, 1981). Infants showed less pleasure and less exploration when mother was reading. Although they were not distressed, they were somewhat subdued, stayed closer to mother, and made fewer bids for her attention.

Most recently, we have been absorbed in researching a phenomenon which we and others have termed "social referencing" (Feinman and Lewis, 1981; Campos and Stenberg, 1982; Klinnert et al., 1983; Sorce et al., 1982). This is an aspect of emotional signaling which begins toward the end of the first year and continues to have major importance during the second year. Social referencing is a general process whereby a person of any age seeks out emotional information from a significant other in order to make sense of an event which is otherwise ambiguous or beyond the person's own intrinsic appraisal capabilities.[8] It is already apparent that social referenc-

---

8. Social referencing could be considered a type of secondary appraisal along the lines of the theories of Arnold (1960), Lazarus (1968), and Bowlby 1969). This is so because it is evoked when prior appraisal processes fail to predict the impact of an event or person.

ing may be especially important at the dawn of self-awareness. Infants then regularly experience more uncertainty about the impact of environmental events in terms of their own safety or in terms of the consequences of their own actions.

In order to study social referencing, our research team has devised a number of experimental situations, including those with an unfamiliar toy (such as a radio-controlled robot), a toy house that collapses when the infant touches it, a stranger's approach, and placement on a visual cliff. In all of these, the infant encounters uncertainty in the midst of exploring a new situation and then references the face of mother or of an experimenter. At this point the adult displays a clear signal of an emotion, and we observe what occurs. Experimental results from all these situations indicate a powerful emotional signaling system. Evidence suggests that the infant is aware of separateness to the extent that he or she (1) registers the dilemma and interrupts ongoing activity; (2) seeks out emotional information from another person about an external event; and (3) makes use of that emotional information in a planful way for guiding subsequent behavior. To illustrate these effects, I summarize a set of experiments with 12-month-old infants in the visual cliff situation (Sorce et al., 1982). The cliff is a plexiglass-covered table divided into two halves, a shallow side in which a patterned surface is placed immediately underneath the plexiglass and a deep side in which a similar surface is placed at a varying distance beneath. The cliff is often used in psychology to test infants' depth perception or wariness of heights (Walk, 1966; Campos et al., 1978), but in this situation we modified the "deep side" to an intermediate depth of 30 centimeters in order to elicit uncertainty. In our pilot work we found that when an infant was placed on the shallow side, the lure of an attractive toy on the deep side typically resulted in an approach toward the center and a pause; this was followed by frequent looks to mother (who stood at the edge of the deep side), but there was no clear avoidance of the depth.

Bolstered by the knowledge that we had constructed an un certain situation, and not a fearful one, we began our experi ments. According to our procedure, when an infant who had been placed on the shallow side of the cliff advanced to the edge of the drop-off, noticed the depth, and looked to mother's face, the latter displayed a facial expression of a given emotion for which she had been trained.

The first experiment compared the effects of mother's expressions of fear and joy. Thirty-six mother-infant pairs were randomly assigned to either condition. Results were unequivocal. All infants included in our experiments referenced the mother's face after looking at the drop-off. When mother posed a fearful expression, none of the 17 infants in this condition crossed to the deep side. In contrast, 14 of the 19 infants who observed mother's happy face crossed! In addition, infants in the fear condition sometimes retreated from the cliff edge and had a demonstrably more negative hedonic tone.

A second study was conducted to see the behavioral consequences of two different-patterned emotional signals—interest and anger. Results again indicated strong effects. When infants referenced mothers who posed anger, only 2 of 18 crossed the deep side; in contrast, when infants looked to mothers' faces posing interest, 11 of 15 crossed.

To understand the effects of social referencing in this situation further, we did two further experiments with 12-month-old infants. A third study investigated infant reactions to mothers who posed sadness. This emotion, although hedonically negative, was not considered relevant in terms of its message as to whether to cross the cliff or not. Six of the 18 infants tested in this condition crossed the deep side. Further, the mean number of references by infants in this group was higher than in any of the earlier conditions, suggesting that the infants were puzzled about the facial signal itself or its meaning in this context.

Our fourth study of this series addressed another issue of context; namely, whether mother's facial expressions of emotion were effective not because of the infant's appreciation of an external situation of uncertainty, but merely because of "unexpectedness." We therefore tested 24 infants with the visual cliff table altered so as to have two shallow sides. All mothers smiled broadly until the infants reached the center of the table, then shifted to a facial pose of fear. In contrast to earlier studies, two-thirds of the infants tested in this condition did *not* look

186   *Robert N. Emde*

to their mothers at all and continued crossing. (Presumably, there was no need to reference since there was no uncertainty.) The 8 babies who did look to mother also crossed the shallow side, in spite of seeing fear in her face; this was in contrast to the lack of crossing in all babies who saw a mother's fearful face in the first study. The findings of the earlier studies, therefore, seem interpretable as a social referencing process—an infant must seek out emotional information from another person in a context of uncertainty for getting information which is of use for guiding subsequent behavior.

I hope this story of one line of experiments has served to vivify this recently uncovered phenomenon which is the subject of current intensive research. In a way social referencing illustrates all of the principles enumerated in this essay. It is a self-regulatory process in a situation of dynamic social interchange in which there is affective monitoring. Further, the development of others, of memory, of anticipation, of causality, and of emotional signaling has reached the point where I think one can see the affective self in a coherent organization. The observer gains a strong conviction that the infant's own emotions are insufficient for guiding action; this becomes apparent as the infant looks to another for emotional information and guidance. But nothing can take the place of being there—of directly observing the dramatic changes which occur in an infant who pauses, puzzles, looks, feels, and alters his or her behavior accordingly. As one observes this repeatedly in large numbers of infants, one feels both their *humanity* and their *individuality*. We share what is common across infants, but no two infants are alike. In this last aspect we encounter what is, perhaps, the basic psychobiological polarity of the affective self.

BIBLIOGRAPHY

ABELSON, R. P. & SERMAT, V. (1962), Multidimensional scaling of facial expressions. *J. Exp. Psychol.*, 63:546–554.
AINSWORTH, M. D., BELL, S., & STAYTON, D. J. (1974), Infant-mother attachment and social development. In *The Integration of a Child into a Social World* ed. M. P. M. Richard. Cambridge: Cambridge Univ. Press, pp. 99–135.
ALS, H., TRONICK, E., & BRAZELTON, T. B. (1979), Analysis of face-to-face

interaction in infant-adult dyads. In *The Study of Social Interaction*, ed. M. Lamb, S. Suomi, & G. R. Stephenson. Madison: Univ. Wisconsin Press, pp. 33–76.

AMSTERDAM, B. K. (1972), Mirror self-image reactions before age 2. *Develpm. Psychol.*, 5:297–305.

ARNOLD, M. (1960), *Emotion and Personality*, 2 vols. New York: Columbia Univ. Press.

BANKS, J. H. & WOLFSON, J. H. (1967), Differential cardiac response of infants to mother and stranger. Read at the Eastern Psychological Association Meetings, Boston.

BASCH, M. F. (1976), The concept of affect. *J. Amer. Psychoanal. Assn.*, 24:759–777.

BERTALANFFY, L. VON (1968), *General System Theory*. New York: George Braziller.

BOWLBY, J. (1969), *Attachment and Loss*, vol. 1. New York: Basic Books.

BRAZELTON, T. B. & ALS, H. (1979), Four early stages in the development of mother-infant interaction. *Psychoanal. Study Child*, 34:349–369.

————— KOSLOWSKI, B., & MAIN, M. (1974), The origins of reciprocity. In *The Effect of the Infant on Its Caregiver*, ed. M. Lewis & L. Rosenblum. New York: Wiley-Intersciences, 1:49–76.

BRONSON, G. W. (1972), Infant's reactions to unfamiliar persons and novel objects. *Monogr. Soc. Res. Child Develpm.*, serial no. 148, vol. 37, no. 3.

BUTTERWORTH, G. (1979), What minds have in common is space. Read at the Annual Conference of the Developmental Psychology Section, British Psychological Society, Southampton.

————— & JARRET, N. (1980), The geometry of preverbal communication. Read at the Annual Conference of the Developmental Psychology Section of the British Psychological Society, Edinburgh.

CALL, J. D. (1980), Some prelinguistic aspects of language development. *J. Amer. Psychoanal. Assn.*, 28:259–289.

CAMPOS, J. J., HIATT, S., RAMSAY, D., HENDERSON, C., & SVEJDA, M. J. (1978), The emergence of fear on the visual cliff. In *The Origins of Affect*, ed. M. Lewis & L. Rosenblum. New York: Wiley, pp. 149–182.

————— & STENBERG, C. (1981), Perception, appraisal, and emotion. In Lamb & Sherrod (1981), pp. 273–314.

CLARKE, A. M. & CLARKE, A. D. B. (1976), *Early Experience*. New York: Free Press.

CONDON, W. S. & SANDER, L. W. (1974), Synchrony demonstrated between movements of the neonate and adult speech. *Child Develpm.*, 45:456–462.

COOLEY, C. H. (1912), *Human Nature and the Social Order*. New York: Scribners.

DAMON, W. & HART, D. (1982). The development of self-understanding from infancy through adolescence. *Child Develpm.*, 53:841–864.

DARWIN, C. (1872), *Expression of Emotion in Man and Animals*. London: John Murray, 1904.

DECARIÉ, T. G. (1969), A study of the mental and emotional development of the thalidomide child. In *Determinants of Infant Behaviour,* ed. B. M. Foss London: Methuen, 4:167–187.

EKMAN, P. & FRIESEN, W. (1975), *Unmasking the Face.* Englewood Cliffs, N.J. Prentice-Hall.

———— & ELLSWORTH, P. (1972), *Emotion in the Human Face.* New York Pergamon Press.

EMDE, R. N. (1980a), Levels of meaning for infant emotions. In *Development o Cognition, Affect and Social Relations,* ed. W. A. Collins. Minnesota Symposi in Child Psychology, vol. 13. Hillsdale, N.J.: Erlbaum, pp. 1–37.

———— (1980b), Emotional availability. In *Parent-Infant Relationships,* ed. P. M Taylor. New York: Grune & Stratton, pp. 87–115.

———— (1981), Changing models of infancy and the nature of early develop ment. *J. Amer. Psychoanal. Assn.,* 29:179–219.

———— GAENSBAUER, T., & HARMON, R. J. (1976), *Emotional Expression ir Infancy. Psychol. Issues,* monogr. 37. New York: Int. Univ. Press.

———— KLIGMAN, D. H., REICH, J. H., & WADE, T. (1978), Emotional ex pression in infancy. In *The Development of Affect,* ed. M. Lewis & L. Rosen blum. New York: Plenum, pp. 125–148.

———— & ROBINSON, J. (1979), The first two months. In *American Handbook o Child Psychiatry,* ed. J. Noshpitz & J. D. Call. New York: Basic Books, pp 72–105.

———— SORCE, J. F., IZARD, C. E., HUEBNER, R., & KLINNERT, M. D. (1982) Adult judgments of infant emotions (in preparation).

ERIKSON, E. H. (1950), *Childhood and Society.* New York: Norton.

———— (1959), Growth and crises of the healthy personality. In *Identity and the Life Cycle. Psychol. Issues,* 1:50–100. New York: Int. Univ. Press.

———— (1968), *Identity.* New York: Norton.

FEINMAN, S. & LEWIS, M. (1981), Social referencing and second order effect in ten-month old infants. Read at the Society for Research in Child Devel opment, Boston.

FRAIBERG, S. (1977), *Insights from the Blind.* New York: Basic Books.

FREEDMAN, D. A., CANNADY, C., & ROBINSON, J. S. (1971), Speech and psy chic structure. *J. Amer. Psychoanal. Assn.,* 19:765–779.

FREUD, A. (1965), Normality and pathology in childhood. *W.,* 6.

FREUD, S. (1900), The interpretation of dreams. *S.E.,* 4 & 5.

———— (1905), Three essays on the theory of sexuality. *S.E.,* 7:125–243.

———— (1915), Instincts and their vicissitudes. *S.E.,* 14:111–140.

———— (1920), Beyond the pleasure principle. *S.E.,* 18:3–64.

FRIJDA, N. (1970), Emotion and recognition of emotion. In *Feelings and Emo tions,* ed. M. B. Arnold. New York: Academic Press, pp. 241–250.

———— & PHILLIPSZOON, E. (1963), Dimensions of recognition of expression *J. Abnorm. Soc. Psychol.,* 66:45–51.

GAENSBAUER, T. J. (1982), The differentiation of discrete affects. *Psychoanal. Study Child,* 37:29–66.

GALENSON, E. (1982), The infantile roots of sexual identity. Read at Sym posium on "Early Life and the Roots of Identity," Univ. California, Los Angeles Extension.

———— & ROIPHE, H. (1971), The impact of early sexual discovery on mood, defensive organization, and symbolization. *Psychoanal. Study Child,* 26:195–216.

GALLUP, G. (1979), Self-recognition in chimpanzees and man. In *The Child and Its Family,* ed. M. Lewis & L. Rosenblum. New York: Plenum, 2:107–126.

GEDO, J. & GOLDBERG, A. (1973), *Models of the Mind.* Chicago & London: Univ. Chicago Press.

GLADSTONE, W. H. (1962), A multidimensional study of facial expressions of emotion. *Austral. J. Psychol.,* 14:95–100.

HALL, C. & LINDZEY, G. (1957), *Theories of Personality.* New York: Wiley.

HIATT, S., CAMPOS, J. J., EMDE, R. N. (1979), Facial patterning and infant emotional expression. *Child Develpm.,* 50:1020–1035.

HOFFER, W. (1949), Mouth, hand and ego-integration. *Psychoanal. Study Child,* 3/4:49–56.

IZARD, C. E. (1971), *The Face of Emotion.* Meredith, N.Y.: Appleton-Century-Crofts.

———— (1977), The emergence of emotions and the development of consciousness in infancy. In *Human Consciousness and Its Transformations,* ed. J. M. Davidson, R. J. Davidson, & G. E. Schwartz. New York: Plenum, pp. 193–216.

———— HUEBNER, R., RISSER, D., McGINNIS, G., & DOUGHERTY, L. (1980), The young infant's ability to produce discrete emotional expressions. *Develpm. Psychol.,* 16:132–140.

JACKLIN, C. N. & MACCOBY, E. E. (1978), Social behavior at thirty-three months in same-sex and mixed-sex dyads. *Child Develpm.,* 49:557–569.

JACOBSON, E. (1964), *The Self and the Object World.* New York: Int. Univ. Press.

JUNG, C. G. (1939), *Integration of the Personality.* New York: Farrar & Rinehart.

KAGAN, J. (1981), *The Second Year.* Cambridge: Harvard Univ. Press.

———— KEARSLEY, R., & ZELASO, P. (1978), *Infancy.* Cambridge: Harvard Univ. Press.

KLINNERT, M. D., CAMPOS, J. J., SORCE, J. F., EMDE, R. N., & SVEJDA, M. J. (1983), Social referencing. In *Emotions in Early Development,* ed. R. Plutchik & H. Kellerman. New York: Academic Press, pp. 57–86.

KOHUT, H. (1971), *The Analysis of the Self.* New York: Int. Univ. Press.

———— (1977), *The Restoration of the Self.* New York: Int. Univ. Press.

KOPP, C. (1982), Antecedents of self-regulation. *Develpm. Psychol.,* 18:199–214.

KRIS, M. (1957), The use of prediction in a longitudinal study. *Psychoanal. Study Child,* 12:175–189.

LAMB, M. & SHERROD, L. R., eds. (1981), *Infant Social Cognition.* Hillsdale, N.J.: Erlbaum.

LAZARUS, R. S. (1968), Emotions and adaptation. In *Nebraska Symposium on Motivation,* ed. W. Arnold. Lincoln: Univ. Nebraska Press, pp. 175–270.

LEVINSON, D. (1978), *The Seasons of a Man's Life.* New York: Ballantine Books.

LEWIS, M. & BROOKS-GUNN, J. (1979), *Social Cognition and the Acquisition of Self.* New York: Plenum.

MAHLER, M. S. & FURER, M. (1968), *On Human Symbiosis and the Vicissitudes of Individuation.* New York: Int. Univ. Press.

————— PINE, F., & BERGMAN, A. (1975), *The Psychological Birth of the Human Infant.* New York: Basic Books.

MATAS, L., AREND, R., & SROUFE, L. (1978), A continuity of adaptation in the second year. *Child Develpm.,* 49:547–556.

MEAD, G. H. (1934), *Mind, Self and Society from the Standpoint of a Behaviorist.* Chicago: Univ. Chicago Press.

MELTZOFF, A. N. & MOORE, M. K. (1979), Interpreting 'imitative' responses in early infancy. *Science,* 205:217–219.

MONEY, J. & EHRHARDT, A. (1972), *Man, Woman, Boy and Girl.* Baltimore: Johns Hopkins Univ. Press.

OSGOOD, C. (1966), Dimensionality of the semantic space for communication via facial expression. *Scand. J. Psychol.,* 7:1–30.

PAPOUSEK, H. (1981), The common in the uncommon child. In *The Uncommon Child,* ed. M. Lewis & L. Rosenblum. New York: Plenum, pp. 317–328.

————— & PAPOUSEK, M. (1979), Early ontogeny of human social interaction. In *Human Ethology,* ed. M. von Cranach, K. Foppa, W. Lepenies, & D. Ploog. Cambridge: Cambridge Univ. Press, pp. 456–489.

————— ————— (1980), Interactional failures. Read at First World Congress on Infant Psychiatry, Cascais, Portugal.

————— ————— (1981), Integration into the social world. In *Psychobiology of the Human Newborn,* ed. P. M. Stratton. New York: Wiley, pp. 367–390.

PIAGET, J. (1936), *The Origins of Intelligence in Children.* New York: Int. Univ. Press, 1952.

————— (1937), *The Construction of Reality in the Child.* New York: Basic Books, 1954.

PINES, M. (1982), Personal communication.

PLUTCHIK, R. (1980), *The Emotions.* New York: Harper & Row.

RANGELL, L. (1967), Psychoanalysis, affects and the 'human core.' *Psychoanal. Q.,* 36:172–202.

REBELSKY, F. (1971), Infants' communication attempts with mother and stranger. Read at the Eastern Psychological Association Meeting, New York.

ROVEE-COLLIER, C. & FAGAN, J. (1981), The retrieval of memory in early infancy. In *Advances in Infancy Research,* ed. L. Libsitt. Norwood, N.J.: Ablex, 1:225–254.

RUSSELL, J. A. & RIDGEWAY, D. (1982), Dimensions underlying children's emotional concept. *Developm. Psychol.* (in press).

SACKETT, G., SAMEROFF, A. J., CAIRNS, R. B., & SUOMI, S. J. (1981), Continuity in behavioural development. In *Behavioural Development,* ed. K. Immelmann, G. Barlow, L. Petrinovich, & M. Main. Cambridge: Cambridge Univ. Press, pp. 23–57.

SAMEROFF, A. J., ed. (1978), Organization and stability of newborn behavior. *Soc. Res. Child Develpm.,* vol. 43.

————— (1981), Personal communication.

_____ & CHANDLER, M. (1976), Reproductive risk and the continuum of caretaking casualty. In *Review of the Child Development Research,* ed. F. D. Horowitz. Chicago: Univ. Chicago Press, 4:187–244.

SANDER, L. W. (1962), Issues in early mother-child interaction. *J. Amer. Acad. Child Psychiat.,* 1:141–166.

_____ (1964), Adaptive relationships in early mother-child interaction. *J. Amer. Acad. Child Psychiat.,* 3:231–264.

_____ (1975), Infant and caretaking environment. In *Explorations in Child Psychiatry,* ed. E. J. Anthony. New York: Plenum, pp. 129–166.

_____ (1980), Polarity, paradox and the organizing process in development. Read at First World Conference on Infant Psychiatry, Cascais, Portugal.

SANDLER, J. & ROSENBLATT, B. (1962), The concept of the representational world. *Psychoanal. Study Child,* 17:128–146.

SCAIFE, M. & BRUNER, J. S. (1975), The capacity for joint visual attention in the infant. *Nature,* 253:265–266.

SCHERER, K. R. (1979), Nonlinguistic indicators of emotion and psychopathology. In *Emotions in Personality and Psychophysiology,* ed. C. E. Izard. New York: Plenum, pp. 495–529.

SCHILDER, P. (1935), *The Image and Appearance of the Human Body.* New York: Int. Univ. Press, 1950.

SCHULMAN, A. H. & KAPLOWITZ, C. (1977), Mirror-image response during the first two years of life. *Develpm. Psychobiol.,* 10:133–142.

SLOBIN, D. I. (1968), Question of language development in cross-cultural perspective. As cited in E. L. Newport (1977), Motherese. In *Cognitive Theory,* ed. N. J. Castellan, Jr., D. B. Pisoni, & J. R. Potts. Hillsdale, N.J.: Erlbaum, 2:177–217.

SORCE, J. F. & EMDE, R. N. (1981), Mother's presence is not enough. *Develpm. Psychol.,* 17:737–745.

_____ _____ CAMPOS, J. J., & KLINNERT, M. D. (1982), Maternal emotional signaling (submitted to *Science*).

SNOW, C. E. (1972), Mother's speech to children learning language. *Child Develpm.,* 43:549–565.

SPENCER, H. (1890), *The Principles of Psychology.* New York: Appleton.

SPIEGEL, L. A. (1959), The self, the sense of self, and perception. *Psychoanal. Study Child,* 16:81–109.

SPITZ, R. A. (1957), *No and Yes.* New York: Int. Univ. Press.

_____ (1972), Bridges. *J. Amer. Psychoanal. Assn.,* 20:721–735.

STENBERG, C., CAMPOS, J. J., & EMDE, R. N. (1983), The facial expression of anger in seven-month-olds. *Child Develpm.,* 54:1814–1819.

STERN, D. N. (1977), *The First Relationship.* Cambridge: Harvard Univ. Press.

_____ (1982), The early development of schemas of self, of other, and of various experiences of "self with other." In *Reflections on Self Psychology,* ed. J. D. Lichtenberg & S. Kaplan. New York: Int. Univ. Press (in press).

TOMKINS, S. S. (1962–63), *Affect, Imagery, Consciousness,* 2 vols. New York: Springer.

_____ & McCARTER, R. (1964), What and where are the primary affects? *Percept. Mot. Skills,* 18:119–158.

TREVARTHEN, C. (1979), Communication and cooperation in early infancy. In *Before Speech,* ed. M. Bullowa. Cambridge: Cambridge Univ. Press.

TURNURE, C. (1971), Response to voice of mother and stranger by babies in the first year. *Develpm. Psychol.,* 4:182–190.

WADDINGTON, C. H. (1962), *New Patterns in Genetics and Development.* New York: Columbia Univ. Press.

WAHLER, R. (1967), Infant social attachments, a reinforcement theory. *Child Develpm.,* 38:1079–1088.

WALK, R. (1966), The development of depth perception in animals and human infants. *Monogr. Soc. Res. Child Develpm.,* 31, 5:82–108.

WOODWORTH, R. W. & SCHLOSBERG, H. S. (1954), *Experimental Psychology.* New York: Holt.

WUNDT, W. M. (1900), *Grundriss der Psychologie.* As quoted in Izard (1971).

The "Stimulus Barrier"

A Review and Reconsideration

AARON H. ESMAN, M.D.

FREUD'S CONCEPT OF THE "PROTECTIVE SHIELD AGAINST
stimuli" (*Reizschutz*) has long been the object of considerable
interest on the part of developmental psychologists and psychoanalysts. It seems germane to the concerns both of those who
wish to study the effect of traumatic events on personality development and neurosogenesis and of those whose focus is on
normative infant development and early interaction patterns.
There have been a number of systematic reviews in the past
(Benjamin, 1965; Martin, 1968; Gediman, 1971), but, apart
from passing consideration by Shapiro and Stern (1980), none
that has considered the concept in the light of those recent
studies of infant behavior which have demonstrated a high
level of sensory receptiveness in the newborn. In this essay I
shall therefore attempt just such a review, seeking to place the
stimulus barrier concept in a modern framework and to assess
its relevance to current views of early development.

HISTORICAL BACKGROUND

As noted, a number of investigators have reviewed the literature on the subject of the protective shield; I shall therefore cite
here only the most salient references in sketching the historical
progression of the concept as it has evolved since Freud introduced it in *Beyond the Pleasure Principle* (1920). There he spoke
of the infant, by analogy with an elementary organism, as:

Professor of Clinical Psychiatry, Cornell University Medical College; faculty member, New York Psychoanalytic Institute.

194 Aaron H. Esman

This little fragment of living substance . . . suspended in the middle of an external world charged with the most powerful energies; . . . it would be killed by the stimulation emanating from these if it were not provided with a *protective shield against stimuli* [my italics]. . . . *Protection against* stimuli is an almost more important function for the living organism than *reception of* stimuli. The protective shield is supplied with its own store of energy [p. 27].

We describe as 'traumatic' any excitations from outside which are powerful enough to break through the protective shield [p. 29]; traumatic neurosis [is] a consequence of an extensive breach made in the protective shield [p. 31].

Freud appears, thus, to have conceived of "external" stimulation as potentially noxious to the infant, whose energies were necessarily devoted to coping with the demands of the "internal" stimuli generated by inescapable biological needs. Toward the menacing external world it turned a protective psychobiological rind, which, he later suggested (1938), represented an anlage of the later developing ego. "From what was originally a cortical layer, equipped with the organs for receiving stimuli and with arrangements for acting as a protective shield against stimuli, a special organization has arisen which henceforward acts as an intermediary between the id and the external world. To this region of our minds we have given the name of *ego*" (p. 145). The merging of psychological and biological constructs that characterizes Freud's observations on this matter should be noted; he refers on the one hand to a "region of the mind," and on the other to a "cortical layer equipped with the organs for receiving stimuli." It is just this merging of levels of discourse that has contributed to much of the confusion surrounding the protective shield concept.

A further source of this confusion is Freud's apparent ambiguity about the exclusionary nature of the protective shield's function. Though, as indicated above, he often seems to regard it as total, in other passages he seems less categorical. Thus:

. . . its outermost surface . . . functions as a . . . membrane resistant to stimuli. In consequence, the energies of the external world are able to pass into the next underlying layers, . . . with only a fragment of their original intensity; and these layers can devote themselves . . . to the reception of the amounts of stimulus which have been allowed through it. [But then:] the outer layer has saved all the deeper ones . . . unless, that is to say, stimuli reach it which are so strong that they break through the protective shield [1920, p. 27].

[And also:] an external protective shield against stimuli whose task it is to diminish the strength of excitations coming in [1925, p. 230].

At the same time, it is unclear whether he saw the protective shield as an active agency "supplied with its own source of energy" and selectively warding off classes of stimulation, or whether he viewed it as a passive structure, shielding the helpless and vulnerable neonate so far as possible against all external stimuli. Rapaport (1951) seems to have understood it in the former sense: "The stimulus-barrier scales down the intensity of external stimuli to a degree which the organism can manage" (p. 694).

Spitz (1955, 1961) echoed and elaborated Freud's views. He, too, maintained that the neonate perceived only internal stimuli; the sensorium was "uncathected: "in the neonate the threshold of the stimulus barrier is so high that the incoming stimuli simply do not penetrate unless they literally break through the protective layer, swamping the organism with unmanageable quantities of excitation" (1961, p. 632). He maintained that "excitation is generalized, and will flow now into one or another neural pathway. When it happens to hit the sensorium of the particular sector being stimulated, a response will be obtained in that sector, but the next time such a response may not occur" (p. 633). Spitz does not consider state variables here, although, as Wolff (1966) later showed, these are crucial in determining response patterns. Spitz regarded the neonatal stimulus barrier as a "prototype" of repression (but see Benjamin's view below).

Escalona in her developmental research dealt on a number of occasions with the stimulus barrier concept. In the now classic paper on special sensitivities, Bergman and Escalona (1949) seemed to view the stimulus barrier as an essentially passive threshold structure with, in the authors' metaphor, individually varying degrees of "thickness" and of "sensitivity" to various modes of sensation. Those children with "thin" innate stimulus barriers are prone, they suggested, to compensatory precocious development of (presumably active) protective ego structures that are "brittle" and nonadaptive; i.e., they are "predisposed" to severe psychopathology. Later, however, Escalona (1963) speaks of two "inactive infants" who "at times ceased responding to [social stimulation], as though they were able to erect a stimulus barrier" (p. 223). These infants were, however, 26 weeks old, so that their presumed capacity to generate an active stimulus barrier might reflect early defensive capacities not available to the neonate. Still later, Escalona (1968) disavowed this approach to the assessment of early stimulus-response patterns: "In previous publications we and others have attributed differences in perceptual sensitivity to differences in the sensory threshold. For many reasons we now consider this view of the matter as untenable. It is impossible to differentiate threshold from response by behavioral methods. If an infant . . . fails to respond, it is impossible to know whether the stimulus failed to enter the nervous system or whether it was perceived but not responded to overtly" (p. 25f.).

Benjamin (1965) reviewed the stimulus barrier concept systematically, in the light of then-available neurobiological data concerning infant development. Basing his conclusions largely on EEG studies, he formulated a two-phase conception of the stimulus barrier. During the first postnatal period he found a low level of sensitivity to stimulation, which increased after 3 to 4 weeks. "Our findings point to the conclusion that the so-called internal 'stimulus barrier' or protective shield against stimulation is . . . a purely passive mechanism due to relative lack of functional connections" (p. 60). In his view, a more active mechanism develops later: "Our impression is that this capacity [to shut out stimuli actively] exists to a slight degree as early as 8–10 weeks and matures rapidly thereafter" (p. 58). Freedman et al. (1970) similarly speak of a "primordial physiological stimulus barrier, i.e., one which cannot be considered defensive in a psychological sense" as opposed to "infantile patterns of concrete experience which both precede and . . . determine the character of later psychic defenses" (p. 315). It is in the intermediate period of vulnerability between the disappearance of the passive neonatal barrier at 3 to 4 weeks and the emergence of the "active defensive barrier" at 8 to 10 weeks that the mother takes on crucial importance as a buffer or protective shield against overwhelming noxious stimuli. Benjamin challenged Spitz's view that the neonatal stimulus barrier is developmentally related to later defensive operations, but he maintained that the later active stimulus barrier has direct continuities with, and represents a developmental precursor of, these mechanisms. Benjamin also stressed the fact that at all times, the stimulus barrier is only relatively effective and subject to "penetration."

Mahler has made extensive use of the stimulus barrier concept in her work on infantile psychosis as well as in her conceptualizations of normal development. In 1965, she said, "In the normal autistic phase, as well as in the symbiotic phase, the mother complements the more or less deficient innate stimulus barrier, performing the vitally important ego functions that the infant's primitive ego cannot execute and serving as a buffer against excess stimulation" (p. 559f.). Here, the stimulus barrier seems to be conceived of as a passive and relatively ineffectual structure, but in another communication (Panel, 1967) she seems to see it as an active agency: the "'stimulus barrier' or 'protective shield' has . . . from the first, a receptive, selective, and *adaptive* organizing function as well, that is, a positive aspect. . . . It determines, or rather guarantees, an appropriate intake of optimal levels of stimulation ('stimulus nutriment')" (p. 132). More explicitly, Mahler and McDevitt (1980) say, "We may infer that the stimulus barrier which existed during the first month no longer automatically keeps out external stimuli during the second month. However, by means of a sensory-perceptive peripheral boundary, a protective, but also a receptive, positively cathected, stimulus shield now begins to form and to envelop the symbiotic orbit of the mother-child unity" (p. 397). Here the authors seem to share Freud's idea of an innate, passive, exclusionary barrier; this is replaced by a more active, selective one, as the sensorium is "cathected." Further, Mahler echoes the propositions advanced by Brody and Axelrad (1966), who suggested not only that the protective shield serves an active, adaptive screening function, but also that, in contrast to Freud's original formulation, it responds both to external and internal stimuli: "where *either* internal or external stimuli are too exclusive in their impact on a young infant, the protective shield is *either* organically unsound, or for some dynamic reasons fails in *either* its receptive or its protective functions, there will be an impairment of the infant's ability to differentiate between inner and outer excitations, and in his capacity to experience a balance of passive and active accommodation to stimuli" (p. 224). Shevrin and Toussieng (1965) also suggest a stimulus barrier "with respect to *internal* stimuli or *cravings*" which are not necessarily drive derivatives.

The most recent systematic review of the concept is that of Gediman (1971). She, in concert with Leopold Bellak, conceives of the stimulus barrier in rather broader terms than earlier writers, identifying it as a "complex ego function rather than a simple sensory or perceptual threshold" (p. 243). She, too, considers nugatory the "inner-outer" controversy; since the neonate is *ex-hypothesi* incapable of making this distinction, one cannot consider the stimulus barrier as operating in response to it. Along with Benjamin and others, she challenges the validity of the Nirvana principle, which served as the neurobiological underpinning for Freud's view of external stimuli as inherently noxious (see also Compton, 1972). In Gediman's view, the stimulus barrier is not merely a protective shield in the infant, but an evolving adaptive ego function that incorporates both threshold and response factors, plays a significant organizing role throughout life, and may, like other ego functions, be definably impaired in psychopathology. Martin (1968), too, reviewed the stimulus barrier concept in the context of evolving ego processes; he spoke of the stimulus barrier *function* of various ego activities, suggesting that the development of attention and of concept formation served to exemplify ways in which ego functions, by narrowing or focusing the perceptual and cognitive fields, reduce vulnerability to excessive or intrusive stimulation. It is not clear in either of these formulations how, in the adult, the stimulus barrier is to be distinguished from the defensive armamentarium—or, indeed, whether the latter is not subsumed under what to Gediman is a more embracing structure.

As an aspect of his continuing concern with the concept of trauma, Furst (1978) has also considered the role of the stimulus barrier. He speaks of "constitutional variations in reac-

tivity . . . demonstrable in the first days of life . . . first manifested solely at the autonomic level" (p. 347). He comments
favorably on Gediman's suggestion that in the adult the stimulus barrier is a "complex ego function" evolving from these
rudimentary biological mechanisms.

In a few cases the stimulus barrier concept has been employed within a clinical framework—usually, by stretching it
beyond its limits. Thus Loeb (1976) speaks of "adolescents who
find it impossible to feel because of the strength of their stimulus barrier [and] who may use hallucinogenic drugs to enable
them to experience feelings" (p. 216f.). Such *descriptive* use of
the concept bypasses a vast array of issues such as object relations (internal and external), primitive defense mechanisms,
passivity/activity balance, etc., which might serve better to explain the clinical phenomena in question. Similarly, Fish (1963)
speaks of how the "increasing 'stimulus barrier' may be seen in
the infant's developing ability to tolerate fatigue and pro-
prioceptive stimuli without showing overflow excitation, and in
his developing ability to focus and maintain attention on specific aspects of the environment" (p. 268). Here the concept is
ballooned out to encompass a wide range of developing capacities that make it virtually coterminous with the early stages of
ego formation.

RECENT INFANT OBSERVATION STUDIES

The past two decades have witnessed an explosion of research
in early infant development.[1] These studies, sparked by Wolff's
(1966) demonstration that the neonate is highly responsive in
certain defined states of consciousness (particularly "alert inac-
tivity"), have greatly enlarged our understanding of the fore-
stages of infantile cognition and have, specifically, required extensive revision of views of the infant's perceptual capacities
and therefore of the concept of the stimulus barrier.

In her comprehensive review of current knowledge of fetal
development, Graves (1980) cites evidence that "avoidance-in-
hibitory reactions ontogenetically precede the approach-appe-

1. Much of this literature has been critically reviewed by Lichtenberg
(1981).

titive reactions toward stimulus and surpass the latter in effectiveness. . . . We may also view the early avoidance reactions as
neurobiological prototypes to later psychological stimulus barrier or protective shield. . . . It may well turn out that fetal and
neonatal protective barriers form . . . a continuity, but fail to
show a genetic correlation with later *psychological* barriers" (p.
253; my italics).

On the other hand, there is a growing body of data that
suggests, as Emde and Robinson (1979) put it, that "the newborn is active and seeks to optimize exposure to informative
aspects of his visual world" (p. 86). They cite Roffwarg et
al.'s (1966) suggestion that "the young organism [is] pro-
grammed not so much to shut out stimulation but to seek it
because it [is] needed for neural growth" (p. 78). Further, there
is evidence that the newborn infant has discriminatory capacity
in a variety of sensory modalities. Brazelton (1980) describes
how the newborn, like the fetus, responds to sound stimulation:
"when the same sound is presented repeatedly to the in utero
fetus [or to the neonate], he can gradually shut down on any
response; i.e., he behaves as if he does not hear the noise when
one judges this from changes in fetal heart rate. However, if
the sound is changed to a new pitch, he again attends to it,
showing an ability for sound discrimination" (p. 205).

Brazelton has, in fact, made major contributions to our growing awareness of the neonate's capacity to receive and regulate
sensorial experience. Not only is the "newborn equipped with
the capacity for processing complex visual stimulation," but his
"capacity to shut out repetitious disturbing visual stimuli pro-
tects him from having to respond. . . . Just as he is equipped
with the capacity to shut out certain stimuli, he demonstrates
the capacity to alert to . . . to follow . . . a stimulus which appeals to him. . . . In a noisy, overlighted nursery, the neonate
tends to shut down on his capacity to attend, but in a semi-
darkened room . . . [he] can be brought to respond to the
human face as well as to a red or shiny object" (p. 213f.).[2]

2. This last observation would seem to be consistent with that of Haith
(cited in Emde and Robinson, 1979) that the newborn engages in organized
visual scanning in darkness.

Brazelton's descriptions are so evocative, impressive, and germane that one feels obliged to quote *in extenso:*

As a newborn lies undressed and uncovered in the nursery, his color begins to change with mottled uneven acrocyanosis of his extremities as he attempts to control loss of body heat. He begins to shiver, then to cry and flail his limbs in jerky thrusting movements in an effort to raise his own temperature. In the face of such enormous demands, as one speaks gently and insistently into one ear, his movements become smoother, . . . his eyes move smoothly to the side from which the voice is coming. His head follows with a sudden smooth turn toward the voice, and he searches for the face of the speaker. He fixes on the eyes of the examiner and listens intently for several minutes. If the examiner moves his face slowly to the baby's midline and then across to the other side, the newborn will track him, his head and eyes smoothly turning in an 180° arc. This complex interaction of visual, auditory, and motor behavior to respond to a human stimulus is managed by the neonate despite the enormous physiological demands of being undressed and unrestrained in a cold, overstimulating nursery. If one ignores the importance of this capacity as he evaluates the neurological and physiological integrity of the neonate, he misses the implication of the powerful effect of the cortex on the autonomic and physiological systems in the neonatal period [p. 213].

One would also, it seems clear, miss the implication of the infant's responsiveness to—indeed, his hunger for—external stimulation.[3] It is only in pathological states, such as autism, that this receptivity is lost. As Kootz and Cohen (1981) point out, "The autistic child is constantly engaged in the rejection of sensory stimulation. . . . Autistic children may, in fact, be hyperreactive to external stimulation but limit their reaction by limiting sensory intake" (p. 698). (This formulation is, of course, consistent with Bergman and Escalona's previously cited ideas about "special sensitivities" and "lowered stimulus barrier" in the psychotic child.)

Similarly, Als et al. (1976) describe a group of underweight

---

3. For a discussion of ethological and neurophysiological bases of these observations, see Als (1983) and Als and Duffy (1980).

full-term neonates who show poor responsiveness and inability to "lock into" social stimuli, and who give the overall impression of stress when handled. Of such an infant they say, "One feels that he is overwhelmed by the environment . . . he wants to be left alone" (p. 599). These definably deviant infants show clear defects in their capacity to process stimulus input and appear to attempt to cope with this deficit with a massive reflex shutdown process; i.e., they appear to show the kind of global active stimulus barrier which Freud and Spitz postulated for the normal neonate.

In their overview of affective development in the first year of life, Shapiro and Stern (1980) consider the role of the stimulus barrier. Like the others cited, they challenge Freud's view of the infant as stimulus-avoider in the light of much recent evidence of his propensity to seek stimuli. They propose to reconcile the two views, however, by considering "the need to regulate both the amount and quality of stimulation of the infant within a range that is optimal to his given constitution . . . there appears to be a constitutional barrier to further [i.e., overwhelming] stimulation and a need for protection that is provided by the mothering individual" (p. 124). The stimulus-seeking behavior is, they suggest, in the service of object attachment, while stimulus-avoiding or modulating behaviors are seen as precursors both of defense and later individuation.

DISCUSSION

From this survey it becomes clear that, like many of his terms, Freud's concept of the protective shield suffers from a considerable measure of ambiguity. In his own work and that of his students and followers, the term (or its analogue, stimulus barrier) has come to have the following meanings:

1. An innate, passive, wall-like shield whose function is to maintain a minimal level of excitation by warding off or attenuating external stimuli ("threshold"), but which may be "penetrated" by stimuli of extreme intensity. This is essentially the classic view enunciated by Freud, predicated, as stated earlier, on the notion that external stimuli are noxious insofar as

they tend to raise the level of "excitation" beyond the fragile neonate's level of toleration. This passive shield is conceived of as nonselective; "penetration" induces a "traumatic" state of excessive and undischargeable tension. It is clear that, in the light of currently available observational data and current conceptions of central nervous system function, this view is untenable. It is tempting to correlate this notion of the universal and obligatory threshold with the well-established fact (Freedman, 1980) that myelinization of sensory tracts and nerve roots is rudimentary at birth and is not completed until 4 to 6 months of age. Unfortunately for this thesis, the normal neonate not only perceives but can discriminate among and respond to a variety of "external" stimuli to which he does not show catastrophic or "traumatic" reactions; indeed, he may, as both Emde and Brazelton point out, be soothed by them. "It would seem likely," Salem and Adams (1966) have stated, "that neuronal assemblies begin to function before the appearance of the first myelin" (p. 400).

2. An innate, active, protodefensive mechanism with the same essential aims. The same objections apply here as well. Although Brazelton and others have shown that the neonate can actively exclude (or, better, show avoidant responses to) certain kinds and intensities of stimulation, it is clear that a selective process operates, and that this protodefensive process, whether or not developmentally continuous with later psychological defenses, is not universal or categorical, is strongly correlated with state variables, and does not serve to keep "excitation" at minimal levels. Benjamin's idea of a two-phase mechanism in which a developing active barrier supersedes an innate passive one rests on the same apparently invalid assumptions. Benjamin places the onset of active shutting out of stimulation at 8 to 10 weeks—whereas both Emde et al. (1971) and Brazelton and his associates have demonstrated the existence of this capacity in the neonate. Thus the break between the "passive" and "active" barriers postulated by Benjamin appears to have been an artifact of his primary method of observation (EEG studies). Similarly, such recent studies of neonatal behavior cast doubt on Furst's (1978) view that the manifestations of

the stimulus barrier appear initially "at the autonomic level"; it is clear that the voluntary muscular system is actively involved as well.

3. An innate, selective, maturing screening mechanism that admits stimuli of certain types and intensities under certain conditions, but excludes others on the basis either of quantitative or qualitative considerations. This appears to be the conception most descriptively consonant with the current state of knowledge. Certain modalities of perception are clearly available to the neonate, deployed differentially according to state, intensity of stimulation, inherent appeal of the stimulus, tolerance or habituation processes, etc. Lack of response to stimulation cannot, therefore, always be understood as failure of the stimulus to "penetrate" the barrier, just as response should not be taken as evidence of "penetration."

Shapiro and Stern (1980) have, as noted, suggested that perceptual experiences most likely to yield active approach and following responses will be those that are most likely to promote object attachment. An alternative, or at least complementary view, however, and one favored by Brazelton (1982) and by Als and Duffy (1980), treats the brain and the mental apparatus as information-processing systems, and suggests an inherent tendency to seek and respond to stimuli that will activate and promote this function. In this view, infants from birth will seek out and respond to those stimuli which they can assimilate and to which they can accommodate, achieving ever higher levels of integration and control as they mature. Thus if one wishes to reify these patterns, the innate protective device of which Freud spoke is best seen, not as a shield or barrier, but as a screen, admitting those stimuli most consonant with adaptive needs and excluding those that overtax adaptive capacities. It is here that the universally recognized role of the mother as buffer and facilitator becomes crucial—not simply as a prosthetic substitute or replacement for a constitutionally inadequate or maturationally declining shield, but as a source of appropriate stimuli and of protection from inappropriate ones at each stage of the infant's development.

4. Finally, it has been suggested that the stimulus barrier is an evolving configuration of threshold and response patterns

that undergoes maturational and developmental progression and that manifests itself throughout life. With this definition one arrives at a totally different notion of what the concept refers to. As suggested earlier, it is difficult to see how this broad expansion of the term's referent aids in conceptual clarification. It subsumes, in addition to innate structures, a range of defensive attributes and action tendencies that are at a considerable remove from Freud's fundamental idea. It is a notion that may have clinical utility in personality assessment, but its heuristic status with respect to the study of development is, I believe, scant.

CONCLUSIONS

Freud's notion of the "protective shield against stimuli" was a characteristically brilliant effort to conceptualize the means available to the infant for maintaining homeostatic balance. It was, however, rooted in a functional theory of the brain and the nascent mental apparatus that is inconsistent with current knowledge and is, therefore, no longer tenable. It is a view that is also inconsistent with current ideas about the relationship between the infant and his object world. A revised formulation that sees the regulation of stimulus intake within the framework of object attachments and information-processing, structure-building concepts seems more heuristically valuable for current psychoanalytic developmental theory. The metaphor of a "stimulus screen" rather than of a "stimulus barrier" seems most appropriate to this viewpoint.

BIBLIOGRAPHY

ALS, H. (1983), Infant individuality. In *Frontiers of Infant Psychiatry*, ed. J. Call & E. Galenson. New York: Basic Books, pp. 342–353.
_____ & DUFFY, F. (1980), The behavior of the premature infant. In *Infant at Risk*, ed. T. B. Brazelton & B. M. Lester. New York: Elsevier (in press).
_____ TRONICK, E., ADAMSON, L., & BRAZELTON, T. B. (1976), The behavior of the full-term but underweight newborn infant. *Develpm. Med. & Child Neurol.* 18:590–602.
BENJAMIN, J. D. (1965), Developmental biology and psychoanalysis. In *Psychoanalysis and Current Biological Thought*, ed. N. Greenfield & W. Lewis. Madison: Univ. Wisconsin Press, pp. 57–80.

BERGMAN, P. & ESCALONA, S. K. (1949), Unusual sensitivities in very young children. *Psychoanal. Study of Child*, 3/4:333–352.

BRAZELTON, T. B. (1980), Neonatal assessment. In Greenspan and Pollock (1980), pp. 203–233.

——— (1982), Personal communication.

BRODY, S. & AXELRAD, S. (1960), Anxiety, socialization and ego formation in infancy. *Int. J. Psychoanal.*, 47:218–229.

COMPTON, A. (1972), A study of the psychoanalytic theory of anxiety. *J. Amer. Psychoanal. Assn.*, 20:3–44.

EMDE, R. N., HARMON, R. J., METCALF, D. R., KOENIG, K., & WAGONFELD, S. (1971), Stress and neonatal sleep. *Psychosom. Med.*, 33:491–498.

——— & ROBINSON, J. (1979), The first two months. In *Basic Handbook of Child Psychiatry*, ed. J. Noshpitz. New York: Basic Books, 1:72–105.

ESCALONA, S. K. (1963), Patterns of infantile experience and the developmental process. *Psychoanal. Study of Child*, 18:197–244.

——— (1968), *The Roots of Individuality*. Chicago: Aldine Press.

FISH, B. (1963), The maturation of arousal and attention in the first months of life. *J. Amer. Acad. Child Psychiat.*, 2:253–270.

FREEDMAN, D. A. (1980), The effect of sensory and other deficits in children on their experience of people. *J. Amer. Psychoanal. Assn.*, 29:831–868.

——— FOX-KOLENDA, B. J., & BROWN, S. L. (1970), A multihandicapped rubella baby. *J. Amer. Acad. Child Psychiat.*, 9:298–317.

FREUD, S. (1920), Beyond the pleasure principle. *S.E.*, 18:7–66.

——— (1925), A note upon the 'mystic writing pad.' *S.E.*, 19:227–234.

——— (1926), Inhibitions, symptoms and anxiety. *S.E.*, 20:87–178.

——— (1938), An outline of psycho-analysis. *S.E.*, 23:144–208.

FURST, S. S. (1978), The stimulus barrier and the pathogenicity of trauma. *Int. J. Psychoanal.*, 59:345–352.

GEDIMAN, H. K. (1971), The concept of stimulus barrier. *Int. J. Psychoanal.*, 52:243–257.

GRAVES, P. L. (1980), The functioning fetus. In Greenspan & Pollock (1980), pp. 235–256.

GREENSPAN, S. I. & POLLOCK, G. H., eds. (1980), *The Course of Life*, 1. Bethesda: N.I.M.H.

KOOTZ, J. P. & COHEN, D. J. (1981), Modulation of sensory intake in autistic children. *J. Amer. Acad. Child Psychiat.*, 20:692–701.

LICHTENBERG, J. D. (1981), Implications for psychoanalytic theory of research on the neonate. *Int. Rev. Psychoanal.*, 8:35–52.

LOEB, L. (1976), Intensity and stimulus barrier in adolescence. *Adol. Psychiat.*, 4:255–263.

MAHLER, M. S. (1958), Autism and symbiosis. *Int. J. Psychoanal.*, 39:77–83.

——— (1965), On early infantile psychosis. *J. Amer. Acad. Child Psychiat.*, 4:554–568.

——— & McDEVITT, J. B. (1980), The separation-individuation process and identity formation. In Greenspan & Pollock (1980), pp. 395–406.

MARTIN, R. (1968), The stimulus barrier and the autonomy of the ego. *Psychol. Rev.,* 75:478–493.

PANEL (1967), Development and metapsychology of the defense organization of the ego. R. S. Wallerstein, reporter. *J. Amer. Psychoanal. Assn.,* 15:130–149.

RAPAPORT, D. (1951), Toward a theory of thinking. In *Organization and Pathology of Thought.* New York: Columbia Univ. Press, pp. 689–730.

ROFFWARG, H., MUZIO, J., & DEMENT, W. (1966), Ontogenetic development of the human sleep-dream cycle. *Science,* 152:604–619.

SALEM, M. & ADAMS, R. (1966), New horizons in the neurology of childhood. *Perspectives in Biol. & Med.,* 9:385–419.

SHAPIRO, T. & STERN, D. (1980), Psychoanalytic perspectives on the first years of life. In Greenspan and Pollock (1980), pp. 113–128.

SHEVRIN, H. & TOUSSIENG, P. W. (1965), Vicissitudes of the need for tactile stimulation in instinctual development. *Psychoanal. Study of Child,* 20:310–339.

SPITZ, R. A. (1965), The primal cavity. *Psychoanal. Study Child,* 20:215–240.

———— (1961), Some early prototypes of ego defences. *J. Amer. Psychoanal. Assn.,* 9:626–651.

WOLFF, P. H. (1966), *The Causes, Controls and Organization of Behavior in the Neonate. Psychol. Issues,* monogr. 17. New York: Int. Univ. Press.

Acknowledgment. I wish to express my appreciation to the members of the Study Group on Infant Psychiatry of the New York Psychoanalytic Institute, chaired by Drs. E. Galenson and H. Roiphe, for stimulating the researches that generated this paper and for their thoughtful critical discussion.

Self-Preservation and the Care of the Self

Ego Instincts Reconsidered

E. J. KHANTZIAN, M.D. AND JOHN E. MACK, M.D.

WE NEED NOT LOOK BEYOND THE PAST TWO DECADES TO FIND ample evidence around us in society and our clinical work of threats to human survival and of self-destructiveness. Despite the fact that ego psychology and object relations theory have become part of the bedrock of psychoanalytic practice and theory, much of our understanding of survival and self-destructiveness continues to be influenced by Freud's early writings. The complex functions relating to self-preservation, self-protection, and survival are relatively neglected in contemporary psychoanalytic literature despite the special urgency of these matters for many of our patients. It is, in fact, surprising in view of the current interest of mental health workers in disadvantaged individuals and families, for whom survival issues including basic protection from real dangers are conspicuous, that so little attention has been given in psychoanalytic theory to the psychology of self-preservation.

The influence of the early psychoanalytic literature is evident in reductionistic formulations which consider such problems as accident proneness, violent or impulsive behavior, weight dis-

Dr. Khantzian is Associate Professor of Psychiatry, and Dr. Mack is Professor of Psychiatry, Harvard Medical School at The Cambridge Hospital; members of the Boston Psychoanalytic Society and Institute, Inc.

turbances, substance (drug and alcohol) abuse,[1] and other forms of self-neglect in terms of explicit pleasure-seeking and/or unconscious self-destructive motives. Such formulations fail to consider adequately how these problems are just as often a result of deficiencies or failure in ego functions that serve to warn, guide, and protect individuals from hazardous or dangerous involvements and behavior.

In this presentation we advance a point of view that places greater emphasis on structural and developmental factors to account for certain forms of human self-destructiveness. We describe a complex set of functions that we have designated as "self-care." We believe that failures and impairments in the development of these functions better explain a range of troubled human behaviors. Although denial, conscious and unconscious self-destructiveness, psychological surrender, and other determinants can explain some human self-destructive behavior and impulsivity, we have been equally impressed that the personality structure and character pathology of certain individuals leave them vulnerable and susceptible to various dangers that result in personal injury, ill-health, physical deterioration, and death. We believe such people are often not so much compelled or driven in their behavior as they are impaired or deficient in self-care functions that are otherwise present in the more mature ego. Exploring the components and elements of the functions that comprise self-care not only has heuristic value for a better theoretical understanding of human development and adaptation, but is equally important for understanding and managing destructive behavior in clinical work, particularly in the treatment of impulse and behavior problems.

Self-care as a developed system of functions includes the following elements:

1. A libidinal investment in caring about or valuing oneself—sufficient positive self-esteem to feel oneself to be worth protecting

---

1. While we first encountered deficiencies in self-care in drug and alcohol abuse (Khantzian, 1974; Wurmser, 1974), the interaction of genetic and psychological factors in these problems is so complex that they require separate treatment.

2. The capacity to anticipate danger situations and to respond to the cues which anxiety provides
3. The ability to control impulses and renounce pleasures whose consequences are harmful
4. Pleasure in mastering inevitable situations of risk, or in which dangers are appropriately measured
5. Knowledge about the outside world and oneself sufficient for survival in it
6. The ability to be sufficiently self-assertive or aggressive enough to protect oneself
7. Certain skills in object relationships, especially the ability to choose others who, ideally, will enhance one's protection, or at least will not jeopardize one's existence.

In this report "self," as used in "self-care" and "self-preservation," refers to the broader meaning of self pertaining to the entire person. Self-esteem and self-regard also are related to self-care. Unless otherwise specified, however, we are concerned primarily with understanding and explaining the structures and functions that serve the survival of the self or person as a total organism. We also distinguish self-care functions related to protection and survival from self-soothing. Self-soothing activities maintain subjective states of comfort and well-being and will be discussed only briefly.

BACKGROUND

Before he evolved his structural theory of the mind, Freud attempted to encompass what we would now consider fundamental functions of the ego within his theory of instincts. Self-preservation, self-care, self-protection, and the like were originally grouped together by Freud as self-preservative or ego instincts. He referred to these as "instincts which serve the preservation of the individual" as opposed to "those which serve the survival of the species" (1913, p. 182). When Freud elaborated his views on narcissism he regarded the ego instincts as the nonlibidinal aspect of narcissism. Ultimately, Freud rejected this distinction and viewed self-preservation as itself erotic in a narcissistic sense: "the instinct of self-preservation is certainly of an erotic kind, but it must nevertheless have an aggressiveness at its disposal if it is to fulfil its purpose" (1933b, p. 209). Thus we see Freud virtually to the end of his life seeking to conceptualize self-preservation within the framework of his instinct theory, even though in 1938 he finally said, "the ego . . . has the task of self-preservation" (p. 145).

Notwithstanding Freud's final admonition that self-preservation was a task for the ego, subsequent psychoanalytic investigators have continued to stress instinctual factors to account for much of human behavior that is dangerous to the self. Works by Menninger (1938) and Tabachnick (1976) are representative examples that illustrate this continuing trend. Menninger believed that Freud's hypothesis of a death instinct could best account for the varied and manifold forms of human self-destructiveness, such as asceticism, martyrdom, invalidism, alcohol addiction, antisocial behavior, and psychosis. He considered such problems as forms of "chronic suicide" and accounted for these tendencies by human aggression turned on the self. Tabachnick came to similar though not identical conclusions in his studies of automobile accidents. He distinguished two types of victims in his study, one group (20%) in which the victims were depressed, and another group (80%) in which the victims were action-oriented but not depressed. Although he identified different features and dynamics in these two groups, he concluded that a "death trend" was common to both groups as a result of tremendous rage and aggression turned on the self. Citing the work of Dunbar (1943) and Alexander (1949) who believe that action-oriented characters are involved in multiple accidents, Tabachnick suggests that a "death or self-punitive trend" might be involved in action orientation. However, Tabachnick concedes that the accident can be an unintended result of conflict in action-oriented characters. In our opinion, such formulations fail to consider sufficiently how the active pursuit of danger, bravado, fatalism, and action substitute for less well-developed, sustaining, stabilizing, and self-preservative functions. These compensatory character traits flourish in lieu of more stable self-care (ego) functions and processes that most often protect human beings from their own self-destructive inclinations.

The functions that are responsible for self-preservation,

standing in opposition to self-destruction, have been ascribed to the life or ego instincts, and more generally to the ego. Although an adaptational, ego-psychological view subsumes self-preservation in human existence, there is little in the psychoanalytic literature that specifically identifies or explains the functions and mechanisms that are involved in assuring human survival and self-care.

In concluding remarks in his classic work on the ego and adaptation, Hartmann (1939) observes that although "emphasis on the ego apparatuses may delineate more precisely our conception of the 'self-preservative' drives . . . we have so far treated [them] like a stepchild" (p. 107). His ideas about the role of the ego apparatus, the part it plays in general adaptation, and its specific role in survival remain central to our understanding of the capacity for self-care and self-protection. In a subsequent paper, Hartmann (1948) allows that both sexual and aggressive drives contribute to the development of psychic function and ultimately serve purposes of self-preservation. He also states that the reality, pleasure, and Nirvana principles and the repetition compulsion can under certain circumstances subserve self-protective functions. He concludes, "it is the functions of the ego, developed by learning and by maturation—the ego's aspect of regulating the relations with the environment and its organizing capacity in finding solutions, fitting the environmental situation and the psychic systems at the same time—which become of primary importance for self-preservation in man" (p. 84). It is surprising how little psychoanalysis has expanded upon or advanced Hartmann's thinking in delineating more specifically the component structures and functions that serve survival.

A review of the literature on self-preservation reveals that a number of psychoanalysts are aware of how little we know about its development and the importance of gaining a better understanding of this much neglected area of human adaptation. Glover (1933) appreciated how children early in their development both depended on external objects for self-preservation and also could experience real threat to their survival as a result of external dangers, injury, and aggression. Loewenstein (1940) stated bluntly, "the self-preservative instincts have

hitherto been greatly neglected" (p. 388). He felt that the so-
called self-preservative instincts were not instincts at all (especially not connected with the death instinct), but that they
must be seen in relation to the whole development of the ego.
In commenting on Loewenstein's work, Zetzel (1949) underscores the importance of the survival instincts and the role of
anxiety in relation to real external dangers. Rochlin (1965) indicates that "instincts of self-preservation" are present earlier
than has been supposed and that small children manifest early
concerns about death and self-preservation. Mahler (1968) observes, "the function of, and the equipment for, self-preservation is atrophied" in the human species (p. 9). Most modern-
day psychoanalysts would agree with this observation, but little
systematic attention has been given to how the "function of,
and equipment for, self-preservation" develops and operates to
protect the self from danger and harm. Recent theoretical and
clinical work focusing on child development, narcissistic disturbances, affects, impulsivity, and substance abuse has helped,
nevertheless, to illuminate how the capacity for self-preservation or self-care develops.

Winnicott (1953, 1960) and Mahler (1968) have stressed the
importance of the quality and quantity of nurturance and care
in the earliest phases of the mother-infant relationship. The
ways in which this maternal care is administered has important
implications for the development of self-care. The works of
Winnicott and Mahler share an emphasis on *optimal* nurturance
that avoids extremes of deprivation and indulgence and enhances the capacities of the ego to tolerate delay, frustration,
and distress. As a result of this process the parent's nurturing
and protective functions are incorporated into the child's ego
capacities in the service of maintaining adequate self-esteem,
ego defense mechanisms, and adaptation to reality. By implication the "good enough mothering" and care obtained from the
environment during preoedipal development contributes significantly to the individual's eventual capacity to take care of
himself or herself.

Through the analysis of narcissistic transferences, Kohut
(1971) reconstructed how failures in parental (particularly ma-

ternal) care leave certain individuals ill-equipped to maintain and regulate their self-regard and self-esteem because of impairments in ego-ideal formation. He stressed failure in maternal empathy and traumatic disappointments in idealized parental figures as central determinants in narcissistic disturbances. Among the consequences of such disturbances are: (1) the external living out of a search for omnipotent, idealized objects that are admired or admiring for achieving a sense of well-being; and (2) the failure to transform through minute internalizations in the preoedipal developmental period various functions of the parents that ultimately contribute to the ego apparatus of the individual. Kohut only touches on the implications for self-preservation of such internalization processes, indicating that the analyst might have to "alert the patient's ego . . . *in the interest of self-preservation*" to certain impending dangers (p. 158). His emphasis, however, on the deficits in self-esteem and on failures of internalization in the formation of psychic structure is quite germane to our concept of how the capacity for self-preservation and self-care is acquired from parental figures, particularly from those aspects of parental care that have provided protection and vigilance as the developing and growing child explores his or her environment.

The works of Tolpin (1971) and Sandler and Sandler (1978) are germane to the concept of self-care in that they consider the part early object relations play in the development of psychic structure. They provide a basis for considering what constitute the precursors and components of the capacity for self-care. Tolpin focuses on the part that transmuting internalizations play as a means through which the infant may develop protective, caring, and anxiety-signaling functions. Sandler and Sandler stress how wish-fulfilling relationships with early objects become the basis for incorporating a sense of well-being and safety.

These reports converge to indicate that the various functions required for self-protection and self-care have their origin in the child-caretaker relationship as well as in maturational processes of both drives and ego. For this reason they are best studied from a developmental perspective.

DEVELOPMENTAL PERSPECTIVE

Freud (1916–17) clearly appreciated children's initial ignorance of danger and the parents' role in helping them to acquire a capacity to avoid harm:

> It would have been a very good thing if they [children] had
> inherited more of such life-preserving instincts, for that would
> have greatly facilitated the task of watching over them to pre-
> vent their running into one danger after another. The fact is
> that children . . . behave fearlessly because they are ignorant
> of dangers. They will run along the brink of the water, climb
> on to the window-sill, play with sharp objects and with fire—in
> short, do everything that is bound to damage them and to
> worry those in charge of them. When in the end realistic anx-
> iety is awakened in them, that is wholly the result of education;
> for they cannot be allowed to make the instructive experience
> themselves [p. 408].

Anna Freud's (1965) description of the developmental line
from irresponsibility to responsibility in body management
comes close to some of the processes that concern us in relation
to self-care. She reminds us that the satisfaction of essential
physical needs, such as feeding and elimination, are only gradually taken on by the child. According to Anna Freud, the slow
assumption of responsibility for self-protection occurs in con-
secutive phases that involve (1) a shift in the expression of
aggression away from the body (e.g., biting and scratching)
toward the external world; (2) an increasing orientation in the
external world whereby cause and effect and the control of
dangerous wishes are understood; these ego functions together
with the narcissistic cathexis of the body "protect the child
against such external dangers as water, fire, heights." But, she
then observed, "there are many instances of children where—
owing to a deficiency in any one of these ego functions—this
advance is retarded so that they remain unusually vulnerable
and exposed if not protected by the adult world" (p. 77); (3) the
child's voluntary endorsement of rules of hygiene and physical
requirements—normally the latest acquisition.

Once established, superego functions naturally play a part
throughout one's life in protecting the self. In striving to do

"the right thing," "following the rules," and consistently obeying internalized parental admonitions and prohibitions, one is less likely to encounter danger or harm. Too severe or rigid superego representations seem at times paradoxically to inspire dangerous risk-taking, as if the child were trying to escape the hold of a restrictive conscience by seemingly heedless activity. However, self-protection or preservation which relies too heavily upon superego strictures is personally costly and likely to limit severely a variety of ego functions and satisfactions. The superego aspect of self-care needs to be distinguished from the complex combination of adaptive and self-caring ego activities which are the primary focus of this paper.

The capacity for self-care relates to the broader question of how infants and small children develop the capacity for self-regulation in general. Greenspan (1981) has identified three levels, or stages of learning, in the formation of psychic structures which subserve self-regulation. In the first stage learning is largely somatic or imitative, dependent on the global fulfillment of body needs by the caretaker. In the second or contingent stage, beginning at 6 to 8 months, affective exchanges with the object become more organized; although imitative modes may still predominate, internalization through identification with elements of the interaction with the parent occurs. In the third phase, beginning at 14 to 18 months, representational learning and more complex affect management and self-regulatory behavior takes place.

Sifneos et al. (1977) hypothesize that psychosomatic disorders are related to developmental failures in self-regulation. It is possible that the inability of such patients to recognize and verbalize their feelings grows out of failures of self-regulation in the somatic or preverbal period. Along these lines, Krystal and Raskin (1970) and Krystal (1977) have identified developmental disturbances and traumatic regressed states in substance abusers, concentration camp survivors, and sufferers from psychosomatic illness that we believe are related to self-care disturbances. Such individuals are unable to identify or verbalize their feelings and use them as guiding signals. Similarly, they also suffer because of impairments in self-comfort, self-soothing, and ultimately self-care. Because of difficulties in including these basic life-maintaining and affective functions in their self-representation, they turn outside themselves for care and self-governance.

The complex functions of self-care and self-protection which we are considering take shape largely during the period of representational learning. Precursors of these functions begin to develop during the somatic and contingent stages. It is possible that older children and adults, who have a good capacity for self-soothing or self-nurturing but poor ability for self-protection, may have identified strongly with nurturant qualities of caretakers during the somatic and contingent periods, while failing later to internalize the more complex representations out of which caretaking and self-protection are structured.

Mahler's (1968) observation of toddlers are consistent with those of Anna Freud and highlight the early appearance of such vulnerability in certain children. Using the case of Jay, Mahler explores how the mother's failures in attending and remaining vigilant as the toddler physically separates from her and explores his environment result in the child's becoming oblivious to dangerous situations. Mahler describes Jay's inability to exercise restraint of his impulses and a recurrent tendency to invite danger as a result of disorientation in space, lags in reality testing, and a tendency to overlook obstacles in his path. Mahler traces some of the origins of Jay's incautious behavior to his mother who maintains a troublesome and bizarre distance and fails to protect Jay's body as he carelessly moves about. Jay obviously was precocious in his locomotor development and was therefore in even greater need of a mother functioning as an auxiliary ego to anticipate and protect him from harm.

One of us (E.J.K.) had the unfortunate opportunity to witness a case in which a similar combination of a child's advanced motor skills and aggressive exploratory behavior and the parents' lack of vigilance led to the child's death. Bill, an 18-month-old, very active, likable, black child, was the son of a patient participating in a methadone maintenance program. He frequently attended his father's group therapy sessions because the baby's mother worked at a full-time position as a secretary. The parents were an attractive couple who cared deeply about each other, but the father's long-standing addiction to opiates left him discouraged and brooding and his wife depleted.

During the father's group sessions Bill would actively bolt around the large conference room in which the meetings were held. He was noted to pick up anything on the floor that appeared "mouthable," whether edible or otherwise, and put it in his mouth. He frequently stumbled, banging various parts of his body, usually his head. He seemed to sustain his bumps and bruises with impunity, cried rarely, and often appeared to be amused by the looks of shock and startle of the adults in the room. Unfortunately, his father usually was not one of those who was alarmed by and concerned about Bill's behavior and injuries.

Around 10 o'clock one morning Bill was discovered to be cyanotic and apneic in his crib. He was rushed to the hospital and placed on artificial life-support systems. He succumbed 10 days later. Subsequent to his admission the staff reconstructed that the child had gone to the refrigerator the previous evening and had drunk a mixture of fruit juice and methadone belonging to his father. Because of the gradual onset of action, Bill had played normally for a while and had then been put to bed by his mother. Unfortunately, neither parent realized that the child had ingested what for him was a lethal dose of narcotics.

In view of the many real dangers in the environment, it is a wonder that children do not more often suffer serious injury and death. That most children escape serious harm suggests how well most parents take care of them, as a result of which they may rather early acquire a capacity to anticipate and avoid danger. The works of Stechler and Kaplan (1980) and Virginia Demos (personal communication to John E. Mack) suggest that, beginning in infancy, a subtle balance exists between the parents' permission for the child to take initiative, to risk and explore, and the parents' protective function, which keeps the risks within reasonable bounds or creates for the child a self-protective representation.

Using video tapes, Demos has documented a range of responses of mothers to the exploratory initiatives of their children. Some mothers allow a rich exploration of the environment up to the point of danger and then set appropriate limits in a finely tuned pattern of interactions. Others show little interest in the child's undertaking and interact only minimally with the child. Gradually, through reciprocal interactions between the small child and his caretakers in the context of explorations of the outside world, the child acquires mental representations of danger, the capacity to anticipate harm, and the ability to renounce unduly risky sorts of gratification.

The acquisition of the capacity for self-care is promoted by intricate, often subtle, reciprocal communications between a child and his parents. For example, at the age of 22 months, Chris appeared to all who encountered him as a rather reckless, wild boy. He would carom from one piece of furniture and one person to another, sometimes glancing up at his mother with devilish glee before heading off on a new, cyclonelike path. Taking a certain delight in the child's rambunctious, explorative nature, the mother would tolerate a great deal of such activity, but as tensions would mount, she would after awhile "just blow." When he reached the limits of her tolerance, or was in any danger of hurting himself or destroying property, she would make clear in unequivocal terms that "that was it." He was to stop and to go no further. In fact, Chris developed an interest in rock climbing and went on expeditions in which a group would scale precipitous cliffs. His father, a circumspect and thoughtful man, worried about these ventures. He did not stop Chris, but he insisted that there be adequate adult supervision, that Chris learn everything he could about mountain climbing, and that he use proper equipment at all times.

Chris's parents did not simply put a stop to his behavior or demand that he control his impulses. Each parent in her or his way took pleasure in the child's motor skills, his explorations of the world around him, and his mastery of new challenges. They clearly valued him *and* his efforts at self-development. But, recognizing the danger involved, they set clear limits, thereby conveying the message: we love you and deeply respect that you wish to express yourself and your aliveness and to learn about the world. But we want to protect you, and we do not want you to be hurt or to damage anything else. So we will limit the risks that you will be allowed to take. We wish to get across to you that we love and value you enough to protect you, that you are a being worth protecting.

There is clear evidence that Chris incorporated these messages, which became part of his self representation and ego functioning. He learned to master, first as a 2-year-old, and later in childhood and adolescence, the challenges he undertook. Chris was a boy who from early on liked to "do it my way." The thrust toward mastery, from which he derived satisfaction and considerable self-esteem enhancement, characterized Chris's functioning. Although he clearly was overcoming fears in relation to danger, his activities were not primarily defensive in their function.

We can see in Chris's case, and that of many children like him, that the function of self-care is intimately related to the development of self-esteem. The capacity for self-care grows in the context of a loving parent's communication that he or she values the child and therefore considers the child *worth taking care of*. The child incorporates this message and comes to value himself enough to protect himself from injury. A complex of functions—expressing pleasure in motor exploration, anticipating danger, setting limits upon oneself when danger is discerned, postponing or modifying the activity to make it safer and more secure—all these depend on valuing oneself enough to invest in self-caring. Small children and adolescents who, in contrast to Chris, take excessive risks and engage in dangerous rebellious behavior show an absence of self-care functioning. Such behavior may be indicative of pseudomastery. Exaggerated risk-taking is accompanied by denial of fear, which is not mastered. In such instances the self as subject undervalues the self as object and permits undue risks to be taken. True mastery is associated, as in Chris's case, with relatively little self-destructive risk.

A distinction should also be made between self-care, in the sense of taking care of, looking after, or protecting oneself, and self-comforting or nurturing.[2] Many individuals are quite capable of soothing themselves, being "good" to themselves with food, alcohol, music, or even hypochondriacal behavior. Such individuals may readily stay home from work with minor illnesses or make frequent trips to the doctor. But self-comforting activity of this sort may not be associated with a genuine

2. Personal communication from Dr. Henry Krystal.

capacity to look after oneself realistically or to guard against excessive risks and dangers.

Yet, even if a reasonably good capacity for self-care has been acquired, it is, like other ego capacities and functions, subject to erosion and regression, as the following case demonstrates. Walter was a 12-year-old black boy, who, by his own admission, was ordinarily conscientious and always tried to do what his parents wished. He had been admitted to the hospital after accidently burning his legs while starting a power lawnmower. He described in some detail how he usually would carefully wipe off any residual gasoline and then pull the starter rope to the motor. On this occasion he somehow had neglected to do this. When he started the motor, it suddenly burst into flames. During his hospitalization the psychiatric liaison service was asked to see him because of his excitability and exaggerated sensitivity to pain. The two psychiatrists who saw him learned that there were two small children at home, a sister, aged 2, and a baby brother, a few months old. With a mixture of pride and irritation, Walter described how his parents looked to him as a big brother for assistance in taking care of his younger siblings. He also indicated that he had had his own room until he had been displaced from it by his baby brother. In the course of the evaluation Walter revealed that his usual attentiveness and caution with the mower had not been present because of anger, irritation, and preoccupation with his changed status in the family.

While in this case the boy's immaturity in combination with specific conflicts and stresses led to what one hopes was a temporary lapse in self-protection, there are other cases in which the capacity for self-care develops unevenly. A 28-year-old single, professional woman in analysis functioned in a highly capable fashion, handling the stressful, at times physically threatening, requirements of her job with unusual intelligence and skill. Working in a field close to that of her highly competent father, she could "look after" herself most effectively. Since age 4 she had suffered from moderately severe attacks of asthma, which continued in her adult life. Her view of her capacity to handle the illness was unrealistic, and as a result she sometimes used poor judgment. On several occasions during the analysis she had permitted asthma attacks, for which there was a clearly effective medical regimen, to reach the point where breathing was severely compromised and her life threatened. The asthma had been heralded in childhood by a severe attack which brought the patient to the point of coma before its nature was discovered in the hospital. The asthma became the arena in which an anxious struggle occurred between the patient and her mother. Constantly fearful for her daughter's safety, the mother held her in an intimate bond, anxiously protecting her and conveying the message that true autonomy was threatening to the *mother's* survival. The patient failed to develop independent skills in self-care in relation to her health, relying on others to rescue her when asthmatic attacks reached crisis proportions. Sometimes she wistfully communicated to her analyst her longing for a "self-management company." The patient's parents also had failed to protect her as a small child from the violent assaults of her troubled older brother. As a consequence she was drawn to the religiously observing Roman Catholic family next door, who, in their elaborate system of rituals directed by an all-powerful God, seemed to have a way of providing protection from harm for small children.

Specific fantasies, growing out of disturbances in narcissistic development, may interfere with self-protection and self-care. Most important of these are wish-laden, grandiose ideas of protection that interfere with the capacity to guard oneself from danger. There may be the idea, for example, that no harm can befall one, that no matter what risks are taken, a powerful being will look after, protect, or come to the rescue. Often this fantasy is acted out dangerously in trying to rescue others. In these instances the "rescuee" represents the endangered self of the rescuer. The vulnerability and absence of self-care become manifest in the consequences which befall the rescuer, often at the hands of the rescuee, in the course of misguided though "well-meaning" rescue operations.

The study of children who are accident prone, injure themselves, and become involved in dangerous activities offers an opportunity to understand some of the predispositions and vulnerabilities which result in impairments in self-care. Such vulnerabilities in children also allow for comparisons with children, such as Chris, who are not so inclined and enable us to consider what forces compel accidents and self-injury. But even more important, they provide an opportunity to consider the psychological structures and functions that ordinarily stand in opposition to or protect against danger and harm. Several reports (Frankl, 1963, 1965; Lewis et al., 1966; Malone et al., 1967) provide vivid examples and vignettes of children and adolescents who suffer injuries and accidents. Although these reports shed light on important determinants that compel the dangerous activities and behavior of certain individuals, they consider only in passing, if at all, the factors that more usually protect against injury and accidents. As in the case of the adult literature on accident proneness, these reports tend to place undue emphasis on drive theory and aggressive instincts, to the exclusion of other considerations (e.g., structural and maturational deficiencies), in accounting for self-injuries and destructive behavior.

Reviewing problems of self-preservation and accident proneness from a developmental perspective, Frankl (1963) presents many compelling accounts of accidents and injuries sustained by normal and disturbed children and adolescents. She seems to appreciate that among healthy children the caring and protective functions of the parents (or substitutes) are gradually taken over by the child in the course of normal development. The failure to take over these functions leaves the children more susceptible to harm and is the result of deprivation of object love and a lack of cathexis of the child's body. However, in her subsequent discussion and formulations, she repeatedly attributes accidents in childhood and adolescence to conflicts relating to impulsivity, superego representations, and (unfused or defused) aggressive instincts turned on the self. Her observations are graphic and clear, but suggest alternative mechanisms and interpretations. She presents, for example, the case of Eric, who was 14 years old when he put his eye out with a dart by pulling on a string that he had attached to the dart as a means of retrieving it (p. 477f.). Frankl interprets this unfortunate accident as the result of the boy's turning aggressive feelings against himself. She supports this interpretation with Eric's own admission that the self-injury was a form of attack on the parents aimed at disappointing and hurting them and making the prospects of success in school less likely. Most striking in Eric's case and Frankl's other cases is the absence of elements of caution, worry, anticipation, or other self-protective measures.

In a study exploring the determining factors involved in accidental ingestion of poisons by children, Lewis et al. (1966) carefully evaluated developmental factors and family influences in 14 children (7 boys and 7 girls ranging in age from 14 to 43 months). These children were compared with a control group, for whom it was assumed that the availability of poison and the child's ability to explore the environment were the same. The most important factors in the accidental ingestion were developmental characteristics (e.g., motor skills, exploratory and imitative behavior, degree of negativism) in the child and the quality of the mother-child relationship at the time of the accident. The latter in particular involved the way the mother organized the family environment, which in this study appeared to have been seriously disrupted within a year before the poisoning event in the majority of the cases. Two factors loomed large as disorganizing influences on the families of the children: (1) a recent birth or death of a sibling; and (2) a loss of adult support for the mother. In this study, spatial or physical elements in the environment invited an accidental ingestion by children who displayed high exploratory activity, superior motor skills, but poor impulse control. These factors combined with a "maternal depletion" that was present in all the cases in which the ingestions occurred. The depletion state consisted of a relative exhaustion of the mother's psychic or emotional resources as a result of inadequate support or a sudden decrease in assistance from other adults upon whom she depended, most usually the husband or the mother's mother.

Lewis et al.'s (1966) observations and conclusion underscore the importance of the mother's caring and protective functions in preventing dangerous behavior in children. Their work has implications for understanding how lapses in the early mother-child relationship and maturational lapses contribute to later vulnerabilities in self-care. The authors suggest that most children do not ingest poison because in the usual closeness of the mother-child relationship the child senses and anticipates the mother's disapproval of a dangerous act and responds to her guidance to avoid danger. In contrast, when the mother suffers from depletion states as a result of loss or stress, she is less attuned to the child and the positive bond of care and mutual attachment is disrupted. The child is then guided more by the wish to satisfy his own explorative curiosity and/or negativistic pleasure rather than the pleasure of pleasing mother. The authors stress that the timing for the establishment of such functions as motor skills, impulse delay, anticipation, and reality sense, all of which require some degree of inner guidance, varies from child to child. We would add that the establishment of these and related functions early in life is crucial for assuring ego capacities for self-preservation and self-care later on.

Studies of children from extremely disrupted environments, such as urban slums or poorly run orphanages, provide dramatic evidence of how experiences from such backgrounds can seriously warp, distort, and impair survival skills at an early age. Using a nursery school as a socializing and therapeutic setting, Malone et al. (1967) observed the disabilities of a group of children who came from disorganized lower-class families in an urban slum of Boston. In particular, their findings about the children's motor activities and appearance vividly demonstrate what we have referred to as impairments and deficits in self-care. The children "seemed to lack any self-protective measures, being careless with the use of their bodies and seemingly not trying to prevent injuries . . . [and] accidents and injuries were usually not accompanied by expressions of appropriate affect" (p. 57). A general lack of body care, heedlessness, and absence of caution were evident as they "carelessly careened around the room stumbling and bumping into things, tipping over chairs or toys and falling off the climber, slide or wings" (p. 140). The authors stress that such behavior was even more significant in view of these children's otherwise good to advanced motor skills (p. 140f.). Malone et al. poignantly describe how the teachers actively had to intercede and substitute their own protectiveness and caution to avoid injury. But through repeated intervention, instruction, and growing attachment to the teachers, the children seemed to exercise growing caution and to learn to request assistance. Strikingly, the authors also observed reversion and regression to incautious behavior as a consequence of parental separation, harsh punishments, or parental criticism.

Frankl (1963) describes similar findings in children from residential nurseries who had suffered discontinuities in early mothering and subsequent relative deprivation of object love and unsatisfactory care. She indicates that there was a much higher incidence of accidents in children who received unsatisfactory residential care. She contrasts these with children raised in nurseries where they felt greatly valued and appreciated by the staff and where accidents were unheard of or could not be recollected. Frankl invokes the mechanism of aggression turned on the self to explain the injuries sustained by the children who suffered discontinuities in object love and care.

Those who try to explain the behavior of children from extreme environments often fail to distinguish between self-neglect and self-hatred. In fact, Anna Freud (1965) makes this distinction when she differentiates maturational defects from "turning aggression on the self" (p. 76), the latter being a defense mechanism adopted by the ego in conflict situations. Although aggression may play a part in self-destructiveness and accidents in children, we believe that there is more involved than aggression turned on the self or a self-punishment motive. It is likely that aggression in these cases brings about ego disorganization, which in turn causes the individual to become less able to exercise the judgment, control, synthesis, reality testing, and related functions that otherwise assure adequate self-care and protection.

We conclude this section by presenting an example of normal children at play in whom elements of self-care were evident at a relatively early age. The play situation provided a glimpse of one child's appropriate fearfulness and inhibition of impulsive action in the face of what surely constitutes a most common challenge to self-protective aims. Three children aged 6, 9, and 10 were happily running around in a backyard. The two older children decided to climb a tree in which there was a makeshift platform-treehouse about 12 feet high. They appeared to do this with skill and ease. A noticeable change in the lighthearted tone of the play could be observed at the point when the older boys began to challenge the younger boy on the ground below to join them. As the boys' challenges escalated to taunts and teasing, the younger boy at first became unhappy and tense, then more obviously fearful, and began to cry. Despite the two boys' continued derision, the younger boy refused to join them. Notwithstanding the obvious intense pressure of his playmates and his own shame about his inability to keep up with them, he seemed to respond more to his own fear and apparent awareness that he did not possess his playmates' strength, coordination, and skill to climb the tree.

Our observations of this realistically fearful boy, as well as the cases we cited where such fear was absent, indicate that the functions for self-care and self-protection begin to develop early in life and may operate (or be deficient) in young children. The capacity for self-care is complex and involves multiple affective and cognitive processes, component functions, mechanisms of defense, ego functions such as signal anxiety, reality testing, judgment, control, delay, and synthesis, as well as relatively stable superego functions. Cognitively, self-care involves a capacity to perceive, realistically assess, integrate, and attend to relevant cues in the environment. Affects are used as a guide for appropriate action, or as signals to institute defense mechanisms or avoid potentially harmful or dangerous situations. Gradually, in the context of experienced parental protectiveness, the child assumes the process of self-protection and care and incorporates those family and societal rules which help to insure his safety. When present, these functions operate automatically or deliberately to guide us away from danger or, once in trouble, to guide us out of difficulty. It is the collective action and interaction of these cognitive and affective processes that we refer to as the ego function or capacity for self-care.

Self-care functions become internalized through the ministrations of the caring and protection of parents. In the earliest phases of development self-care begins with incorporative processes in which the nurturing role of the mother contributes to a rudimentary sense of harmony and security (Meissner, 1979). In subsequent periods internalization of the caring and protective qualities of the parents occurs as the child, under their watchful eyes, encounters and explores the environment. If the parents' attendance to and care of the child are good, the developing child acquires a capacity to care for himself or herself and to protect against and anticipate harm and danger.

CONCLUSIONS

We have reviewed a number of reports that document and ' interpret a range of human problems involving self-injury and harm, including impulsivity and accidents in children. Most of these accounts lay heavy emphasis on drive theory and a motivational psychology that places aggressive drives at the heart of most forms of human self-destructiveness. In this presentation we have considered the functions which ordinarily stand in opposition to these destructive trends and how normal self-care and self-protection develop.

As with most human functions and reactions, problems of survival and self-destructiveness are multiply determined. Much of human destructiveness, including the self-directed form, may of course be compelled, defensive, or specifically motivated. In seeking to identify and understand impairments in survival skills and self-care, we have stressed a developmental perspective focused upon how early nurturing attitudes and the caring and protective functions of parents, particularly the mother, are internalized and transformed into positive attitudes of self-regard and adequate structures and functions assuring self-care and self-protection.

We have shown that self-care capacities are closely associated with positive self-esteem, for the developing child must internalize the conviction that he is a being of value, that he is worth protecting, before he can care for himself. We have noted the dysjunction which sometimes occurs between self-soothing or self-nurturing and the full capacity for self-protection or self-care, suggesting that the former function may grow out of earlier more somatically based experience, while the latter depends on more highly structured representational learning.

This report can only be considered preliminary in attempting to explain the complex relationships between self-regard, self-care, and human self-destructiveness. Although self-care functions are fundamental for survival, they build upon an earlier sense of well-being and harmony within the self. It is most likely from such early subjective states that we derive a sense of optimism and "aliveness." When this rudimentary sense is lacking or violated, despair and feelings of "deadness" may later result (Kohut and Wolf, 1978; Friedman, 1980).

In the developmental model we have presented, self-preservation is contingent upon the establishment of particular structures and ego functions. Furthermore, self-destructiveness results as much from lapses and failures in self-care and protective functions as it is specifically motivated, overdetermined, or driven. Further reports and explorations in this area must ultimately consider self-care functions in dynamic interaction with other operative factors. We have only touched, for example, upon how basic attitudes about the self, starting with beginning self-awareness and self-experiences, are crucial for making one feel that the self, and ultimately existence, is worth preserving. We need to understand further how early failures in the development of a cohesive sense of self and the resultant search for self-comfort and self-worth become so overriding, that matters of self-care and survival often remain tragically subordinate, secondary, and underdeveloped. We also need to consider how anger, rage, depression, aggression, or other affect states erode or interfere with established self-care functions. We need to explore especially how conditions of depletion, anergia, and inertia associated with intense affective states may cause a lapse or regression in self-care. Further study is needed, for example, of the extent to which self-care functions become relatively immutable and autonomous once established or, in contrast, may under particular circumstances that burden or threaten the ego become temporarily or permanently lost.

BIBLIOGRAPHY

ALEXANDER, F. (1949), The accident prone individual. *Pub. Health Rep.*, 64:357–361.

DUNBAR, F. (1943), *Psychosomatic Diagnosis*. New York: Hoeber.

FRANKL, L. (1963), Self-preservation and the development of accident proneness in children and adolescents. *Psychoanal. Study Child*, 18:464–483.

———— (1965), Susceptibility to accidents. *Br. J. Med. Psychol.*, 38:289–297.

FREUD, A. (1949), Aggression in relation to emotional development. *Psychoanal. Study Child,* 3/4:37–42.

―――― (1965), Normality and pathology in childhood. *W.* 6.

FREUD, S. (1913), The claims of psycho-analysis to scientific interest. *S.E.,* 13:165–190.

―――― (1916–17), Introductory lectures on psycho-analysis. *S.E.,* 16:243–463.

―――― (1933a), New introductory lectures on psycho-analysis. *S.E.,* 22:5–182.

―――― (1933b), Why war? *S.E.,* 22:197–215.

FRIEDMAN, L. (1980), Kohut: a book review essay. *Psychoanal. Q.,* 49:393–422.

GLOVER, E. (1933), The relation of perversion-formation to the development of reality sense. *Int. J. Psychoanal.,* 14:486–504.

GREENSPAN, S. I. (1979), *Intelligence and Adaptation.* New York: Int. Univ. Press.

HARTMANN, H. (1939), *Ego Psychology and the Problem of Adaptation.* New York: Int. Univ. Press, 1958.

―――― (1948), Comments on the psychoanalytic theory of instinctual drives. In *Essays on Ego Psychology.* New York: Int. Univ. Press, 1964, pp. 69–89.

KHANTZIAN, E. J. (1974), Opiate addiction. *Amer. J. Psychother.,* 28:59–70.

―――― (1978), The ego, the self and opiate addiction. *Int. Rev. Psychoanal.,* 5:189–198.

KOHUT, H. (1971), *The Analysis of the Self.* New York: Int. Univ. Press.

―――― & WOLF, E. S. (1978), The disorders of the self and their treatment. *Int. J. Psychoanal.,* 59:413–425.

KRYSTAL, H. (1977), Self representation and the capacity for self care. *Annu. Psychoanal.* 6:209–246.

―――― & RASKIN, H. A. (1970), *Drug Dependence.* Detroit: Wayne State Univ. Press.

LEWIS, M., SOLNIT, A. J., STARK, M. H., GABRIELSON, I. W., & KLATSKIN, E. H. (1966), An exploration study of accidental ingestion of poison in young children. *J. Amer. Acad. Child Psychiat.,* 5:255–271.

LOEWENSTEIN, R. M. (1949), The vital or somatic instincts. *Int. J. Psychoanal.,* 21:377–400.

MAHLER, M. S. (1968), *On Human Symbiosis and the Vicissitudes of Individuation.* New York: Int. Univ. Press.

MALONE, C. A., PAVENSTEDT, E., MATTICK, I., BANDLER, L. S., STEIN, M. R., & MINTZ, N. (1967), *The Drifters,* ed. E. Pavenstedt. Boston: Little, Brown.

MEISSNER, W. W. (1979), Internalization and object relations. *J. Amer. Psychoanal. Assn.,* 27:345–360.

MENNINGER, K. A. (1938), *Man Against Himself.* New York: Harcourt, Brace.

ROCHLIN, G. (1965), *Griefs and Discontents.* Boston: Little, Brown.

SANDLER, J. & SANDLER, A.-M. (1978), On the development of object relationships and affects. *Int. J. Psychoanal.,* 59:285–296.

SIFNEOS, P., APFEL-SAVITZ, R., & FRANKL, F. (1977), The phenomenon of 'alexethymia.' *Psychother. Psychosom.,* 28:47–57.

STECHLER, G. & KAPLAN, S. (1980), The development of the self. *Psychoanal. Study Child*, 35:85–105.

TABACHNICK, N. (1976), Death trend and adaptation. *J. Amer. Acad. Psychoanal.*, 41:49–62.

TOLPIN, M. (1971), On the beginnings of a cohesive self. *Psychoanal. Study Child*, 26:316–352.

WINNICOTT, D. W. (1953), Transitional objects and transitional phenomena. *Int. J. Psychoanal.*, 34:89–97.

———— (1960), Ego distortions in terms of true and false self. In *The Maturational Processes and the Facilitating Environment*. New York: Int. Univ. Press, 1965, pp. 140–152.

WURMSER, L. (1974), Psychoanalytic consideration of the etiology of compulsive drug use. *J. Amer. Psychoanal. Assn.*, 22:820–843.

ZETZEL, E. R. (1949), Anxiety and the capacity to bear it. *Int. J. Psychoanal.*, 30:1–12.

Struggling against Deprivation and Trauma

A Longitudinal Case Study

SALLY PROVENCE, M.D.

OVER A PERIOD OF SEVERAL YEARS, MARIANNE KRIS AND I
spent many hours discussing this case and preparing it for possible publication. From that document which covered the first 3
years of a child's life, this report of the first 15 months has been
condensed for presentation. The ideas presented reflect Marianne Kris's thinking as much as my own. The story of Anne, a
normal infant at birth, is one of an infant struggling against
deprivation and trauma resulting principally from problems in
the mother-child relationship. This is the same child about
whom Ernst Kris wrote the paper, unfinished at his death and
later published under the title, "Decline and Recovery in the
Life of a Three-Year-Old" (1962). In several other papers, too,
aspects of the development of this child have been described
(Coleman et al., 1953; Provence, 1965). Anne educated the
Yale Child Study Center research group in memorable ways:
she and her mother captured our sympathy, challenged and in
some respects frustrated us as clinicians, and presented us with
issues and opportunities for thinking, speculating, and examining psychoanalytic propositions which have had an enduring
influence.

Professor of Pediatrics, Child Study Center, Yale University, New Haven,
Ct.; faculty, Western New England Institute for Psychoanalysis.
Presented as the First Annual Marianne Kris Memorial Lecture at the
meeting of the Association for Child Psychoanalysis, Denver, Colorado,
March 21, 1982.

This presentation is intended to illustrate with data from the first 15 months of Anne's life: (1) how observations of infant behavior and the dyadic interaction can be used to examine propositions of psychoanalytic developmental psychology and stimulate refinement of theory; (2) the rich opportunity provided by service-centered investigations and the participation of a multidisciplinary group of investigators in advancing understanding in child development; (3) most of all it is intended to convey something of Marianne Kris's intense interest in the preverbal period of childhood and her reactions to the data of this case.

CASE REPORT

Anne and her parents were part of a study in which parents having their first child were offered pediatric care, social work services, and, when children reached age 2, attendance in our nursery school in exchange for their participation.[1] It was Ernst Kris's view that a service-centered approach offered unique opportunities for gathering data, which could be looked at within the broad framework of psychoanalysis. The investigators were experienced clinicians in pediatrics, social work, early childhood education, psychology, and psychoanalysis. For each family there was a team of service providers augmented by observers who were not involved directly with the families. The frequent, regularly scheduled contacts and those stimulated by the needs of the family generated a very large amount of data on each child. That the report of this case reflects some of the interests and preoccupations of the Yale group will be apparent, but it was also expected that the issues and concerns presented by Anne would be of interest to all child analysts and to other early childhood specialists.

As a newborn, Anne A. was described by the observers as an unusually pretty and well-formed infant who ate and slept well and was normal in every way. She was responsive in all sensory modalities and was especially alert visually. A moderately active infant who nestled easily into the arms of the adult, she was

1. For a more detailed description of this study, see Ritvo et al. (1963).

promptly quieted when restless by being held and cuddled. Neuromotor behavior was slightly immature as judged by the type and organization of movements, but there were no abnormal findings. She responded with expectably increased activity when stimulated from without and when uncomfortable for any reason. It may have been partly due to Anne's being such an attractive, ideal baby girl that it took so long to realize the depth of her mother's disappointment and the deficits in the mothering. There were several clues which we registered but largely disregarded at first: in the lying-in period, Mrs. A., who had earlier verbalized her wish for a boy, denied disappointment in the birth of a girl, but her criticisms were significant. She had a small perineal tear, and complained "the baby tore me apart." This was the first of many comments over the next 2 years in which she characterized the infant as aggressive and damaging to her, and this statement anticipated the battle ahead. On the first day she found the baby beautiful but by the second day began to refer to her as unattractive and seemed jealous that her husband considered the baby beautiful. She had expressed a wish to breast-feed, but by the third day it was apparent that this involved too great a conflict for her, and she gratefully accepted the pediatrician's suggestion that she shift to bottle feeding. She was convinced that she could not manage breast feeding when she went home; she also said that she was afraid that her large breasts would smother the baby. Mother and baby went from the hospital to the home of Mrs. A.'s brother out of town where they remained for 3 weeks during which time things went well. This was the first of several periods over the years when the beneficial influence of Mrs. A.'s sister-in-law upon her capacity to function in the maternal role was apparent. Mother and child returned home when Anne was 30 days of age. The pediatrician on a routine home visit at that time found the infant in good condition and Mrs. A. managing reasonably well except that she found the night feedings very trying. Anne's father seemed especially adoring of her. We were to learn much later that when he took care of her, which was unfortunately rare during the first year, he was more nurturing than the mother and unambivalent in his love for her.

The first visit to our center for a well-baby examination oc-

curred when Anne was 2 months of age. Mr. and Mrs. A. had
been on vacation for one week, leaving Anne with the sister-in-
law mentioned above. Mrs. A. expressed surprise that she
missed the baby, though she had enjoyed the vacation. Our
staff described Anne as alert and responsive with an excellent
balance of receptivity and reactivity and an unusual ability in
perceptual discrimination. She smiled responsively to the face
of adults and visually followed both persons and toys. She reacted to social stimulation by cooing and other vocalizations.
Neuromotor organization and motor development were normal but were not as impressive as her advanced perception,
social development, and the early phases of language. It
seemed reasonable to propose at this time that this alertness
and type of responsiveness to persons indicated a good capacity
and a readiness to form an attachment to the mothering person. She was especially responsive to her mother's voice and
face. These qualities appeared to reflect both the biological
preadaptedness of the human infant as a social being and good
progress in the development and specificity of Anne's object
relations. All observations led us to believe that Anne was an
unusually well-endowed infant. However, at this 2-month visit
we first noted Mrs. A.'s problems in holding and cuddling her
baby. She was observed to give the infant the bottle while holding her at a distance across her lap, minimizing body contact. In
this feeding behavior she looked competent but not contact-
seeking.

She reported that she did not pick up the baby often or hold
her more than very briefly for fear she would spoil her. She
said that the baby liked being talked to better than being handled, a statement that clearly reflected her own style and preference in mothering. Nevertheless, as the pediatrician noted,
Anne was still cuddly and responded with signs of comfort and
pleasure when held by someone who enjoyed contact with her.
What was learned later of Mrs. A.'s attitudes toward tender
physical contact suggests that here she projected her own needs
and preferences onto the baby. In addition, as we gradually
knew her and her problems better, it appeared that her avoidance of physical contact with the baby may also have been an
effort to control the sadistic impulses stimulated at times by

holding the baby close to her; thus her behavior also had a protective function. Marianne Kris was insistent on this point when others of us were inclined to be critical of the mother's way of holding Anne. Later, when Mrs. A. felt under increased stress, her ability to control these impulses diminished and at times broke through with unhappy consequences for Anne. This kind of observation, easily made by those who observe mothers and infants, is an example of the value, for preventive work, of trying to distinguish early between a new mother's awkwardness due to inexperience and avoidance of physical closeness due to serious psychological problems.

In regard to feeding, Anne, though somewhat small, sucked well, was easily comforted, and took adequate amounts of formula in spite of Mrs. A.'s awkwardness in holding her. By 2½ months she could get thumb to mouth easily when in prone, and her mother put her in this position so that she would sleep through the night without a feeding. At this time, however, she cried lustily when hungry, clearly registering her need, and Mrs. A. reported that she kept Anne waiting for her feedings as long as half an hour since she rarely anticipated Anne's need and could not quickly prepare the bottle. In contrast, at 3 months Anne was sucking her thumb for as long as half an hour in the early morning, appearing contented. This observation, which became more meaningful in the light of later development, suggests that the hunger, that is, the physiological need, was present, but the baby had made some kind of adaptation to the mother's habitual lack of promptness in feeding her since when she saw the bottle she would, as Mrs. A. said, "suddenly become voracious" and take it hungrily. In some respects this behavior resembled that of deprived institutional infants in whom crying from hunger diminished after a few weeks, apparently because the need was not responded to at the time it was felt and expressed (Provence and Lipton, 1962). In Anne there are two possible interpretations of the significance of the diminished signaling of hunger: (1) as a result of some satisfying feeding experiences she may have replaced the bottle with the thumb, possibly having hallucinatory gratification for a time; but this was not accompanied by behavior that suggested anticipation of a gratifying experience to come; (2) thumb sucking may have been an autoerotic activity *without* the hallucinatory gratification and pleasure normally derived from the ministrations of the mother that lead to more energies cathecting the outside. In Anne these mental images were not so readily formed and the energies not so readily mobilized because the gratifying experiences were so meager. The diminished signaling suggested a disturbance in the budding object relationship.

In contrast with this early morning behavior, at other times during the day Anne at age 3 months cried intensely when hungry. It later became clearer that Mrs. A. was unable to make any feeding fully satisfying and pleasant for Anne. She could not mobilize herself to feed the baby at the first signs of hunger and gave the bottle only after Anne's crying was prolonged and intense. Her behavior often placed too great a strain on the baby's capacity to tolerate tension. This continued in one form or another throughout the years of our contact. Another example of Mrs. A.'s ambivalence toward Anne was seen at this 3-month visit when she dressed the baby nicely for the social worker and enjoyed showing her off but left her strapped on the bath table and was unresponsive to her crying.

At the 3½-month clinic visit Anne was fretful at first and appeared to be reacting to her mother's tension. Mrs. A. said she feared Anne would not perform well on the developmental test, a statement that emphasized her need to have Anne be intelligent and to behave well and was representative of many others we heard later on. At this visit she revealed that the baby's crying upset her very much and that she had been screaming back at her. In the pediatrician's presence, however, Mrs. A. was able to be more comforting and tender with Anne; she was better able to suppress her negative reactions in the presence of other adults than when alone with the baby. At the same time there were indications of her rivalry with Anne for attention from her husband and from a woman neighbor.

Anne was described at 3½ months by the pediatrician as petite, well-nourished, and adequately developed. All signs of the relative neuromuscular immaturity described earlier had vanished. Prone behavior and head control were good. The beginnings of purposive reaching and grasping were visible, as was hand play. Anne initiated social contact with her mother by smiling spontaneously at her and only at her during this session. She initially reacted to the sight of the physician by crying but subsided and smiled when her mother came near and talked to her in comforting tones. There was no doubt that she distinguished between familiar and unfamiliar persons and that her mother's presence made her feel more comfortable. It was significant—and sad—that Mrs. A. was unable to see that Anne responded more positively to her than to others even when it was pointed out to her. She insisted that Anne smiled "at everyone" and especially warmly to the neighbor mentioned above. While Anne's progress in discrimination and in recognition of her mother was excellent, the first slowing down in language development and in playful social reactions was apparent in her performance on the developmental tests. Language development had progressed only 3 weeks in the 6-week interval, a significant observation in view of the rapid development evident on the first test. While she did coo, chuckle, and vocalize responsively, her responses were less robust and output of vocalization was diminished when compared with the norm and with herself 6 weeks earlier. Moreover, though we were not aware of its significance at this time (3½ months), the earliest signs of discrepancy between the maturation of the motor apparatus and its functional use began to be visible, i.e., what Hartmann et al. (1946) referred to as a distinction between maturation and development. Anne was not utilizing fully the motor abilities available to her through maturation; she was not as active in reaching out and in changing position as she could have been given her level of maturation. There was also a relatively low investment of interest in toys. These observations—the muting or dampening of language and social responses, the relatively low investment in toys and the discrepancy between maturation and function—are identical with, though less severe than, the picture reported in a group of infants institutionalized due to severe deficits in the nurturing environment (Provence and Lipton, 1962). It also appeared that the mother's screaming at Anne exercised an inhibiting influence on the baby's vocal expression. Thus one could propose that both a diminution of positive communication and stimuli and the presence of negative stimuli began to have an adverse effect on the baby's development and behavior. I want to stress, however, that at this time we were not aware of the significance of Anne's behavior. Moreover, because she still looked good, in general, and Mrs. A. balanced some of her negative statements about Anne with positive ones, we were not impressed with any great difficulty. She was pleased that Anne fit so well into her schedule and was so good. While it appeared that Mrs. A.'s relation to the infant was not a mature one, contained many narcissistic elements, and had not yet extended to include an empathic consideration of the child, her feelings of pride and pleasure were not yet outweighed by the negative feelings.

At the 4½-month visit Anne was still well-developed in some respects. She was appealing and adequately nourished. She was irritable and anxious, and it was difficult for her mother to comfort her. There was much body tension, only slowly relieved by being held on her mother's shoulder. But there were more prominent signs of disturbances in her development, clearly suggesting problems in the mother-infant relationship. There also was a change in the thumb-sucking behavior that we interpreted as significant: the infant who had previously sucked her thumb selectively and with apparent pleasure and relief of tension was now sucking her whole fist instead. This shift suggested some disorganization of a previously acquired level of one aspect of early ego development and organization. Our speculation was that it was caused by the mother's aggressive behavior toward the child which had already begun, although we had only hints of it at this time. We had two thoughts about Anne's behavior: (1) the mother's slowness in response to the child's need for feeding overtaxed the infant's capacity to tolerate tension and produced regression in an area of early ego development. Here Hoffer's (1949) ideas about hand, mouth, ego integration, and body ego are relevant; and (2) the directly expressed behavior—abruptness of handling, yelling, and spanking—of the mother toward the child may have stimulated an early aggressivization of the mouth-hand contact. Tension discharge as reflected in hand-mouth activity, was less effective than it had been earlier. Still, the predominant impression of the infant was of alertness to her environment and responsiveness to people, including frequent visual contact with the mother.

It was during the period from 5 to 8 months that we increasingly gained the impression of serious problems between Anne and her mother, and Anne's decline became clearly manifest, though it did not reach its greatest depth until the end of the tenth month. Early in the fifth month Mrs. A. was disturbed by what she considered an unnecessary frequency of feeding and asked permission to give more solids to lengthen the interval between feedings. (We learned only later that from Anne's early infancy Mrs. A. had been reading as she fed her, being unable to muster interest in her.) It was during the fifth month, too, that Mrs. A. first confessed with some guilt that she was spanking the baby when the child's crying made her "feel wild inside." Mrs. A. was depressed and unable to find pleasure in caring for the baby; she could not enjoy feeding her or make the feeding experience and undoubtedly also other experiences gratifying for the baby; she was stimulated by the crying to sadistic action (spanking) and not to tenderness.

At the 6-month visit a delay in motor development was visible but not dramatic: Anne was unable to maintain her trunk erect when placed in sitting position and did not roll, although she did make some efforts to change position and to reach out to others. She could reach out and grasp toys with adequately coordinated arm movements, and the grasping patterns were evolving normally. She played with her hands and feet, behavior suggesting progress in investment and awareness of the body self. However, she manifested even less interest in play with the toys than she had before; she reacted to the sound of the bell and to some other noises by closing her eyes, as though shutting out the stimuli—an unusual reaction and perhaps an adaptation to the provocative, tension-producing elements in the maternal behavior. She was reported to be taking long daytime naps in addition to sleeping 12 hours at night, suggesting a diminished interest in the outside. However, she was amiable and responsive both to the pediatrician and to her mother and seemed to find pleasure in social contact, showing that when comfortable she could enjoy others. Language continued to be somewhat depressed as reflected principally in the minimal use of vocalization in the social interchange. This did not indicate a delay in the maturational timetable since the vowel sounds and changes in tonal range of the voice expected at this age emerged normally, as did the capacity for discriminatory acoustic attention. The problem was in those aspects of early language development that are dependent upon satisfactory interaction with the maternal figure. This again is similar to our findings on institutional infants in whom the amount of vocalization was sparse and minimally used in social interaction, while the underlying maturational steps necessary for the formation of words and the elaboration of sounds had proceeded adequately. In Anne, as in the institutional infants, the interference with speech can be viewed as a disturbance in ego development reflecting trouble in the object relations.

Anne's decline[2] in all aspects of development was rapid during the next 8 weeks, and by the time she was 7¾ months old her misery and depression were prominent. Language was her most retarded sector averaging 6 weeks below the norm for her age. Gross motor achievements were more delayed than before, and muscle tone was described as poor for the first time. Movements were observed to be less skillfully modulated than in a healthy child of her age; either they were quick and poorly controlled or wcrc quite slow. They also were relatively less goal-directed than they had been earlier, and she was less active in changing position to move toward a toy or person. Maturational patterns in respect to fine motor development had continued to evolve normally, but the use of the apparatus was increasingly deviant: her characteristic behavior with the test materials was to approach, flick, grasp briefly, and release quickly. She showed more vigor in getting rid of objects than in obtaining them. This was accompanied by an apparent preference for stimulation of low intensity and a tendency toward withdrawal. Even so there was some progress in her use of toys. For example, she did pick up a cube in each hand and "match them," that is, brought them together in the midline combining them as she observed her own activity, a normal pattern of her age. It is of interest that at the same age she was observed to match the cubes, she did not play pat-a-cake, a game that makes use of the same neuromotor organization. The pat-a-cake

2. This decline was in rate of development, i.e., less progress was made than before. There was no loss of previously acquired functions.

game, however, requires an additional ingredient, namely, the social stimulation of the adult with playful mutual imitation between adult and infant. This observation we viewed as another example of the disturbance in Anne's social relationships.

A dramatic example of the disturbed relationship between mother and child which dismayed all who saw it at this 7¾-month visit was that Anne cried repeatedly at the approach of the mother but could be comforted by the pediatrician and, in addition, responded with more pleasure to her than to the mother. Mrs. A. revealed that she was depressed, dissatisfied, lonely, bored, and angry at her husband. She had gained a great deal of weight, and this intensified her feelings of depression. While she felt dissatisfied as wife and mother and wished for a part-time job, she would not let herself consider it and expressed a conviction that a mother should stay home and take care of her own baby. She felt immobilized and trapped— and indeed she was by her psychological problems. After she saw a younger child who was better developed, she wondered whether Anne was mentally defective and could not be reassured by the pediatrician. She felt guilty about her behavior toward the infant but was unable to modify it. Anne showed an unhappy tension and had screaming spells of 10 or more minutes, which the mother reported were connected with her own moods, especially her "blue Mondays." Anne's hyperattentiveness to acoustic and visual stimuli, her increased anxiety, and particularly her distress at the approach of the mother suggested a heightened cathexis of the world in regard to danger. An anxious apprehensiveness pervaded her behavior. She also was quite fearful of strangers—a source of anxiety that was to stay with her for many months to come. This was paralleled by a relative impairment of libidinal attachment, inferred from her tenuous contacts with the human object, her relative incapacity to play, and her low investment in toys. In the observers' view of the mother-child couple at this time (around 8 months), the libidinal tie was weak and the infant seemed miserable, depressed, and overwhelmed.

The staff, extremely concerned about mother and child, tried to help Mrs. A. with the daily demands and needs of the child and with suggestions for herself. The pediatrician saw them weekly at home during the 8th month, talked with Mrs. A., and made recommendations about the care of the baby. While eager to be seen, Mrs. A. was only minimally able to use the advice given. It should be said here that the relationship between Mrs. A. and the pediatrician remained good in the sense that the doctor felt sympathetic and tried to be supportive and helpful, and Mrs. A. trusted her and was obviously grateful in a rather childlike way. At the same time the observations of the child's impaired development and of the disturbed mother-child interaction in the face of all attempts to help reflected the severity of the mother's problem in nurturing her infant. For example, at a home visit when Anne was 8 months old, Mrs. A. showed the pediatrician how she went through the recommended play period and massage. She was aware of being bored and could verbalize her boredom, but was unaware of the cursory and cold quality of her contact with Anne. There were even fewer experiences that were mutually pleasurable. Anne's crying and the mother's loss of control resulting in the spanking scenes were more frequent. In contrast to the mother's feeling about the infant's unreasonable demandingness, it appeared to observers that Anne had made considerable adaptation to the nongratifying and threatening environment: she accepted being alone for long periods without making strong demands. When fretful she quieted down if brought to the room where her mother was working or reading. It was as though an accommodation had been arrived at in which for several hours a day being in the mother's presence meant there was not complete abandonment; at the same time the distance (i.e., the lack of close physical involvement) may have protected against the danger of spanking. Here was an adaptation that was self-protective in the short term, but cut Anne off from the interactions needed for more favorable development.

The time span from 9 to 12 months was one in which Anne's greatest depression, withdrawal, and misery were seen. However, the tide also began to turn during this period, and we saw the first glimmer of improvement in the baby's development and in Mrs. A.'s mothering. When Anne was 9 months of age, Mrs. A. reported that eating and sleeping were both quite satisfactory, and she felt things were better in general. Mrs. A., following the doctor's suggestion, now ate when the child did and as a result seemed able to make the meal more pleasant for Anne. The spanking scenes set off by the child's crying were still going on, however, and Mrs. A. characterized herself as a person who would "spank hard but would also love hard." As an example of the spanking, Mrs. A. reported that Anne cried on being left in the carriage in the grocery store so she had had to carry her around as she shopped and had spanked Anne's hands to "give her something to cry about."

In spite of the reported improvement, Anne's performance on the developmental test at 9 months showed a greater decline in rate of development. She was anxious and apprehensive but was somewhat more comfortable when on her mother's lap. Her test performance was characterized by its unevenness: there was evidence of advanced, heightened discriminatory capacities, which had some positive implications for cognition, but her attitude toward almost everything that occurred during the session was one of anxious expectancy. She seemed to obtain only meager satisfaction from any of the toys. Language was again her lowest area of functioning, being 7 weeks under age. She was able to obtain mild enjoyment from the peek-a-boo game but did not initiate it, nor did she respond to other social games such as pat-a-cake, so-big, bye-bye. The absence of the kind of playful social interaction so prominent in normally developing infants at this age was especially poignant. Anne had pulled to a standing position for the first time the night before the visit, much to her mother's delight, but she still sat very poorly and with rounded back. She could crawl on her belly but not on all fours. Her weight was below the 3 percentile; her body was thin and muscle tone poor. *She was an infant failing to thrive.* There were no other significant findings on the physical exam, which included a number of laboratory studies directed at her poor growth and developmental delay. A few days after this visit, at the psychiatric consultation arranged for her, Mrs. A. recapitulated her account of her blue spells and seemed aware that her 2-month period of feeling particularly depressed might have influenced Anne. However, she was unable to accept the idea of psychotherapy, voicing her conviction that psychologists and psychiatrists were for people who could not help themselves and that some hard times in life were to be expected. She told both the pediatrician and the social worker about her fear of psychotherapy: she felt that a friend had become more ill as a result of treatment. A few days later Mrs. A. and Anne went to visit at the home of her brother and sister-in-law. This visit with its supporting influence, and probably also Mr. A.'s increased attention, seemed to give both mother and infant a new lease on life. They stayed for 2 weeks, and on returning home Mrs. A. reported that being with them had made her feel better and that things were all right between her and Anne now. Friends and neighbors had come in, and Mrs. A. had relished the adult company and the chance to talk. She was looking forward to spending a month at the shore during the summer. Anne had been able to enjoy her cousin, who had played with her a great deal.

At the 10½-month visit Anne was described as a pretty little girl who gave the impression of physical and psychological fragility. She was able to smile occasionally at the examiner when the contact was kept to a minimum and at a distance but became extremely anxious when touched or handled, crying in a way that was distressed and despairing. Her smile differed from earlier ones in that it often had the quality of a grimace, which markedly diminished her attractiveness. Motor development had improved slightly. She could move from sitting position to prone and could creep on all fours, but there was an impairment of the ego's utilization of motility in that she did not use her ability to creep to move away from something she did not like. In such situations she could only cry in a distressed way, suggesting an interference in her coping behavior. In our setting she was hardly able to play at all. Approaches to toys were tentative; she could manipulate them comfortably only if they were presented very slowly. She regulated this in part by refusing to deal with more than one object at a time, often turning away or discarding one. This and other similar observations revealed her difficulty in coping with multiple stimuli. She did not do well with nonverbal problem-solving tasks on the test apparently both because she was not sufficiently interested and because she tended to break down into distressed crying the moment any obstacle was introduced. She was mostly silent during the session except when crying; there was no imitation of sounds; while she vocalized an occasional "dada" or "baba," there was no specificity in their use, i.e., they were not names for her parents. Language was 15 weeks below average at this time. Her contact with the examiner and with her mother appeared weak and poorly sustained and needed to be kept at low intensity to avoid upsetting her. While in some respects Anne's development, especially the developmental profile, resembled the deprived infants in the institution there were significant differences. As Ernst Kris (1962) commented,

> Her behavior differs from them in several essential respects. Her bad nutritional status, the frantic crying spells, and the marked, at times hardly controllable fear of the strangers are not part of the syndrome of children in the institutions mentioned before (Provence and Lipton). . . . We see features in Anne's behavior which reach an intensity that forces us to consider them as symptoms. These symptoms are, we suggest, not due to lack of stimulation, but rather to a specific kind of provocative overstimulation which was bound to produce mounting tension in the child without offering appropriate avenues of discharge [p. 203f.].

I would add here, it was the combination of deprivation and provocative overstimulation that caused such intense psychological discomfort and interference with many aspects of development. While Mrs. A. was less worried about mental retardation and there was a beginning upward trend in some areas, Anne's development and behavior continued to reflect the disturbance in the relationship. Mrs. A. showed a little more awareness of Anne's unhappiness and made more of an effort to comfort her. A new social worker began to see Mrs. A. when Anne was 11 months of age, and some of her observations having the advantages of independence and freshness were of special interest. At a home visit, Mrs. A. received Miss J. courteously and was obviously eager to talk about herself. She appeared to want very much to do the right thing for her child but did not know how and asked rather pathetically, "Miss J., how *do* you play with a baby?" The social worker was struck by Anne's silence and her isolation, her subdued and passive appearance and behavior.

Toward the end of the first year Anne became less apathetic and more actively complaintive. Her mother said that she was crying intensely ("screeching") at night in her crib and at times during the day. Here Mrs. A. chose a word and used a tone that unmistakably conveyed her anger at the child. Anne's appetite had again dropped off, and Mrs. A. was finding her very trying, complaining that Anne wanted constant entertainment. While Anne's tension and despair were abundantly manifest as before, there was now also anger in her cry, the first time this had been noted in the records. During the well-baby visit just before her first birthday Anne cried almost constantly for an hour and was not comforted by anything the mother or pediatrician could do. Bottles, toys, Mrs. A.'s talking to her or holding her on her lap were to no avail. The crying had a desperate, intensely unhappy quality. Ernst Kris (1962) wrote about it as follows: "The effect of the child's crying on all observers was lasting, as if they had witnessed a tragic experience. They found themselves watching a child who could not be reached or comforted, but was left to her own uncontrollable despair" (p. 212). While anxiety and fatigue probably played a part, the intensity and duration of the crying were most unusual, and the mother's incapacity to provide comfort was startling. Mrs. A.'s own anxiety, frustration, and exasperation over the continual crying mounted; finally she seemed only with the utmost effort able to avoid spanking Anne who at last fell asleep as her mother and the doctor talked. It was reported that Anne now went to sleep at night holding her bottle in one hand and rubbing the soft tail of her bunny over her face, later to wake up and cry as mentioned before.

At the same time (11–12 months) Anne's environment had in some ways become more favorable. The family was at the shore, and her father was around much more. Relatives had visited on several occasions, and Mrs. A.'s mood had lightened. Anne had obviously had much more in the way of positive, pleasant nurturing experiences than for many months. We assume that this experiential change as well as the endogenous forces of maturation combined to produce improvement in several areas of development. As Anne's apathy and depressed mood were increasingly replaced by manifestations of rage, the active conflict between mother and child emerged. We took this to be one sign of improvement. At other times at home she appeared sweet and docile. These contrasting states—the overt conflict between them and Anne's conformity—were seen more clearly in the second year.

At the end of Anne's first year she was characterized as a developmentally impaired and psychologically disturbed infant. Over the months that had elapsed we witnessed, with delayed recognition, the impact of Mrs. A.'s problems upon her well-endowed and attractive baby. Our first knowledge of the disturbance in nurturing was stimulated by observations of the child's declining growth rate and performance in several dimensions of the developmental tests. As we became alerted to the situation through the baby's condition, we gradually learned much more from Mrs. A. about her feelings of boredom, loneliness, unattractiveness, depression, anger, and sadistic tendencies. Anne's developmental delays and disturbed behavior produced by her mother's incapacity to nurture her adequately further heightened Mrs. A.'s own difficulties and made the situation between them even more unfavorable.

The story of the second year contains its own drama in which both Anne and Mrs. A. remained recognizable, but there were shifts of emphasis dictated by maturation and changes in the interaction. At around Anne's first birthday Mrs. A. expressed pleasure in her for the first time in many months, saying that she was a very different child from the "negative thing" she had been. Now she was so much more of a person; Mrs. A. felt she could talk to Anne who was beginning to understand. Anne could walk with two hands held and crept expertly on all fours. She was observed to creep about the house with considerable interest and pleasure in the activity. With the full mastery of creeping and the early steps in walking, Anne appeared sturdier and more vigorous. This was perhaps the first time she was capable of moving out on her own to explore her surroundings or actively to move away from her mother. She remained quite fearful of strangers. The crying at night had stopped, but she was continuing to wake several times. She would search for and find her bottle in the crib and go back to sleep with it and her bunny. There seemed to be no doubt about the attachment to

and the comfort-giving value of the bottle. Anne's fondness for
the bunny and the way in which she used it gave it, we believed,
the characteristics of a transitional object. Later (at 18½ months)
concomitant with increased expression of anger and hostility in
her interchanges with her mother and with other children, she
also used the bunny as a target of aggression, ferociously biting
its ears as well as using it as a comforter. Between 13 and 18
months the bunny seems to have lost some of its transitional-
object qualities for at 18 months and beyond Anne appeared to
use the bunny much more as the recipient of displaced ambivalent feelings for the human objects. At age 13 months Anne
had improved markedly in her general development as measured on the developmental tests, but her anxiety was still abundantly manifest. Part of the pediatrician's description follows:

> Anne was tested on her mother's lap where she seemed uneasy,
> fearful, and frequently turned toward her mother in her anx-
> iety. I approached her very cautiously and slowly and felt she
> was distracted by the smallest sort of change. Conversation
> between her mother and me seemed disturbing to her, even
> when we lowered our voices to a soft murmur. She was most
> comfortable and used the materials most freely when nothing
> was being said. On two occasions, a telephone bell was heard
> faintly in the distance and both times she responded with a
> distressed expression and tensing of her body. There was little
> vocalization, and her approach to objects was very tentative. I
> gave her the ball, and we rolled it back and forth two or three
> times. At this her face lighted up, she smiled broadly, turned
> toward her mother, and clutched her briefly. She then turned
> back to the ball, and the game continued for several minutes.
> She looked very happy, smiled and laughed, and for the first
> time gave the impression of having made a positive human
> contact.

Anne was terrified, however, at the approach of her ball-game
companion for the physical examination. The improvement in
her development can best be illustrated by giving some comparisons: gross motor development had increased 19 weeks in the
12-week interval since the last complete test. She could walk with
one hand held, cruise at the crib rail, and creep adeptly. She
could pick up small objects with great precision, and eye-hand
coordination was good. Language development showed the

most spectacular improvement—a gain of 25 weeks, that is, almost 6 months. She had 4 words, including mama and dada as names for her parents. She recognized the names of a few familiar things in her surroundings. These were all quite spectacular and encouraging gains. On the deficit side, the tentativeness of her approaches remained, as did the persistent attitude of anxious expectancy and relatively low investment of toys. Although she did play with toys more than she had for several months and used them with more signs of interest and understanding of their possibilities, she was quickly discouraged by obstacles. Coping efforts as described by Lois Murphy (1974) were still poorly developed for her age, as was mastery motivation (competence) in Robert White's (1959) sense.

When the social worker saw Anne at 15 months, Miss J. was very impressed with the improvement in her. Anne not only walked about the house with great pleasure but laughed a great deal, initiated a peek-a-boo game with Miss J., and was very invested in social interaction. Mrs. A. reported that now she could teach Anne and demonstrated by having Anne perform with her blocks, books, and other toys. This was the first unmistakable evidence of a teacher-pupil relationship between mother and child, a role that was obviously more comfortable for Mrs. A. than meeting dependency needs. Since Anne could fulfill some of the mother's demands to be intelligent, she appeared to become a source of greater narcissistic gratification to her mother, Miss J. put it very well:

> I think that Anne's activity and behavior and signs of learning have made things much better between her and her mother. Mrs. A. can take an intellectual delight in Anne's achievements, can fulfill the role of teacher and guide, and can respond to a child who is not the helpless infant making demands upon her emotional giving. In spite of the much greater and happier interchange between the two, I had the impression that Mrs. A. had not changed to any great extent but that Anne was now satisfying something in her and she could therefore be more responsive to Anne.

One can speculate that Anne's ability to walk exerted a beneficial influence in three ways: she could now go away from her mother or seek her out as she felt inclined and therefore had some control over the contact; the greater mobility was also a help in enriching her everyday experiences; to the mother it may also have meant that the child was not so fragile anymore.

I will leave the story of Anne here—at 15 months, though our work on the case summary was continued to the end of our contact with the family when Anne was 3½ years old. Perhaps I should say, to lighten some of the gloom I may have created, that in the second and third years Anne improved in ways that were almost as dramatic as her decline had been. I think it is correct to say that by the time she was 3½, though problems were easily discernible, those who did not know her well would not have imagined how desperately unhappy and impaired she had been in the last half of the first year. As we followed her development closely through her attendance in our nursery school, continued home visits, and pediatric contacts, both the substantial improvement and the areas of stress and difficulty were apparent.

DISCUSSION

The observations of Anne and her mother have provided us with rich opportunities to examine propositions of psychoanalytic child psychology. The story of Anne is an especially fine reminder of the interdependence of drive and ego development and of each of these with object relations. Indeed, to the extent that we disregard any one of them, we oversimplify the task of trying to understand the development of the psychic life of this child and others.

In this case the disturbance in the object relationship was reflected most vividly and dramatically in the mother-child interaction and in the infant's behavior. The mother was at times comforting, but the child experienced a great excess of unpleasure, frustration, hunger for physical and psychological nourishment, physical and psychological pain, and eventually awareness of danger and fear. Deprivation and trauma coexisted here: nurturing in the positive sense was deficient in many respects. Especially noxious to the infant's development was the chronicity of the traumatic elements in the situation. Ernst Kris would refer to Anne's experience, I think, as strain trauma, a condition in which the child's heightened vulnerability fairly continuously influenced how each day was experienced. The disturbance in the object relations caused trouble in ego and drive development and organization as well. In regard to the autonomous functions of the ego, after a favorable beginning, problems of one kind or another were seen in motility, speech, intelligence, capacity for delay of discharge, and in the organizing function. Perception was heightened in respect to danger from the human object and at times impaired in regard to inanimate objects in her environment. Memory, especially for anxiety-producing situations, was very sharp.

While Anne made some active efforts to cope with adverse experiences and one was occasionally encouraged by glimmers of good functioning (efforts at active mastery, withdrawal or avoidance in the face of danger, seeking comfort from adults, comforting herself), it appeared that the deficits in the nurturing environment and the provocative, painful overstimulation were too overwhelming to favor the beginning development of stable defenses.

Libidinal and aggressive drive development was adversely affected singly and in their relationship to each other. This is inferred from the many observations of characteristics of the infant's early ego development and her interaction with her environment. The disturbance in body ego was among the first findings. There are many references after the fourth month to what impressed us as an interference with libidinal cathexis of the object, the self, and of emerging ego functions. What we interpreted as an imbalance between aggressive and libidinal drive development began to be especially prominent early in the second year. Behavioral signs of aggressive drive development and discharge increased at the end of the first year, concomitant with improvement in Anne's development in other areas. While there were signs of more positive elements in Anne's relationship with her mother and more nurturing from her father, emerging functions in the second year reflected, we believe, an undercathexis with libidinal energies and an overcathexis with aggressive energies. The discharge of aggression through motor activity was responded to by painfully experienced counteraction from the mother, leading to a more complicated situation in which identification with the aggressor, inhibition of aggression, and turning aggression against the self were prominent.

Finally, when we looked at affect development and expression, again we saw in early infancy the expected normal repertory and differentiation: the responsive and spontaneous social smile, contented pleasure, the ability to cry lustily when hungry or otherwise uncomfortable. By 3½ months Anne showed fretful crying in reaction to her mother's tension but still often expressed feelings of pleasure—albeit in a less robust way than was true of her earlier. She was alert and interested in her surroundings and responded with obviously good feelings to many stimuli. In months 5 and 6 we saw crying spells which seemed to express anxiety and an unhappy tension, but at other times Anne was amiable and able to enjoy social contact. Expression of affect through noncrying vocalization was diminished. By the 7¾-month contact two new descriptors were used by the investigators: Anne's *misery* and *depression* were prominent. *Severe* anxiety to the stranger, and at times to the mother, was manifest. Between 9 and 11 months the terms "acute anxiety," "despairing cry," "severe distress," "unhappy tension" as well as "withdrawn," "subdued," and "apathetic" were used to describe her. When she was just under a year, it was noted that she was less apathetic; that though one heard in her frantic crying spells the despair and misery heard earlier, *anger, rage* and *protest* now also seemed present. In the expression of anger, rage, and protest Anne's repertory of feelings and their intensity differed markedly from the institutional infants of her age who, by comparison, were much more restricted and bland. The change in Anne was seen as improvement. Creeping and walking with support were accompanied by expression of pleasure. She seemed better able to discharge tension and also, at times, to comfort herself. At 15 months there were more interchanges between Anne and her mother, especially in the teacher-pupil relationship in which Anne seemed to take considerable pleasure.

To recapitulate, looking at the expectable manifestations of developmental progress as observable behavior, we saw in the beginning a healthy, normal, well-functioning baby. As Anne's development declined in rate, signs of difficulty appeared in every area: motor development, speech, nonverbal problem-solving and social behavior were impaired. Sleeping, eating, and physical growth were disturbed at one time or another, as was her interaction with her environment, both human and inanimate. Descriptively, and through the eyes of any parent or professional, Anne's delayed development, depression, and misery would give cause for concern.

Viewing the data on Anne from the perspective of psychoanalysis, I have tried here to specify the interference with and disturbances in healthy personality development during the first 15 months. At one time or another after the 4th month signs of trouble in object relations, libidinal and aggressive drive development, and in various aspects of ego development can be measured or inferred from the data. Anne's affective experience can be assumed to be a complex mixture of positive and negative experiences, with an excess of painful or disorganizing events. Recovery began to take place when several factors converged—further maturation in Anne, some change in Mrs. A.'s perception of her child, and improvement in the family's living situation.

It is difficult to interrupt the story here, for the data of the second and third years have their own fascinations and challenges to understanding. Perhaps a future report will continue the story.

BIBLIOGRAPHY

COLEMAN, R. W., KRIS, E., & PROVENCE, S. (1953), The study of variations of early parental attitudes. *Psychoanal. Study Child*, 8:20–47.
———— & PROVENCE, S. (1953), Environmental retardation (hospitalism) in infants living in families. *Pediatrics*, 11:285–292.
HARTMANN, H., KRIS, E., & LOEWENSTEIN, R. M. (1946), Comments on the formation of psychic structure. *Psychoanal. Study Child*, 2:11–38.
HOFFER, W. (1949), Mouth, hand and ego-integration. *Psychoanal. Study Child*, 3/4:49–56.
KRIS, E. (1962), Decline and recovery in the life of a three-year-old. *Psychoanal. Study Child*, 17:175–215.
MURPHY, L. B. (1974), Coping, vulnerability and resilience in childhood. In *Coping and Adaptation*, ed. G. V. Coelho, D. A. Hamburg, & J. E. Adams. New York: Basic Books, pp. 69–100.
PROVENCE, S. (1965), Disturbed personality development in infancy. *Merrill-Palmer Q.*, 11:149–170.
———— & LIPTON, R. W. [COLEMAN] (1962), *Infants in Institutions*. New York: Int. Univ. Press.

RITVO, S., MCCOLLUM, A. T., OMWAKE, E., PROVENCE, S., & SOLNIT, A. J. (1963), Some relations of constitution, environment, and personality as observed in a longitudinal study of child development. In *Modern Perspectives in Child Development,* ed. A. J. Solnit & S. Provence. New York: Int. Univ. Press, pp. 107–143.

WHITE, R. W. (1959), Motivation reconsidered. *Psychol. Rev.,* 66:297–333.

Infants of Primary Nurturing Fathers

KYLE D. PRUETT, M.D.

"Love is the standard issue—only the objects change"
ELVIN SEMRAD

MANY OF THE RECENT ATTEMPTS TO CORRECT THE SCIEN-tific neglect of the father-infant relationship are plagued by the nagging *déjà vu* of old questions inviting, yet evading, new study. Still, increasing numbers of reports in the literature by serious analytic thinkers (Cath et al., 1982) and careful researchers (Lamb, 1976, 1981; McKee and O'Brien, 1982; Parke, 1979; Parke and Sawin, 1980; Pedersen et al., 1980) struggle with the meaning and nature of contemporary paternity. And why now? Surely the extensive use of birth control in the present century has been a compelling factor in the father's (re)emergence, as the choice to become a parent could now be consciously controlled by *both* parents. In addition, the ongoing turmoil within the nuclear family; the increasing access to the work force enjoyed by, if not forced upon, women; the slow but progressive softening of sexual stereotypes—all have invited, indeed compelled, the father of the young child, and those who study them, to reexamine his role as nurturing parent in his own right.

A group of special interest consists of fathers who not merely

Associate Clinical Professor of Psychiatry, Child Study Center, Yale University, New Haven, Ct.
Based in part on papers presented at the American Academy of Child Psychiatry, Chicago, Oct. 23, 1980, and Dallas, Oct. 15, 1981.

257

participate in the care, or supplement the mother's nurturing, for their children, but in fact serve as the primary nurturing objects in their infants' lives, functioning as what one ambivalent man dubbed himself—a "father-mother."

The literature that does exist on father-infant interaction is quite recent and generally focuses on the unique role of the father in the infant's life, often in the form of descriptive study of the father's sensitivities to babies and young children in general. In a laboratory setting, Frodi and Lamb (1978) monitored the psychophysiological responses of mothers and fathers while watching a video tape of the smiling and crying of an infant. The patterns of autonomic arousal and reported irritation to crying or unpleasant emotions, and autonomic relaxation to smiling, were indistinguishable for male and female parent in all studies. The authors conclude that their evidence refutes the conclusions by Harlow (1958), Lorenz (1966), and others that there are innate biological hormonal mechanisms which are responsible for the females' superior responsiveness to babies, and ultimately for the woman's greater involvement with the child. Instead, the authors postulate that social pressures are probably stronger than biological influences in determining the sensitivities of fathers to their infants' needs. These findings, when coupled with research by Brazelton et al. (1979) and others, indicating the extremely active role of the infant in shaping his own environment, lead one to assume that the father's role, even when not primary, has been vastly underestimated.

It has been frequently noted (Ferholt and Gurwitt, 1982) that fathers are often not interviewed directly by mental health professionals, pediatricians, or educators, and that the mothers are usually asked to describe their spouses and the father-child relationship, giving only indirect and subjective reports of such interaction.

Kotelchuck (1976), in a laboratory setting using strangers as stressors, concluded: "Children can and do form active and close relationships with their fathers during their first years of life. Children do not innately or instinctively relate only to their mothers. The presumed uniqueness of the mother-child relationship appears ephemeral. The child's response to either parent in experimental situations is clearly more a function of the nature of the parent-child interaction than of a biological predisposition" (p. 343). Regarding the unique impact of the father on child development, Biller (1974) suggests that mothers and fathers react differently to their infants' attempts at exploring the environment. He notes that fathers encourage their babies' curiosity and urge them to attempt to solve cognitive and motoric challenges, thereby fostering their sense of mastery over the environment. Mothers engage in more conventional and toy-mediated acts of play. Fathers initiate more physical, rough-and-tumble, idiosyncratic forms of play, an observation also made by Burlingham (1973) and Greenacre (1966). Fathers are more likely to pick up their infants and play with them, whereas mothers most often pick them up to engage in caretaking activities. Finally, Maccoby and Jacklin (1974) and Bloch (1978) have pointed to the father's role in sexual differentiation, as he appears more interested than the mother in clearly delineating and promoting sex-typical behavior.

It is generally agreed in the literature that fathering as a process serves most importantly through fostering autonomy and the enhancement of individuation and independent functioning. Yet, it is also clear that such an "unattachment theory" per se is of limited use in assessing father-infant relationships, as it fails to acknowledge the very early mutual regulation by both infant and parent of the dyadic process. Greenspan (1980) introduces the term "dyadic-phallic stage" of development for this complex interaction as it "connotes the importance of the relationship between drive organization, levels of ego functioning, and levels of object relations in both interpersonal and internalized dimensions" (p. 593). Analyzing video tapes of father-infant and mother-infant interactions, Yogman et al. (1977) conclude that the qualitative differences between mothers and fathers may not be based purely on the infant's familiarity with the parent, but instead on the father's unique handling style: "It is tempting to speculate that infants may be predisposed to seek an appropriate balance of both arousing and well-modulated stimulation from the caregiving system."

The literature is particularly sparse in its attention to the primary caretaking father. Even the prevalence of primary caretaking fathers in the population of intact families remains unknown, although it is assumed to be rare. In contrast, material relating to father absence continues to burgeon, adding to the unfortunate impression that absent fathers may be psychologically more significant than present father.

Nevertheless, interesting material is emerging. Some recent reports have focused on limited comparative behavioral assessment of primary and secondary caretaking fathers and their various interactions with infants. Field (1978) reports that primary caretaking fathers interact with their infants in certain ways that resemble secondary fathers, while in other ways they are similar to primary caretaking mothers. Lamb et al. (1982) have collaborated in the study of the characteristics of maternal and paternal behavior in families where the father has spent more than a month as a primary caregiver in the infant's first 16 months of life (see also Lamb, 1981).

Generally stated, most of the research supports the view that fathers are capable of unique and important contributions to the development of their infant's personalities and skills. Parke and Sawin (1977) have noted that fathers are able to feed their newborns as effectively as mothers, handling the small, irritating problems and disruptions of daily feeding with skill and empathy. Dealing with a research population of 8 to 12 months, these authors also report that if fathers are more involved in the daily care of their babies, the infants tend to be more socially responsive and generally able to withstand stressful circumstances better. In a study of 5- to 6-month-old infants, Pedersen et al. (1980) suggest that the more active the fathers are with the infants, the higher are the cognitive and motor skills measured by the Bayley Mental Development Index.

In a large study of 300 infants ranging in age from 6 to 24 months, Kotelchuck (1976) concludes that the infants are able to withstand stress better if fathers are involved in caretaking tasks such as bathing and dressing.

With few recent exceptions, however, most of the literature remains focused on the father as supplemental, not primary, parent and can only hint at the myriad complexities when the father serves as the main nurturing object. Consequently, the following questions quickly form. What are the babies of such fathers and mothers actually like? How does attachment evolve between such fathers and their infants? How do the fathers, *ne* the couples, decide to parent in this fashion, and what are the contributing psychological factors? Are there certain vulnerabilities, conflicts, special pleasures, or opportunities unique to this caregiving arrangement?

DESCRIPTION OF CLINICAL STUDY

In order to answer these questions I began a prospective clinical inquiry focused both on the development of infants being raised primarily by their fathers, and the fathers doing the raising. The study addresses itself to: (1) the development of infants in intact families (ranging in age from 2 to 24 months); (2) the psychodynamic characteristics of these fathers; (3) their nurturing patterns; and (4) their relationships to the infants' mothers. Two similar groups were investigated a year apart, the first consisting of 9 two-parent families, the second assembled a year later, comprised of 8 families. The families were recruited primarily from general pediatric practices in the Greater New Haven area and ranged broadly across the socioeconomic spectrum from welfare, blue- and white-collar, to professional status. The criterion for admission to the study was that although the parenting might be shared with the mother, the fathers must (in the referring clinician's judgment) bear the major responsibility for, and the commitment to, parenting. The arrangement need not necessarily be considered long-term, and might consist of a working mother, student father, or so-called "dual-career" family. Whatever the arrangement, it allowed for the formation of a primary affectional tie or bond between the father and infant. Although not by original design, the infants available for study were all firstborn into lower or middle-class families and consisted of 5 male and 4 female infants in the first group, and 5 female and 3 male in the second group.

Using retrospective analytically oriented interviewing techniques, I first saw the fathers at home while they were caring for their infants. Extensive histories were taken and naturalistic observations were recorded of the father-infant dyad in the process of typical "male care." After the initial interview, the babies were examined in a laboratory setting at the Child Development Unit of the Yale Child Study Center, using the Yale Developmental Schedules to assess in detail their developmental competence in gross and fine motor performance, adaptive problem-solving, language skills, and personal-social function. A final interview was then conducted, again preferably at home, and usually the most extensive, with both mother and father to take a marital history and to record further naturalistic observations about the family triad.

CASE MATERIAL

Material from two representative father-infant pairs from the second group and data from a family studied in the initial group now in follow-up are presented.

CASE 1

Mr. and Mrs. N., ages 24 and 22 respectively, had been married for 2½ years when they decided it was time to begin their family. They described their relationship as "not full of a lot of sex, so it was good we did not have to work too hard to make Nina." Nina was a product of a full-term pregnancy, weighing 2800 grams, and was delivered by Caesarian section because of pelvic disproportion. Mr. N. reported that "the pregnancy wasn't an awfully happy time for me. I had dreams of being afraid of my wife, that she was going to somehow hurt me."[1] Mr. N. wanted to become involved with the pregnancy but could not really "find a handle on it." He had attempted one such "handle" by measuring his wife's increasing abdominal girth at weekly intervals, keeping a chart and tape measure affixed to the back of the bathroom door. Meanwhile, he in-

---

1. Several of the fathers in both groups reported disquieting dreams about being in physical danger from their wives, and in one instance specifically focused on the genitals, during the end stages of the pregnancy. See also the case reported by Gurwitt (1976).

creased his own weight-lifting and body-building exercises, a favorite form of tension discharge and physical mastery since adolescence. He did not attend the birth, and had not planned to, even had it not been a Caesarian section. After Nina came home, he felt intruded upon by his daughter, and preferred not to help his wife with child care at the beginning of a 12-week maternity leave from her accounting firm.

When his wife had said soon after the delivery that she was uncertain whether she really wanted to leave her career to stay home and mother this child, he was surprised to find himself rather casually offering to look after the baby. He reasoned that he could run his marketing business from home, "for a while," with the use of telephones, a secretary, and an occasional visit to the office.

After 6 weeks at home, his wife was ready to return to work. Mr. N., in talking about his daughter, said, "Suddenly at about 9 weeks, I figured her out. My wife never seemed to be able to, so I was reluctant to admit it at first. But Nina became crystal clear to me. The 'intruder' feelings left, and I began to feel overwhelmed with the wish to raise her in my own image, to develop her the way that I wanted her developed. It may sound crazy, but I started to almost look forward to her waking up at night!"

At first, when his wife returned to work, he was often anxious: "What would happen to me? I didn't want to watch the TV soaps and go stupid, so I went out and bought a copy of the *Wall Street Journal* and it helped."

Since that time, Mr. N. continues to "read" his daughter well. He feeds her in his own fashion and, like most of the fathers in the first group, does not depend on a mental image of "what my wife would do" to guide him in the care of Nina.

Initially, he experienced some guilt about his successful parenting of his daughter, and would attempt to "back off" whenever his wife returned from work. Nina, however, usually responded instantly to such withdrawal, and would fret or whine plaintively while he was trying to prepare dinner.

Mr. N. takes much pride in Nina and he being "very much alike." He reports that his sister-in-law describes them as being like twins, "both crazy," referring to a shared, mildly hypo-manic personality style that leads them both to prefer intense levels of social interaction.

Nina's mother, unlike the majority of the mothers in the study, had chosen not to breast-feed and returned to work after 12 weeks. She described her husband as a "softee," reporting that *she* had to help her daughter end a sleep disturbance at 9 months, by insisting that Nina "cry it out in bed."

Mr. N. spontaneously reported that he has felt more accept-ed and valued by his family of origin since he has fathered this infant. His own father, of whom he remembers little, had died in a trucking accident when he was 6 years of age. He had been unable to visit his father's grave for 17 years until he took Nina one afternoon to the cemetery to "introduce them."

At the time of the developmental testing, Nina, then 11 months old, was a vigorous, bright-eyed, smiling, well-scrubbed little girl who leaned forward immediately from her father's arms to examine my moustache, which bore some likeness to her father's. She looked back and forth between the two faces for a moment, looked at the door to the examining room, and ordered a peremptory "Go." She came to the testing room with no hesitation, clearly expecting and trusting to be dealt with amiably. She squirmed out of her father's arms onto the floor, as soon as she got next to the examining high chair. Though 44 weeks at the time of the testing, she exhibited a 52- to 56-week profile in her personal-social and language functions. She would clap her hands in an excited fashion, breaking into a broad smile whenever she successfully achieved a testing item. Her adaptive skills were equally advanced, but it was her play that was most precocious, exhibiting a broad range of skills with the unfamiliar toys presented to her in the testing situation.

CASE 2

Mr. M., 27, and Mrs. M., 25, had been married for 4 years and felt that if they did not have a child soon, they might never be parents. Mr. M. was ready first, while his wife was anxious because she felt that, unlike her own mother, she would not be a "good enough mother." Nevertheless, they comforted one another through the conception process. Their daughter Mary, weighing 2300 grams, was born 4 weeks early, after a difficult final trimester characterized by mild toxemia and a sleep disturbance in the mother, caused by repetitive nightmares about the baby. During this same time, Mr. M. was also dreaming about having a baby, but was uncomfortable about telling his wife about his dreams because they were pleasant. He reported a significant increase in his daily milk consumption early in the second trimester (also reported by 4 of the 9 fathers in the first group). He had looked forward most of his life to being a father, "or at least to being *there*" more than his career military officer father had been for him. He had always found himself interested in, and drawn to, young children. His career is in fact in a field related to pediatric health care delivery.

Mrs. M., a school nurse, was quite devoted to her career. They decided early in the pregnancy that because of Mr. M.'s more flexible work schedule, he would be responsible for most of the child care during the week, and that they would split the care of their daughter on weekends.

Mr. M.'s feeling when he first saw his daughter was that she was "perfect in every way" (even though she had some mild neonatal jaundice). She was born in the summer, and the mother had 6 weeks before she was to return to work. During that time, Mr. M. felt that "he was the play machine" and his wife was "the milk machine." Mrs. M., like the majority of mothers in both groups, continued to breast-feed whenever possible after she had returned to work.

Even prior to the mother's return, the father felt that his daughter was becoming "his." Mary had first smiled for him, and fed more easily and completely for him. Both he and his wife felt that their daughter "worked harder for him at eating." By the fifth month, the mother commented, "You are more like brother and sister than father and daughter." She remarked that they were "both morning people," and seemed to have almost identical eating cycles and sleep patterns. During the summer and school vacations, Mrs. M. increased the amount of time she spent with Mary, while Mr. M. purposefully tried to distance himself from his daughter. He was often troubled during such times by an unwelcome envy of his wife's nurturing of Mary, preferring the image of a wife who remained a working, competent, "more interesting person." He reported that often his erotic attraction to his wife lessened when he withdrew to the position of secondary parent, and that when she did return to work, it was as though "she became more sexy to me."

Mr. M. was among the 4 fathers in both groups who reported that they had begun on occasion to find themselves sitting down to urinate. It seemed that such a pattern began as a necessity, because holding an infant in one's arms impedes accurate elimination into the toilet bowl. However, this "habit" still lingered on for several months after their babies had become quite mobile.[2]

At 10 months, when Mrs. M. had to end one of the joint-nurturing periods because of the resumption of school, Mary began clutching one of her mother's hair curlers day and night. Within 36 hours of the mother's return to work, Mary returned to primarily choosing the father for comfort or need fulfillment. Although the mother was troubled by the clarity and force of this return to the father, she was comforted by the ease with which her daughter and husband related, as it evoked pleasant memories of her relationship with her own father.

Mrs. M. noted other gradually emerging similarities between her husband and daughter, besides their being "morning people." They enjoyed similar musical styles, had like tastes in food, and had certain body movements in common. Such observations raised the possibility that they had begun to achieve a kind of biorhythmic synchrony, a phenomenon I shall examine later.

On developmental assessment, Mary, though a premature infant, demonstrated at 10 months a skill with the manipulation of the test items more appropriate for a 12-month-old child. She was walking competently, and there was a tenaciousness to her curiosity. She exhibited a pleasure-filled drive toward the more novel materials which riveted her attention. Striking attributes of this little girl were her visual acuity and her intense

2. James Herzog (personal communication) reports the same finding in his own clinical investigation of fathers of young infants.

interest in the visual details of the environment around her, qualities highly valued by both her parents.

CASE 3

The final case vignette is a brief description of the follow-up of a now 19-month-old male toddler who continues in the same father-mother care pattern established at the third week of life. The mother works full-time as a court clerk, and the father as a sign painter out of the studio in his home.

Henry's mother describes him as growing up "much too fast." At follow-up, he was no longer being breast-fed. Henry had weaned himself at 10 months when the mother "shrieked when he bit down hard on my nipple. We both sat there looking at each other, stunned and horrified, but that was the last time he would ever take the breast." Henry has continued to develop vigorously, in the same precocious pattern which had been obvious in his previous testing, only now his language was even more highly developed. His parents described him as using his father as the primary source of nurturance and "fueling," to borrow Mahler's term, and turning exclusively to his father when tired or distressed.

At the time of Henry's first developmental assessment, I observed Henry then 8 months and his father taking a meal together. I shall describe it in some detail, because it is representative of the reciprocity most of the father-infant pairs had achieved. Henry sat next to his father in his high chair, feeding himself with his fingers proudly, if exhibitionistically, from the high-chair tray. A game evolved in which he would wait for his father to raise food to his own mouth before Henry would follow suit with his food. He stayed in touch with his father vocally as well, by humming as he chewed, pausing only when his father conversed with him. Henry would respond with a "Dada, Dada" when his father would "chit-chat" during the meal. When he was finished with his finger meal, Henry held his arms up in anticipation of being picked up by his father and held for the bottle portion of the feeding. He nestled quickly against his father's chest, and sucked vigorously on his bottle, maintaining an intense, almost longing eye contact with his father for a few moments. He then felt for his father's hand, transferred the bottle into it, and began looking about the room while exploring his father's shirt buttons or face. His father followed his gaze and spontaneously labeled and named the objects at which he assumed Henry was looking. Henry would "coo" responsively between swallows until sated. He ended the feeding himself by pushing the bottle away and struggling to sit up. His father agreed that dinner was over and put Henry down, who then crawled off to investigate the observer.

When I saw Henry again for the first time after an additional 11 months, he was carrying a stuffed kangaroo under one arm, and a fluffy elephant under the other as he toddled animatedly about his new house. I was informed by his father that these were his constant companions since the summer vacation had ended a month previously. The animals are less in evidence on the weekends, when both parents are home together. On such weekends he tends to wander around the house in his father's shadow, and will ask "Mommy, Whazzat?" whenever he hears a noise in another part of the house obviously made by his mother. When he is in his mother's company, he will not ask about his father's presence in the reverse circumstance. Though the family had just moved into new living quarters, Henry and the father had adjusted easily and had anticipated the move with pleasure. There was little of the regression usually seen at such disruptions of the typical environment in children of this age. The mother described herself as adapting less well to the change, feeling depressed about leaving their old home.

Just prior to the move it seemed that, though Henry spent the bulk of his time with his father, he had begun to prefer his mother, and more or less to disregard his father unless distressed. At those times, he would climb onto his father's lap, resting quietly against him, and then, when satisfied, toddle off in an exploring fashion to do something with his mother. Could the mother be emerging as an important figure in helping to lead the child out of an intimate, symbiotic tie with the father? Did the possession of two transitional objects, a kangaroo and an elephant, indicate the blessing or the curse of having two parents so committed to one's well-being?

DISCUSSION

"Engrossment" clearly falls short of describing what these men feel for their infants. Greenberg and Morris (1974) use this word to describe the sense of "absorption, preoccupation and interest by the father in the new infant," but it is shallow and wanting in the context of these descriptions. Instead, there seems to be more active and encompassing incorporation of these infants into the psychic life and structures of these men. There appears to be a very literal "taking in" of these babies by the fathers as a profound psychological event, metaphorically analogous to the physiologic incorporation by the mother of her growing fetus.

The fathers themselves often had difficulty believing that they had become so immensely significent to their own infants. A 4-month-old female in the first group stopped eating for two days and developed a week-long sleep disturbance after her father had shaved off his beard. She became irritable and inconsolable and avoided her father's gaze when he attempted to comfort her. She would accept her mother's presence and comforting, but only briefly. It was only after a neighbor had failed to recognize him outside his apartment that it occurred to him that this might be the source of his daughter's distress.

The finding of a prevalence of absent grandfathers in both groups suggests that some of these fathers' attachment to their infants may be abetted by the wish to repair some their own perceived paternal nurturing deficits through active mastery. Jacobson (1950) says that a man's "readiness to assume the responsibility of a father [is] based on identifications with his own father" (p. 144).

The nurturant role itself, however, seems most clearly rooted in the father's identification with his mother, not his father. Such involvement through *actively* caring for the baby seems rooted in a comfortable identification with his own nurturing mother. The *passive* identification with the loved infant, obvious when Mr. M. speaks of Mary becoming "his," may ease or aid resolution of the father's disappointment and grief over *his* own father's nonnurturance.

Although father absence or remoteness certainly promotes identification with the mother, it seems unnecessary to invoke a neurotic explanation regarding these fathers' choices. Such choices do, however, seem more strongly fueled by maternal than paternal identification. In fact, the bulk of the clinical material suggests an increasing comfort over time in the identification with their own fathers, as these men internalize and master their primary nurturing roles. The competitive envy of their wives' ability to breast-feed that afflicted some of the fathers may stem more from breast, rather than womb, envy, as the maternal *role* is coveted, not its organs.

Though it has been suggested that these fathers represent a highly select population, I think that there may be something rather idiosyncratic about the marriages themselves. It seems as unique for the mother to yield the primary nurturing role in these couples as it does for the father to assume it. A fertile area of future inquiry lies in the motivation of such a decision by these women, and their own sources of nurturant identifications. How and why have they decided to relinquish the destined traditional role? Do these couples in fact choose each other because of what they intuit about their nurturing qualities?

Most of the families began life with their infants with a 4- to 6-week period in which the mother was often the primary, or at least coequal, caretaker of the infant. The mothers would then typically return to work or career. Are these fathers so deeply attached to their infants (and vice versa) because they are the ones who have never really left their infants? Interestingly, it is during the same time span, around the second month of life, that the fathers may benefit from, or feel attracted by, a general "biodevelopmental shift," described by Emde (1980), who says:

> This shift involves attentiveness, orienting, reflex changes, and encephalographic alterations that permit increasing periods of time in quiet, alert states. Though endogenous smiling may begin prior to 6 weeks, it is now joined by exogenous (elicited by external stimulation) smiling. Such basic physiologic beginnings may now be seen as the precursors to psychosocial organization. Indeed, the biodevelopmental shift itself is a sign that

a new "organizer" has taken hold, heralding that *affect* can serve an increasing role in conscious social regulation [p. 91; my italics].

Inadvertently, the prevalent informal maternity-leave arrangements unwittingly, but decisively, brought the father into the infant's life at this critical biodevelopmental period.

Such early primary father-infant attachment seems to be more than the fruit of respite from parent duty in the first 6 weeks. In a recent study of Caesarian section–delivered infants where the father was more deeply involved in early attachment behavior than the mother, Field and Widmayer (1980) found that the father was closer to, and had a more positive view of, the infant's personality. These fathers also demonstrated a greater range of caregiving activities and more flexible responsiveness to distress than the fathers of vaginally delivered infants.

Well into the second year of the study, I continue to find no evidence, though the majority of both groups is still young psychosexually, that the gender identity of these children is in any way in jeopardy, nor have I found any evidence to support contentions reported elsewhere that the fathers' sexual identifications are compromised. To wit: in a controversial Australian study, Russell (1978) reported that deeply involved fathers of preschoolers were more "feminine" than traditional fathers, whereas their spouses tended to be more "masculine" than more traditional mothers. Though ready access to unconscious material is necessarily limited by the method of data collection in this study, I saw no evidence, manifest or covert, of any deviance in gender identity. Nevertheless, it may be postulated that primary caregiving fathers may have less fully "disidentified with mother" (Greenson, 1968) in establishing their own masculine identity. In addition, though it is now more socially acceptable for a father to raise his babies, this practice is still a somewhat aberrant custom carried out by a small minority, and protest does appear inherent in such choices. If it does, what is the protest, and does it matter to the child and his or her development?

Unlike the fathers described by Lamb (1976) and others,

these men show no special or exclusive interest in the sexual
differentiation or stereotyping of their infants. We may speculate that when given the opportunity, true empathic nurturing
eclipses that more peripheral role assigned or allowed the sup-
plementary father. Alternately, will the absence of this role as
clear sexual differentiator, so often assigned to the father, pass
to the mother? And if so, or if not, what will the implications be
for oedipal resolutions later in life?

Those children from the first group now old enough to be
engaged in the separation-individuation struggles of the second year of life evidence other intriguing patterns. Of the original 9, 5 of the fathers still are the primary caretakers, although
some are now supplementing the care of their children with
various combinations of day or child care. Henry was more rule
than exception, as the mothers seem to be beginning to fulfill
the role of "uncontaminated other" as Mahler et al. (1955,
1975) call the supplemental parent fathers in their description
of the resolution of the rapprochement crisis. For Henry and
his colleagues, it seems that it is the *mother* who may serve the
critical role of helping the child relinquish the early symbiotic
unity with the father. Abelin (1980) describes the father in the
classic rapprochement resolution as "the knight in shining armor beckoning from outside the symbiotic orbit" (p. 152). Instead, do these children experience the mother as the "queen in
flowing raiment" beckoning from outside the father-infant
symbiotic orbit?

On the basis of these clinical descriptions it is reasonable to
speculate that these father-infant pairs may evidence a kind of
biorhythmic synchrony that is reminiscent of the psychobiological rhythmicity described by Sander (1969) in his study of
mother-infant pairs. Greenacre (1966) reminds us that "the
father . . . is never as close and constant in bodily relationship
with the young infant as the mother . . . must be. Nature has
seen to that" (p. 747). Although the mother's body may have
been the original prenatal metronome, these infants seem to
have increased their repetoire to include a rhythmic synchrony,
or cadence, with the father's body as well. Does this suggest that
there is an innate potential in *all* human beings regardless of
gender identity to establish such intimate reciprocity in and
through the nurturing of one's own infant?

Within each group, some objective aspects of development and behavior were compared to help formulate further research questions. Even though no statistically valid conclusions could be drawn because of the very small sample size, some observable differences between male and female infants were noted. Five pairs of infants and pretoddlers were roughly matched for age and socioeconomic grouping and data collected in four developmental categories: (1) Reaction to separation from the father. Here girls tended to protest affectively, both behaviorally and verbally, somewhat earlier (6 to 10 weeks earlier) than boys.[3] Might this lead us to speculate that fathers tend to bind their daughters to them more tightly than their sons, experiencing them as less rivalrous, but also as identified with the father's wife-lover? (2) Reaction to strangers. The reverse held in this comparison, with the boys showing clear reaction to the approach of strangers at a somewhat earlier age than girls (4 to 8 weeks earlier). Interestingly, none of the children was described by their parents as being *afraid* of strangers— "interested," "curious," "subdued," "cautious," but never fearful. (3) Developmental milestones. No significant differences were described. (4) Overall levels of activity-motility. Again, no appreciable differences were noted.

CONCLUSIONS

I summarize what can be said on the basis of the observations made in this study: (1) Children raised primarily by men can be vigorous, competent, and thriving infants who may be especially comfortable with and interested in stimulation from the external environment. (2) These men are capable of forming the intense reciprocal nurturing attachments so critical in the early life of the thriving human organism. (3) The choice and the style of caretaking are drawn from deep within the father's own adaptive narcissistic wish to nurture and be nur-

---

3. Hide-and-seek games, the ritualized rehearsal for separation mastery, was, not surprisingly, initiated with the fathers, and played most intently, though not exclusively, with them. Greenacre (1966) describes this as the child "dosing himself and her [mother (father)] with his needs for separateness" (p. 748).

tured, and the derived style is not merely that of a mother substitute, "wife-mirror," or *in loco matris*. (4) The father's nurturing style is a distillate of selected identifications and disidentifications with the important objects in his own life. Such nurturing capacities do not, therefore, seem to be wholly determined by genetic endowment or gender identity.

Yet many of the questions in this study beg further inquiry. One of the more intriguing questions raised by the assessment of the infants is why these babies are developing so well. Most of the babies seemed to have a heightened appetite for novel experience and stimuli. Need we invoke a particular style of care and interaction common to such father-infant dyads, for example, "robust and stimulating," to explain these findings? Or is this merely the male counterpart to what Escalona (1963) describes in her discussions of maternal style as the "active mother-active infant" dimorphism? Or is it the libidinal commitment by *two* parents instead of one and a quarter, or one and a half to the infant's well-being and growth (e.g., the majority of mothers breast-fed, often at great inconvenience to themselves)?

Or does such parenting carry an extra valence because, unlike the mother's, it has not been the father's lifelong role identity or expectation to nurture, raise, and take responsibility for his baby? Instead it is a choice, not a fate, which can inherently be presumably *un*chosen as well, without the self-devaluing denial of a lifelong role expectation.

As a conscious choice, it of course implies an integration of deeper libidinal currents with more superficial, cognitive constructs. One toddler in the first group was observed to deal with this embarrassment of nurturing riches by wandering into the living room after dinner with her blanket; after careful scrutiny of both mother and father, she declared, "I want you" as if to announce the resolution of some internal debate, and crawled into her father's lap.

From this tentative perch, the long-range impact on the infants can hardly be divined, yet there are hints at some important benefits. The more democratic or shared the rearing, the broader the flexibility and range of subsequent object choice offered such children. The fluidity of the important objects certainly must offer the ego a wider range of acceptable choices, identifications, and pleasurable interchanges. It remains to be corroborated by further research whether such fluidity outweighs the loyalty conflicts in choosing among important objects, as demonstrated by the blanket-toting toddler described above.

A subtle either/or dichotomy about who in particular serves as the primary love object seems to drift into discussion of such material which can distract us from the more complex theoretical questions inherent in this investigation. Do these babies thrive because of an unusually rich, fertile mosaic between primary and secondary love objects? Does the ego harbor as one of its autonomous functions a kind of integrating mechanism which permits a successful mosaicism? The majority of infants in this investigation seem to have mastered the integration of these different attachments to the primary love objects in a way that enhances their overall competence.

Finally, there is obviously a great distance to go in understanding and articulating the factors that are at work in these immensely complex relationships. It is safe to say, however, from this vantage point that our more traditional ways of understanding why fathers become involved with their infants seem both shallow and simplistic in the face of these families' stories. "Womb envy," "the urge to create," "the wish for immortality," as sole or primary motivations for such fathers would not provide the libidinal fuel to carry a father through the second week of 4 A.M. feedings, to say nothing of colic or diarrhea. The beginning evidence instead portrays an exquisite reciprocity of such attachment with their infants and toddlers. It seems, after all, the child *is* father to the man, and maybe the mother as well.

BIBLIOGRAPHY

ABELIN, E. L. (1980), Triangulation. In *Rapprochement*, ed. R. Lacks, S. Bach, & E. J. Burland. New York: Aronson, pp. 151–169.
BILLER, H. B. (1974), *Paternal Deprivation*. Lexington, Mass.: Heath.
BLOCH, R. (1978), American feminine ideals in transition. *Feminist Stud.*, 4:101–126.

BRAZELTON, T. B., ET AL. (1979), The infant as a focus for family reciprocity. In *The Child and Its Family*, ed. M. Lewis & L. A. Rosenblum. New York: Plenum, pp. 62–80.

BURLINGHAM, D. (1973), The preoedipal infant-father relationship. *Psychoanal. Study Child*, 28:23–48.

CATH, S. H., GURWITT, A. R., & ROSS, J. M., eds. (1982), *Father and Child*. Boston: Little, Brown.

EMDE, R. N. (1980), Toward a psychoanalytic theory of affect. In *The Course of Life*, ed. S. I. Greenspan & G. H. Pollock. Washington: N.I.M.H., 1:63–113.

ESCALONA, S. K. (1963), Patterns of infantile experience and the developmental process. *Psychoanal. Study Child*, 18:197–244.

FERHOLT, J. & GURWITT, A. R. (1982), Involving fathers in treatment. In Cath et al. (1982), pp. 557–568.

FIELD, T. (1978), Interaction behaviors of primary vs. secondary caretakers fathers. *Develpm. Psychol.*, 14:183–184.

——— & WIDMAYER, S. (1980), Developmental follow-up of infants delivered by Caesarian section and general anesthesia. *Infant Behav. & Develpm.* 3:253–264.

FRODI, A. M. & LAMB, M. E. (1978), Sex differences and responsiveness to infants. *Child Develpm.*, 49:1182–1188.

GREENACRE, P. (1966), Problems of overidealization of the analyst and analysis. In *Emotional Growth*, 2:743–761. New York: Int. Univ. Press, 1971.

GREENBERG, M. & MORRIS, M. (1974), Engrossment. *Amer. J. Orthpsychiat.*, 44:520–531.

GREENSON, R. R. (1968), Disidentifying from mother. *Int. J. Psychoanal.*, 49:370–374.

GREENSPAN, S. I. (1980), Analysis of a five-and-a-half-year-old girl. *J. Amer. Psychoanal. Assn.*, 28:575–603.

GURWITT, A. R. (1976), Aspects of prospective fatherhood. *Psychoanal. Study Child*, 31:237–271.

HARLOW, H. F. (1958), The nature of love. *Amer. Psychologist*, 13:673–685.

JACOBSON, E. (1950), Development of the wish for a child in boys. *Psychoanal. Study Child*, 5:139–152.

KOTELCHUCK, M. (1976), The infant's relationship to the father. In *The Role of the Father in Child Development*, ed. M. E. Lamb. New York: Wiley, pp. 329–344.

——— ZELAZO, P. R., KAJAN, J., ET AL. (1975), Infant reactions to parental separations when left with familiar adults. *J. Gen. Psychol.*, 126:255–262.

LAMB, M. E. (1976), The role of the father. In *The Role of the Father in Child Development*, ed. M. E. Lamb. New York: Wiley 2nd ed., 1981, pp. 1–61.

——— (1981), Characteristics of maternal and paternal behavior in traditional and nontraditional Swedish families. *Int. J. Behav. Develpm.*, 5 (in press).

——— FRODI, A. M., ET AL. (1982), Varying degrees of paternal involvement in infant care. In *Parenting and Child Development,* ed. M. E. Lamb. Hillsdale, N.J.: Erlbaum, pp. 117–138.

LORENZ, K. (1966), *On Aggression.* London: Methuen.

MACCOBY, E. & JACKLIN, C. (1974), *The Psychology of Sex Differences.* Los Angeles: Stanford Univ. Press.

MCKEE, L. & O'BRIEN, M., eds. (1982), *The Father Figure.* London: Travistock Publications.

MAHLER, M. S. & GOSLINER, B. J. (1955), On symbiotic child psychosis. *Psychoanal. Study Child,* 10:195–212.

———— PINE, F., & BERGMAN, A. (1975), *The Psychological Birth of the Human Infant.* New York: Basic Books.

PARKE, R. (1979), Perspectives in father-infant interactions. In *Handbook of Infant Development,* ed. J. D. Osofsky. New York: Wiley, pp. 110–130.

———— & SAWIN, D. B. (1977), The family in early infancy. Read at Society for Research in Child Development, New Orleans.

———— ———— (1980), The family in early infancy. In *Father-Infant Relationship,* ed. F. A. Pedersen. New York: Praeger, pp. 44–70.

PEDERSEN, F. A., ANDERSON, B., & KAIN, R. (1980), Parent-infant and husband-wife interactions observed at five months. In *The Father-Infant Relationship,* ed. F. A. Pedersen. New York: Praeger, pp. 65–91.

RADIN, N. (1980), Child rearing fathers in intact families. Read at Conference on Fatherhood and Social Policy, Haifa.

RUSSELL, G. (1978), The father role and its relations to masculinity-femininity and androgeny. *Child Develpm.,* 49:1174–1181.

SANDER, L. W. (1969), Regulation and organization in the early infant-caretaker system. In *Brain and Early Behavior,* ed. R. Robinson. London: Academic Press, pp. 311–332.

YOGMAN, M. (1983), Development of the father-infant relationship. In *Fathers,* ed. H. Fitzgerald, B. Lester, & M. Yogman. New York: Plenum (in press).

———— DIXON, S., TRONICK, E., ALS, H., & BRAZELTON, T. B. (1977), The goals and structure of face-to-face interaction between infants and their fathers. Read at Society for Research and Child Development, New Orleans.

THE SIBLING EXPERIENCE

The first five papers in this section are expanded versions of a preliminary report of the Sibling Study Group,* of which Marianne Kris was a key member. They are based on presentations made at the Annual Meeting of the Association for Child Psychoanalysis, Boston, on March 28, 1980. The last paper, an independent study, demonstrates some of the vicissitudes of the sibling experience in adult life.

*The study was sponsored and funded by the Psychoanalytic Research and Development Fund.

The Sibling Experience

Introduction

ALBERT J. SOLNIT, M.D.

SYSTEMATIC CLINICAL STUDIES OF SIBLING EXPERIENCES have not been carried out with a focus on healthy or progressive development. Traditionally, in psychoanalysis, the advent of a younger child has been viewed as traumatic to the older sibling. Most of the reports regarding siblings, especially the psychoanalytic clinical studies, have placed the main emphasis on sibling rivalry and on the burdens to a first child when the second child enters the family. To some extent, as in most clinical research, the attention has been given to what is "noisy," i.e., what is associated with deprivation, conflict, or distortion; whereas those children who develop well and progressively are relatively "noiseless"; they do not demand or invite our clinical and theoretical scrutiny.

Utilizing data and theoretical propositions formulated during the Yale Longitudinal Study and the Psychoanalytic Study of a Family, we propose in these reports to examine the sibling experience with an emphasis on those aspects that promote growth and development. In order to provide a manageable frame of reference, we initially limited ourselves to a family with two children, 4 and 2 years of age. In this way we could identify assumptions, observations, and formulations some of which would be valid in principle for families with more than two siblings, with differing ordinal positions, and with a variety of age differences. At the same time, there will be differences

Sterling Professor of Pediatrics and Psychiatry, School of Medicine, and Director, Child Study Center, Yale University, New Haven, Ct.; faculty, Western New England Institute for Psychoanalysis.

associated with ages and numbers of siblings, as well as their respective ordinal positions that cannot be adequately accounted for by the focus of this report.

Even with only two siblings, there are four possible combinations of sexual differences and similarities (boy:boy, girl:girl, boy:girl, girl:boy). However, we concentrate more on what are the common threads shared by such siblings regardless of their biological, sexual differences.

Although we do not emphasize deviant sibling experiences, we are sharply aware that normative or development-promoting sibling experiences include a wide range of relationships and conflicts that constitute the vicissitudes of a progressive development. Thus, we describe and discuss the continuum of sibling companionship, rivalry, and socialization; and the envy, jealousy, and hatred between siblings as well as the resentment and reassurance that children feel when parents take good care of their siblings.

Our emphasis is placed on how the various sibling experiences contribute to each child's capacity to confront and resolve interpersonal, intrapsychic, and developmental hurdles and conflicts. In order to maintain a sharp focus we concentrate on situations in which there are two siblings with a largely healthy relationship. This, of course, implies predominantly positive parent-child and parent-parent relationships. It would be difficult, if not impossible, to maintain the focus of the study if important and deserved attention were given (as it can be in future reports) to situations in which there are more than two siblings; or to pathological sibling relationships; or to the differences best explained by the ordinal position of boys and girls in regard to age and sex. As Neubauer has suggested, "One can get lost in the large universe of the sibling experience."

By normative sibling experience we refer to the relationship between two children cared for and wanted by the same parents or parent in the same sociophysical environment. Usually, the siblings have the same biological parents and therefore each child has a unique genic makeup stemming from a common genetic pool. However, it is not the blood tie that determines the primary relationships of parents and children, or of siblings; rather it is the continuity of hour-to-hour, day-to-day experiences that form the interactional patterns of closeness, rivalry, collaboration, envy, admiration, and community of interests that characterize sibling experiences and the primary parent-child psychological relationships in which they are embedded.

Sibling experiences are always significantly shaped by two interacting, profound dynamic forces. Operating simultaneously and in influential, reverberating patterns, there is, first, the nature of the mutual relationships of parents and child; and second, the child's developmental capacities and preferences that are formative in sibling relationships and experiences. Whether expressed in rivalry or cooperation with, envy or admiration of, or by affection or hatred for the sibling, the nature of the parent-child relationship and the child's developmental level are two major intersecting axes along which to gauge and understand the quality of the sibling experience.

The parent-child relationships are expressed in terms of mutual attachments, identifications, and empathic resonances. The child's developmental level which plays its part in these relationships cannot be assessed or understood without our taking into account the sociocultural environmental context and interpersonal relations. In the absence of parents, sibling relationships are often the only abiding ones. Then they are more sustained and continuous than those of the children to specific adults. In such instances the sibling relationships must be protected and supported. Siblings left alone, as in war, natural catastrophe, or abandonment by parents, are often in high-risk situations since the sibling relationship is the most that is left for such children, even though it is not adequate by comparison to having a permanent adult caretaker. In these instances the sibling relationship is burdened with and challenged by tasks that belong to the dynamics of a child-adult relationship.

In noting this characteristic of sibling relationships, we also call attention to the signal importance of the community of interests and experiences shared by siblings. This points to the greater developmental closeness of siblings, and to the greater developmental distance between parents and children. Developmental distance refers to a wide range of tolerances and capacities, including levels of excitation, frustration, and conflicts as well as capacities for regulation, anticipation, planning, and adaptation. The developmental closeness of siblings enables them to play, fight, love, and compete in a manner that usually is protective because their physical, emotional, and intellectual strengths and weaknesses are more proportionally matched than are those of children and their parents. For a child to play, fight, love, and compete with an adult requires the adult to control and limit his or her strength, and as an auxiliary ego to lend such ego resources to the child in ways that promote the child's sense of safety, well-being, and identification with the adult. Since the child is born helpless, usually to parents expecting and wanting him or her, the child-parent bond is basic. The ties between siblings usually are viewed as derivative of this primary child-adult relationship.

These considerations also enabled us to formulate the concept of developmental distance and space, taking into account the relevance of partially shared developmental space. In our study we originally concentrated on 2-year-old and 4-year-old siblings because we wanted to focus on siblings who are close to each other in their developmental tasks, capacities, tolerances, and intolerances. When siblings are separated by more developmental space, they may be living in widely separated developmental epochs (e.g., a 2-year-old and his 9-year-old sibling). Such siblings may still have a closer community of interests than either of them has with an adult, but their ease in communicating, empathizing, and identifying with each other is not nearly as great as in siblings who are developmentally close to each other.

In this way we call attention to the significance of the developmental space between brothers and sisters as a major factor that normatively influences how the sibling experience is formed and unfolds.

In preparing these papers for publication, however, we have gone beyond this initially circumscribed scope. Each contributor raises questions and points to issues infrequently discussed in relation to the sibling experience. While we do not treat these problems extensively, they are meant to highlight areas and issues that require further exchanges of views and more intensive study.

The Psychoanalytic Literature on Siblings

ALICE B. COLONNA AND
LOTTIE M. NEWMAN

AT FIRST GLANCE THE PSYCHOANALYTIC LITERATURE ON SIB-
lings seems to be sparse. There are only very few papers in
which sibling appears in the title. In contrast to other important
topics, there has never been a panel or symposium on siblings.
Yet, Freud wrote a good deal about their importance—in his
case studies, dream analyses, and applied papers. It is therefore
especially surprising that "sibling" is not even mentioned in the
index of the *Standard Edition* (although Siberia is), nor is "birth
of sibling." "Brothers and sisters" and "relations between"
them have 5 entries. Nor do brothers, sisters, or siblings appear
in the indices of a large number of general texts on psychoanalysis.

In fact, Freud's discovery that intense hostile feelings between siblings are "far more frequent in childhood than the
unseeing eye of the adult observer can perceive" (1900, p. 252)
was quite momentous. It was part of what he discovered about
the child's inner world—the intensity of conflicting emotions.

I

In "Dreams of the Death of Persons of Whom One Is Fond,"
which Freud regarded as typical dreams (1900), he discussed

Alice Colonna is a research associate, Child Study Center, Yale University,
New Haven, Ct.; faculty, Western New England Institute for Psychoanalysis;
Lottie Newman is lecturer, Child Study Center, Yale University, New Haven,
Ct.

the relation of children to their brothers and sisters most extensively. He said, "Many people . . . , who love their brothers and sisters and would feel bereaved if they were to die, harbour evil wishes against them in their unconscious, dating from earlier times; and these are capable of being realized in dreams" (p. 251).

In his dream book as well as in many subsequent papers, he placed particular emphasis upon the feelings of the older child toward the new sibling. In the following passage, Freud points out how closely this discovery is linked to that of the oedipus complex.

> When other children appear on the scene the Oedipus complex is enlarged into a family complex. This, with fresh support from the egoistic sense of injury, gives grounds for receiving the new brothers or sisters with repugnance and for unhesitatingly getting rid of them by a wish. . . . A child who has been put into second place by the birth of a brother or sister and who is now for the first time almost isolated from his mother, does not easily forgive her this loss of place; feelings which in an adult would be described as greatly embittered arise in him and are often the basis of a permanent estrangement [1916–17, p. 333f.].

In *The Interpretation of Dreams,* Freud cites many examples of the hostility toward younger siblings, both from his own practice and observations as well as those supplied by others.[1] He repeatedly mentions the child who "was told that the stork had brought a new baby. He looked the new arrival up and down and then declared decisively: 'The stork can take him away again' . . . [Little Hans said firmly,] I don't *want* a baby sister!" (p. 251f.).

Freud gives several examples of the intensity of these hostile feelings, which usually take the form of death wishes. These exacerbate the child's reaction to the death of a sibling. In his paper on Leonardo (1910b), Freud makes several allusions to incidents in the life of Leonardo and Goethe in which the child experienced disruption and threat to closeness with his mother. Goethe, who in his recollection mentioned neither the birth nor the death of a younger brother, had a memory of having "slung crockery out of the window," which Freud explains as a "magi-

---

1. In footnotes added to subsequent editions.

cal act against a troublesome intruder" (p. 182f.).[2] This screen memory, he found, was common enough to serve almost as a universal, symbolic metaphor and was paralleled by other reactions patients showed at the death of a sibling.

While the trauma of the birth of a sibling was described in a number of cases, Freud also saw the resentments and hatreds that came from the younger to the older child. In a general way, what he learned from his patients gave him a picture of the inner life of children very different from the Victorian view of innocence and idealized love between siblings. As Freud (1900) portrayed it, "The elder child ill-treats the younger, maligns him and robs him of his toys; while the younger is consumed with impotent rage against the elder, envies and fears him, or meets his oppressor with the first stirrings of a love of liberty and a sense of justice" (p. 250). Elsewhere Freud (1916–17) cites Shaw's observation: "As a rule there is only one person an English girl hates more than she hates her mother; and that's her eldest sister" (p. 205).

Taking the existence of these early hostile and rivalrous feelings for granted, Freud proceeded to describe their vicissitudes. He linked them to character formation and neurogenesis. For example, in 1917 Freud described a patient who after the birth of a sibling at age 4 "became transformed into an obstinate, unmanageable boy, who perpetually provoked his mother's severity. Moreover, he never regained the right path" (p. 149).

He also traced out the impact of siblings on the child's relation to parents and their influence on later object choice, both normal and deviant.

In "A Child Is Being Beaten" (1919), the sibling relationship is examined from the aspect of the erotic masochistic fixation which may develop. In the female cases described,

> The child being beaten is never the one producing the phantasy, but is invariably another child, most often a brother or a sister if there is any. . . . '*My father is beating the child . . . whom I hate*' [p. 184f.].
>   If the child . . . is a younger brother or sister . . . it is de-

2. In 1917, Freud also discussed Goethe's childhood recollections and the fact that he did not mourn his brother.

spised as well as hated; yet it attracts to itself the share of affection which the blinded parents are always ready to give the youngest child, and this is a spectacle the sight of which cannot be avoided. One soon learns that being beaten, even if it does not hurt very much, signifies a deprivation of love and a humiliation. And many children who believed themselves securely enthroned in the unshakable affection of their parents have by a single blow been cast down from all the heavens of their imaginary omnipotence. The idea of the father beating this hateful child is therefore an agreeable one, quite apart from whether he has actually been seen doing so. It means: 'My father does not love this other child, *he loves only me*' [p. 187].

Freud (1922) also discusses how poor sibling relationships (which stem from problems in the mother-child situation) may form part of a homosexual development. He mentions

. . . several cases in which during early childhood impulses of jealousy, derived from the mother-complex and of very great intensity, arose [in a boy] against rivals, usually older brothers. This jealousy led to an exceedingly hostile and aggressive attitude towards these brothers which might sometimes reach the pitch of actual death-wishes, but which could not maintain themselves . . . these impulses yielded to repression and underwent a transformation, so that the rivals of the earlier period became the first homosexual love-objects . . . after a short phase of keen jealousy the rival became a love-object [p. 231f.].

Similarly, in the case of a homosexual woman, Freud (1920) refers to the way the patient displaced her oedipal feelings from her father to her older brother, toward whom in early childhood she had felt intense rivalry and penis envy. In her adolescence the birth of a younger male sibling had a profoundly disturbing effect on her sexual development, causing her to make the shift toward homosexual object choice.

Numerous other quotations could be cited to show that the older child experiences siblings as intruders. In the chapter on symbolism in dreams (1916–17, p. 153), they are referred to as small animals or vermin. On the one hand, these feelings are seen by Freud as representative of the child's egoistic and omnipotent state which needs to undergo many changes to reach adult maturity. On the other hand, Freud generally places great emphasis upon the fact that it is the way in which the individual deals with his conflicts, problems, and feelings that determines normality or neurosis in adulthood. Freud always assumes that civilized, mature adults have come to terms with their infantile wishes, though the price paid for it may be their suffering from a neurosis. Yet, that this is not an inevitable outcome is demonstrated in passages relating to the development of great writers and artists. Leonardo, for example, was able to sublimate his intense longings for his mother (whom he had to share with others) into a desire for knowledge and passion for research.

Freud repeatedly made it clear that curiosity stemmed essentially from the child's desire to find out where babies come from—a desire decisively stimulated by the arrival of a new sibling.

> The threat to the bases of a child's existence offered by the discovery or the suspicion of the arrival of a new baby and the fear that he may, as a result of it, cease to be cared for and loved, make him thoughtful and clear-sighted. And this history of the instinct's origin is in line with the fact that the first problem with which it deals is not the question of the distinction between the sexes but the riddle of where babies came from [1905, p. 194f.].

Freud's emphasis on these initially negative feelings to siblings and the fact that living with them is difficult may convey the impression that he believed there were disadvantages in a person's having siblings.[3] Apart from the intellectual stimulation mentioned above, however, Freud clearly described some other specific developmental advantages. For example, he points to the impetus which the arrival of a sibling may give to the girl's "maternal instincts" if the "gap in time is sufficiently long" (1900, p. 252). He suggests that a younger sibling may also provide stimulus, particularly for the girl, who needs a

3. This may be suggested by the frequently quoted passage in which Freud (1917) said that a man who "has been his mother's undisputed darling . . . retains throughout life the triumphant feeling, the confidence in success, which not seldom brings actual success along with it" (p. 156).

push to move away from her preoedipal desire for union with her mother and the wish to give her a baby. Disappointment of this wish plays an important part in enabling her to make this developmentally necessary turn away from the mother toward the father (1931, p. 239). Elsewhere Freud describes the changes which take place in this respect:

> As these brothers and sisters grow up, the boy's attitude to them undergoes very significant transformations. He may take his sister as a love-object by way of substitute for his faithless mother. Where there are several brothers, all of them courting a younger sister, situations of hostile rivalry, which are so important for later life, arise already in the nursery. A little girl may find in her elder brother a substitute for her father who no longer takes an affectionate interest in her as he did in her earliest years. Or she may take a younger sister as a substitute for the baby she had vainly wished for from her father [1916–17, p. 334].

In several places Freud referred to the mechanisms by which the child's negative reactions are transformed and linked them to specific phenomena. Examples of displacement and sublimation have already been cited. Reaction formations, reversals, and identifications are other important pathways leading to a sense of fairness, group feelings[4] and special justice.

> . . . for a long time nothing in the nature of . . . group feeling is to be observed in children. Something like it first grows up, in a nursery containing many children, out of the children's relation to their parents, and it does so as a reaction to the initial envy with which the elder child receives the younger one. The elder child would certainly like to put his successor jealously aside, to keep it away from the parents, and to rob it of all its privileges; but in the face of the fact that this younger child (like all that come later) is loved by the parents as much as

4. Similar mechanisms are responsible for clan feelings and may form the basis for the Ashanti rule that "your brother or your sister, you can deny them nothing" (Radcliffe-Brown and Forde, 1950, p. 275). The achievement of the prescription always to be available to one another, or other rules like it, may, on the one hand, be based on an identification with the mother's protective, indulgent stance and, on the other, be an extension of the individual's egoistic omnipotence to family, clan, or nation.

he himself is . . . , he is forced into identifying himself with the other children. So there grows up in the troop of children a communal or group feeling, which is then further developed at school. The first demand made by this reaction-formation is for justice, for equal treatment for all. . . . If one cannot be the favourite oneself, at all events nobody else shall be the favourite. This transformation—the replacing of jealousy by a group feeling in the nursery and classroom—might be considered improbable, if the same process could not later be observed again in other circumstances. . . . What appears later on in society in the shape of . . . 'group spirit' does not belie its derivation from what was originally envy. . . . Thus social feeling[5] is based upon the reversal of what was a hostile feeling into a positively-toned tie in the nature of an identification [1921, p. 119ff.].

He also elaborated (1914) on the way in which family life, with parents and siblings, serves as a kind of child-size arena for learning to function in the wider world to which earlier attitudes, though transformed, are carried over.[6]

For psycho-analysis has taught us that the individual's emotional attitudes to other people, which are of such extreme importance to his later behaviour, are already established at an unexpectedly early age. The nature and quality of the human child's relations to people of his own and the opposite sex have already been laid down in the first six years of his life. He may afterwards develop and transform them in certain directions, but he can no longer get rid of them. The people to whom he is in this way fixed are his parents and his brothers and sisters. All those whom he gets to know later become substitute figures for these first objects of his feelings. . . . These substitute figures can be classified from his point of view according as they are derived from what we call the 'imagos' of his father, his mother, his brothers and sisters, and so on. His later acquaintances are thus obliged to take over a kind of emotional

5. See also Freud (1923); "Even to-day the social feelings arise in the individual as a superstructure built upon impulses of jealous rivalry against his brothers and sisters" (p. 37).
6. Toman (1976) has used this idea for his statistical investigations of the influence of the sibling position on choice of partner and the success of marriages.

heritage; they encounter sympathies and antipathies to the production of which they themselves have contributed little. All of his later choices of friendship and love follow upon the basis of the memory-traces left behind by these first prototypes [p. 243].

In summary, Freud clearly described the importance of the sibling relationships, in several instances linking them to the oedipus complex. He described the initial envy, rivalry, and jealousy the older child feels when he or she is "displaced" in the mother's affections, but he also described the changes and transformations of these feelings and their impact on later relationships—both normal and pathological. Since so many of Freud's discoveries derived from his clinical observations of patients, it is not surprising that the emphasis on the role of siblings in the formation of neurosis seems to predominate.

II

Freud's discovery of early sibling rivalry inspired much research testing the validity of his findings. We single out just a few representative studies.

David Levy (1937) described extensive research objectively testing the intensity of the older child's anger and resentment toward the new baby. Levy offered the child toys which depict an older child observing an infant sibling at his mother's breast. The child's responses were recorded after the experimenter gave the stimulus words, "The mother must feed the baby." In another experimental group, phrases aimed at eliciting further hostility were spoken, such as "The nerve of that baby or nasty baby at my mother's breast." Elaborations of patterns depending on the age and development of the child were then observed as well as reaction formations, defenses against aggressive impulses, and the wish to be the baby. These findings dramatized the existence of sibling rivalry.

Several other studies investigate the effects of the birth of a sibling on the mother-child interaction (Taylor and Kogan, 1973; Dunn and Kendrick, 1980; Dunn et al., 1981; Kendrick and Dunn, 1982). They all conclude that marked changes in the interaction between mother and firstborn child occur after the birth of a sibling.

It was perhaps the evidence compiled by these studies as well as the analysts' own continuing efforts[7] that have been instrumental in changing child care practices. It is now commonplace for parents to prepare children for the arrival of new siblings, as the vast pediatric literature suggests, and to take a certain degree of jealousy and rivalry for granted.[8] While these changes have undoubtedly brought more candor and openness into the parent-child relationship, we do not know conclusively whether they have also materially influenced the sibling experience itself.[9]

III

Freud and psychoanalytic authors following him have been criticized for stressing only the negative aspects of the sibling experience. Bank and Kahn (1980) state that in Freud's case histories and writings most of his references to siblings are negative. In the case of the Wolf-Man, they contend, it was the sister who seemed to have a more negative impact than the parents: "It was she who first inspired his phobia of wolves by frightening him with picture books. It was she who seduced him sadistically, who rebuffed his sexual advances as he matured, who made him feel inferior because of her brilliance. And it was she who lorded over him the parents' tendency to shower her with attention and money" (p. 495). In the case of Little Hans, the authors regard the questions that Freud taught

7. For example, Mary O'Neil Hawkins (1946) and Buxbaum (1949) in publications written for parents. These attempts were so successful that only a few years later Fraiberg (1959) was concerned about "the right to sibling rivalry" being "so firmly entrenched in the modern family that parents show a tendency in their own behavior to protect those rights" rather than helping the child "find civilized solutions" (p. 280f.).

8. See, e.g., a study by Legg et al. (1974) on how a group of parents prepared their firstborns for siblings and on the coping mechanisms employed by the older children.

9. We have not come across a single case study in which the analyst reports whether or not his patient as a child was prepared for the arrival of a sibling.

Hans's father to ask as selectively pressing Hans toward the negative side of sibling ambivalence. They also state that "siblings in *Totem and Taboo* get along only because they are working out oedipal guilt" (p. 497). While some of the claims of these authors are exaggerated, especially that "Freud's own status as a sibling predisposed him to select only negative phenomena in the sibling relationship" (p. 497), their criticism is more applicable to the literature following Freud than to Freud himself.

In the work of Melanie Klein siblings are mainly objects which interfere with the intense enactment of possessive, introjective strivings directed toward the maternal person. Envy plays the major role in feelings toward siblings. For Winnicott, too, the sibling is of interest essentially in the child's fantasies and anxieties about being replaced.

Many of the early analysts made and recorded observations of their own children illustrating the intense negative reaction of the older to the birth of a sibling and confirming the existence of sibling rivalry. In addition, there are innumerable case studies associating the role of the birth of a sibling with the pathogenesis of the older child's neurosis. In many instances, a patient's symptomatic behavior appeared for the first time when a sibling was born or is traced back to this event. To document this statement would require a survey of all analytic case studies in which patients had siblings. It might in fact be more interesting to single out those case reports in which the birth of a sibling was not implicated in an adult patient's neurosogenesis.

The literature on child analysis, too, is replete with references to the traumatic impact of a sibling's birth and its link to a variety of disturbances and disorders. Lundberg (1970) described the extent to which the analysis of a 3-year-old was dominated by reactions to the birth of a sibling. This event was implicated in Little Hans's phobia as well as in that of Frankie (Bornstein, 1949). Sperling (1952) refers to the intensification of oral-sadistic impulses, severe sleep problems, and anorexia following the birth of a brother when her patient was 26 months old. And Bornstein (1953) presents the case of an obsessional child, whose fear of death developed shortly after the birth of her younger sister, the girl's "uncertainty and doubt in regard to life and death [being] the nucleus of her neurosis" (p. 314).

Gauthier (1960), who observed his own children, also refers to the birth of a sibling as a traumatic event, but he stresses the variety of ego mechanisms called into play in coping with this trauma and "the possibility for *growth* . . . and for formation of *character-traits*" (p. 84).

Nagera (1969) describes a more unusual reaction to the birth of a sibling. He mentions several children who responded to this event by creating an imaginary companion. One adult patient, the fifth of 7 children, converted his initial jealousy of his younger brothers into a fatherly attitude to them. While the younger brothers at first enjoyed his attention, they refused to be ordered around by him as they grew older. In his attempt to regain control and prevent the loss of his favorite brother, he once hit the latter in a "blind" rage and subsequently revived his imaginary companion brother fantasy, which he had first developed at 18 months when his next younger brother was born. From the age of 8 to 10 years his fantasied, now blind little brother never left his side.

Depending upon their findings in individual cases, analysts also attempted to show that the time at which a sibling is born is significant. It seems, however, that there is no ideal or best time, because almost all developmental phases have their special hazards. For example, Jacobson (1950) states that among her male patients, she found "an intense and persistent envy of female reproductive ability—an envy which is often disguised by a seemingly normal masculinity—only when a younger sibling had been born at the peak of their castration conflict" (p. 142). In the case she describes, moreover, the patient's overconcerned attitude to his own daughter is linked to the oversolicitous reactions to a sister born during this man's adolescence. Greenacre (1950) elaborates on the "Medea complex," which is noted when a younger sibling is born before the older child is 15 or 16 months of age (see also Greenacre's remarks in Symposium [1954, p. 39]). And Mahler (1966) points out that the birth of a sibling during the rapprochement phase greatly complicates the latter. She cites a child whose heightened ambivalence expressed itself in "pernicious withholding of feces. The 'baby-stool' equation seemed to be unequivocal in her behavior and in her verbal material" (p. 165). The degree to which a girl's penis envy and a boy's castration anxiety is intensified by the birth of an opposite-sexed sibling during the phallic phase is a well-accepted clinical finding.

The problems of younger siblings are most often referred to in terms of mutual sexual exploration and seduction experiences. While Freud had stressed the latter especially in his very early writings on hysteria, he regarded them as essentially traumatic influences. In contrast, Maria Bonaparte (1953) wrote that for a girl seduction by her older brother may have a beneficial effect, "applying a corrective to his sister's oedipal frustration, as well as teaching her to change her object and return to lovers of her own age, which is biologically desirable, since every succeeding generation must make its life together. In the same way, the sister, as a substitute for that unsatisfactory initiator into sexuality, the oedipal mother, may play an analogous part for her little brother" (p. 136).[10]

On the other hand, an analytic case report of brother-sister incest (lasting for 4 years) was presented by A. Reich, who viewed the incestuous relation as part of the patient's abnormal development and saw its origin in the chaotic social environment, the many sexual seductions to which her patient had been subjected as a child, and the little love she was given.

The question of the effect of sexual seduction was further gone into in the 1954 Symposium on "Problems of Infantile Neurosis." Discussing Greenacre's contribution, Anna Freud referred to the commonly held opinion that seductions are "harmless when they occur between partners who are on the same level of libidinal development. . . . It is different where a much younger child is exposed to sexual stimulation from a much older one. When this happens, the seducer only discharges his libidinal urge in a phase-specific form; the seduced one finds himself caught in a situation where the sexual re-

10. See also Ritvo (in Lindon, 1967). Experiments on the influence of siblings on the child's sexual development and sexual identity have been reviewed by Sutton-Smith and Rosenberg (1970).

sponse of which he is capable does not fit the sexual approach which has been made to him. Dr. Greenacre describes very convincingly how such events either hasten maturational processes or throw them into confusion" (p. 29).

In reply to Waelder who questioned whether seduction was damaging to the younger child, Anna Freud said that she felt "alarmed" when she saw "a helpless infant of the oral or anal stage who has to submit to the curiosity, the aggressions, and the sexual advances of an older child" (p. 62).

The usefulness of this view is borne out by a case presented by Paul Kramer (Panel, 1962). He relates a young man's compulsive masturbation, which utterly lacked satisfaction and only engendered intense guilt and shame, to "a traumatic history of sex play" with his 2-year-old sister (p. 95).[11]

Abend (1978) believes that the routinely encountered material of adult patients which indicates erotic interest of siblings in each other may not always be simply a more readily accessible derivative of incestuous wishes that are indistinguishable from the effects of the oedipus conflict. He describes two cases, both younger siblings, whose preference in love partners was influenced by an unconscious attachment to a sibling who had been exhibitionistic and seductive in early childhood. The object choices of both patients were made on the basis of resemblances to their siblings rather than to the opposite-sex parent.

Ritvo, too, comments on the influence of the sibling relationship on adult psychosexual functioning, but adds, "Although the family life of siblings prepares in many ways for marriage and the establishment of a new family, the unconscious revival and repetition in the marital relationship of intense conflicts [from childhood] . . . may be poorly adaptive and frequently are the bases of marital problems" (in Lindon, 1967, p. 25). Jacobson (1950) pointed to a specific problem that occurs when husband and wife become prospective parents. In both "infantile unconscious equations of the expected baby with . . . the sibling rivals may be revived and become the unconscious carrier of various narcissistic expectations and fears" (p. 145).

---

11. Lewin (1952) discusses the variety of ways in which "sister" may be represented in dreams and phobic symptoms.

While the influence of sibling position has been studied extensively, there are only scant references to the role of the number of siblings. Eissler (1963) points out that those who have many siblings only "gradually and after a long period of steady analytic work establish the exact sequence of siblings." When asked the number of children their parents had, such people reply by giving the number of their siblings. "This error is deeply rooted in the child's narcissism, but it also betrays an act of denying that the child is one among many" (p. 703).[12]

One sibling relationship has received very little attention—perhaps not only in the literature. There are no in-depth studies of the reactions of healthy children to their physically ill or handicapped siblings.[13] Colonna (1981) learned how blind children used their sighted siblings and often wondered about the impact this had on them. A physically ill or handicapped child usually requires special care and attention, and the healthy sibling is often enlisted to help or asked to show special consideration. We know that some mothers may concentrate their devotion on the ill child and neglect the healthy ones; others may turn away from the "damaged" child, who is boarded out as quickly as possible and hardly ever mentioned again. Thus, the attitude of the parents as well as the nature of the sibling's illness must influence the healthy brothers and sisters in special ways. Clearly, this is an area requiring further study.[14]

A series of papers examines the impact of the parents' pathology on two siblings who were in analysis at the Hampstead Clinic (Kennedy, 1978; Hurry, 1978; Sherick, 1978). Kennedy stresses that the effect of severe parental pathology on the de-

12. Could this be one of the reasons for the "omission" of siblings from so many analytic books?

13. Severe psychological pathology in siblings, on the other hand, has received attention. See the studies by Lidz et al. (1963, 1965) of siblings of schizophrenic patients.

14. The only papers we could find are by Bergmann and Wolfe (1971), Gath (1972), and Binger (1973). One special issue made possible by modern medicine has been investigated by Basch (1973). He describes some of the conflicts and reactions of patients who are the recipients of kidneys donated by their siblings. The emphasis is on the recipient, however, and not on the donor.

veloping child will depend on his or her sex, position in the family, and the particular role the child is assigned; and "that one sibling's intrapsychic perception of a sister/brother relationship can be rather different from that of the other" (p. 119). The older child's life was dominated by her being the "battleground and scapegoat" of both parents. She regarded her little brother primarily as a hated phallic usurper and rival, though she could at times be maternal toward him. "As he grew into a phallic boy she increasingly turned into the hostile, 'castrating' envious older sister that we have learned to recognize as a dangerous influence on the developing masculinity of a small boy" (Kennedy, p. 120). The younger sibling was frightened by his mother's outbursts of anger with his sister but also vicariously gratified by the punishment she received. He was the preferred child, but nevertheless envied her. In fantasy play he most often portrayed her as a "groany" older boy, perhaps because he recognized her penis envy.

The impact of parents on the sibling relationship is usually discussed in terms of favoritism, special preferences, and unconscious expectations of the parents for particular children. When siblings are discussed in relation to the parents, on the other hand, they are traditionally viewed as stand-ins for the parents—as objects to whom both positive and negative feelings are displaced and transferred, resulting in a "'double' of the oedipus complex" (Fenichel, 1931, p. 212). The issue of whether or not the sibling relationship is only a second edition of the relationship to the parents[15] does, of course, have a direct bearing on how sibling vs. parent transferences are viewed and interpreted in the analytic situation. We were amazed that we could not find a single paper dealing with siblings in the transference, though there are undoubtedly buried references to it in case reports. Nor, for that matter, did we come across papers dealing with "analytic" siblings. What one does find are reports of a patient showing interest in or being jealous of the analyst's other patients, which is usually interpreted as reflecting the

---

15. Some of the authors of the following papers in this volume question his view.

wish to be the only one. (This theme is of course mentioned frequently in the analyses of children.) But is this really all that can be said about sibling transferences?

An actual reversal of the parent-sibling relationship is pointed to by Rappaport (1958). He cites N. Lionel Blitzsten about the confusion created in children when grandparents live in the same household. "Then the grandparent is invested with the prerogative of the parent, while the real parent is relegated to the position of the child's older sibling" (p. 522).

Analysts have studied another real event that has an impact on the sibling experience—the loss of parents. Anna Freud and Sophie Dann's studies of concentration camp children (1951) demonstrate the drawing together and increased closeness of children raised together (see also Adams, 1981). Pollock (1972, 1978) has elaborated on aspects of loss both of parents and of siblings and discussed how this related to the creativity of well-known writers and artists. An early case report (Mason-Thompson, 1920) describes how the youngest of three sisters reversed her exaggerated affection for her older sister into violent hatred after their father's death when she was an adolescent. Shambaugh (1961) presents a case study of a latency boy whose jealousy of his younger sister became intensified after their mother's death. "She became a vehicle for expressing his own unacceptable affects as well as the target of his projected sense of guilt and blame" (p. 516). Most reports comparing the reactions of siblings to the death of a parent (Scharl, 1961; Barnes, 1964; Rochlin, 1965; Furman, 1974), however, stress the factors determining the differing reactions to this event but say very little about its influence on the sibling relationship itself.

In studies of partial loss of a parent following divorce, Judith Wallerstein found that siblings tended to support each other and that children with siblings adjusted better than only children. Heinicke and Wertheimer (1965), investigating temporary loss of parents, found that when siblings are placed together in a residential nursery, they will initially comfort each other. After a few days, however, "these sibling relationships do not fully meet the needs of the child, nor do they eliminate the hostile impulses" (p. 195).

Studies of sibling loss itself tend to emphasize the intensification of guilt. Musatti (1949) gives a clinical illustration of the way the child who gave up the position of the last-born to the newcomer gets it back after the brother's death.[16] Berman (1978) describes a case in which the death of a sibling in childhood organized a profound unconscious sense of guilt and a repetitive need for self-punishment, which also manifested themselves in the patient's analysis in the form of a negative therapeutic reaction. Hilgaard (1969) views some depressive and psychotic states as anniversary reactions to the death of siblings in childhood. Pollock (1970) discusses patients who replaced a sibling who had died prior to their birth. These children not only react to the overcompensatory safety measures usually instituted by their parents but also identify with their parents' guilt. And in a psychological study of the pioneer of modern archaeology, Niederland (1965) emphasizes sibling loss as one of the factors contributing to Schliemann's professional choice. He was born very shortly before the death of an older brother whose name he was given.

Greenacre (1959) presents a particularly interesting case of a little girl who lost her older brother when she was 14 months old. Although she was too young to understand, her behavior indicated that "she was probably missing the body contact with him," which she tried to re-create with a teddy bear, attempting "to animate the bear and convert him into the lost brother." After one of her father's absences, she was puzzled upon his return and addressed him by the name of the lost brother. When she was 3 years old she formed an intensive relationship with a younger sister who had been born in the meanwhile, making her a "captive audience." The younger child seemed "in a state of happy bondage." When a third sister was born, the oldest child, "who had gone through a season of elation in the reinforcement of herself in the applause of her sister, had again become a sober child" (p. 157f.).

16. Several contributors to studies of hospitalized children (Oremland and Oremland, 1973) suggest that siblings of dying children be allowed to visit them because the reality may be less overwhelming than their fantasies and private fears.

This vignette highlights not only the reactions to the death of a sibling, but stresses points rarely found in the literature: the changes in sibling relations and the enthralled reactions of younger siblings to their elder ones, as well as the loss the younger child experiences when the older one goes off to school. The middle girl had been inconsolable when she lost her playmate.

It is surely no coincidence that the reports that include loving companionship between siblings derive from observational rather than analytic case studies. For example, Balint (1963) describes his view of play between siblings:

> Where the age difference between two sisters is not very great, say about two years, as a rule it is the older sister who is openly feminine, usually somewhat narcissistic, whereas the younger sister has to develop more bisexually. If they sing, it is the elder who sings the melody in soprano and the younger who accompanies her either in mezzosoprano or contralto. If they dance, it is the elder who is the woman while the younger has to learn to dance both ways, like a woman and like a man. [Invariably the elder insisted upon playing the "Cinderella" role, while assigning that of Prince Charming to the younger] [p. 226f.].

Ritvo and Solnit (1958) mention a child's "highly advanced fantasy role play as one means of coping with the new sibling and the separation from the mother" (p. 70).

Mahler et al. (1975) give an interesting example of a 22-month-old boy whose mother had a difficult relationship with him. He benefited in many ways from the close tie to a brother 16 months older than himself. This and similar examples highlight instances in which the relationship between mother and child may contain severe pathology but in which siblings can gain some help from each other.[17]

Ritvo cites the example of a family of 4 girls in which the

---

17. In a Dialogue (1976) on "The Role of Family Life in Child Development," Peter Neubauer wondered whether a child would turn to a sibling when the parent is inadequate. Anna Geerts thought that the "absence of the mother with siblings of different sex, but close in age, increases rivalry and stimulates sex games between siblings as a substitute for masturbation" (p. 404).

younger 2 were twins. The parents, because of their neuroses, were unable to carry out their nurturing and protective functions. Each of the older sisters adopted one twin and stood in a parental relationship to them. He points out that here the older sibling was not only an object of displacement from the oedipal relationship but served as a substitute for the parent (in Lindon, 1967).

It was in fact Ritvo who most extensively discussed the positive aspects of the sibling relationship. He stressed that siblings can be an obvious source of enjoyment; they provide rich opportunities for elaboration of fantasy and discharge in mutual play; they stimulate each other in mutual learning and teaching.[18] To this E. J. Simburg (in Lindon, 1967) added that siblings form the model upon which other peer relations are based, a point first made by Freud in his letters to Fliess.

Recognizing the importance of the sibling relationship, Goldstein et al. (1979) stress the need for courts to "avoid separating siblings. Children raised together have a common background and experience that usually is characterized by companionship, rivalry, and mutual support in times of common threat or need. Staying together enables children to support each other by buffering the traumatic family breakup. It provides children with a sense of ongoing community, the continuity that strengthens them in coping with felt threats to future security and self-esteem, and with guilt feelings and associated defensive reactions" (p. 32).

In this context, the special closeness that twins develop should be mentioned. However, the numerous and important studies of twins have not been included in this survey because the special problems inherent in twinship require a review of their own.[19]

With the changes in theoretical formulations, psychoanalysts

18. Social siblings such as children raised in a kibbutz who share these common experiences usually not only show increased loyalties but also "a marked incest taboo" (Neubauer, 1965, p. 26).

19. Nor have we attempted to cover the papers or books in which analytic findings concerning siblings are applied to eminent writers (e.g., Eissler, 1963; Kiell, 1983), biblical figures (e.g., Grinberg, 1963) and other literary documents (e.g., Dalsimer, 1982).

have looked with greater interest at the impact of early experiences, identifications, and object relations on subsequent developmental phases, but the role of siblings during latency[20] and adolescence has not been specifically studied.

For instance, much has been written by analysts and nonanalysts concerning the development of cognitive functions during the latency years. The notion of family loyalties, values, and sense of fairness; ideas relating to past, present, and future—all take clearer forms during latency. This is also the period when relationships change and interests and skills are chosen. Yet the impact of the sibling experiences on these developments is hardly ever mentioned, except for an incidental reference by Frijling-Schreuder (1972) to the way in which one child may "forbid himself the field of interest which another sibling allows himself to develop and vice versa" (p. 187).

It is especially surprising that there is so little in the psychoanalytic literature on the role of siblings during adolescence. Even those who have most extensively written on adolescence (e.g., Blos, Erikson, Anna Freud) do not assign a specific role to the sibling relationship in adolescence and appear to view it as deriving solely from the relationship to the parents.[21]

This has been true of other analytic writers as well who throughout a patient's life cycle rarely view the sibling relationship as a genuine object relationship in its own right.[22] Yet, Erikson's (1950) concept of the life cycle as a continuum may provide some perspective on the ways sibling relations change during various phases in the life of the individual, for example, how they will be affected by the marital choices of each sibling,

20. It is of interest that in her classic papers on latency Bornstein (1951, 1953a) does not refer to the role of siblings.

21. So does Friend (1976), but he adds that the "sibling subsystem of adolescents appears [to be] more fluid than the adolescent of the adult recollection in analysis" (p. 382).

22. The imbalance in viewing the sibling relationship, however, has been corrected in some recent books by psychologists. Bank and Kahn (1982) include a chapter on the sibling twosome in adolescence and adulthood in their book on the sibling bond, in which they discuss sibling identifications and loyalties as well as bonds sustained by aggression. And Lamb and Sutton-Smith (1982) look at the sibling relationship across the life-span.

or the manner in which siblings share in the task of caring for their parents when this becomes a necessary reversal of the childhood situation.

SUMMARY

This survey has covered Freud's writings on the role of siblings; the research, mostly by analysts, stimulated by his views, and the changes in child-rearing practices inspired by them; and the writings of analysts since Freud. Our review has been selective rather than comprehensive in the attempt to highlight aspects which, though embedded in clinical experience, are infrequently focused upon.

Every analyst of both children and adults knows that siblings play an important role in the life of those who have them.[23] Many hours are devoted to this theme in the analyses of patients, but the literature does not accurately reflect this. Even though Freud described other aspects of the sibling relationship, the overwhelming emphasis in the psychoanalytic literature is on rivalry between them, the detrimental effect of the birth of a sibling as well as sex play and mutual seduction, and their role in symptom formation. Rarely is there any mention of the constructive role of siblings, of enjoying play with them, or of their closeness in childhood and later as adults. That conflictual aspects predominate in analytic case reports is expectable, but the relative neglect of the sibling experience as a topic deserving study in its own right is surprising. If one compares the extensive literature on the parent-child relationship, the role of early object relations, and the many reexaminations of the oedipus complex, for example, with the few papers focused directly on siblings, it becomes apparent that the reasons for this neglect require an explanation.

This report is submitted in the hope that once analysts are alerted to looking for the complex and positive elements and intricacies in the sibling experience, they will also report on cases where the sibling relationship was not directly implicated

---

23. Nor are the fantasies of only children about their lack of siblings insignificant (see especially Arlow, 1972).

in a patient's neurosis or where, after initially being involved in conflict, the rivalry and envy underwent important transformations into object love.

BIBLIOGRAPHY

ABEND, S. M. (1978), Sibling love and object choice. Abstr. *Psychoanal. Q.*, 47:660–661.
ADAMS, V. (1981), The sibling bond. *Psychol. Today*, June, pp. 32–47.
ARLOW, J. A. (1972), The only child. *Psychoanal. Q.*, 41:507–536.
BALINT, M. (1963), The younger sister and Prince Charming. *Int. J. Psychoanal.*, 44:226–227.
BANK, S. P. & KAHN, M. D. (1980), Freudian siblings. *Psychoanal. Rev.*, 67:493–504.
————— ————— (1982), *The Sibling Bond*. New York: Basic Books.
BARNES, M. J. (1964), Reactions to the death of a mother. *Psychoanal. Study Child*, 19:321–333.
BASCH, S. H. (1973), The intrapsychic integration of a new organ. *Psychoanal. Q.*, 42:364–384.
BERGMANN, T. & WOLFE, S. (1971), Observations of the reactions of healthy children to their chronically ill siblings. *Bull. Phila. Assn. Psychoanal.*, 21:145–161.
BERMAN, L. E. A. (1978), Sibling loss as an organizer of unconscious guilt. *Psychoanal. Q.*, 47:568–587.
BINGER, C. M. (1973), Childhood leukemia—emotional impact on siblings. In *The Child and His Family*, ed. E. J. Anthony & C. Koupernik. New York: Wiley, 2:195–211.
BLOS, P. (1962), *On Adolescence*. New York: Free Press.
BONAPARTE, M. (1953), *Female Sexuality*. New York: Int. Univ. Press.
BORNSTEIN, B. (1949), The analysis of a phobic child. *Psychoanal. Study Child*, 3/4:181–226.
————— (1951), On latency, *Psychoanal. Study Child*, 6:279–285.
————— (1953a), Masturbation in the latency period. *Psychoanal. Study Child*, 8:65–78.
————— (1953b), Fragment of an analysis of an obsessional child. *Psychoanal. Study Child*, 8:313–332.
BUXBAUM, E. (1949), *Your Child Makes Sense*. New York: Int. Univ. Press.
COLONNA, A. B. (1981), Success through their own efforts. *Psychoanal. Study Child*, 36:33–44.
DALSIMER, K. (1982), Female adolescent development. *Psychoanal. Study Child*, 37:487–522.
DIALOGUE (1976), The role of family life in child development. *Int. J. Psychoanal.*, 57:403–409.
DUNN, J. & KENDRICK, C. (1980), The arrival of a sibling. *J. Child Psychol. Psychiat.*, 21:119–132.

—— —— & MACNAMEE, R. (1981), The reaction of first-born children to the birth of a sibling. *J. Child Psychol. Psychiat.*, 22:1–18.

EISSLER, K. R. (1963), *Goethe.* Detroit: Wayne State Univ. Press.

ERIKSON, E. H. (1950), *Childhood and Society.* New York: Norton.

FENICHEL, O. (1931), Specific forms of the oedipus complex. In *Collected Papers*, 1:204–220. New York: Norton, 1953.

FRAIBERG, S. (1959), *The Magic Years.* New York: Scribner's.

FREUD, A. & DANN, S. (1951), an experiment in group upbringing. *Psychoanal. Study Child*, 6:127–168.

FREUD, S. (1900), The interpretation of dreams. *S.E.*, 4 & 5.

—— (1905), Three essays on the theory of sexuality. *S.E.*, 7:123–244.

—— (1910a), Five lectures on psycho-analysis. *S.E.*, 11:1–56.

—— (1910b), Leonardo da Vinci and a memory of his childhood. *S.E.*, 11:59–137.

—— (1914), Some reflections on schoolboy psychology. *S.E.*, 13:239–244.

—— (1916–17), Introductory lectures on psycho-analysis. *S.E.*, 15 & 16.

—— (1917), A childhood memory from *Dichtung und Wahrheit*. *S.E.*, 17:145–156.

—— (1919), 'A child is being beaten.' *S.E.*, 17:175–204.

—— (1920), The psychogenesis of a case of homosexuality in a woman. *S.E.*, 18:145–173.

—— (1921), Group psychology and the analysis of the ego. *S.E.*, 18:67–143.

—— (1922), Some neurotic mechanisms in jealousy, paranoia and homosexuality. *S.E.*, 18:221–232.

—— (1923), The ego and the id. *S.E.*, 19:3–66.

—— (1931), Female sexuality. *S.E.*, 21:221–243.

—— (1950), *The Origins of Psychoanalysis.* New York: Basic Books, 1954.

FRIEND, M. R. (1976), The role of family life in child development. *Int. J. Psychoanal.*, 57:373–384.

FRIJLING-SCHREUDER, E. C. N. (1972), The vicissitudes of aggression in normal development, in childhood neurosis, and in childhood psychosis. *Int. J. Psychoanal.*, 53:185–190.

FURMAN, E. (1974), *A Child's Parent Dies.* New Haven & London: Yale Univ. Press.

GATH, A. (1972), The mental health of siblings of congenitally abnormal children. *J. Child Psychol. Psychiat.*, 13:211–218.

GAUTHIER, Y. (1960), Observations on ego development. *Bull. Phila. Assn. Psychoanal.*, 10:69–85.

GOLDSTEIN, J., FREUD, A., & SOLNIT, A. J. (1979), *Before the Best Interests of the child.* New York: Free Press.

GREENACRE, P. (1950), Special problems of early female sexual development. *Psychoanal. Study Child.*, 5:122–138.

—— (1959), On focal symbiosis. In *Emotional Growth*, 1:145–161. New York: Int. Univ. Press, 1971.

GRINBERG, L. (1963), Rivalry and envy between Joseph and his brothers. *Samiksa*, 17:130–171.

HAWKINS, M. O'NEIL (1946), Jealousy and rivalry in brothers and sisters. *Child Study,* Summer, 103–105, 127.

HEINICKE, C. M. & WESTHEIMER, I. (1965), *Brief Separations.* New York: Int. Univ. Press.

HILGAARD, J. R. (1969), Depressive and psychotic states as anniversaries to sibling death in childhood. *Int. Psychiat. Clin.,* 6:197–211.

HURRY, A. (1978), The analytic treatment of two siblings. *Bull. Hampstead Clin.,* 1:121–134.

JACOBSON, E. (1950), Development of the wish for a child in boys. *Psychoanal. Study Child,* 5:139–152.

KENDRICK, C. & DUNN, J. (1982), Protest or pleasure? *J. Child Psychol. Psychiat.,* 23:117–129.

KENNEDY, H. (1978), The analytic treatment of two siblings. *Bull. Hampstead Clin.,* 1:119–120.

KIELL, N. (1983), *Blood Brothers.* New York: Int. Univ. Press.

KLEIN, M. (1961), *Narrative of a Child Analysis.* New York: Delta.

LAMB, M. E. & SUTTON-SMITH, B. (1982), *Sibling Relationships across the Life Span.* Hillsdale, N.J.: Erlbaum.

LEGG, C., SHERICK, I., & WADLAND, W. (1974), Reaction of preschool children to the birth of a sibling. *Child Psychiat. Hum. Develpm.,* 5:3–35.

LEVY, D. M. (1937), *Studies in Sibling Rivalry.* New York: American Orthopsychiatric Association.

LEWIN, B. D. (1952), Phobic symptoms and dream interpretation. *Psychoanal. Q.,* 21:295–322.

LIDZ, T., FLECK, S., ALANEN, Y. O., & CORNELISON, A. R. (1963), Schizophrenic patients and their siblings. *Psychiatry,* 26:1–18.

———— ———— & CORNELISON, A. R. (1965), *Schizophrenia and the Family.* New York: Int. Univ. Press.

LINDON, J. A., ed. (1967), A psychoanalytic view of the family. *Psychoanal. Forum,* 3:13–65.

LUNDBERG, S. (1979), Envy and despair in the life of a three-year-old. *Bull. Hampstead Clin.,* 2:3–15.

MAHLER, M. S. (1966), Notes on the development of basic moods. In *Psychoanalysis—A General Psychology,* ed. R. M. Loewenstein, L. M. Newman, M. Schur, & A. J. Solnit. New York: Int. Univ. Press, pp. 152–168.

———— PINE, F., & BERGMAN, A. (1975), *The Psychological Birth of the Human Infant.* New York: Basic Books.

MASON-THOMPSON, E. R. (1920), The relation of the elder sister to the development of the Electra complex. *Int. J. Psychoanal.,* 1:186–195.

MUSATTI, C. L. (1949), Death of a little brother. Abstr. *Int. J. Psychoanal.,* 30:196.

NAGERA, H. (1969), The imaginary companion. *Psychoanal. Study Child,* 24:165–196.

NEUBAUER, P. B., ed. (1965), *Children in Collectives.* Springfield, Ill.: Thomas

NIEDERLAND, W. G. (1965), An analytic inquiry into the life and work of Heinrich Schliemann. In *Drives, Affects, Behavior,* ed. M. Schur. New York: Int. Univ. Press, 2:369–398.

OREMLAND, E. K. & OREMLAND, J. D., eds. (1973), *The Effects of Hospitalization on Children*. Springfield, Ill.: Thomas.

PANEL (1962), Masturbation. I. M. Marcus, reporter. *J. Amer. Psychoanal. Assn.*, 10:91–101.

——— (1983), Psychoanalytic inferences concerning children of divorced parents. M. H. Etezady, reporter. *J. Amer. Psychoanal. Assn.*, 31:247–258.

POLLOCK, G. H. (1970), Anniversary reactions, trauma, and mourning. *Psychoanal. Q.*, 39:347–371.

——— (1972), Bertha Pappenheim's pathological mourning. *J. Amer. Psychoanal. Assn.*, 20:476–493.

——— (1978), Childhood sibling loss and creativity. *Annu. Psychoanal.*, 6:443–481.

RADCLIFFE-BROWN, A. R. & FORDE, D. (1950), *African Systems of Kinship and Marriage*. London, New York, & Toronto: Oxford Univ. Press.

RAPPAPORT, E. A. (1958), The grandparent syndrome. *Psychoanal. Q.*, 27:518–538.

REICH, A. (1932), Analysis of a case of brother-sister incest. In *Psychoanalytic Contributions*. New York: Int. Univ. Press, 1973, pp. 1–22.

RITVO, S. & SOLNIT, A. J. (1958), Influences of early mother-child interaction on identification processes. *Psychoanal. Study Child*, 13:64–91.

ROCHLIN, G. (1965), *Griefs and Discontents*. Boston: Little, Brown, pp. 51–53.

SCHARL, A. E. (1961), Regression and restitution in object loss. *Psychoanal. Study Child*, 16:471–480.

SHAMBAUGH, B. (1961), A study of loss reactions in a seven-year-old. *Psychoanal. Study Child*, 16:510–522.

SHERICK, I. (1978), The analytic treatment of two siblings. *Bull. Hampstead Clin.*, 1:135–146.

SPERLING, M. (1952), Animal phobias in a two-year-old child. *Psychoanal. Study Child*, 7:115–125.

SUTTON-SMITH, B. & ROSENBERG, B. G. (1970), *The Sibling*. New York: Holt, Rinehardt & Winston.

SYMPOSIUM (1954), Problems of infantile neurosis. *Psychoanal. Study Child*, 9:16–71.

TAYLOR, M. K. & KOGAN, L. I. (1973), Effects of birth of a sibling on mother-child interactions. *Child Psychiat. Hum. Develpm.*, 4:53–58.

TOMAN, W. (1969), *Family Constellation*. New York: Springer.

WINNICOTT, D. W. (1964), *The Child, the Family and the Outside World*. New York: Penguin.

Parents and Siblings

Their Mutual Influences

MARIANNE KRIS, M.D. AND SAMUEL RITVO, M.D.

THE SIBLING EXPERIENCE IS PART OF THE HUMAN INSTITU-
tion of the family. The family, in all its variations—nuclear,
extended, or alternative types—has biological roots in the infant's long period of dependence on the adult for survival, no
matter how active or competent the newborn may be. The
forces which hold the family together include rational or pragmatic ones as well as the powerful affective and psychological
ties which are intertwined with them. The latter, however, also
give content and intensity to the psychic conflicts within the
family. This is the setting in which the most enduring love ties
are formed and in which the most abiding hatreds arise.

If the family is to serve its socializing, adaptive function, it
must fulfill the same condition in both the sibling relationship
and the parent-child relationship, namely, the relationships
must be aim-inhibited in terms of the sexual and aggressive
drives. As Freud (1930) pointed out, one price paid for this
demand of civilization is repression and neurosis.

While the sibling experience is not essential for normal development and a significant portion of the population does not
have it, the psychic life of those who do have that experience is
profoundly influenced by it throughout their lifetime. The sib-

Dr. Kris was a senior research associate, Child Study Center, Yale Univer-
sity; faculty, New York Psychoanalytic Institute and Western New England
Institute for Psychoanalysis. Dr. Ritvo is Clinical Professor of Psychiatry,
Child Study Center, Yale University, New Haven, Ct.; faculty, Western New
England Institute for Psychoanalysis and New York Psychoanalytic Institute.

311

ling relationship contributes to characteristic qualities and features of the personality which may be both enriching and constricting.

The sibling relationship has two dimensions which need to be distinguished for purposes of study, though in actuality they are always interconnected and cannot be entirely separated. One dimension is the relationship of the siblings to each other as peers, the other is the relationship of the siblings in regard to the parent or parents. These complex, mutual relationships have an impact throughout the life cycle.

THE IMPACT OF PARENTS ON THEIR CHILDREN'S RELATIONSHIPS

No one doubts the crucial role of parents in influencing their children's interaction. From psychoanalytic clinical observations of children and adults and from direct observations of parents and children we have extensive knowledge of how parents convey their own expectations for how the siblings should relate to each other. Specific aspects of the children's experience with each other are colored by both the conscious and unconscious wishes and fantasies of their parents. These wishes and fantasies are communicated by suggestion and coercion, through words, gestures, facial expressions, encouragements, prohibitions, threats, rewards, and punishments. Parental behavior may operate to promote positive feelings and relationships between siblings or may foster difficulties between them. (Obviously, there are determinants other than the parents, too, the importance of which will differ in each individual situation.)

It is nearly universal for parents initially to harbor an idealized image of the future of the firstborn and later, when the second child is expected, of their children's future relationship with each other. This idealization is in conflict with a fear of the impending competitive demands of the children on them. Even under the best conditions, such an idealized fantasy must meet with disappointment. When there is pathology in the parent's personality, there will ensue a diminished capacity to cope with the disillusionment of the fantasy as well as with the increased reality demands. We usually see and focus on pathology more readily than on what we call "normal." Pathological situations may provoke the wish for change, whereas lack of symptomatology does not, and we therefore tend to spend little time with it. It is only in recent years that we have turned our full attention to normal development with all its variations and complexities. Freud, though, was always interested in normal development, constructing much of it from pathology.

When the firstborn has a good constitution, received appropriate nurturing, and has developed into a healthy 2-year-old, he or she will then be faced with many adaptive tasks. The motivation for tackling these tasks is provided in part by inner maturational needs and in part by environmental demands. If development is to proceed undisturbed, the child must receive a great deal of support from a positive relationship with the caretaker. The better the parents' ego capacities, the better will be their influence on the child's unfolding personality.

Until the time of the birth of the second child, the firstborn takes for granted, as his birthright, the caretaker's almost complete attention to him. When the second child has become a reality, everything changes. In fact, even during the pregnancy the firstborn already experiences disappointments regarding the diminution of full attention. The mother is frequently indisposed during the first months and less agile during the latter ones. Emotional reactions also play a part in the mother's withdrawal of attention from the child to her inner needs. At the same time, in a positive attempt to help, the mother usually tries as well as she can to prepare her child for the changes that will be brought about by the new baby. But a 2-year-old's capacity to understand or anticipate his or her feelings is very limited. Even if the child is older, these explanations leave the child much room for fantasies. After the baby's birth, the older child faces the painful reality that the time the mother has available for him or her is even more diminished. Furthermore, due to her fatigue following delivery, the mother's attention is diminished as well.

Viewed from the mother's side, her task is in many ways very difficult indeed. Her caretaking responsibilities not only are doubled, but are also complicated by the simultaneous and differing needs of her two children. In addition, the older child often regresses and naturally becomes more demanding and harder to satisfy than before. The mother often responds to these demands with irritability.

These external demands on the mother are augmented by an internal psychological dilemma that she has to deal with: will she be able to love two instead of one, and how will she manage to love them differently? Her capacity to resolve this problem is crucial for the future development of each of her children as well as for their future relationship with each other. This capacity is to a great extent determined by the mother's own childhood experiences with her parents and siblings.

If one looks at the other child and his new situation, one is bound to find that he will direct his negative reactions to the mother as well as to the newborn. Although the mother usually strives to remain constant in her love for the older child, this may still be doubted, especially and characteristically by the ambivalent 2-year-old, who may even go so far as to question whether he still is a member of the family. He may view the newborn as a replacement of himself and thereby become the outcast. The most frequent initial response of the older one is the suggestion to the mother quickly to get rid of "it." "It" does not yet belong to the human race, and is neither male nor female; "it" is only a nuisance.

One of the most common first responses of the parent to the older child's wish to get rid of the baby is a strong emotional "No!" This forceful "no" may be more significant than is usually recognized. If the "no," the negation of the child's suggestion, is pronounced by a parent with empathy for the other person—here the 2-year-old—the child can try to master the task of accepting the permanence of the baby's presence. The motivation for attempting this task lies in the firstborn's urgent desire to keep the mutually loving relationship with the mother. The parents may succeed in assuring the firstborn that in spite of his or her present negative feelings to the infant, who will be a permanent member of the family, the baby may eventually be even welcomed by him or her into the family.

In a less well-balanced parent, the "no" may be filled with aggressive overtones that can have a devastating effect on the child. Such a change, from the friendly parent to an aggressive one, is blamed not only on the parent but again to a considerable extent on the newcomer. This blame is then added to the child's original hostile feelings which had been caused by the experience of frustrating deprivation. This additional weight of reactive aggression may endanger the opportunity that usually exists for growth of positive feelings toward the younger one.

The parents' aim of a well-related sibling pair also can achieve fulfillment through the child's normal use of identification. The most important person with whom the child, even the little boy, identifies at that early stage is the mother. It is one of the most influential factors in this situation that the mother's behavior toward the baby serves as a model of identification for the older child. Clearly, it is necessary for the positive outcome of this identification that the mother possess the tenderness and sensitivity to the needs of the infant as well as to the first-born. If the older sibling succeeds in that step of identifying with the tender mother, the positive reaction from both parents will encourage him or her to further attempts of positive contact with the younger one. At first this "good behavior" will be due more to the need for approval from the parent than to real positive feelings for the baby. Nevertheless, it provides the foundation for other positive experiences which might derive from the direct interaction between the children and which can serve to build a more realistic positive relationship between them. For example, the older child frequently tries to make the baby smile and is highly pleased when he or she succeeds. The usual hero worship of the older child by the younger one gives gratification for a time to both siblings.

In addition to the direct aims of the parents to guide their children's mutual relationship, the quality of their nurturing of each individual child certainly also has an impact on the sibling relationship. Parental guidance in this respect ought to focus on the way the child's attitudes to himself, to the parents, as well as to outsiders develop. This task demands from the parent, in addition to the qualities mentioned before, the capacity for fairness in a deeper sense, which must be based, besides other factors, on a secure and stable self-image and healthy self-respect. These will enable the parent to provide each child with a similar inner setup and thereby facilitate respect for other persons, including the siblings. In addition, the parents' sense of fairness must rest on good reality testing, allowing them to perceive differences between people in general and, of course, between their children. The capacity for empathy will naturally enhance good reality testing. Moreover, flexibility must be available so that the parents can do justice to the many different situations they will encounter.

The parents' differentiated and selective partiality becomes even more important as the infant grows and with each new developmental achievement becomes increasingly capable of invading more areas that until then were the older's own domain. As much as the newborn must at first be protected against the older's unneutralized aggression, the situation is reversed with the advancing maturation of the baby. The older one now needs to know that his possessions—usually the goal of the younger one—and his or her place in the family is defended by the parents against the intrusion of the little one. We know how often the charm of the infant seduces the parents to excuse the aggression and destructive tendencies toward the older sibling. Yet, it is obvious that the infant must at that time begin to curb these still uncontrolled impulses. If the parents handle such situations properly, it helps each child to feel secure and enables each to turn an otherwise aggressive interaction into a more positive mutual experience.

The quality of fairness, as we have described it, must be distinguished from a tendency rigidly to equate every action in relation to "the children," which would to some degree negate their individuality or their difference in age and sex, as, for example, when parents ritualistically give the same toy to both children. If, for instance, there is reason to celebrate one child's achievement by a gift, such parents feel obliged to give a gift to the other child too and automatically give precisely the same to both. They might give a book, which would be a good present for the child who is interested in reading; the other child, then, will also get a book, although a ball might be more to his liking. In order to be "fair," it would not only have to be a book, but a book of the exact same size and price. It is not really the inappropriate gift itself but the parents' anxious attitude and defenses against their own sibling rivalry that make their action counterproductive. Instead of fulfilling their conscious aim to encourage the positive sibling relationship, such "equal" treatment leads to the opposite—it heightens sibling rivalry. One of the mothers in our longitudinal study expressed her reaction to the rigidity of her own mother very well, saying that she wanted to treat her own children as individuals. She would never do what *her* mother had done—to dress her and her older sister alike, as if they were twins. In reality, there are many factors that can distort the parents' impartiality to their children; for instance, a special positive or negative overattachment of the parents to *their* siblings, the quality of which may be transferred to their own children. For example, with the birth of a second child, a father quickly transferred his affection from the first child, originally the "apple of his eye," to the second. The first, now the *older* sister, became identified by him with his own, much hated older sister. Parents also may either reject or prefer a child because of his or her sex, an attitude which may increase the hostility between the children.

Another important quality of the parents that helps facilitate good sibling relationships is their relative freedom from ambivalence. Parents with basic problems of ambivalence readily cause similar disturbances in their children. In order to relieve their own inner tension, they may unconsciously split their conflicting feelings and project the now separated emotions to their children; as a result, one child is experienced as the good one and the other as bad. In such a case, we can well imagine the emotional reaction of each child and the outcome of their feelings for each other.

In addition, parents can be of great help to the siblings' relationship by stimulating the interests of their children in an informal way. For instance, one of the mothers in our longitudinal study, being artistically inclined, showed her children with genuine pleasure how to draw and paint. All three daughters, more or less gifted, developed enormous enjoyment in these activities. The best way for a parent to stimulate a child's interest is to choose an area which is libidinally cathected by the parent. This helps each child to sublimate drive energy as well as fosters good shared experiences, resulting in more generalized good feelings for and with each other.

Last, but not least, the quality of the relationship between the parental couple is of the greatest significance for the quality of the relationship between the siblings. Again, the modes of parental interaction form an important model for the children to follow. Feeling to some extent excluded from the parental closeness, the children have the tendency to form their own close sibling unit with friendly feelings to each other. If, on the contrary, a fighting parental relationship prevails, *this* model can just as readily be taken on by the children and will add to the aggressive atmosphere in the home. On the other hand, we know of cases in which the siblings, following the break-up of the parental unit, tended to strengthen their ties to each other in order to counteract the total dissolution of the family.

THE IMPACT OF THE SIBLING RELATIONSHIP ON INSTINCTUAL DRIVE DEVELOPMENT

In the age relationship we have chosen the children are close enough so that they can have both a progressive and regressive effect on one another. As we address ourselves to the instinctual development, we can find in the sibling experience additional stimulation in the development of the libidinal drives as well as aggressive strivings in various forms and combinations. For purposes of systematic exploration, though not clinically realistic, we shall separate these more rigidly than they in fact occur in order to keep a sharp focus on the differentiated involvement of the drives. We are increasingly aware that the psychosexual stages, though they are organized in a progressive and hierarchical fashion, have a much greater latitude in the timetable of their appearance and dominance than we formerly thought. In the early years, they can be appropriately thought of as open systems responsive to stimulating and inhibitory influences. One important feature of the instinctual drives in the sibling relationship in young children is that the aggressive drives are stimulated for the older one first. In the beginning the newcomer is often experienced as an intruder who is observed and experienced as receiving directly the familiar and pleasurable gratifications and attentions which cannot be given to both at the same time by one adult. At that time the infant is not an immediate source of pleasure to the older child; so there is no way the newcomer can be a love object in any form, and there is no motivation for inhibiting the aggression or the wish to cast out the newcomer. This comes only gradually, as mentioned, at first out of the fear of losing the adult's love, and then out of identification with the adult's attitude to the infant, and, finally, in response to the infant's admiration of the older sibling. This is the archetype of the sibling experience, which sets the stage for the aggressively charged rivalry, envy, and jealousy with which the ego has to find ways to come to terms. Eventually, through reaction formation and the influence of the superego, these aggressive, intruding tendencies may evolve into nurturing, protective, loyal relationships.

On the libidinal side, the siblings eventually offer one another excitement and pleasure via their mutual play in which all the pregenital partial instincts are involved and by no means in an orderly progressive manner, but with rapid shifts from one modality and erogenous zone to another. This is one of the chief ways that the siblings become libidinal and aggressive objects for one another. The psychoanalytic literature abounds with observations in childhood and in reconstructions in adult analyses of the shaping effects of these infantile sexual relationships on object choice and the conditions of pleasure in adult sexual life. One can clinically distinguish a number of significant variations. For instance, the younger child may be stimulated precociously on a psychosexual level which is out of synchrony with the level of ego organization that is normally concomitant with that psychosexual stage. The younger may be forced by the older and stronger into the role of a passive or helpless partner. In another variation, the older child may be drawn into a regressive position by a younger child, resulting in progressive drive and ego organization.

For example, a child in the third year may react with regression to seeking and demanding oral gratifications which he might otherwise be prepared to relinquish when he sees an infant in the first year enjoying and being indulged in oral gratifications. By the same token the anal-sadistic phase in the older child may be prolonged or intensified when a younger child comes into that phase. Such vicissitudes in the sibling relationship may contribute to the disruption of the normally expectable sequence of phase dominance, or may distort the usual timing of psychosexual stages. We must also note that siblings may play together and each behave in a manner consonant with the stage of his or her development without moving progressively or regressively toward one another. A child in the latter part of the second or in the third year may behave very possessively in relation to a toy, asserting "It's mine" when a younger child picks up and plays with it, whereas the younger child shows no such possessive interest. We may ask what is the longer-term significance of these mutual influences on drive development? The most likely outcome is that they influence the fixation points in the individual's psychosexual development. They also contribute to the personality and character traits.

INFLUENCE OF THE SIBLING EXPERIENCE ON EGO DEVELOPMENT

The influences of the sibling experience on the ego can be considered from two points of view. We can look at functions of the ego which have a greater degree of relative autonomy from the drives such as cognition, physical skills, competencies, capacity for play. We can also examine those qualities of the ego, e.g., the defensive structure, which develop more closely in relation to the instinctual drives, psychic conflict, and object relations. In the autonomous type, the sibling relationship, while not a *sine qua non* of development, offers the opportunity for the enrichment of play experience which is a nutriment for skill, imagination, and fantasy. The position of the older one as the first explorer of new experiences outside the home and family may offer appeal to qualities of leadership, teaching, and responsibility. For the younger the relationship offers the possibilities for preparation and trial action, observation and vicarious participation.

When we consider the influence of the sibling experience on those qualities of the ego which develop in closer relationship to the drives, namely, the defensive and inhibitory features of the ego, we find that the effects of the aggressive drive for the older child are more prominent and significant in the beginning than the libidinal. The intruder arouses the aggression of the older sibling toward both the parents and the newcomer. Thus, for the 2-year-old the sibling experience may be one of the earliest direct expressions of hostility. Out of the fear of the loss of the parents' love the child accepts the parents' restraints and prohibitions on some expressions of aggression. Thus the sibling experience is a determinant in shaping the defensive structure which the child begins to erect against the aggression directed toward the object, the sibling. Severe inhibitions of aggression and assertiveness which can become difficult character traits may have their origins in these features of the early sibling experience.

The child's love of the mother and the fear of losing her love on the one hand and the aggression mobilized by the loss of her to the newcomer on the other hand contribute to the ambivalence of the child toward the mother. This experience may also be elaborated as a narcissistic injury which may exert a continuing influence on the evolving image of the self.

In some families one child may be chosen out of unconscious or preconscious motivations by the parents as the evil or satanic child, who then, with the implicit permission and encouragement of the parents, also becomes the victim of the sibling's aggression. In the normal course of events, however, the sanction of the parents provides an impetus to the process of defense and inhibition. One can observe clinically in some siblings that the massive inhibition of aggression as well as the need to avoid and flee intense libidinal attachments to members of the family contribute to the alienation from them and a difficulty in maintaining close and warm relations with members of the family, while they are better able to form affectionate relations outside. This may represent in part a transference from the sibling relationship.

The Impact of Siblings on the Oedipus Complex and Adult Object Relations

The sibling relationship has a rich interaction with the oedipus complex beginning in the preoedipal period of early childhood and extending to parenthood. The sibling realtionship in the preoedipal period establishes a second triangular relationship between the child himself, the sibling, and the parents, besides the child's own triangle with the parents. These triangles, in which the child experiences and develops ways of coping with conflicts over jealousy, envy, love, and hate are different from the triadic relationship of the oedipal period in which the child not only has to contend with the conflicts in his relationship with each of the parents but also has to cope with his conflicts over the parents' relationship to one another. The fantasies, defenses, preferred modes of discharge, and responses to parental authority become organized and contribute to the features of the oedipal phase, in which ambivalence, rivalry, and envy are central issues. In other words, some of the same issues are dealt with in both the preoedipal and oedipal phases, but the outcome of the preoedipal modes of coping affects the ways in which the child confronts the oedipal issues. The child who experiences intense rivalry, envy, and jealousy of the sibling in the preoedipal period is more prone to intense conflict over the same feelings in the oedipal phase.

In the oedipal period the sibling relationship offers opportunities to repeat many features of the sibling relationships with the parents and vice versa. By reversal from passive to active, by elaboration and sublimation in fantasy and play, the sibling may be a substitute for the parent, a substitute who may be more malleable than the parent in the child's efforts to seek adaptive resolutions to the oedipal conflicts. Where there is a large age gap between siblings (unlike the cases to which we originally confined our study), an older sibling can be a less conflictual alternate or substitute parent figure and offer opportunities for resolution of the oedipal conflict which are constructive and healthy. For example, as Freud (1916–17) pointed out, the love of an older brother may enable the girl to keep her female sexuality alive through latency when she has repressed her femininity because of a severe oedipal disappointment. A much younger sibling also can serve as a substitute object for the girl's sublimated wish for a child in the oedipal period.

We believe that the sibling relationship is always a factor in the choice of a marital partner because it involves overcoming the incest barrier against the peer generation which derives from the sibling relationship and thus ultimately from the oedi-pal incest barrier. For example, a young man whose phobic neurosis in childhood was organized around the birth of his sister chose as his wife a young woman who represented his sister in a number of ways. However, one important feature was reversed.Not he, but his wife was phobic. His attitude to-ward her phobia was compounded of maternal and elderly brotherly features—he was solicitous and protective. For in-stance, he would never make appointments which kept him away from her when she would be home alone and most prone to attacks of anxiety.

The attitudes of a parent toward a child may be powerfully determined by the relationship with a sibling in the context of the oedipus complex. We earlier mentioned a father who wel-comed his first child and had a loving interest in her, despite his disappointment over not having a son. He turned away from her totally when the second daughter was born. The second child then represented the son for him, and the first child became his detested older sister. This constellation re-created the family of his childhood. His older sister was his father's favorite. He felt she received undeserved advantages and a disproportionate share of the family's limited resources. He was bitter that she had deprived him of his father's love and held her responsible for the deprivations which affected his life prospects. He identified his eldest daughter with this sister. The child became the target of critical feelings and never re-gained her original position with him. In adolescence, the daughter was consciously aware that her father identified her with his older sister and she had resigned herself to the realiza-tion that she would never have a close, loving relationship with him. Fortunately, she was able to make a marriage in which the relationship with her husband was warm and close. In this in-stance the positive transference to the male analyst in child-hood (ages 3 to 5 and 7 to 10) and the analyst's availability as an alternative to the father and as a new object made an important contribution to the preservation of a positive attitude toward her own femininity.

The sibling relationship has an impact on how the adult will function as a parent to the child. This could be observed in the relationship of two adult siblings to their own children. The older sibling had a strong unambivalent affection for his own first child and had an aversive response to the coming of a second child. The younger sibling, a sensitive, patient parent with the first child, was unaware of his impatience and poor tolerance for the child's hostile attitudes toward the younger sibling. Only after it was interpreted could he recognize that it was difficult for him to empathize with the feelings of the older sibling, but he could readily identify with the younger child as the target of the older child's attacks. In effect, the parent's functional capacity in this area was specifically affected by his own childhood sibling experience which could exert its effects unconsciously on the next generation.

BIBLIOGRAPHY

FREUD, S. (1916–17), Introductory lectures on psycho-analysis. *S.E.*, 15 & 16.
———— (1930), Civilization and its discontent. *S.E.*, 21:59–145.

The Importance of the Sibling Experience

PETER B. NEUBAUER, M.D.

WHEN WE CONSIDER THE ROLE OF SIBLINGS WE PROBABLY think immediately of the ordinal position of siblings and its effect on the child and of sibling rivalry. I shall begin by citing a vignette from Anna Freud's book, *The Ego and the Mechanism of Defense* (1936), because it illustrates a number of points.

> She was the middle child of several brothers and sisters. Throughout childhood she suffered from passionate penis envy, relating to her elder and to her younger brother, and from jealousy, which was repeatedly excited by her mother's successive pregnancies. Finally, envy and jealousy combined in a fierce hostility to her mother. But, since the child's love fixation was no less strong than her hatred, a violent defensive conflict with her negative impulses succeeded an initial period of uninhibited unruliness and naughtiness. She dreaded lest the manifestation of her hate should cause her to lose her mother's love, of which she could not bear to be deprived. . . . As she entered upon the period of latency, this anxiety situation and conflict of conscience became more and more acute and her ego tried to master her impulses in various ways. In order to solve the problem of ambivalence she displaced outward one side of her ambivalent feeling. Her mother continued to be a love object, but, from that time on, there was always in the girl's life a second important person of the female sex, whom she hated violently. This eased matters: her hatred

---

Director of the Child Development Center in New York, Clinical Professor of Psychiatry at the Psychoanalytic Institute, New York University, and John B. Turner Lecturer, Columbia University.

325

of the more remote object was not visited with the sense of guilt so mercilessly as was her hatred of her mother. But even the displaced hatred was a source of much suffering. As time went on, it was plain that this first displacement was inadequate as a means of mastering the situation. . . .

The patient then entered on a process of projection. The hatred which she had felt for female love objects or their substitutes was transformed into the conviction that she herself was hated, slighted or persecuted by them. . . . But the use of this mechanism left upon her character a permanent paranoid imprint, which was a source of very great difficulty to her both in youth and adult years [p. 44ff.].

Here we see the role of the sibling position and the influence of envy and jealousy. We also see that these important factors are subject to continuous changes during the developmental phases, leading to changes of defenses and symptoms and influencing personality organization and character formation.

The vignette highlights envy and jealousy, but we also know that in the child's early years—the focus of our study—rivalry plays an important role. While these three affects undoubtedly are related and in fact mutually influence each other, I believe there are advantages to differentiating them, as I have shown in my 1982 paper (which was partly based on this sibling study). In order to avoid using these terms interchangeably, I shall define them on both dynamic and genetic grounds and test the validity of these definitions on the basis of clinical data.

Rivalry is the competition among siblings for the exclusive or preferred care from the person they share. This definition stays close to the original meaning of the word, for rivalry was the fight for the access to the river, that is, for the supply of the basic nutrients of water. Rivalry also involves competition, an ongoing struggle for the exclusive possession of the object. Rivalry is therefore not an intent or a wish but an act; if the wish to compete is not acted upon, we will observe undue defenses or reaction formations.

Envy refers to the wish for the possession of attributes that a parent or sibling has, such as penis, strength, breasts. Thus, envy is located on many levels of development—from the wish to incorporate, to the envy of possessions, to phallic competition with castration anxiety. If envy is the insistent wish to gain what is realistically unattainable, then we assume that reality testing is challenged, that fantasies and wish fulfillment have a power which will have a serious effect on psychic structure.

It should at least be mentioned that Melanie Klein assigns a major role to envy in the child's relation to the mother and specifically relates envy to aggression. As my definition indicates, I assume that envy occurs on various levels of development and is subject to changes in successive phases. Nor do I believe that envy is part of the interaction prior to the evolvement of the ego as a psychic structure.

Jealousy is the competition with a sibling or parent for the love of the person whom they share. Underlying it is the fear of the loss of the object's love. Jealousy therefore is close to the phallic-oedipal organization.

Both rivalry and jealousy are defined in the context of triadic relationships, while envy is an expression of the diadic relationship and does not directly focus on a third person.

Observing these phenomena as they emerge and following them through the various steps of development, we can see the extension of each in the arena of differentiated function and how each links itself with the other in many forms and combinations. Rivalry easily leads to jealousy, and it is precisely this continuity which makes their differentiation valuable. As we discern the forerunner of jealousy, we can study the effect of unresolved rivalry on jealousy. Proceeding in this way, we avoid the interchangeable use of the terms and therefore do not obscure genetic considerations.

These concepts can be further clarified if they are viewed from the perspective of the developmental line extending from fear of the loss of the object, fear of the loss of the object's love, to castration fear. Rivalry corresponds to the period of fear of loss of the object, but rivalry is more than separation fear. Rivalry is characterized by an increased longing for the object and by acts to eliminate the other person who wishes to share the primary object. The competition may accentuate and intensify the relationship to the primary object with increased libidinal and aggressive strivings toward both the primary object and the rivals.

It may be a crucial moment in the life of the child when rivalry is given up, when the child feels abandoned and turns away from the exclusive tie to the object. We know from the analyses of adults and children that reaching such a turning point has a permanent influence on the child's subsequent psychic functioning, which may express itself in a variety of ways. It may lead to detachment and isolation, or to a premature search for substitutes, or to substantial gains in individuation and differentiation.

As the term penis envy indicates, envy originally relates to a body attribute. Similarly, envy of breasts, hair, color of eyes refers to physical conditions. As was true of rivalry, these envious wishes may stimulate competition, but they may also increase fear of loss of body integrity. Later on the envy of physical attributes may be extended to envy of talents, strength, intelligence, and any characteristic that the other person possesses, regardless of whether it is realistically possible to obtain them.

The following observations, easily made, seem to be examples of envy. A young brother seemed intent on destroying whatever his older sister possessed and wished to take away whatever she seemed to have, but then he really did not know what to do with her possessions. This is quite different from rivalry, though the desire to possess something may underlie it. Another case is that of a girl who after the birth of a brother desperately longed for a doll in a shop window which she passed every day. Eventually the doll was given to her, but at once she tired of it and discarded it.

Does envy contribute to the slow differentiation of outside and inside (e.g., if we regard the breast as an external object and the wish for oral incorporation and possession as arising from internal sources)? Is there a developmental line which indicates a progression in the formation of the body image and in the corresponding formation of the object image? The pervasive desire to acquire and possess may actually help in establishing the permanence of objects. One can observe toddlers playing next to each other, each with exactly the same toy, but they are continually intrigued by the toy being used by the other child. We will surely also link this to the oral and anal strivings and the correlation between envy and greed. However, the frustration, exploration, and mastery of such envy can be supportive of progressive development.

If we think of young children who wish for attributes of mother or father or older sibling, we realize that they may believe their wishes to be unobtainable because they cannot yet grasp that by growing up they eventually will be able to obtain them. Thus envy could be a desire for something a person *thinks* may never be reached.

Freud (1925) assumes that the castration anxiety is related to the perception of anatomical differences during the phallic phase. Today we have evidence that these differences are noticed earlier and that envy may be observable before the phallic phase. These prephallic experiences could then influence the role and the intensity of penis envy and castration fear. Earlier sibling reactions which reflect envy influence the outcome of the castration complex in girls, and for this reason alone it is useful to differentiate envy from jealousy. Freud (1931) proposes that the *beginning* of the castration complex in girls leads to the positive oedipal position, while the positive oedipus complex in boys is terminated by the castration complex. It is important to follow the lines of development of envy more carefully in order to learn more about the differences in the development of boys and girls.

It is clear that, in addition to the interaction between siblings, we have to consider the influence of parents. The response of siblings to the preferred child highlights this important aspect because rivalry, jealousy, and envy are increased. The story of Joseph is an example; he was the preferred child, the one who was the most intelligent and best dressed. We can also study the character of the preferred child, Joseph's avoidance of rivalry, his guilt and his wish to share that which he could give away with siblings. Does the preferred child struggle to maintain his position with his parents by avoiding rivalry, or is this his "hidden" rivalry? Does he avoid sibling envy, or does he look for those attributes which he does not have; Joseph was the intelligent one, he may have envied the strength of his siblings. In addition, this story tells us of the lasting bonds between siblings, for Joseph saved them all.

Differences in the evolvement of rivalry, jealousy, and envy may depend upon whether the child is an older or younger sibling. The sibling position may be significant. When the only child becomes the older child, he or she moves from a central position of interest and care to one which requires sharing. The younger child will, in the first years of life, take the circumstances of his environment as he finds them for granted, without having to experience a sudden shift, but he will also be exposed to the older sibling's attacks on him. The older child, while feeling displaced, may later enjoy the younger's admiration, which the latter rarely experiences to the same degree.

Rivalry can emerge within the context of the existing fabric of parent-child relations and is not dependent upon the birth of a sibling. Furthermore, the younger child's turning toward and finding pleasure in the older sibling may start the younger on the road of a positive relationship, while the older sibling will begin by viewing his sibling as an intruder, especially if they are only 2 years apart.

When John was 4 years old, he had many fights with his 22-month-old younger brother, Michael, for it appeared to him that Michael was preferred. Whenever John was comforted or approached by his brother, he pushed him away. At 7 years of age John wanted to live in the cellar, but he was afraid that his mother would lock him in or out. He was aware of his anger toward his mother and brother, but not quite of his projection. This constellation of fear of loss of mother's love and jealousy affected his oedipal struggle. Here we can see the sibling jealousy not only as a displacement from the oedipus complex but also as an earlier condition which in turn influences the oedipal, libidinal and aggressive organization. This was further accentuated by the father's emotional absence from his family which left the center to rest on the mother-sibling negotiations.

The triadic aspect has a different psychological impact on the older and the younger child; and the road which is taken in the rivalry between them seems to follow different directions so that eventually a measure of equality between siblings can be found. The younger child's libidinal attachment to the older can be contrasted with the stimulation of aggressive strivings in the older child. The circumstances of whether one rejects or is rejected may have an influence on drive distribution and super-ego development.

If I am correct in these assumptions, then this difference in rivalry will then also affect the characteristics of envy and jealousy. This is to say, the nature of envy—of wishing to have something from someone one admires, rather than from someone one feels negative about to begin with—may affect the coping with these problems as expressed in imitation and identification or disengagement and separation. As to jealousy, I would suggest the notion that when a child admires the older sibling, he or she will assume that the parents will also love that older sibling. The child will have a different response when he or she predominantly resents the younger sibling who continues to have the love of the parents.

In the psychoanalytic literature the traumatic reaction to the birth of a sibling is mentioned most often. I believe we would agree that the story begins earlier, during pregnancy. As the mother's body changes, the child may make an identification with her, express the wish to carry a baby too, and his envy can be stimulated as well. Dependent on the parents' attitude during this period, the expectation of a playmate can result in disappointment when the unresponsive sibling is born. When the mother disengages herself from her firstborn child, aggression against the not yet born newcomer may already arise and the child may turn to the father for comfort. Thus we can observe envy and rivalry, which later on may also include jealousy. The parental fantasies, their wish for the same- or opposite-sex child will set the stage for the older child's future reactions.

I have referred to the child's displacement of the sibling experience to the phallic-oedipal correlation or of his relationship with the parents to the sibling. The question has been raised whether this displacement presents advantages which allow the working through of conflicts or under what conditions they burden the already existing conflicts by intensifying them. Here I just mention another displacement, namely, that to the relationship with peers.

B. was a child who, in the latter part of the first year, showed much mouthing with an intense urge for oral incorporation.

This attitude was paralleled by her equally intense visual incorporative approach. She was quite vocal, but when her sibling was born, this activity was greatly reduced. She became receptive rather than motor-active and did not reach out socially. She also took a long time to show her aggression, but when she did, she was quite forceful. She tended to be verbally rather than physically aggressive, but when her anger against her sibling was sufficiently strong, she had an enormous outburst.

B. had always had a strong yearning for her mother's love and affection, a longing which she did not show easily and covered by her wish for the teacher to function as a mother substitute. When her sibling was born, the teachers were concerned that B. was truly deprived of maternal attention, but later the mother turned her affection back to B.

B.'s preferred activity in the classroom was painting, which was related to her mother's interest. Most of the contacts of her otherwise quiet behavior described were between her and her "substitute siblings." There was rivalry between her and her peers in regard to the possession of toys, but her reaction in these situations was less intense than that to her sibling. This replay on a reduced scale may be the significant factor. Similarly, she observed the teacher's reaction as she did that of her mother.

In the nursery group, B. had a calming, quieting influence on the other children, except for a boy toward whom B. showed much aggression in her fantasy games. This could be explained by the fact that he preceded her in the treatment with the same therapist—he had become a "transference sibling"; but she also assumed that as a boy he would be preferred by the analyst who, like her own father, would prefer a boy. As she saw this boy playing very actively, sometimes hyperactively, in the nursery school, she attempted to compete with him by adopting his way of playing in the therapy room in order to be loved by the therapist. Here, too, she was receptive, visually incorporative, and then "imitative." Her behavior with this boy with whom she had to share the therapist contrasted with that during the earlier period, when she had not made a strong attachment to any of the nursery school children.

I have so far stressed the singularity of the sibling experience with reference to rivalry, envy, and jealousy, which may give the impression that the sibling experience is the primary condition for the occurrence of these phenomena. But there is evidence that rivalry, envy, and jealousy also are evoked in a child who has no siblings and that they emerge in the context of the relationship to the parents. One could go a step further and assume that these reactions, with different shades of emphasis, also are characteristic of only children raised by a single parent. These situations raise the question how the sibling experience adds to and modifies the outcome of these powerful affects. Furthermore, they would allow us to examine three inferences:

1. Envy and jealousy are basically related to the feeling of conflict and dissatisfaction the child experiences with the primary psychological parent. Rivalry more closely reflects the child-to-child reaction.

2. The child's need to experience the parent as omnipotent and omniscient is at the same time universally expressed in those residues of infantile wishes and expectations that we observe as rivalry, envy, and jealousy and other "sibling experiences."

3. The need for acquisition and possession underly rivalry, envy, and jealousy.

In general, discussions of rivalry, envy, and jealousy are based on the implicit assumption that the child forms an exclusive primary relationship; that is to say, that early bonding and attachment, rather than being selective, occur only with the "primary objects." All other secondary relationships are then viewed as a spin-off of this relationship, carryovers from, or displacements of it. As Anna Freud and Sophie Dann (1951) put it, "According to the results of child analysis and reconstruction from the analyses of adults, the child's relationship to his brothers and sisters is subordinated to his relationship to the parents, is, in fact, a function of it. Siblings are normally accessories to the parents, the relations to them being governed by attitudes of rivalry, envy, jealousy, and competition for the love of the parents" (p. 166).

In our study group, however, we also considered the possibility that children might form relationships with their siblings that are not merely a reflection of their relationship to the parents but have special characteristics unique to the sibling relationship. That this may be the case was suggested by the following observations:

1. Children have a special empathy with one another for they still share a similar psychic organization when there is only a small age difference between them. They easily tune in to one another with respect to drive manifestations and fluctuations between progression and regression. In twins one refers to the twinning relationship, which is codetermined by mirroring of the same images and similar dispositions. Yet, some of the factors of twinning cannot be totally excluded from the regular interaction systems among siblings.

2. Experimentation, displacement of aggression, sexual curiosity, and sex play can provide special, shared nontraumatic experiences that go far beyond the identification with the parents they share.

3. As the siblings go through various phases of development, they can try changing attitudes and interaction systems on each other; models of identification can be established; and processes of differentiation will occur.

4. On the basis of infant observations which document that infants respond differentially to various people early in life, we can assume that infants form significant relationships quite early. I believe that out of these various interactions a primary relationship emerges gradually, depending upon the libidinal cathexis offered the child by the objects and the choice which the child makes according to his own disposition and needs.

It is most interesting to review "An Experiment in Group Upbringing" by Anna Freud and Sophie Dann (1951). The children who were orphaned during the war had formed a primary group relationship; only later did they accept, step by step, an attachment to significant adults. The children clung to the group as others may cling to a parent. "They had no other wish than to be together and became upset when they were separated from each other, even for short moments. No child would consent to remain upstairs while the others were downstairs, or vice versa, and no child would be taken for a walk or on an errand without the others. If anything of the kind happened, the single child would constantly ask for the other children while the group would fret for the missing child" (p. 131).

While these phenomena were observed in very special circumstances—the children all had spent their first years in a concentration camp—one must consider the possibility that even under less severe circumstances the child will seek out various objects when the mother, inevitably, is unable to provide the full libidinal gratification or the sensory and affective interaction the child desires. On the basis of the gratification obtained from these objects, the child will form significant attachments of various intensity, in addition to the one with mother, and all of these will serve his further development. We certainly have come closer to acknowledging that fathers play a significant role in this respect; similarly, siblings undoubtedly play a significant role, which deserves further exploration.

I shall briefly comment on two such areas in which the rivalry, envy, and jealousy experienced and modified in the sibling relationship play a significant role: (1) their potential effect on character formation; (2) their influence on object choice.

1. In the early period of psychoanalysis it was understood that character deviations were closely linked to the inability to resolve libidinal-phase conflicts. Greediness or phallic competition, exhibitionism or overcontrol with compulsive features were seen to be consequences of these conflicts. I believe it would be fruitful further to explore the role of rivalry, envy, and jealousy as they are deposited within the character structure, particularly when the sibling interaction does not lead to modifications and changes, or when the correlates of rivalry, envy, and jealousy as experienced with the parents reinforce the sibling constellation.

Drawing on our analytic experiences with children and adults, we can say that unresolved rivalry, envy, and jealousy not only leave their imprint on a person's character but also are related to specific character disorders. While earlier psychoanalytic, nosological outlines considered oral, anal, and phallic character disorders, one can also use rivalry, envy, and jealousy as one of the features to characterize a personality deviation without assigning to either one of them the primary organizing role in the development of pathology or even implying that rivalry, envy, or jealousy plays a primary causative role in the specific symptomatology. Penis envy, for instance, may be part of the whole phallic complex, castration anxiety, phobic phenomena, omnipotence; but, as can be seen, it involves a clustering of factors around envy.

It has been suggested that sibling group functioning on various levels of development will assist in the modification and resolution of rivalry. I doubt, however, that group functioning has the same influence on the resolution of either envy or jealousy.

2. Psychoanalytic findings indicate the significant role of early object relations in a person's later choice of love object. Such choices frequently betray the link to specific characteristics of both parents. But the choice of a marital partner is often influenced by others than the parents; partners may be selected on the basis of resemblances to siblings; or the psychic representation of the sibling may lead to the choice of a love object having opposite qualities, thereby indicating the importance of this influence. Naturally, we always consider the impact of parents, their preference, but we also seek the "matching" aspect which makes a tie between two people more intense.

These are just a few examples of the importance of the sibling relationship that has to be examined in greater detail. One needs to follow more carefully not only the phase-specific influences on the sibling relationship, but also how it changes in the course of development and throughout the life cycle.

BIBLIOGRAPHY

FREUD, A. (1936), The ego and the mechanisms of defense. *W.*, 2.
────── (1965), Normality and pathology in childhood. *W.*, 6.
────── & DANN, S. (1951), An experiment in group upbringing. *Psychoanal. Study Child*, 6:127–168.
FREUD, S. (1924), The dissolution of the oedipus complex. *S.E.*, 19:173–179.
────── (1925), Some psychical consequences of the anatomical distinction between the sexes. *S.E.*, 19:243–258.
────── (1931), Female sexuality. *S.E.*, 21:225–243.
NEUBAUER, P. B. (1982), Rivalry, envy, and jealousy. *Psychoanal. Study Child*, 37:121–142.

Development-Promoting Aspects of the Sibling Experience

Vicarious Mastery

SALLY PROVENCE, M.D. AND
ALBERT J. SOLNIT, M.D.

AS INDICATED IN THE INTRODUCTION AND THE OTHER PA-
pers, the sibling experience is not universal, nor is it a requirement for a full expression of the human potential in the developing child. However, the sibling experience, an opportunity
for enrichment and practice of social exchange, can promote or
be supportive of a progressive development and touches on
universal developmental tasks and accomplishments. In this paper we emphasize in theory and illustrate by observations of
interactions how siblings can influence each other in positive
ways. Developmental progress does not take place in a straight
line. There are frustrations, regressive reactions, and disappointments. Overall, the mastery of developmental tasks and
environmental challenges enables children to bear the frustration of initial failures and disappointments when instant success
is not available. If there is developmental progress over time,
children can tolerate some sadness and the conflicts associated
with initial disappointment followed by compromise solutions.
Despite inevitable transient setbacks, the momentum of developmental progress enables children to acquire self-esteem re-

Dr. Provence is Professor of Pediatrics, Child Study Center, Yale University, New Haven, Ct.; faculty, Western New England Institute for Psychoanalysis. Dr. Solnit is Sterling Professor of Pediatrics and Psychiatry, School of
Medicine, and Director, Child Study Center, Yale University; faculty, Western New England Institute for Psychoanalysis.

serves as well as to cope with inner demands and environmental stresses and with conflicts between the individual child and his concerned parents.

Utilizing a composite format, we shall describe some typical patterns of sibling experiences of young children.

OBSERVATIONS

Mark, age 4½, and his 2½-year-old sister Susan were the children of 30-year-old, well-educated, middle-class parents living in a small city. Mark attended morning nursery school three times a week, while Susan went with her mother on one of these days to a small play group of three other 2-year-olds. Mark was driven to school by his father and called for by his mother and Susan. Their mother, whose professional training led to a belief in the importance of the early years of life, decided to interrupt her career until her children were older—a decision apparently reached with minimal ambivalence, supported by her husband, and approved by her parents and his. This was a reasonably harmonious household; husband and wife were free of major psychological problems, were mutually respecting and loving of one another and committed to being good parents.

The material we have selected from the lives of Mark and Susan has the major purpose of highlighting some of the usual developmental phenomena in the sibling relationship. Our emphasis will be on observable behavior with speculations about its connections with the inner life.

It seems probable that at 2½ Susan was less conflicted about Mark's existence than he was about hers. For one thing, she was born into a family that included her brother as well as her parents, so that from the very beginning he was a part of the environment to which she adapted; he was one of the persons with whom she began to form a relationship from early on. When Susan was born, Mark was just 2 years of age, a healthy, attractive child, well cared for and undoubtedly highly valued by his parents. While he was most closely attached to his mother, he also accepted the care of his father. Under the careful preparation of his parents for the advent of the second child, Mark seemed at first enthusiastic about it, though it was clear he was at times puzzled over the changes in his mother and about what it was that was being so joyfully anticipated by his parents and members of the extended family. The birth of a cousin 4 months before Susan was born helped his parents to explain, as best they could, to this 2-year-old.

One might expect that Mark's view of the baby, once she became real and was brought home from the hospital, included but was probably not limited to the following: he no doubt saw her as an intruder, disrupting the state of exclusiveness he had enjoyed in being the only child. Susan's presence and his gradual realization over time that she was in the family to stay and not returnable to the hospital were daily reminders of the changed state of affairs. A child of 2, of course, most likely already would have developed some awareness of his lack of complete exclusiveness in that there would have been a growing awareness that others—father, grandparents, and perhaps the mother too—had needs, interests, requirements, and privileges running counter to his immediate wishes and self-centered attitudes.

The presence of a sibling, however, makes the realization unavoidable, both cognitively and affectively. One aspect of the sibling's presence is the older child's view of the new baby as the one who gets or takes away what he values—time, attention, and love of the parents; the sibling becomes a competitor reacted to with feelings of anger, envy, and rivalry.

In his behavior and such speech as he had, Mark complained that Susan was dirty, that she couldn't play ball, that she was *always* eating, that she should be sent away, that his mother was mean not to stop what she was doing with Susan and attend to him, all very expectable at his phase of development. For a while, after he had been stopped a few times from "patting" her too hard, he took to closing his eyes when he walked by her crib. Mark's reactions and wishes, in substance and mode of expression, reflected the security of his relationships with his parents, the dominance of libidinal ties, and a tolerance of his own anger and aggression in the reassuring context of the baby's being well cared for and safe.

His negative reactions did not tell the whole story. On the other side and running parallel was the older child's attraction to the infant. Susan aroused a variety of interests in Mark at a time when there was already considerable curiosity about other persons, events, and material objects. He expressed a certain fascination in his scrutiny of her, with the way she moved or the sound of an explosive bowel movement, or her contented vocalizations after being fed or the way she smacked her lips. He noted the absence of a penis and missed no chance to watch a bath or diaper change. Already he had the exposure to comforting and upsetting reminders and echoes of his own earlier infancy. This might be paraphrased as "You mean I was like that a long time ago?"

Along with the rivalry, competitiveness, and intellectual interest aroused by seeing Susan being cuddled, fed, diapered, bathed, and so on, there were other events in Mark's psychological life. He appeared to reexperience his own past in some respects. He enjoyed hearing from his mother how she had taken care of him as an infant. This reexperiencing probably added not only to his self-awareness but to his awareness of continuity in the relationship to his parents. For a 2-year-old experiencing the usual developmentally expectable conflicts (which, though beginning to be internalized, still are mainly with the mother), such a reexperiencing and identification with the baby might also be a comfort, reassuring the child about his value to his parents. In addition, his urge to internalize attitudes and characteristic behavior of his parents, i.e., to identify with them, plays a part. At this age such identification is a very strong tendency and will include identification with their nurturing or nonnurturing attitudes toward the new baby. During the first 6 to 9 months of Susan's life Mark became the self-styled expert on what she wanted or needed and at times reproachfully demanded that his parents attend to her promptly. Perhaps this was an indication of a defense against his hostility as well as an identification with Susan's helplessness and wish for gratification.

It is probable that a 2½-year-old, while clearly distinguishing himself from his infant sibling and from others, interprets her behavior as being an expression of needs, feelings, wishes, and attitudes that are identical or similar to his own. Thus he may interpret quite freely, as Mark did, what he assumes to be the causes of the younger child's distress, pleasure, etc. Only gradually does there develop an appreciation that the younger child might feel anything differently.

Another factor in the experience of the older sibling is that when an infant begins to smile, reach out, and move about, her social attractiveness to the older sibling is enhanced. To some extent this enhancement is due to a narrowing of the differences in behavior between infant and older sibling, but even more significantly it conveys in a reassuring and still burdensome way to the 2-year-older brother that his sister is not as helpless as earlier and that she may be responding to him. By the time Susan was 6 months or so of age, for example, Mark discovered that he could make her smile, laugh, chortle, and act excited; he seemed aware that he was an object of fascination to her. Her manifest pleasure in watching his activities and antics gave him pleasure. By his actions, he could also turn her tears into smiles at times. It is probable that at his age he would interpret her beaming smiles, excitement, and interest as unalloyed approval, something he got neither from himself nor his parents in such pure form at this time.

Her positive responses toward him, which continued over time, probably assisted him in dealing with his negative feelings and facilitated the development of loving feelings toward her. Then, too, as is usual, behavior of an older child suggesting a certain affection or generosity toward the younger meets with parental approval, and so it was for Mark. Shame at hateful behavior toward the sibling, which the 2-year-old experienced, also heightened motivation to behave in more approved ways, and parental approval added to Mark's approval of himself.

To turn to the relationship between Mark and Susan at 4½ and 2½ years: Susan's behavior toward Mark reflected both expected phase-specific and highly individual attitudes, feelings, and psychological development. In accordance with what one might expect of a 2½-year-old, at times she seemed to adore her older brother; he could do no wrong. She complied with his directions and requests. She found his toys and activities fascinating, she tried to imitate much of what he did, often things that were beyond her capabilities. Frequently she mirrored his pleasure and pride as he mastered a new task, coped successfully with a familiar challenge, or acquired another skill. At such times she indirectly, vicariously, empathically joined him in his mastery. At other times she was intolerant of him, appeared envious, tried to take possession of his toys, and did not relinquish them gracefully. Without apparent provocation or with minimal provocation at times she became angry and aggressive, trying to push or bite him if he transgressed the variable limits of her tolerance or was simply *there* when she became upset for any reason.

Mark was often patronizing in manner toward Susan, as he demonstrated his superior knowledge and competence in a variety of ways. At such times he patiently instructed her or called her dumb, encouraged her responses to his demonstrations, or went off to do better things with his time. One element in his ridiculing the little girl probably was his own castration anxiety. When Mark and Susan were with neighborhood children, he might join in teasing her, but was often protective of her. He behaved with a mixture of pleasure and furtiveness at her open interest in his penis and sometimes could not decide whether to close the bathroom door or not. Both children engaged in excited gigling on occasions when they saw each other nude. Mark both enjoyed calling Susan's attention to his erect penis and covered it protectively if she came too close. When angry with Susan, Mark, as he had learned to do, usually first scolded or instructed her in proper behavior, but at times revealed the precariousness of that kind of control by pushing or hitting her. Yet he had made peace, at least in part, with his earlier resentment of her. Some of the time, they were companions and allies—companions in play, allies in acts of mischief or in anger against their parents. They seemed frequently to understand each other more quickly than the adults understood either of them. Perhaps the older child was still close enough to the feelings and perceptions of the recent past to identify and empathize with the younger, who in turn found the older child much more comprehensible than the adults.

From these observations one can examine the advantage of a partially shared developmental space or overlapping of developmental periods. Such a theoretical or potential advantage is realized only if the parents' reactions and the nature of their attachments to each child are supportive of the advantage. Lest we be misunderstood to be advising, on the basis of these psychoanalytic inferences, that ideally parents should have their children close together, we hasten to point out that many other factors are involved in any particular preference regarding family planning. For example, there were also the disadvantages for Mark and Susan that their closeness developmentally often encouraged regressive behavior, individually and together. Such regressive behavior at times was appropriate and supportive of development. At other times, depending to a large extent on parental reactions, the regressive behavior tended to get out of hand, exceeding what would be development-promoting, especially for Mark. Thus when siblings share developmental space, the temptation to utilize regressive behavior for its discharge satisfaction rather than for its elaboration of each child's physical, emotional, and intellectual experiences (and for its qualities of resting before moving ahead) can be disadvantageous.

At times Susan and Mark were noted to help each other, their behavior being modeled after that of the adults. Susan's helping Mark involved primarily taking toys or other playthings to him, or remembering to ask for a cracker for him, or trying to pat or hug him when he was hurt or upset, or saying something intended to be comforting such as "Mommy's coming." Mark was more versatile, of course. He was strong enough to help Susan up when she fell. He cautioned her about danger; he could hold her hand and insist that she stay with him if asked to walk her into the house from the car, etc.

They sometimes enjoyed imaginative play together, though there were substantial differences in the level and complexity. Often they were able to tolerate each other's demands, attacks, expectations, and rising levels of excitation since they were developmentally close to each other; that is, they were reasonably close to each other in how they perceived, tolerated, and responded to common experiences. We do not suggest that the experience is identical, only that their developmental closeness gives them an easier access to each other's mental activities than is likely to occur when siblings are, for example, 6 to 8 years apart. As they played "house," or dress-up, or hide-and-seek, or sheriff and prisoner, the roles were assigned and the play directed by Mark, and Susan either went along with it or objected. In each, however, one could observe the pretending.

Their play together provided both a safety valve and an arena in which to practice and improve their ability to get along with each other and, it is assumed, with others. Even their direct aggression toward one another, enacted in a play context, tended to be taken less seriously both by themselves and the adults than when it occurred outside the play. Of course, at their ages, any playtime could suddenly deteriorate into a scene when one child was hurt, angered beyond his tolerance or disappointed. Then the support of the adults was necessary in order to sustain the play, when it was appropriate. An agreement between siblings of Mark's and Susan's ages that they are "just playing" goes far to reassure them that their hostile, acquisitive, greedy, exhibitionistic, noisy, controlling, sadistic, and sexually exciting behavior does not endanger them too much. The younger child worries mainly about parental disapproval, and contends with a few internalized conflicts; the older must contend with those more complex feelings and fantasies that characterize the oedipal phase. Progress in the socialization of sexual and aggressive drives was reflected in Mark's and Susan's behavior, a process which begins largely through identification with socialized, nurturing, and reasonable parent figures.

The anecdotes to follow are samples of behavior of Mark and Susan, all around the time they were 4½ and 2½ years.

1. Mark very much wanted to play with a new toy given to Susan by their father who had just returned from a trip. It was a plastic toy with fluid and colorful shapes inside, capable of being shaken into all sorts of fascinating arrangements. He wanted to look it over and see how it worked, and it seemed a much better gift than the car his father had brought to him. His first approach was direct, "Let me have it," which Susan refused, holding tightly to the toy and yelling loudly, "No! Mine! Mine!" At the sound of the mother's voice in the next room asking what was going on, Mark turned loose and said, "Okay stingy," glowering at Susan who looked defiant. Mark then turned his back on Susan and played busily with his own toy

putting it through various maneuvers in an animated way. Susan, attracted by her brother's activation of and obvious enjoyment of the car, tried to join him and take over the car and the activity, setting aside her new toy. Mark fended her off for a while as he continued his activity, then said, with calculated magnanimity, "Okay, you can have it," gave the car to her, and unobtrusively picked up Susan's new toy. He played quietly with it, looking enormously pleased with himself, fully aware that he had outmaneuvered her. Their mother, coming into the room, observed the scene, reflected upon Mark's manipulation of the situation, but decided to do nothing since it was a peaceful scene. She wondered whether and at what moment Susan would notice and object. Such exchanges, manipulations, and compromises are the stuff of daily socialization. The extent to which such behavior is encouraged or discouraged by the shared life styles and values of the family and is reinforced or discouraged by the community's customs and laws is quite variable. The interchange between Mark and Susan was not only fun for the time being, there also were many points at which Susan and Mark understood and empathized with each other in this play that indicated exploratory and practicing gains for each.

2. Outdoors Mark was demonstrating to Susan how well he could throw a ball in the air and catch it, repeating as he did so, "Look at me, Susan. Whee!" Susan watched admiringly for a minute or two, then wanted to try it. Mark tried to engage her in a game of catch, which did not work because Susan could not yet throw and catch well enough. Mark's at first benevolent coaching was replaced by disgust, and he criticized Susan for being a baby and a girl at that. He went back to his solitary game as Susan dissolved into a storm of angry tears and went into the house to her mother, crying, "My ball! My ball!" At this point it was an open question what Susan would do: she might seek her mother as someone who could get the ball for her or might blame her mother for everything and hit her; she might neither complain about Mark nor hit her mother but kick over the dog's water or squeeze the cat too hard. Or she might seek and accept comfort quickly from her mother and find something else to do; or return to the yard and Mark to try again,

attracted by the activity and tenaciously determined to be a part of it.

3. Mark was walking along a low stone wall demonstrating his superior motor skill and balance. Susan followed him, trying to imitate. Their father watched from across the yard with some dismay, not knowing whether to call out or not. Mark said, "Look at me, Dad!" Susan fell from the wall onto the grass, looked surprised and began to cry. Mark looked startled, then anxious. The father reached Susan, picked her up, hugged her and said, "You're all right, baby." Mark said, "I didn't do it," but looked troubled and walked away. Susan continued to sob, it appeared more because she felt injured and frustrated than because she was in physical pain. There was obviously some enjoyment of her father's attention as well. When he put her down, she clambered back onto the wall where Mark had resumed his walk. The father said sharply, "Both of you get off the wall." Susan began to cry. Mark glowered but complied and, taking Susan by the hand, said, "Come on Susan, we'll go in and see Mommy and get some juice." She went along willingly. They were relieved by their father's setting limits; they united against his sharp tone to neutralize what might have been mortifying; they exploited the advantage of having two parents; they exercised a sharing of experiences that could become an investment in the future: mutual understanding and loyalty to each other.

4. Susan and Mark were in their pajamas after having their baths. As Mark began to run and leap about the room with Susan in gleeful pursuit, their mother tried to slow them down anticipating that the excitement would culminate in disaster. She picked up Susan who cried angrily for a few seconds, then subsided as her mother cuddled and talked to her. To Mark who was eyeing the scene while he tossed a sofa pillow into the air, then to the floor, and jumped on it, she said, "Mark, you could climb up on the kitchen stool and get your dishes and Susan's from the cabinet while I put her in her high chair." She gave Mark a special smile and he decided to come along. He asked about his father who was out of town, "Is Daddy coming home tonight?" When she responded, "Not until tomorrow," he inquired, with a show of generosity, "Would you like for me

and Susan to sleep with you?" expecting, no doubt, that if he included Susan there was a better chance of success. When told that would not be necessary, he reminded her that his dad would take him to his office on Saturday and let him use the adding machine. Susan said, "Me too"; and after Mark said angrily, "No you're not!" and was about to repeat it, he intercepted a disapproving look from his mother, who said, "Don't bedevil her, Mark," and they went back to eating their supper. Later Susan asked, "Mommy, what is devil?"

In these observations one can see the power and subtlety of oedipal longings and conflicts. In offering to bring Susan with him to mother's bed, Mark was able to express his longing more subtly, more acceptably, and with less anxiety than if he had made the request for himself alone; at the same time Susan's presence provided him with both a buffer against his disappointment and a scapegoat for his anger. Such compromises would appear to enable Mark to avoid the anxiety of the direct oedipal temptation, at the same time as they pave the way to a resolution of the conflict by facilitating the positive identification with his father. Here we emphasize the transformation of rivalry and jealousy into development-promoting reactions as well as the appearance of these affects and attitudes in the sibling experience during the oedipal period.

When their father came in from a 5-day trip, Mark, Susan, and their mother were at the airport to meet him. Mark was fascinated by the jets landing and taking off, and asserted his intention to be a pilot. Susan, somewhat intimidated by the crowd and the noise, stayed mostly on her mother's lap, looking at the people and commenting on their suitcases, hats, etc. At one point she asked anxiously about a small dog being transported in a pet carrier. As their mother said, "There comes Daddy," Mark and Susan suddenly looked shy, did not run to meet him, and only the greeting from his wife made him feel very welcome. As they got into the car for the drive home, Susan suddenly threw herself into her father's arms, clung tightly, and asked, "Daddy, where you went?" Mark wanted to know, "What did you bring me?" When his father, only half-jokingly said, "*That's* a great welcome," Mark looked out the window. When his wife said, "We all missed you," the father responded, "I missed you—all of you, too." Still holding Susan, he caught Mark's eye, smiled, and said, "I have lots to tell you, son, about what I saw in San Francisco." Mark looked more comfortable and began to tell his father about what he had been doing. Later in the evening after Susan had preempted their father's lap for what seemed a long time, Mark and his father found a way to displace her to give Mark his turn. Mark reminded his father about the promised trip to the office. This happening not only suggested the unfolding power of children identifying with each parent in differing and characteristic ways but also indicated that internalization was at a more differentiated level in Mark than was yet possible for Susan.

5. Susan and her mother had a difficult morning and Susan was in a stormy mood. In contrast to her usual behavior, Susan protested when her mother said it was time to pick up Mark at school, tried to refuse her car seat, and kicked at her mother, who told her to stop it. She was quiet during the ride but refused to be cajoled into a better mood by her mother's efforts to get her interested in what they were passing. When Mark got into the car, his mother said, "You'd better watch your p's and q's. Susan's in a bad mood." Mark, who had had a fine morning, said sympathetically, "What's the matter Susan?" smiled at her and showed her his painting. Susan seemed to brighten immediately, and the drive home and lunch were quite pleasant. Later in the day, the mother recalled that Susan had asked for Mark several times during the morning.

DISCUSSION

The capacity of siblings who are approximately 2 years apart—in close developmental proximity—to form a positive relationship tends to be underemphasized for two reasons. The relationship is taken for granted when it proceeds relatively smoothly despite transient flurries of rivalry and age-appropriate conflicts. Secondly, even the sibling's normative rivalry, envy, and jealousy create difficulties that are more memorable for their parents than the predominant friendliness, loyalty to each other, and ability to form a united front in response to an external threat or discomfort. Such frequent mutual support and acceptance of each other enable siblings to form a community of interests that can strengthen their confidence in each other and in themselves as brother and sister. Such an attachment is a source of feeling more secure in the continuity from the past into the future. It also provides someone more like oneself in size, functions, tolerances, and interests with whom to explore one's world, to practice one's intimate personal engagements, and against whom one can define oneself.

Although the sources of challenge and discomfort are quite different, siblings who are developmentally and personally close also are helpful to each other when maturational changes and other inner demands create difficulties for each of them. Such demands as those of the instinctual drive thrusts (aggressive and libidinal), appetitive longings, yearning for exclusiveness with one of the parents; at a later time the threats of a punitive conscience (superego); the fear of loneliness; the uncertainty of the future; and the struggle for the ability to feel comfortably alone in the presence of others—all these often are met more comfortably or confidently when a child is in a mutually positive, resonant relationship to a close-enough sibling. That is, coping with and mastering these inner demands often can be strengthened by the support and example of and the interaction with a sibling, especially an older one.

At the same time, the advantage of developmental closeness is often more than canceled out by parents feeling exhausted and under too much sustained pressure when there are two children with such similar dependency needs. For these parents it seems like an unrelenting demand for more than twice the energy, toleration of sleeplessness, patience, and postponement of taking care of the adult needs than if they were caring for only one child at a time.

There are two major threads that could be followed clearly in our study of the healthy sibling experience, i.e., *in the context of positive parent-child relationships.* They are: (1) developmental closeness and overlapping of siblings may favor the establishment and elaboration of a quiet but effective empathic communication, verbal and nonverbal; (2) each child, the younger and the older, in differing and differentiated ways, is able to share indirectly in the experiences of the other. Empathically, they can broaden their experience by sharing in what their sibling experiences, at the same time as they do not fully experience it.

It is the empathic relationship between siblings that enables them to share many of their experiences and vicariously to increase their practice for mastery. It is clear that Mark and Susan often used their empathic relationship (not always affectionate or friendly) to broaden their experiences. Although empathy does not assure this extension of experiential events, it is a prerequisite for such opportunities for one person to use another person's experience as a "practice-run" or "trial action" without having to be directly involved. The well-accepted phenomenon in twins of understanding of each other without speaking or explicitly communicating with each other is an example of this interaction at an extreme rarely achieved by singleton siblings.

On the other hand, efforts to comfort and communicate with one another are more frequent between young children than has been appreciated. Even toddlers are capable of discerning and responding to the need of another child in a tender, effective way, as in the following example. David and Leslie, age just 2, knew each other very well from their long association in our daycare center. One morning, Leslie, on arriving at the center, was irritable and did not respond to the teachers' efforts to comfort her. David busied himself in finding a toy he knew Leslie especially liked, though it was no favorite of his own. Her face brightened and her fretting stopped as he handed it to her with an affectionate smile.

Empathy is the "projection of one's own personality into the personality of another in order to understand him better"[1] or "the capacity for participation in another's feelings or ideas." The sibling experience provides repeated opportunities to elaborate and practice the capacity for empathy. There is little doubt, however, that the basic capacity for empathy is established in the parent-child interaction and relationship. This special form of sensing and knowing another person's feelings and thoughts is inextricably interwoven with the child's ability to internalize and to identify with parental attitudes and expec-

1. Webster's *New Collegiate Dictionary*, p. 373.

tations as a fundamental process for each child to unfold his or her own unique personality. Sibling relationships and experiences reflect and can elaborate the quality and intensity of this aspect of the primary child-parent relationship.

Viewed from the perspective of these observations and theoretical propositions, the sibling experience, when it is mainly positive and facilitating of the unique development of each child, becomes a powerful secondary stage on which children, directly and vicariously, have opportunities to rehearse as well as to act out the scenes of their inner lives. These sibling experiences also prepare children intellectually and emotionally for what lies ahead, those scenes and acts that characterize the drama of a life fully and well lived.

The Revival of the Sibling Experience during the Mother's Second Pregnancy

JANICE ABARBANEL, Ph.D.

PREGNANCY IS A PHASE IN THE LIFE OF A FAMILY DURING which parents and existing children prepare for the birth of a new family member and anticipate new roles and relationships. In the case of a second pregnancy, one of the key parental tasks is to prepare the firstborn for his or her new sibling.

The quality of the mother's interaction with her firstborn during the second pregnancy will depend to a significant degree upon the mother's own childhood relationships. The mother who is producing a sibling for her first child is closely attuned to her own childhood sibling experience and to the way her own parents handled such sibling issues as rivalry, competition, friendship, caring, and sharing. Even before the birth, the developing fetus affects the mother's relationship to her firstborn, which in turn colors the child's attitudes toward the sibling.

This paper focuses on pregnant mothers and female toddlers, examining how the second pregnancy challenges the mother's relationship to her firstborn toddler daughter. I shall

Graduate of the Graduate Center for Child Development and Psychotherapy, a program jointly sponsored by the Los Angeles and Southern California Psychoanalytic Institutes. Presently affiliated with the Regional Center for Infants and Young Children of Washington, Maryland and Virginia.

A shortened version of this paper was presented in Cannes, France, at the Second World Congress of the World Association for Infant Psychiatry, March 1983.

explore how the mother's own sibling experience is revived during the second pregnancy, as both she and her firstborn await the arrival of the new baby. I shall demonstrate how this reawakening of the mother's sibling experience during the second pregnancy affects her relationship with her first child and the quality of her preparation of the firstborn for the new baby. The main case I shall present portrays a mother whose unresolved sibling rivalry inhibited her ability to be psychologically available to her toddler and may in turn have adversely affected her toddler's attitude to the newborn sibling. I shall also present material from another mother-toddler pair in which the revival of the mother's sibling experience helped the mother prepare her daughter to anticipate the new baby with pleasure.

The psychoanalytic literature on pregnancy repeatedly addresses the impact of the pregnant woman's relationship with her own parents upon her future feelings about herself as woman and mother (e.g., Bibring et al., 1961; Benedek, 1970; Colman and Colman, 1971). I have found nothing in the literature, however, discussing the significance of the mother's own sibling experience during pregnancy or the effects of this experience on the ongoing relationship with the firstborn child. Indeed, there is very little literature on second pregnancies altogether. Much of what exists on second pregnancies appears in popular magazines (e.g., Viorst, 1979; Weiss, 1981a, 1981b; Weissbourd, 1981) or in books on parenting with sections on sibling rivalry (e.g., Barber and Skaggs, 1977; Daniels and Weingarten, 1982). The subjects of timing and spacing of children, preparing the firstborn for the second, and handling issues of envy and jealousy are covered in a general fashion.

Psychoanalytic case reports, starting with Freud's, abound with references to children whose problems were exacerbated by a sibling's birth, and to adults whose pathology could in part be traced to unresolved preoedipal issues heightened by the birth of a sibling (e.g., Freud, 1909; Bornstein, 1949; Erikson, 1950, pp. 53–58; Jacobson, 1950; Blum, 1978). However, the relationship of the mother's own sibling history or her ordinal position to her capacity to parent her child during a pregnancy has not been explored.

Marianne Kris, in both the longitudinal and family studies at the Yale Child Study Center, noted the frequency with which parents view their children in terms of their own sibling experiences. That is, often the first child represents a sibling, while the second child may represent the self as one wished to be. Which sibling a child represents can change in the course of the children's development: in some instances, for example, the oldest daughter may always represent the same sibling; in others, these patterns may change with the birth of new children (Kris, 1972).[1]

Others have noticed that it is common for expectant parents "to identify with a baby in the same position in the birth order as they" (Colman and Colman, 1971, p. 39). This identification may have a significant effect on the attitudes toward the pregnancy and toward the firstborn. If, for example, the mother is a second child and sees herself as the growing fetus, then the firstborn child would represent the older sibling. Depending on her childhood relationship with that sibling, the pregnant mother may anticipate a kind of repetition of her own sibling relationship with all its emotional content.

It is widely accepted that pregnancy is a time when a woman revives conflicts in her relationship with her own mother, as she moves toward becoming a mother herself (Bibring, 1959; Colman and Colman, 1971; Kestenberg, 1976). It is logical to assume that during a second pregnancy this process of revival and reintegration of family relationships would have another focus—the mother's relationship with her own siblings. Although this phenomenon has not been thoroughly explored in the literature, the case materials that follow present two variations in the way in which the maternal sibling experience affects the mother-toddler relationship during the second pregnancy.

This paper presents material drawn from an intensive study of the relationships between pregnant mothers and daughters.

1. Freud, too, had noted this phenomenon as early as 1911. Responding to a question from Jung, Freud said, "He [Martin] is not his mother's favourite son; on the contrary, she treats him almost unjustly, compensating at his expense for her overindulgence towards her brother, whom he resembles a good deal, whereas, strangely enough, I compensate in my treatment of him for my unfriendliness towards the same person" (McGuire, p. 394).

I followed through the course of the pregnancy four mothers whose firstborn daughters were each between 12 to 24 months old at the onset of their mothers' pregnancy. Three of the mothers "suggested" themselves in their inquiries into the parent-toddler program I was then directing. They were eager for a social experience for their children, and each mentioned in passing that she was newly expecting. The fourth mother was referred by one of the other three. As it happened, the four mothers who volunteered had girls.

I visited each mother and toddler at home twice each month during the pregnancy. In the weeks before delivery, I visited each home once a week. I made at least two postpartum visits to each home.

I described my role to the mothers as that of participant-observer. I said I was interested in how families experience a pregnancy, particularly how the child develops during this period and how the mother reacts to the changes. During these home visits, the mother and I sat in the playroom, the kitchen, the den, or any place selected as comfortable for the child to play about. Usually, each mother brought up topics of conversation based upon the week's events. The focus on the pregnancy tended to produce material about family history, marriage, siblings, parenting, and the child's development. In addition, of course, I observed the mother-daughter interplay during the hour of my visit. I generally took down a few notes or summaries of dreams, and then reconstructed each session later in the day.

Hence, the clinical material contained in this paper is not from the analyses of these mothers, but from my bimonthly visits in their homes.[2] However, since I was spending so much time with these mothers and toddlers, both made relationships with me. The mothers sometimes sought my guidance or advice, and the children sometimes played with me. I expected that the nature of each mother's and each child's relationship to

2. Because of the scope of the study and my own time limitations, I did not systematically gather material about the fathers. I did have occasional opportunities to speak with the fathers during the course of my home visits, but I did not conduct individual interviews.

me would give me additional data with which to assess the functioning of mother and child.

CASE ILLUSTRATIONS

MRS. C. AND CAREN

I met Mrs. C. as she sat in a circle of mothers on the first morning of the parent-toddler group. She was quiet during most of the discussion, which offered each mother a chance to introduce herself and say something about her goals in joining such a group. Mrs. C. sat a bit apart from the others, looking down at the rug and seeming sad and preoccupied.

Toward the end of the mothers' time together, Mrs. C. started to cry and to talk. She said she was crying because this was Caren's first day of "school." She felt that this day meant that Caren had "grown up." This comment seemed out of place, because Caren was the only toddler in the group who was not yet walking: at 14 months, Caren was not the youngest child in the group, but she appeared so because she still crawled.

Mrs. C. began to talk about Caren. Caren had not been an easy baby, and now that she had started "school," there seemed to be no more baby time possible. Mrs. C. said that she had "missed her chance" with Caren. While Mrs. C. was talking, Caren did not gravitate to her mother's lap as had other toddlers, even though Mrs. C. made some efforts to pull Caren toward her when Caren scooted by. Caren resisted this "return," and Mrs. C. did not pursue her daughter. Mrs. C. remained immobile in her place in the circle while Caren wandered about the room. Several times, the staff had to rescue Caren from obstacles, like table edges and other children's feet.

One week later, at the second meeting of the parent-toddler group, Mrs. C. arrived with Caren walking. Everyone was surprised to see such a sudden transition. Even though she was a new walker, Caren walked with the skill of a toddler who had been upright for months. During the mothers' group time, Mrs. C. revealed that her second pregnancy had been confirmed during the past week. She did not herself note the coincidence of Caren's walking and the new pregnancy, but another mother pointed this out, adding, "Now when the baby comes, you won't have two babies. It looks as though Caren has decided to grow up."

Mrs. C. talked more this second session. Her first remarks were about her sister. "Marcie is 14 months older than I am. I was told that Marcie started walking the day I was brought home from the hospital. Having a sister so close is not my reason for having my kids close in age. The main reason is that I want to go back to work as a photographer, and in my field you cannot be out too long." I was struck by Mrs. C.'s verbal negation of her own family situation which she was unconsciously reconstructing.

Mrs. C.'s Family History[3]

Mrs. C.'s parents worked together in a successful home furnishing business. "Mom was never home on Saturdays and Dad was even less available. I recall waking up in the middle of the night, seeing my father working with papers for his business."

Mrs. C.'s sister Marcie was born when their mother was 20. Mrs. C. was born 14 months later. Both girls were the result of breech deliveries. "My mother used to complain of bad backaches which she said were due to the deliveries: that is, we caused her a lot of pain. I remember her ill at home with pain, and sometimes she would go into the office when she was not well. In her mid-30s, my mother had a hysterectomy, in an emergency situation related to a tumor in her uterus. I recall that my father had one of the first vasectomies, though I'm not sure why."

Mrs. C. felt that her mother never took much pleasure in her daughters. "She seemed like a longed-for, unavailable person." She described numerous fights that she provoked with her mother during her childhood: "I used to be perfect at school and then I would come home and fight with my mother. This was the only way I could get her attention."

Mrs. C. often described herself as coming from a line of

3. While I summarize the relevant material here, I should emphasize that the material, including that about the relationship to the older sister, came up spontaneously during our interviews.

strong working women. Her maternal grandmother, now 72, had many successful businesses in her career. Mrs. C. clearly admired her mother and grandmother for their strengths as professionals. "If I wasn't going to have another child, I could see starting back to work now, since Caren seems ready for more school-type activities and does not need me so much." When Mrs. C. showed me some of her photographs, she said, "I feel like I have to get involved in my work or I will think about how overwhelming this next child will be. Work will give me something to do until the birth."

Mrs. C.'s model of mothering was her own mother. Her mother's distance and unavailability to her now seemed to be Mrs. C.'s way of being with Caren. Although Mrs. C. recalled yearning for closeness with her mother, she emphasized in her own parenting her wish to be independent of Caren.

Mrs. C.'s sister Marcie was 14 months older than Mrs. C. The sisters' closeness in age must have overwhelmed their mother, who had little interest in being with her growing daughters. The two girls turned to each other as playmates: "Marcie always treated me like a little sister, telling me what to do. She'd always be the Mommy and I the baby." At the same time, the two sisters were rivals for their mother's limited affections.

According to Mrs. C., Marcie was the "normal" sibling, perfect and easy. Her mother resented having a second child so close to Marcie, and Mrs. C. felt that her own pessimism and her sense that she was always "second best" stemmed from her mother's attitude toward her daughters. Mrs. C. felt that her birth had interfered with her mother's career ambitions. Her mother's inconsistency with her probably reflected her ambivalence about her children. "Sometimes I felt that Marcie and I were treated as one person, kind of blended, and I reacted to this."

Mrs. C. often repeated how she tried to do the opposite of Marcie whenever possible. She fought with her mother, while Marcie remained cool and distant. Mrs. C. was the better student at school, but would come home and make life miserable for her mother. She described numerous bladder infections and subsequent hospitalizations to have her urethra enlarged during her early childhood and adolescence. She recalled blanking out in an amusement park when she spiked a fever and passed out from a urinary infection. "Childbirth was nothing compared to the pain I experienced as a child. I think some of the illnesses were attempts to get my mother's attention. I only had her when I was ill."

During Mrs. C.'s second pregnancy, Marcie became pregnant with her first child. Mrs. C. occupied each of her meetings with me with some material about Marcie, information often couched in a tone of rivalry. In the sections that follow, I shall present some examples of Mrs. C.'s descriptions of her sister, and how her feelings and responses to Marcie became represented in Caren, the "older sister" in Mrs. C.'s expectant family.

The Second Pregnancy

During the first trimester, Mrs. C. mentioned casually to Caren that there would be a new baby in the house, but there was no dramatic announcement and the parents did not further discuss the news with Caren. It appeared from the outset that the pregnancy would not be a shared experience which Mrs. C. would assist her first daughter in understanding. Instead, during the early months of the pregnancy, Mrs. C. enrolled Caren in numerous toddler activities: a gym class, twice-a-week swimming lessons, and a preschool program. She explained, "I must help Caren relate to other children. I don't want to lose myself in my children. My mother and grandmother taught me that you should think of yourself first, then your husband, then your kids."

Early in the pregnancy, Mrs. C. reported a dream:

> I was talking to 10-year-old twins who looked Israeli. They were my daughters. They seemed like robots—they were too identical, each had a scar on the right cheek. I asked if they were twins and they said, "No, we are triplets, a brother is on the way."

Mrs. C. described this dream as eerie and scary. She wondered whether a second daughter would be as morose and pessimistic as she remembered herself. The dream seemed to bring up the sibling theme, how Mrs. C. often felt "blended" with Marcie and how destructive this was for her own individuation. Her sense of being a foreigner to her mother and at times feeling "foreign" or "robotlike" in her responses to her daughter are also apparent in the dream. Hinted at too are the rivalry themes which, as Mrs. C.'s pregnancy progressed and she began to create more vividly a "rival" for Caren, became uppermost in her associations and discussions with me.

The most important change in Caren's behavior early in the pregnancy was her walking on the day her mother's pregnancy was confirmed. Mrs. C.'s view was that she was tired, nauseous, and less available to Caren during the early weeks of the pregnancy, so "Caren had to fend for herself." Because Mrs. C. needed to use her limited emotional resources to prepare for the new infant, she withdrew from Caren and found ways to avoid her. For Mrs. C., the revival of sibling issues and unresolved sibling conflicts intensified her treatment of Caren as the hated rival. Her exaggerated withdrawal from Caren seemed a playing out of feelings she herself had experienced as the ignored, "second best" sister. Perhaps Caren's walking at this point was her way of making a dramatic effort to reengage her mother.

During the first trimester, Mrs. C. reported that Caren was having sleep difficulties: Caren refused to go to bed, woke up in the middle of the night unable to relax and demanded to walk. Sleep problems are commonly associated with developmental milestones, especially motor ones such as Caren's new walking. But Mrs. C.'s response to the night waking was not to help Caren relax, reassuring Caren of her availability. Instead, Mrs. C. struggled with Caren, in turn arguing and cajoling her to go to sleep, but to no avail.

Caren expressed her initial reaction to changes that had come about because of the pregnancy rather vividly during one of my visits. Mrs. C. and I walked upstairs to her workroom. Caren followed behind, though not invited by her mother; Mrs. C. did not assist her toddler up the stairs, nor did she look around to check whether Caren had arrived safely at the top. While we talked in the workroom, Caren was banging something in the baby's room. Mrs. C. finally got up to see what was happening and discovered that Caren was dismantling a smoke detector that was in a box on the floor. Mrs. C. removed the box and told Caren to come with us into her room. There Caren proceeded to dump all her clothes from one drawer onto the floor and to hand each piece to me while Mrs. C. sat passively, making minimal verbal or physical contact with Caren. Caren then returned to the next room where she continued her destruction of the smoke alarm. A few minutes later, Caren rejoined us, carrying a small baby seat which she placed in the middle of her room and sat in herself. When Mrs. C. tried to put Caren's dolls on the seat instead, Caren tossed the dolls away and returned herself to the infant "throne." I thought that Caren was communicating clearly her own developmental needs in this episode.

Toward the end of the first trimester, Mrs. C. began to turn over much of the childcare to the housekeeper, who had lived with the family since Caren's birth. On my visit one morning, I arrived to find Mrs. C. on the phone and Caren seated on the kitchen floor screaming. The maid came in, picked her up, and whisked her upstairs to dress her.

I also noted at this time that Mrs. C. seemed to show no pleasure in Caren. She did not talk with her, name things, show excitement, or even "baby talk" to her. Her lack of contact and flat affect were marked. At the end of this visit, Mrs. C. showed me her extensive doll collection, which she kept in a large glass case in the living room. Each doll was preserved, rigid, and still, much like the emotional relationship between Caren and her mother.

At the end of the first trimester, Mrs. C. had several dreams of twins, and reported "superstitious" feelings when she cracked an egg with a double yolk or received a double-apple at a restaurant. These "doubles" seemed related to her feelings about caring for two children, and about her difficulties with her own sibling relationship and its reflection in her relationship with Caren.

At one meeting early in the second trimester, Mrs. C. showed me her family album containing pictures of her family at the time Mrs. C. was pregnant with Caren. As I looked at the pictures, she spoke at length about how she always felt "second best" to Marcie. At the same time, she recalled more details about her relationship with Marcie: about their differences and competition for their parents' attention. She remembered her numerous friends in high school, how social she was, and how she was different from Marcie who always sought out one best friend. Mrs. C. then worried about nursing the new infant, expressing fears that nursing would make the child too dependent and that she would get too attached to the baby.

At my visit when Caren was almost 18 months old and Mrs. C. was 18 weeks pregnant, I found that changes had occurred in the home. Mrs. C. had moved Caren into a new crib, which turned into a junior bed. Mrs. C. did not explain to Caren why she was changing beds, nor did she prepare Caren for the change. Apparently, Caren resisted for several days, whining and fussing, waking up several times a night. Mrs. C. attributed this behavior not to the bed change, but to Caren's teething. (The family pediatrician agreed that the behavior was related to teething.)

At this meeting, Mrs. C. looked exhausted and depressed: "This has not been a good pregnancy—I have not felt myself." There was much talk at this time about Marcie and her competition with Mrs. C. for a "perfect" pregnancy. "Really, I think that Marcie is overinvolved with her pregnancy: she thinks everything is so wonderful, that she will have an easy delivery. Marcie never wanted to have kids and actively considered a tubal ligation early on in her marriage. I think her seeing me with Caren helped change her mind. When Marcie had some spotting early in her pregnancy, I was glad this happened because it made Marcie see that pregnancy is not so rosy. I'm tired of her denying the possibility of so many problems. Since I had Caren, I've *felt* like the older sister, and Marcie's giving me information about pregnancy irritates me—it's as though she has discovered these things and is telling me."

About 6 months into the pregnancy, Mrs. C. reported that she dreamed about delivering a baby 3 months early, and was shaken when she awoke to find she had not really delivered. She said that she wished the pregnancy was over, yet was apprehensive about taking care of two babies. "I realize that even if Caren thinks that other babies are nice, she may not like her brother or sister." Mrs. C. had recently read a lot of books about child care and sibling rivalry. She commented, "I did not realize that the rivalry part of sibling relationships was normal. I thought that sisters were just supposed to get along, and that in my case it was me who was always the bad one. I did everything I could not to be like Marcie. She would smile all the time; I would pout. She played the piano; I took up art and painting. Her birthday came before mine in the calendar year, and I could not understand this."

Mrs. C. rarely spoke to Caren about the pregnancy, about the upcoming birth, or about the "new" brother or sister. Surely, Caren must have felt that there was less room on Mommy's lap, which by the end of the sixth month was rapidly disappearing; but Caren spent little time on her mother's lap anyway. She was very much isolated, possibly clinging defensively to an image of herself as the "baby." Mrs. C. constantly had to keep Caren out of the newly finished baby's room, and punished her for taking the new baby's clothes or toys, which had been set out so long ahead of time. Caren was already being "cut off" from experiencing her family's development. It seemed that Mrs. C. had already established a pattern that would leave Caren out of her mother's relationship with the new baby.

So, as Mrs. C. moved into the last trimester of her pregnancy, she remained caught up in unresolved rivalries with her sister. Marcie's parallel pregnancy heightened the rivalry and served as a focus for Mrs. C.'s preoccupation with sibling themes. At the same time, Mrs. C. persisted in expressing themes relating to cutting off feelings and in avoiding a relationship with her daughter. She preferred to allow others to care for her daughter, while Caren demanded her mother's involvement. Caren's demandingness may have reminded Mrs. C. of her own neediness and unresolved ambivalence toward her mother and sister.

At the beginning of Mrs. C.'s seventh month, she reported a dream about Marcie:

> Marcie delivered a baby boy. She was 2 months early, so she delivered before me. I drove her to the hospital and they said she was 10 centimeters, so she had the baby. Then she and I drove downtown to her husband's office. They began jumping around, very happy. The baby weighed 7 lb. 13 oz.

A month later, Marcie went into premature labor triggered by a urinary infection. Medication and bed rest halted the labor, but there were a few tense days for the family. When Mrs. C. phoned to tell me this news, she seemed most interested in the possibility that her sister might indeed deliver before her.

During Mrs. C.'s eighth month, she seemed especially focused on herself and her own needs. She tended to withdraw even more from Caren and to send her into the housekeeper's care whenever possible. At the same time, she seemed to resent Caren's efforts to separate from her.

Mrs. C. described attending a neighbor's birthday party during which Caren had put two pretzels into her mouth and walked quite fearlessly into the swimming pool. Mrs. C. had panicked, grabbed Caren as she went down the pool steps, and pulled her out. "Caren was fine, just upset that her pretzels were wet. Somehow, she just wandered away from me." After this episode, Mrs. C. had the following dream:

> We were at a pool. A lot of people were around, like a toddler class. A fat lady was in front of me and I couldn't see where Caren was. Suddenly, I got worried and tried to get around the fat lady who was in my way. Finally, I reached Caren, but it was too late. She lay, like in a coma. I woke up frightened.

This kind of dream during pregnancy may not be unusual for a multipara (see Kestenberg, 1976, p. 241, and Mrs. B.'s dream below). What is exaggerated here, however, is Mrs. C.'s withdrawal from Caren. The pregnancy (fat lady) is in the way of their relationship and Mrs. C. is "too late" to reach out to her daughter. The fat lady could also be her pregnant sister Marcie who represents the intense, rivalrous feelings which seemed to inhibit Mrs. C. from being optimally available to Caren.

I talked with Mrs. C. about her toddler's understanding of the new baby. Mrs. C. said that Caren had begun to put some small blocks into her diaper when she went outside to play. She explained this behavior as Caren's identification with her pregnant mother. Also, Caren often said "Baby," but Mrs. C. felt that this was a name for Caren herself, and not some awareness of a separate baby. Mrs. C. did not answer me directly about

Caren's preparation for her sibling. When I repeated the question, she said, "I think she'll be surprised, although my husband has begun mentioning her new baby brother or sister."

Mrs. C. spoke about her desire to have a son: "I feel like I'm carrying a boy; I seem to be a different shape this time, more pointed, not so full around. I'd be surprised if I had a girl, although a girl would be easier since I'm used to girls. A boy would be more fun." Mrs. C. recalled feeling that she and Marcie were blended by her mother; she concluded that having a son would help her parent two different children.

Mrs. C. viewed Caren these weeks as a "nuisance." Her screaming, fussing, and messing up the kitchen cabinets annoyed her and she felt herself losing patience with Caren again and again. "Caren is learning to be independent, though. Sometimes she will push me away and say 'Bye-Bye,' preferring to go with the housekeeper. She can tell when I don't want to be with her, so she'll find something else to do."

Mrs. C. recalled that her own childhood was spent in the constant company of Marcie. "It would have been awful without her." She added, "I think Caren is bored now. She'll like the companionship of a brother or sister." Mrs. C. may have sensed that Caren might get more nurturance from a sibling than from her mother.

In one of our last meetings before the birth, Mrs. C. spoke about Marcie, who now seemed out of danger of delivering early. Marcie was experiencing some edema in her fingers but refused to see her doctor. Mrs. C. commented, "She's afraid to find out there might be more problems. I'd go right away; that's one difference between us."

After these comments about her sister, Mrs. C. proceeded to comment about Caren, "She's been so difficult, always squirming, throwing food when we take her to restaurants. It's really unpleasant being around her a lot of the time." She added, "I'm glad I'm almost finished with this pregnancy and that I will have had my children close together. I've been preparing my husband that this is the last pregnancy, even if it is a girl. Marcie is sure she will have a son, but she looks just like I did last time." The sisters' parallel pregnancies continued to promote these rivalrous, competitive feelings in Mrs. C. Her associations to Marcie and Caren made it difficult to tell about whom she was more concerned.

Postpartum

Mrs. C. delivered a healthy 8 pound boy on her due date. On the day she went into labor, the housekeeper left suddenly, following a buildup of tension around the house. In desperation, Mrs. C. asked her mother to come and care for Caren while she and her husband went to the hospital. Mrs. C. spent two days in the hospital.

I visited Mrs. C. when she was one week postpartum. The household was somewhat chaotic: there was much coming and going and Caren was probably excited, confused, and disorganized by this transition in her life. The new baby was a quiet, calm infant, however. He was an extremely slow eater who proved difficult since he required a full hour to feed properly. Sometimes the baby would fall asleep midfeed, then wake crying because he had not yet finished.

While Mrs. C. was nursing the baby, Caren stood next to her mother, then went to her room to bring back a child-sized baby carriage that her grandmother had just given her. Caren tried to pull the carriage into her brother's room and refused my assistance. The new baby nurse was upset by the clutter and told Caren to take out her toys. Caren pouted, then cried. I suggested to Mrs. C. that Caren wanted to stay around the baby.

As the baby was being changed, Caren edged up to the changing table, and I picked her up so that she could watch her brother. Caren quieted and looked on attentively. I sensed that she wanted to be included in every possible way. Caren asked for "more" when it was my chance to hold the baby, so she and I looked at him together. Caren was gentle, patting his head, pointing to his nose, ears, hair, mouth, and eyes when her mother asked her where these parts were on the baby. Caren laughed happily during this opportunity to be with her brother.

When I visited Mrs. C. at one month postpartum, she said she was overwhelmed by "problems" with Caren. Caren had refused to go to her bed at night, pulling off her diapers and refusing to let either parent dress her. Caren was staying up until 11:00 P.M. Caren's nap schedule was also irregular and there was no correlation between days she napped and days she stayed up late.

My last interview with Mrs. C. and Caren came when Mrs. C. was 6 weeks postpartum and Caren was 2 years old. Prior to my arrival, I had arranged with Mrs. C. to spend part of the session alone with Caren. But Mrs. C. seemed unable to allow me this time with Caren: holding her son, Mrs. C. joined us in Caren's room. Both mother and daughter seemed depressed and low key. Caren avoided me, keeping a straight-lipped face, eyes down. Her language was limited to a dozen words at most. Throughout this visit Caren remained "cranky" and grim-faced, with no smiles for anyone including her mother.

Mrs. C. said she had stopped nursing the baby: "I could not attend to Caren while I was nursing and he took too long to get through a feeding." The baby barely whimpered, sucked his bottle on and off, looked around with a vague interest in his surroundings. Mrs. C. said, "He behaves like I did as an infant. Caren is more like my husband, impatient and demanding. Even his mother thinks Caren resembles him. This baby is exactly the opposite. I think he even resembles the way I looked as a baby."

At the end of the hour, Caren went to her bureau and, saying "Binkie," tried to climb up to grab the jar of pacifiers. Mrs. C., who was feeding her infant, said that Caren would want only the yellow pacifier. I reached the jar for her and let her pick. Caren took out a new, clear pacifier, pulled her yellow blanket off her bed, and stood stiffly next to her mother holding the two items. Mrs. C. paid little attention to Caren, making no room on the couch for Caren to sit next to her. After a few minutes, I suggested that Caren might need to snuggle, and helped her nestle in on her mother's other side. I left Mrs. C. feeding her quiet infant, while Caren tried her best to get comfortable next to her mother.

Discussion

Mrs. C. was very much caught up in her rivalry with sister Marcie. At times, this rivalry seemed a defense against Mrs. C.'s ambivalent, dependent wishes toward her mother, as well as against sexualized aspects of her femininity. So much of Mrs. C.'s identity seemed formed in the shadow of Marcie. In part because of her own mother's withdrawal from Mrs. C., she was mothered by Marcie. This mothering never proved a completely satisfactory substitute, and the girls always were vying for a piece of their mother's availability. Sometimes it seemed as though Mrs. C.'s fighting with Caren represented the fighting she never permitted herself to carry on with Marcie, since she depended too much on Marcie as a substitute mother.

The pressure of the pregnancy seemed to heighten sibling issues for Mrs. C. and increased her unavailability to her toddler daughter. Mrs. C. would rather show me her photographs than her child, for Caren had come to represent just another rival. Mrs. C. seemed to wish not to get too involved with Caren, not to let Caren be too dependent. Perhaps her fear of closeness to Caren represented a fear of her emerging envy of Marcie, feelings Mrs. C. would be unable to deal with.

The intensity of Mrs. C.'s revived sibling conflicts interfered with her ability to be available to Caren during the pregnancy and prevented her from preparing Caren for the new baby. Mrs. C.'s unresolved envy of Marcie suggested that she could not create a good parenting triangle with Caren and the new baby. Her sibling rivalry made her more likely to repeat her own family situation with Caren: she seemed to set up Caren as a rival, repeating her experience with Marcie. Her all-too-easy willingness to let Caren go also suggested a deficit in her ability to be warm and close with her child. Mrs. C.'s second pregnancy was promoting an exaggerated pulling away from Caren, perhaps because she now identified Caren with her older sister Marcie.

Because Mrs. C. had not worked through her own sibling conflicts, she was unable to prepare Caren for the sibling. It seemed likely that Caren's lack of preparation combined with her lack of resolution of rapprochement issues, e.g., her unneutralized aggression, might result in the aggression being displaced to the sibling. One could already see precursors in Caren's aggressive approach to other toddlers and her impulsive, aggressive, chaotic outbursts at home with her mother.

MRS. B. AND BETH

This section briefly describes the second pregnancy of another mother-toddler pair. Although Beth was the same age as Caren at the onset of her mother's pregnancy, her relationship with her mother differed significantly from Caren's relationship with Mrs. C. Mrs. B. brought to her parenting the warmth, reciprocity, and involvement that were missing from Mrs. C.'s mothering of Caren. Mrs. B., too, frequently and spontaneously spoke of her sister, but in her case the revival of the sibling experience had a predominantly positive cast.

Second Pregnancy

Mrs. B. was 2 years younger than her sister Janet. On one visit early in the pregnancy, Mrs. B. described how nice that spacing had been for her sister and herself: "I shared a room with Janet. We would jabber late at night and talk about everything." The sisters often played together. As children, Janet used to play the "mother" and Mrs. B. the "child" in their games. Now, as adults, it seemed that Mrs. B. was the "mothering" sister and that Janet came to her for advice and nurturance.

Mrs. B. talked about their similarities and their differences. Janet was more "dramatic," and had fewer personal relationships. Mrs. B. saw herself as the more stable of the two. "I married at 19, a crazy thing to do at the time, but it was just right and I had to do it. We were married 9 years before we had Beth, and this period was important to both of us. Janet married at 20 and divorced 6 years later." Since her divorce, Janet had been involved in a number of relationships and was still fairly unsettled.

Mrs. B. continued, "Janet acts excited about this pregnancy, but I think she is really jealous. It's not what she says in words, it's just how it feels being around her." Mrs. B. commented that she did not want Janet to be jealous of her, adding, "My life choices have not necessarily been the best ones. I'd like to think that it is fine for Janet to be comfortable in the variety of relationships she chooses."

Mrs. B. planned to have her children 2 years apart, so that

Beth could enjoy the kind of sibling relationship Mrs. B. had had with Janet. Mrs. B.'s pleasure within her family seemed to influence her preparation of Beth for the prospective sibling experience.

On one of my visits in the second trimester, Mrs. B. told me how wonderful a week's vacation with Mrs. B.'s parents and her sister had been. Beth had been easy and a delight to have along. When I arrived for this interview, Beth was playing an elaborate doll game with two dolls. Mrs. B. said these two dolls had become very important companions for Beth during the vacation.

Mrs. B. looked very pregnant. She wondered aloud if she would deliver early. "Sometimes now I get low, feeling too pregnant and wishing that I had more attention from husband and family. I want to say, Hey, I'm pregnant, pay attention to me!" She reported a dream:

> I woke up from the delivery and turned to my parents who were nearby. I asked, "So, what is it?" My mother replied, "It's a girl, isn't that ridiculous?" Everyone around laughed.

Mrs. B. thought that her mother's friendly comment meant, "You now have two daughters like I did." Mrs. B.'s expressed dependency wishes seemed reflected in this dream, as was her identification with her own mother's experience. Also, the dream revealed her wish to repeat her mother's family and to feel secure in the repetition of that experience.

Next, Mrs. B. reported that she had talked with Beth about the "big baby" and the "little baby," both of whom would need mother's attention. According to Mrs. B., Beth had pointed to herself as the "big baby" and to her mother's growing abdomen as the "little baby." Occasionally, however, Beth had seemed confused and pointed to the big belly as the "big baby." From Beth's almost 2-year-old perspective, mother's enlarging belly was surely the big one.

At my next visit, Mrs. B. told me that she had invited Janet to lunch to discuss Janet's present life choices. Mrs. B. wanted Janet to take herself seriously. Apparently, the sisters had had an intimate discussion, and Janet had agreed that she should make some decisions about her work and relationships. Later in the week, Janet had invited Mrs. B. to come to a meditation session at a center she was attending. Mrs. B., who first hesitated to go along, decided at last to join her sister, and discovered that the experience was a pleasant one. She felt she now had a better understanding of Janet's present world.

As Mrs. B. prepared for the baby's birth, she reported a variety of stories she heard at her toddler group about sibling responses to a new infant. "One child regressed a lot upon the baby's homecoming, but after the initial outburst, all seemed fine. Another child seemed unaffected for 6 months, then all hell broke loose. I can't really predict how Beth will handle this. I'll have to take it as it comes." Mrs. B. also observed other families with two children: "One mother I know put her older toddler into a big bed, dumped his bottle, and insisted on grown-up behavior. This boy, months later, seemed whiny and demanding. Another mother in the group was more relaxed, allowing the older child his bottle and his crib. And this toddler was verbal, related well to other children—even though he turned to his bottle occasionally."

During this period, Mrs. B. seemed to be sorting out Beth's needs as the future older sibling, and her own needs as the parent of two very young children. She reported this dream:

> I was outside my house, perhaps across the street, taking care of some other matter which took awhile. Then I remembered that Beth was inside the house alone. I dashed inside, only to discover that all the furniture had been rearranged and that Beth was playing contentedly without me.

She commented that she felt very anxious about Beth's well-being and was quite surprised that Beth was so content without her. The dream suggests Mrs. B.'s preoccupation with the developing fetus and her awareness of Beth's individuation. It reveals Mrs. B.'s sense of loss over the end of Beth's infancy and her relief as the mother of a normally developing toddler (Mahler et al., 1970, p. 263). The rearrangement of the house suggests the coming change in family structure brought on by the new baby's birth.

On my first visit during the third trimester Beth (22 months) took me upstairs to play with her toys. She named a set of bears:

"Mommy bear, Daddy bear, Beth bear, baby bear." We made a house of blocks for the baby bear. Beth pointed to her belly and said, "Mommy, baby inside." I acknowledged this information. Then Beth said, "Beth, baby too." I thought that in the context she meant that Beth had a baby growing inside herself like Mommy did. I asked, "Oh, Beth has a new baby inside too?" Beth said, "Yes," then dashed over to put the bears to sleep. After the bears woke up, I had the baby bear hug the mommy bear and the "Beth bear" watch, then demand a hug too, pushing the baby bear aside. Beth laughed, clapped her hands, and then climbed into her crib to lie down a minute next to another doll. Then, just as quickly, Beth wanted to get out of the crib but refused my help. Only her mother's help would do.

Before I departed, I mentioned to Mrs. B. what Beth had told me about the baby inside her. Mrs. B. said, "When I mention the new baby, she'll often say, 'Beth, baby too.' I thought she meant that *she* was still a baby too, indicating that she was not ready to be replaced as the baby in the house." We laughed at the two interpretations and at the obvious ambivalence of Beth's language. In her words, Beth had simultaneously demonstrated her feelings about being big like a pregnant mother who has babies, and about being little like a cared-for baby herself.

During Mrs. B.'s eighth month, Beth was given a new "big" bed, an attractive, natural-wood bed with 6 drawers underneath. The new bed was placed across from Beth's crib, which was still up and which Beth pointed out was now free for the new baby. When I visited in the middle of the eighth month, Mrs. B. reported that Beth was talking frequently about the new infant. The new bed and the changed-about room made it clear that the baby would soon arrive. Beth began calling herself the "helper," saying that she would teach the baby how to talk and help change its diapers. Beth moved her stuffed animals from the crib onto her new bed, insisting that these were still "hers" and not for the baby. Once Beth began sleeping in her new bed, she refused to return to the crib, although she had tried a few times to squeeze into the baby cradle which was set up in her parents' room. When Mrs. B. asked Beth where the baby was, Beth pointed to her own belly.

One meeting, I arrived at the house prior to Mrs. B.'s return from visiting her mother. Mrs. B. told me that she had asked Beth in the car, "Guess who will be at home when we get there?" Beth answered, "The baby." Beth seemed alert to the imminence of the birth, viewing the baby as a separate entity. Mrs. B. reported that a few days earlier Beth had announced as her mother walked into Beth's room, "Here comes mommy and the baby." Beth had developed a narrative of her own life history: "Beth in tummy, born. Beth big girl now. Baby in tummy now."

Two days before her delivery, feeling exhausted and "miserable," Mrs. B. accepted her mother's invitation for Beth and herself to "move in" and allow her parents to take care of all of them. Her mother's housekeeper would entertain Beth, and Mrs. B. would have time to sleep.

Postpartum

Two days after Mrs. B. and her family moved in with Mrs. B.'s parents, she delivered a son after a long, hard delivery. "He looks just like Beth," she announced to me. When she heard that siblings were allowed into the hospital, Mrs. B. asked her husband to bring Beth into her hospital room and the family had its first hour together with the new baby.

After Mrs. B. left the hospital, she returned to her parents' home to be nurtured by her extended family. When I visited her at one week postpartum, she looked happy and involved with her infant son. She said that when Beth had visited at the hospital that first day postpartum, she had hugged her mother, then had gone with her father to wave at the baby through the window. "Now, Beth tells me what to do to take care of the baby and is upset if anyone but me holds him. She sings around the house, sometimes goes off by herself to read, and is otherwise entertained by my mother."

Beth, however, looked strained, not excited or enthusiastic as I had so often seen her. She did not look at her brother and seemed to avoid getting too close to her mother. The night after the return from the hospital, she woke up and asked to sleep with her parents. (The baby also slept in a cradle next to his parents' bed.) They allowed this, without making much of it.

Beth had also asked her mother repeatedly to hold her and to nap next to her.

Mrs. B. said she was exhausted from nursing every 1½ hours during the first few days. She found her son to be a demanding infant, who was not as easily satisfied as Beth had been at the beginning. She wanted me to know that her sister Janet had stayed with her during the labor, rubbing Mrs. B.'s legs and keeping things calm. Mrs. B. felt this was very supportive. Mrs. B.'s mother commented that Mrs. B. had done a wonderful job preparing Beth for the baby, and Mrs. B. added that she thought our talks helped prepare Beth better than she might have otherwise. Mrs. B.'s mother recalled that Janet had been very protective of Mrs. B. when she was born, acting in ways similar to Beth's behavior.

Discussion

Because Mrs. B. was not overwhelmed by sibling conflicts, she was less preoccupied during her second pregnancy with the rivalries and jealousies that inhibited Mrs. C. from being available to Caren. Mrs. B.'s sibling experience seemed to manifest itself primarily in her attempt to understand Beth (as she tried to understand Janet). Her sensitive ability to prepare Beth for the coming sibling grew out of her empathic feelings for her sister.

Mrs. B.'s view of herself as a mother and her identification with her own mother in an ongoing relationship were major factors in her ability to prepare Beth for the coming sibling. Her support system was extensive. Her mother-in-law was a regular and welcome baby-sitter. Her own mother and father were eager and invited caregivers to Mrs. B., her husband, and Beth. By taking care of Mrs. B. for the few days before her delivery, by attending at the hospital during the delivery, and by making themselves available as auxiliary caregivers in the first postpartum week, Mrs. B.'s parents provided her with an environment within which she could better nurture both Beth and her newborn. The reciprocal relationships she maintained with her parents were ideals which guided her own parenting.

Within this context, Mrs. B.'s positive feelings about her sister Janet helped her to anticipate Beth's sibling with pleasure.

Beth played out a variety of roles in preparing for her sibling: the pregnant mother, the proud sibling welcoming her mother and the baby, the possessive big sister sorting out her toys from the baby's, the tiny baby in the cradle. Buoyed by good feelings about her own sibling, Mrs. B. was available emotionally to help Beth experience these roles.

For Mrs. B. and Beth, the pregnancy involved the whole family. Mrs. B. talked about the baby with Beth, helping her sort out her new role in the family: big sister, mother's helper. Mrs. B. described how the grandparents, aunts, and uncles would be the new baby's uncles, aunts, and grandparents, too. In contrast, Mrs. C. experienced her pregnancy in isolation from her family, and succeeded in isolating Caren from the pregnancy and new sibling as well.

CONCLUSION

Expecting a sibling is one of the major themes of a second pregnancy. A woman often has the wish to re-create her own family so that parenting can feel easier and more familiar through an identification with her own mother's experience. The second pregnancy involves the pregnant mother in a re-opening of her own family history. The mother's own sibling experiences will color her ability to prepare herself and her firstborn for the new sibling.

If, as in the case of Mrs. C. and Caren, the mother's own feelings of sibling rivalry are intense and unresolved, these feelings may be exaggerated during the pregnancy and may adversely affect the first child's preparation for the new baby. On the other hand, the revival of the maternal sibling experience during the pregnancy can create positive feelings enhancing the mother's relationship with the firstborn and their attitudes to the new baby. If, as in the case of Mrs. B. and Beth, the mother's sibling relationship was a generally positive one, she and the firstborn may come to anticipate the birth with pleasure and accept with relative ease the shift in the family occasioned by the birth of the new sibling.

Both Mrs. B. and Mrs. C. were younger sisters with daughters. One might expect variations in the revival of the maternal sibling experience where the mother's ordinal position and the sex of her siblings are different. If, for example, the pregnant woman were an older sister, she might reexperience her own feelings with the imminent birth of a new baby. In one of the families I followed, the pregnant woman was the eldest of three children, with a sister 2 years younger and a brother 4 years younger. In her own family, her parents experienced great conflict with the son, the third born. Through most of her second pregnancy, this woman wished to have a son, motivated in part by feelings that she and her husband would be better parents to a son than were her own parents to her brother. The birth of her second daughter, however, re-created for this woman her own positive sibling experience with her sister and seemed to dissipate for the time being the conflict she felt with her brother.

The age of the child when the mother is pregnant, and the mother's own spacing from her siblings, may also affect the mother-child experience during the second pregnancy. Many parents begin the shift to a four-person family when the first child is a toddler. "Pediatricians have noticed that the most common time for mothers to ask for advice about child spacing is when the first child stops being a helpless, agreeable baby and becomes a mobile, often stubborn toddler. . . . Spacing children two years apart is so common in our culture that people have come to assume, without thinking about it, that a 2 year interval is best" (Rubin et al., 1980, p. 147).

Mothering a toddler is not easy even in the best of times. Mothering a toddler when pregnant is difficult indeed. Parenting a child caught up in the profound changes of the rapprochement subphase of separation-individuation (about 15 to 24 months of age) requires a resilient availability (Mahler et al., 1975). As discussed, the pregnant woman is herself immersed in a heightened period of developmental change, typically wrestling with issues of separation-individuation respecting her own mother, her siblings, her first child, and her unborn infant (Bibring et al., 1961). When a pregnant mother must parent a toddler, the optimal development of the toddler may be compromised.

The ability of the child to anticipate the sibling's birth de-

378 *Janice Abarbanel*

pends in great part on the ongoing relationship between mother and child. The child's behavior is a function of the quality of interaction with the mother, and may reflect normal developmental processes or difficulties in the mother-child relationship. During the pregnancy, the child will try in his or her way to understand the mother's experience, and will become aware that the relationship with mother is changing. The change in the mother should promote a change in the child. Although the particulars will be unique for each mother-child pair, the mother, influenced in part by her own sibling experiences, profoundly influences during the second pregnancy her first child's expectations for and feelings about the new sibling.

BIBLIOGRAPHY

ANTHONY, E. J. & BENEDEK, T., eds. (1970), *Parenthood.* Boston: Little, Brown.
BARBER, V. & SKAGGS, M. (1977), *The Mother Person.* New York: Schocken Books.
BENEDEK, T. (1970), The psycholobiologic approach to parenthood during the life cycle. In Anthony & Benedek (1970), pp. 109–206.
_____ (1973), The emotional structure of the family. In *Psychoanalytic Investigations.* New York: Quadrangle, pp. 224–445.
BIBRING, G. L. (1959), Some considerations of the psychological process in pregnancy. *Psychoanal. Study Child,* 14:113–121.
_____ DWYER, T. F., HUNTINGTON, D. S., & VALERSTEIN, A. F. (1961), A study of the psychological process in pregnancy and of the earliest mother-child relationship. *Psychoanal. Study Child,* 16:9–72.
BLUM, H. P. (1977), The prototype of preoedipal reconstruction. *J. Amer. Psychoanal. Assn.,* 25:757–786.
_____ (1978), Reconstruction in a case of postpartum depression. *Psychoanal. Study Child,* 33:335–363.
BORNSTEIN, B. (1949), The analysis of a phobic child. *Psychoanal. Study Child,* 3/4:181–226.
BRAZELTON, T. B. (1981), *On Becoming a Family.* New York: Delacorte Press.
COLMAN, A. & COLMAN, L. (1971), *Pregnancy.* New York: Bantam Books.
DANIELS, P. & WEINGARTEN, C. (1982), *Sooner or Later.* New York: Norton.
ERIKSON, E. H. (1950), *Childhood and Society.* New York: Norton.
FRAIBERG, S. (1959), *The Magic Years.* New York: Scribner's.
FREUD, S. (1909), Analysis of a phobia in a five-year-old boy. *S.E.,* 10:3–149.
JACOBSON, E. (1950), Development of the wish for a child in boys. *Psychoanal. Study Child,* 5:139–152.

JESSNER, L., WEIGERT, E., & FOY, J. L. (1970), The development of parental attitudes during pregnancy. In Anthony & Benedek (1970), pp. 209–244.

KAPLAN, L. J. (1978), *Oneness and Separateness*. New York: Simon & Schuster.

KESTENBERG, J. S. (1956), On the development of maternal feelings in early childhood. *Psychoanal. Study Child*, 11:279–291.

—— (1976), Regression and reintegration in pregnancy. *J. Amer. Psychoanal. Assn.*, 24:213–250.

KRIS, M. (1972), Some aspects of family interaction. Freud Anniversary Lecture at New York Psychoanalytic Society.

MCGUIRE, W., ed. (1974), *The Freud/Jung Letters*. Princeton: Princeton Univ. Press.

MAHLER, M. S., PINE, F., & BERGMAN, A. (1970), The mother's reaction to the toddler's drive for individuation. In Anthony & Benedek (1970), pp. 257–274.

—— —— —— (1975), *The Psychological Birth of the Human Infant*. New York: Basic Books.

RUBIN, R., FISHER, J., & DOERING, S. (1980), *Your Toddler*. New York: Collier Books.

VIORST, J. (1979), You'll love the new baby. *Redbook Mag.*, July, p. 52.

WEISS, J. S. (1981a), Your second child. *Parents Mag.*, May, p. 47.

—— (1981b), And baby makes four. *Redbook Mag.*, July, p. 27.

WEISSBOURD, B. (1981), Your toddler and your pregnancy. *Parents Mag.*, May, p. 96.

WINNICOTT, D. W. (1960), The theory of the parent-infant relationship. *Int. J. Psychoanal.*, 41:585–595.

PROBLEMS
OF PATHOGENESIS

The papers comprising this section are modified versions of papers presented to the International Scientific Study Colloquium on "The Psychoanalytic Approach to the Nature and Location of Pathogenesis," held at the Hampstead Child-Therapy Clinic, London, on October 30 and 31, 1981.

Problems of Pathogenesis

Introduction to the Discussion

ANNA FREUD

WHEN, AT THE END OF LAST YEAR'S SYMPOSIUM ON THE SU-
perego I suggested "Problems of Pathogenesis" as a further
subject for discussion, I did so under the misapprehension that
we stood more or less isolated with our distrust of many of the
current conceptions in this respect. Since then, however, I had
the privilege of reading a paper on the same subject by Arlow
(1981), which gave me the feeling that we have a potent ally,
and that this should encourage us all the more to bring forward
our own data derived from the observations and analyses of
children.

What I and many others had been waiting for is the kind of
insight and objective appraisal of the many theories which
dominate the analytic field at present. What worried us, as
evidently it worried Arlow, is the present trend to place single
pathogenic determinants at ever earlier phases of life—a quest
which invalidates or ignores every element of Freud's original,
broad, developmental view. It is the essence of this view that the
onset of mental disturbance, and especially of neurotic disorder, is due to conflicting forces within the personality; that it is
nonspecific, i.e., that it has multiple causes; and that it can be
located in all phases of development. In contrast to this view,
many authors today regard the events of the early mother-
infant relationship as the main pathogenic agents, thereby either ignoring the role of conflict or assuming its existence at a
time of life when the personality, according to our views, still is
unstructured. In addition, they ascribe to a single stage of development the power to determine on its own the individual's

future health and pathology, thereby diminishing the importance of all further stages, preoedipal or oedipal, in this respect.

The Interdependence of Developmental Stages

Not that on the grounds of our own material we have reason to
doubt the significance or impact of early happenings. However,
we regard them primarily as laying the base from which further
development proceeds. If anything, we go further in our expectations than those authors who regard the outcome of
mother-infant interaction above all in the light of the vicissitudes of narcissism and object relationship. We, too, assign to
this phase a beginning capacity to distinguish between an inner
and an outer world; the first establishment of a balance between pleasurable and painful experience; the first beginnings
of the body ego; ego nuclei emerging from the more or less
differentiated id. We consider success in these advances essential for initiation of the next phase when with the step from oral
to anal sexuality the further humanization of the infant should
take place. What needs to be negotiated by the individual at this
time is an impressive list of new achievements, such as temporary separation from the mother and individuation as a replacement of the former biological unity; object constancy in
the place of transient need-directed relationships; mental instead of physical outlets for excitation; the beginnings of secondary process thinking; division between id and ego which
allows for organization of the earliest, even if still primitive,
defense mechanisms; beginning control of body functions;
building up of a reality sense; etc. As formidable as these accomplishments are, however, in a longitudinal study of young
children they take on the aspect of mere underpinning for the
moves due to appear together with the step from anality to
phallic sexuality: object constancy as the precursor of the emotional entanglements of the oedipus complex; denial replaced
by repression and other sophisticated defenses; structuralization increased to make room for the addition of the superego;
reality sense extended to include a time sense; and objective
instead of subjective appraisal of the happenings in the external world.

If these very well-known facts are listed here, it is done to give weight to the argument that the demands made on the individual by development are countless, ongoing, extensive, complex, and that at all times they contain numerous possibilities for failure, delay, disharmony, and consequently for pathological involvement. No step forward can be taken without the ground being prepared for it by previous achievement. To name only a few examples: object constancy will not occur if, in the first year of life, in the anaclitic relationship to the mother, frustration rather than need fulfillment has been the order of the day; control of sexual and aggressive impulses will remain defective if in the anal phase the fear of loss of love, i.e., the toddler's attachment needs, have not urged him toward compliance with the mother's wishes; identification and superego formation in the phallic phase will be effective only commensurate with the strength and validity of the child's object relationships during orality and anality.

THE CONCEPT OF THE INADEQUATE MOTHER AS PATHOGENIC AGENT

I criticize above all the lack of data to support the concept of the unempathic mother as pathogenic agent. There are too many diagnostic statements which take the mere fact of later pathology as evidence that the mother must have failed in her task of empathy with the infant—in spite of no relevant evidence being available, or even when the available data speak against it. Equally, if a child shows healthy adaptation in later life, the mother's adequateness is automatically taken for granted, sometimes in the face of an available history which points to the contrary. From our own observations, we can quote the impressive example of a child who was exposed to potentially traumatic abandonment and lack of care in infancy but who nevertheless developed pleasing normal characteristics and adapted healthily to nursery school and school; as well as of children who developed more or less severe pathology, even though in infancy their successful interaction with a concerned and empathic mother had been open to our view.

The statement that an inadequate mother causes pathology by halting or distorting progress may be erroneous or correct, but in any case it is not reversible. Any longitudinal observation shows that even the most perfect mother-infant interaction and developmentally successful first year are no guarantee of future mental health and certainly no safeguard against neurotic symptomatology. There are countless ways in which such early gains can be lost or, even worse, where the initial benefit of the mother-infant harmony can turn into a threat.

To quote from our own data:

1. In our Baby Clinic we have observed more than one infant who developed in an all-around satisfactory manner during part of the first year while cared for by a concerned, empathic mother, but lost all of his gains irretrievably when, prematurely, she returned to full-time work, leaving the child to a less than adequate substitute.

2. We can cite at least a similar number of instances of the opposite kind, i.e., of mothers whose narcissistically based empathy with the infant failed to change into the normally more distant and flexible object relationship and thus outlasted its appropriate time. When this happens, the bond interferes drastically with the separation-individuation moves which are normal for the child in the second year of life.

3. We are seeing infants who, on their side, cannot tolerate an ending to the period of biological unity with their mothers, quite especially in cases where the interaction with their mothers was a total one. Typically after the birth of a sibling with its natural consequences or after the return of a father following a prolonged absence, the drop in intimacy with the mother is experienced as traumatic; this may lead to a withdrawal of object libido, increased narcisstistic cathexis of the body or the self, and in some instances to long-lasting damage to the growing individual's capacity to form valid object relations.

4. We, like all other child analysts, are familiar with instances where a girl's exclusive bond with her mother is prolonged from infancy and proves an obstacle to her turn to the father in the phallic phase, i.e., prevents oedipal attachment. It is well known that the child's ambivalent battle against this crippling tie—her conflict with the repressed death wishes against the mother—forms the background of many of the most persistent school phobias.

5. For the analyst of adults, any revival of the mother-infant attachment in the transference—even if it is only approximate—should be immensely instructive. It reveals that during this early phase the individual is insatiable, totally egocentric, and exclusively governed by the urge for pleasurable need and wish fulfillment. There is no doubt that these primitive characteristics by themselves cause pathological involvement and character distortion if in any form they persist longer than the time normally allotted to them.

THE ROLE OF CONFLICT IN PATHOGENESIS

There are serious problems which arise when, as a reason for pathology, interaction with an object is put in place of clashes between contrasting forces within the personality. In fact, our own efforts have gone in a direction opposite to the authors named by Arlow. Instead of playing down the significance of internal conflict, we have gone out of our way to demonstrate the inevitableness and ubiquity.

1. We have tried to show that in the growing child's battle for impulse control "developmental defect" can take the place of the regressive processes which initiate neurosis. A different rate of growth, or a different endowment in the relative strength of the drives and the ego, creates internal disharmonies which the individual resolves via compromises. These at least resemble neurotic symptomatology, and are, by the way, a fertile breeding ground for future true neurotic development. The best examples of this are certain obsessional manifestations which occur as early as the anal phase and are not due to regression from the phallic stage, as is the case in true obsessional neurosis. This happens if ego maturation is premature, compared with a much slower development of the drives. In contrast, uncontrollable impulsiveness occurs in cases where ego development lags behind drive development or where, for constitutional reasons, ego strength is minimal with an increased, constitutionally given urgency of the drives. In all the instances mentioned, it is disharmony which leads to conflict, and in turn conflict which leads to pathology.

2. We have made, and tried to substantiate, the assertion that

conflict governs the entire process of personality development. That id, ego, and superego are at cross-purposes with each other in the sphere of drive control is basic knowledge. It is less recognized that the same may also be true for the whole range of gradually unfolding ego achievements. I have described this process in detail under the term "developmental lines," i.e., sequences which lead from immaturity to maturity concerning characteristics such as emotional self-reliance, adult object relations, peer relations of equality, control of body functions and motility, development of signal anxiety, secondary process functioning, working ability, etc. (A. Freud, 1965). To look at such developmental gains as the result of smooth maturation seems to me a fallacy. On the contrary, I believe, and have tried to prove, that each step forward in any of these respects represents a hard-won victory in a battle of influences which emanate simultaneously from the inherited constitution, the environment, and the three different agencies within the mind. Thus, in this ego area, too, I see progress as based on compromise formations between conflicting forces. So far as these compromises (fashioned with the help of the synthetic function) are adaptive, they serve progress toward adulthood and mental health. However, as often as not they are nonadaptive in the sense that they halt or limit forward movement. In the latter instance, they give rise, if not to symptomatology, at least to pathological distortions of character and personality (A. Freud, 1981).

Conclusion

I am offering this compressed and abbreviated statement of my own position on pathogenesis to invite discussion. Any contribution which further adds to, widens, or clarifies the subject will be more than welcome.

BIBLIOGRAPHY

Arlow, J. A. (1981), Theories of pathogenesis. *Psychoanal. Q.*, 50:488–514.
Freud, A. (1965), Normality and pathology in childhood. *W.*, 6.
───── (1981), Psychoanalytic psychology of normal development. *W.*, 8.
Symposium (1981), Problems of the superego. *Psychoanal. Study Child*, 37:219–281.

Clinical Notes on Developmental Pathology

CLIFFORD YORKE, F.R.C.PSYCH., D.P.M.

I

IN A RECENT PAPER, ARLOW (1981) POINTED TO THE MULTI-plicity of pathogenic conflicts in childhood and their ultimate fate in terms of adult neurosis. In particular, he emphasized the ubiquity, during the formative years of childhood, of foci and loci of future disturbance, and he rejected naïve and over-inclusive views of pathogenesis. This firm recommitment to a view unpalatable to founders of psychoanalytic fashion, wheth-er ephemeral or not, was particularly welcome and prompted Anna Freud (1983) to discuss, from the standpoint of child-hood development, problems of pathogenesis in an unusually broad, if condensed, review. Her paper brings together much of her thinking on problems of nosology: thinking which is central to her work of the past two decades.

If, for the most part, Arlow wrote from the standpoint of adult *neurosis,* Anna Freud felt obliged to consider other forms of pathological disturbance, such as developmental dishar-monies, as these are encountered in children. It may be useful

Director of the Hampstead Child-Therapy Course and Clinic, London, which is maintained by the Herman A. and Amelia S. Ehrmann Foundation, New York; the Field Foundation, Inc., New York; the Freud Centenary Fund, London; the Anna Freud Foundation, New York; the New-Land Foundation, Inc., New York; the Anne Pollock Lederer Research Institute, Chicago; and a number of private supporters.

In collaboration with Stanley Wiseberg, Hansi Kennedy, George Moran, and other members of the Diagnostic Study Group at the Hampstead Child-Therapy Clinic.

389

to draw on some of the points made by Anna Freud and, in the light of clinical illustration, to ask ourselves how, and in what way, certain diverse developmental disturbances can declare themselves. In attempting such a clarification with any brevity or concision, I find it necessary, in the main, to look to children for my examples.

It is generally agreed that developmental disorders in children, unless they are transient or influenced by treatment, have fateful consequences for adults. Although such disorders may predispose to adult neuroses, they may equally give rise to adult disturbances of a nonneurotic kind. Unfortunately, it may be far more difficult in adults than it is in children to disentangle the various contributants to the presenting pathology.

Nevertheless, it is not always impossible to detect a developmental disturbance in adults even at the diagnostic stage if, as is rarely the case, a detailed serial history from childhood onward is available. Before I turn to child cases, and the main body of the paper, a brief example of a developmental disturbance based on a constitutional drive deficit may serve to remind us of this fact.

Ralph was 21 at the time of assessment. A developmental history was available from the mother. He was, according to her, "lazy from the word go." From birth onward it was difficult to keep him awake, and it was a family joke that, in his childhood, wherever he was found, he would be asleep. Even during his feeds it was difficult to keep him awake. In adult life, he would choose fluid or semifluid nourishment in preference to food which needed mastication. He had been a passive boy who welcomed prolonged mothering; he was still bathed by his mother at the age of 12. In school as in adult life he was devoid of ambition, and never learned to read or write properly, although psychological testing indicated that this was well within his capacity. In his sexual life he was singularly passive, waiting always on the woman's initiative; and his sexual activities were largely prompted by a passive compliance with directions to take part in sex shows for which he was paid. Even then, as in private, he could only undertake active intercourse through the artificial "pep" supplied by methedrine. He never quarreled, argued, fought, or said "no" to anybody. His passivity was almost complete. The diagnostician felt, understandably, disinclined to recommend a couch for him to lie on.

II

It is vital for analysts, whether of children or adults, to try to distinguish between certain phenomena which are designated more often than they are delineated. These include: the preconflictual states in what Glover (1950) has called "the primary functional phase" of development; expectable conflicts, whether internal, external, or internalized, appropriate to each developmental phase; conflicts which issue in neurotic solutions, whether of symptoms or of character; conflicts in which the contesting forces persist alongside each other without adequate resolution and which lack the measure of synthesis achieved in either adaptive or neurotic solutions; reversions along developmental lines as distinct from regressions of structures; developmental deviations; developmental disharmonies; developmental defects; and developmental arrests.

I do not propose to enter into a detailed discussion of all these various terms. Some of them, in any case, have acquired the status afforded by general agreement and are not in need of any reemphasis. Others, however, require some clarification in terms of their clinical applications or degrees of conceptual usefulness. Perhaps we should confine ourselves to certain developmental disorders; and simply take, from one or two striking child cases, a few clinical vignettes, and ask ourselves which of these various disturbances may be illustrated by them. In thus proceeding from the clinical to the theoretical, I begin with the case of Basil.

CASE 1

A discussion of developmental disturbances necessarily involves a consideration of developmental lines. It is no accident that Anna Freud (1963, 1965) took, as a prototype for such lines, the one which leads from dependency to emotional self-reliance and adult object relationships. This line, after all, touches on every aspect of internal and external adaptation.

The question arises whether we can legitimately speak of *deviations* on such a line, as well as arrests and reversions along it. We all know people who, for a variety of reasons, internal or external, fix their affections and focus their instinctual life on dogs, cats, or horses. It is likewise a matter of common observation that inanimate as well as animate objects can play an important part in progressions along this line. For that matter, the child's relationship to his close (animate) objects is often reflected in his attitude to things. Moreover, the latter frequently form a link in transitions of cathexis from subject to object. As in any other developmental evolution, however, difficulties may arise in the course of it which lead by one route or another to varying degrees of adaptive failure. The relationship to inanimate objects may, indeed, for some, turn out in the end to assume a greater prominence than relationships to people.

Basil's case may illustrate this point. He was in psychoanalytic treatment for 8 years, beginning at the age of 9. When he was first seen he was "absorbed in a fantasy world, isolated from other children, and showed no affection. He often threatened to bite or strangle his younger sister. His behavior varied from rigid overcontrol to complete breakdown . . . and unbearable anxiety attacks. Primitive play with urine and feces evoked no shame in him." Bizarre fantasies were apparent in his notions about the body. For example, he once asked: "Why does my nurse not turn her head right round, so that I could use it as a wheel?" (Thomas et al., 1966, p. 530). He described his anxiety about the lavatory: "You never know what will happen when you sit on that hole—everything may fall out and you'd find yourself being a skeleton with nothing but this bit of skin holding you together" (Rosenfeld and Sprince, 1963, p. 629).

His early life was wretched and characterized by traumas, an episode of severe cruelty and starvation, inconsistent love, and violent behavior by the parents toward each other. His own memories were of feeling "all deserted, feeling all alone, and waiting and waiting for *something* or *someone* to turn up" (Kennedy, 1968). He rarely spoke of the good experiences which a fuller anamnesis revealed. In the second week of treatment his analyst provided him with a large toy cash register which conformed with his exact specifications. This cash register became a very important object for the next 3 years; but in the first few months of treatment it was the only valued object in the treatment room, while the therapist was relegated to a role akin to the furniture. It was the first thing Basil looked for when he arrived. He talked to the machine rather than the therapist; a blissful smile appeared on his face when he caught sight of it; he explored it from every single angle with his hands as well as his eyes; and only the register itself seemed to provide him with a measure of contentment and well-being otherwise absent from his life.

Hansi Kennedy (1968) emphasized the manner in which Basil put the cash in at the top of the register and took it out of the bottom in a way which reflected the enrichment of the self and which replenished the feared loss of valued attributes into the lavatory pan. Over the years his interest gradually diminished so that when, at the age of 12, he was given a transistor radio by his mother for Christmas, it immediately replaced the cash register, though it was employed in a radically different way. Whereas the register was used almost exclusively as a need-fulfilling object and source of comfort, the radio was never an unalloyed source of undiluted pleasure and reassurance. It was also a focus of his fantasies and fears; of aggression as well as libido; and it carried both narcissistic and object cathexis in a transitional way. Thus damage to the radio was both feared and brought about; it acted as a conflictual seducer and as the seduced; but displacements from different levels of instinctual development prominently included active and passive expressions of disintegration as well as castration.

In summary, it could be said that Basil found his relationships to real objects unsatisfying, fragmented, disappointing, and, in the end, disillusioning.

I suggest that the foregoing vignette describes a *developmental deviation* on the object relations line. But what is a developmental deviation? In what way does it differ from other forms of developmental disturbances in which forward progress may be halted, slowed up, or reversed in one or more of the structures themselves, or in their interaction with each other or with the outside world? In a developmental deviation at least *one* developmental line is itself "skewed." It is as if forward progress to adaptive way stations had gone badly awry. It could be argued that, in the case of *deficits* and the like, the individual may attempt to reach expectable goals, but is too handicapped to achieve them. In deviations, on the other hand, development proceeds as if certain way stations, and in particular the end points to which the various developmental strands converge, were of a qualitatively different kind. This is not to say that certain *defects, arrests,* or *disharmonies,* as yet undefined in this paper, do not play their part in the genesis of deviations. But however this may be—and it may well be the case with Basil— we believe that Basil's story shows a particularly clear type of deviation on the developmental line of object relations; and that the later steps on this line are permanently influenced in the direction of inanimate objects rather than living people.

To be sure, there are various ways in which a developmental line may be disordered and give rise to a deviation. Certain way stations may be omitted altogether, or be subjected to serial change. This would happen, for example, when the oedipal phase is by-passed so that all subsequent object relations are colored by the omission. Some of these considerations may also apply to Basil. It may be objected that such deviations come about for defensive purposes: this may or may not be the case in any given instance, but the question of definition is by no means thereby affected.

There is another possibility which may account for deviations which involve—as must often be the case—more than one close-ly associated developmental line. The line of object relations development cannot, for example, be divorced from the line which leads from egocentricity to companionship. An advance toward the latter might still be closely accompanied by a mea-sure of arrest in a stage of need fulfillment where close object relations were concerned; so that a degree of apparent social adaptability might be accompanied by an inability to form satis-factory or stable relationships with objects that are close. But let us now take a second vignette, and ask ourselves whether or not it illustrates a different kind of developmental disturbance.

CASE 2

Ling-pi was born shortly after his parents came to this country. He was referred to the Clinic when he was 4 years old. He was the second of three children. His mother described him as an unhappy child with aggressive impulses which at times were overwhelming. He was extremely negativistic toward his mother, often appeared frightened and anxious, and was uncommonly prone to injury. Stuffing with food, subsequent vomiting, and continued enuresis were also mentioned in the referral. We were fortunate in that Ling was already known to us: he had been observed regularly in his home from the age of 2 onward.

At the diagnostic stage, the developmental lines were unusually interesting; and not one of those described in the Profile appeared age-adequate or without some measure of developmental lag or distortion. For present purposes it will be enough to focus only on one of them: the line which leads from irresponsibility to responsibility in body management. Ling's progress along this line was distinctly odd. The first "way station" is reached when aggression is turned outward. Ling certainly directed aggression against the mother from an early age, but it was still, in part, lived out on his own body. In some respects the second "way station" had perhaps been reached; but that, too, was no less odd in its manifestations. For while, indeed, the child had achieved the required advances in ego functioning which characterize that "way station," such as orientation in the external world, understanding of cause and effect, and some appraisal of external danger, he had nonetheless failed to exploit these achievements in the service of control of dangerous and self-damaging impulses.

Subsequent treatment of material, obtained between the ages of 4 and 6, taken together with the developmental observations, revealed how a number of factors—some of them coming together in infancy in hapless interplay, others carried forward from one developmental stage to another in reciprocity—laid foundations for Ling's pathology. To begin with, there was a serious insufficiency of need satisfaction in infancy. The baby's difficulties in feeding, the mother's depression, and her inconsistent and sometimes uncaring handling were important contributants to this insufficiency; and they must have helped to ensure that painful experiences predominated and became organizing and structuralizing factors in the development to come. There was inadequate preparation for instinctual fusion. To all this must be added the mother's continuing externalization of her own aggression upon him. From the very first she had seen his feeding difficulty as a hostile rejection of her; and when, during his second year, Ling became hyperkinetic, she could only see his overactivity as intentionally and frighteningly destructive. There is, of course, no suggestion that the child's hyperkinesis was induced by the mother or that it did not, in itself, make a significant contribution to pathology; but with the emergence of the boy's anal aggression, she could see him only as a monster.

Yet, during this same period, the child's tie to pain began to show itself in an unusual propensity for accidents—accidents partly furthered by the mother's inability to set protecting limits. On several occasions these accidents necessitated medical treatment. When, toward the end of the second year, the mother's third pregnancy became obtrusive, his aggressive behavior and self-damaging activities were intensified. At the same time, attempts at toilet training were instituted; the child went off his food altogether; and he began to smear various things with feces. After the third child was born when Ling was 2¼, he would intermittently stuff himself with food and vomit. He would try to hit the baby with a toy truncheon; and although the mother protested vigorously, she always left the truncheon where he could find it. But he also repeatedly took flying and damaging leaps down the stairs; and he took so few personal precautions in self-protection that, even at 3½ he got a black eye as he watched a cricket ball falling into his face.

With the birth of the baby the mother saw Ling's aggressive behavior toward the newborn as evidence of a "killer." Her fear of the child had already reached pathological proportions. Her attempts to hide from him, together with her refusal or inability to limit his aggressive expression, gave his externally directed aggression an omnipotence which hindered the establishment of any substantial controls. Ling came to see himself as dangerous and unloved; and these self-perceptions were fostered by an ego which, in its intellective functions, was unusually well advanced, and he could readily understand her interdictions. From the standpoint of fantasy play, symbolic thinking, abstract reasoning, and awareness of the world, Ling's ego and its functioning were unusually sophisticated; but it did not serve to establish effective internal checks and controls. Indeed, it did not even allow him to take the step from physical to verbal aggression. Instead, it played its part, together with the mother's externalizations following the birth of the baby, Ling's own unbound aggressive energies, and the mother's interdictions which he subsequently internalized, in presiding at the foundation of harsh superego precursors. This meant that Ling felt less "bad" when he attacked himself, a feeling nurtured by the circumstance that self-injury, and self-injury alone, could attract the mother's concern, or at least the mother's attention. The following sequence thereby developed. He attacked the baby; he felt bad about it afterward; he reduced this feeling of badness by attacking himself or at least by sustaining injuries; and thereafter he received a measure of care from his mother. By itself, of course, this formulation is too simplified; but the detailed observation and treatment notes support the contention that Ling's case shows serious *developmental disharmonies*. There is a disharmony between the advanced part of the ego and superego precursors on the one hand, and the id on the other; there is a disharmony between the superego and the defective part of the ego which was unable to supply sufficient control in response to the former's demands; and the ego itself displayed an internal disharmony between intellective sophistication on the one hand and the most elementary advance toward impulse control and the appraisal of external danger on the other.

Anna Freud (1979) has clarified the concept of developmental disharmonies and has given them this name. She refers to the fact that these disharmonies arise between the mental agencies in the course of development; and she has pointed, as a particularly clear example, to a situation in the anal phase where ego development is substantially in advance of drive development, and from which disparity early obsessional phenomena may result (1983).

It was already evident, from the study of neuroses, that the factor of instinctual regression to a fixation point results in a disturbance of balance between id and ego forces from which, in turn, arises the threat of the return of the repressed. A disharmony is thus created. The ego is obliged to give ground, but in doing so attempts, under the influence of the superego, to maintain something of the standards, attainments, and precepts of the adult ego. The resulting compromise formation is kept in uneasy stability by the synthetic function of the ego, though it is still treated as a foreign body in relation to the rest of the personality. What is synthesized here is the *compromise;* whereas, in the developmental disharmonies, what is synthesized is the *disharmony,* which henceforth becomes part and parcel of the developing personality. What has to be emphasized, in any event, is that a preceding disharmony may equally well predispose to neurosis.

In summary, reasonable harmony between the structures demands some equality in their development; and if, by reason of timing or strength, the structuralization of one agency or its level of development is sufficiently in advance of another to create an appreciable disparity, both will be brought into uneasy compromise, under the influence of the synthetic function of the ego, and a developmental disharmony will arise which will be perpetuated and built into the personality.

We could observe that a *defect* in the ego led, in Ling's case, to a *disharmony* within that structure. In this instance the defect was within the defensive organization. But ego defects may equally be cognitive, perceptual, or whatever; and they may vary from the gross and compound defects of severe mental retardation to circumscribed defects in, for example, reality testing. They often are constitutional or maturational in origin, or arise from the operation of other factors in the process of formation of certain ego structures and functions. But we can also speak of constitutional deficits in the drives, and perhaps maturational ones as well. It may be precisely such a defect which was in Ralph when, as a neonate, he was altogether passive and incapable of sucking at the breast with any vigor. It is also common practice to speak of superego defects, though these can only arise during the formation of that structure. Such a defect might show itself, for example, in an undue selectiveness in the admissibility of instinctual trends which are otherwise equally damaging in terms of adaptation.

Let us now turn, for the last clinical illustration, to a rather puzzling case.

CASE 3

Jane's birth was uncomplicated, but problems over feeding began as soon as mother and child returned from the hospital. Jane would fall asleep almost as soon as she was put to the breast, but would awake screaming the moment she was put in her cot. The mother felt physically exhausted and unable to cope with her. Mother and baby were admitted to the hospital when breast feeding was supplemented by the bottle. A satisfactory regime was established, but broke down again as soon as the child returned home. Improvement was gradual until weaning was accomplished and solids were introduced.

Jane's difficulties in feeding amounted, for the mother, to willful and hostile refusal. She said of her daughter, "I tried to do all the right things but could not stand this thing making demands on me" (Berger and Kennedy, 1975, p. 283). She referred to Jane's "shyness" and called it a "symptom" and found these supposed characteristics as hurtful to her pride as the child's supposed "lack of intelligence" at the age of 14 months. She was unable to deal with her daughter's needs.

Indeed, the baby was late in achieving normal milestones, and even the staff of the Well-Baby Clinic, which Jane attended almost since birth, thought she was backward. When she was 3 she was referred to the nursery school in the hope that this would help her. At the same time her brother Dan was born; but the mother was unable to understand Jane's jealous reaction to Dan's arrival, her mother's feeding and evident approval of him. Jane looked to the father in vain for better mothering.

In the nursery school she displayed excessive autoerotic activity and generally retarded behavior. She was clumsy, vacant, drooling, and smelly; and she was considered to be as miserable as she was unlikable. Intellectual retardation was suspected; and the staff was astonished when, on testing, Jane was found to be of high average intelligence.

At this point the child was taken into analysis. Transference manifestations and fantasies during treatment strongly suggested that Jane had complied with the mother's devaluing image of her. There was evidence that the mother's defensive externalizations were accepted and internalized by the child. Her image of a damaged self was later reinforced by conflicts centering on penis envy. Jane's wish to be a boy had been reinforced when her mother displayed obvious affection for, and pleasure in, Dan. The fact that the father was unable to be an adequate oedipal object further compounded Jane's inability to make any substantial developmental advances.

In analysis, however, she made good progress. Within 2 years her view of herself was considerably more benign and she could express the fantasy that, when she was very little, she had been "a pretty baby in blue socks."

When Jane was a baby, our observers noted a degree of resignation which suggested undue placidity from the beginning and which may have laid the foundations for the continued acceptance of the role assigned by the mother. Such an acceptance may have been the only way in which Jane felt she could retain contact with an otherwise "unavailable" mother; while, conversely, any protest against the mother's imposed view of herself may have been felt to jeopardize whatever feelings of security she may have possessed. But any freedom from anxiety in the face of fears of loss and even abandonment may have been purchased at great cost; and the price was pseudobackwardness.

Both Jacob Arlow (1981) and Anna Freud (1983) have spoken of the manner in which some analysts have attributed all pathology to inadequate, ineffective, or plainly "bad" mothering. No doubt, these analysts would have a field day with a case like Jane's, but the maternal influence alone cannot be held responsible for Jane's disturbance. Her passivity at the breast, and the readiness with which she accepted and internalized the mother's externalizations, point to a certain reciprocity of internal and external influences in the developmental process.

What, then, is the nature of the clinical puzzle offered by a case of this kind? What is the nature of Jane's disturbance? Descriptively, it is tempting to suggest that, at the time of referral, there was serious developmental delay, if not virtual arrest. But the results of the IQ testing showed that appearances were in some important respects misleading; important areas of progress coexisted side by side with apparent retardation, thus leading to a clinical, and perhaps conceptual, paradox. This paradox—of striking developmental delay and maturational progress *in the selfsame areas*—was not, perhaps, fully revealed until the child came into treatment. Certainly, innate givens and the lack of environmental facilitation had interacted in such a way that a major degree of pathological structuralization was, at first sight, suggested. As an account of pathogenesis, this statement is incomplete; and it is not enough to say that the child's potentialities were not brought out during the early stages of development, and that the abnormal interaction between mother and child ensured that the latter's functioning remained at a retarded level.

Something more has to be added if we are to account more fully for the fact that a *behavioral delay* goes hand in hand with a *developmental capacity* which has itself moved forward without achieving *manifest* progression. What we have witnessed can only be an *inhibition* in the service of a pathological relationship. Once a fresh, important, and intensive object relationship became available to the child and, indeed, established, a basis was laid for rendering the inhibition unserviceable. Even so, it is doubtful whether much could have been accomplished had not other factors been operative. The mother was given help in loosening, from her side, the pathological attachment; and fresh peer and teacher relationships, in what would normally be regarded as a latency phase, all played their part in reducing the ego inhibitions and in modifying the ego ideal which had helped to keep them in being. In due course the child made striking progress, and is today a successful and well-adapted young woman. What we were dealing with was not, then, a true developmental arrest but, as Berger and Kennedy (1975) stated, a "pseudobackwardness," albeit of a very particular kind.

Finally, this attempt to clarify certain terms, as these are applied to developmental disturbances, is in no way inclusive. A striking omission is the concept designated as "developmental dissolution" or, more correctly, dissolution of developmental achievements. In this case, however, the omission is deliberate. For although such terms as "superego dissolution" and "ego dissolution" are in widespread use, it would be important, for example, to consider how, and in what way, the latter differs from "ego regression" inasmuch as this, too, involves loss of ego functions. In any case, the concept of "dissolution" touches too closely on many problems posed by adolescent and adult psychosis to permit adequate discussion within the present context; and it seems more appropriate to set it aside for consideration elsewhere.

BIBLIOGRAPHY

ARLOW, J. A. (1981), Theories of pathogenesis. *Psychoanal. Q.*, 50:488–514.
BERGER, M. & KENNEDY, H. (1975), Pseudobackwardness in children. *Psychoanal. Study Child*, 30:279–306.
FREUD, A. (1963), The concept of developmental lines. *Psychoanal. Study Child*, 18:245–265.
―――― (1965), Normality and pathology in Childhood, W., 6.
―――― (1979), Mental health and illness in terms of internal harmony and disharmony. W., 8:110–118.
―――― (1983), Problems of pathogenesis. *Psychoanal. Study Child*, 38:383–388.
GLOVER, E. (1950), Functional aspects of the mental apparatus. *Int. J. Psychoanal.*, 31:125–131.
KENNEDY, H. (1968), Some thoughts on the role of the inanimate object in a borderline child. Read at the Hampstead Clinic.
ROSENFELD, S. K. & SPRINCE, M. P. (1963), An attempt to formulate the meaning of the concept "borderline." *Psychoanal. Study Child*, 18:603–635.
THOMAS, R. ET AL. (1966), Comments on some aspects of self and object representation in a group of psychotic children. *Psychoanal. Study Child*, 21:527–580.

CLINICAL CONTRIBUTIONS

First Class or Nothing at All?

Aspects of Early Feminine Development

E. KIRSTEN DAHL, Ph.D.

PENIS ENVY "DOES NOT HAVE ITS PRIMARY ROOTS IN OBJEC-
tive anatomical realities . . . penis envy frequently has its origin
in the dyadic relation between mother and daughter and is a
symptom reflecting the child's difficulties in identifying with
and achieving differentiation from a mother who is experienced as jealous, intrusive, or castrating" (Lerner, 1976, p.
275).

As early feminine development has been reexamined during
the past decade (Blum, 1976; Fliegel, 1973), the concept of
penis envy has come under particular scrutiny. Some authors
propose that it be viewed as a metaphor for other developmental issues. My own clinical experience contradicts this; for the
very young girl, penis envy is best understood as a central and
complex fantasy configuration through which the girl struggles
to understand and come to terms with the fact of genital
differences.

This paper presents selected material from the first year of
treatment of a 4½-year-old girl to illustrate the complexities
and demonstrate the vicissitudes of feminine preoedipal development, especially the oscillations between various positions
before the final oedipal organization is achieved. The centrality
of the girl's preoedipal attachment to her mother, the difficulty
with which this is relinquished, and its contributions to the
vicissitudes of feminine development are examined.

Assistant Professor, Child Study Center, Yale University, New Haven, Ct.
I wish to acknowledge my great debt to Dr. Robert Evans who not only
supervised my work but read critically each draft of this paper.

Freud was convinced that detailed study of the little girl's preoedipal attachment to her mother, with its oral, anal, and phallic wishes expressed in the pursuit of active and passive aims, is crucial for the understanding of female sexuality. The renunciation of her mother in favor of her father as primary love object follows a circuitous route. Freud (1925, 1935, 1933) emphasized the hostility involved in this turning away from the mother, which he traced to a number of sources, especially the inherent ambivalence of the mother attachment and early narcissistic injuries. One of the narcissistic blows is the girl's discovery that she is not equipped with a penis, a circumstance for which she blames her mother. When she finds that her mother is equally lacking in what she perceives as vital equipment, the little girl reacts with contempt, devaluing her mother as a love object: her mother then becomes a ready target for all of the previously accumulated hostility (Freud, 1933). It is only when she renounces her active phallic strivings toward her mother as primary love object that the little girl enters the oedipal phase.

It is generally agreed (Nagera, 1975) that for girls the oedipus complex unfolds in two stages: the first is the *phallic*-oedipal in which sexuality is essentially masculine and active, with the mother as object and the father as rival. The second is the true oedipus complex in which the girl has largely renounced her phallic sexual strivings in favor of more receptive, feminine ones, with her father as object. Both of these stages are thought to have their corresponding inversions. Edgcumbe and Burgner (1975) have argued that there is a distinct *preoedipal* phallic-narcissistic phase which precedes the phallic-oedipal period. This preoedipal phallic phase is distinguished by the drive derivatives of exhibitionism and scopophilia used in the attempt to gain the admiration of the object. This phase must be understood as preoedipal in that there is no real appreciation of triangular relationships; the fantasies emphasize the dyad, with little role differentiation between self and object and drive derivatives are from earlier psychosexual phases.

CASE ILLUSTRATION

Clarissa W. was 4½ years old when she began four times a week therapy; her mother sought treatment for Clarissa because of her persistent elective mutism outside the family. At the end of the treatment Clarissa appeared to be solidly launched into latency. Although the analysis was brought to a successful conclusion after 3 years, I have chosen material from the first year because it most clearly demonstrates the little girl's lengthy and circuitous preoedipal journey and the gradualness with which the final oedipal configuration is reached.

BACKGROUND

Mrs. W. reported that Clarissa was bilingual: she spoke English to her American father and Hungarian to her Hungarian mother. At school Clarissa spoke not at all. She was extremely anxious and uncomfortable about going to school, where she performed poorly and was socially isolated. There were two other complaints: since the age of 24 months, Clarissa had refused to allow anyone except her mother to see her toes, although there was nothing physically wrong with them. During the past 6 months, Clarissa had become preoccupied with thoughts of death, especially her mother's.

Clarissa was an unexpected, but much wanted, first child. Although Mrs. W. was happy to be pregnant, it was an emotionally difficult time for her as her beloved stepfather was dying. Mrs. W. reported that from the moment of Clarissa's birth, she felt extremely close to her because she was a girl— "we share our sex," and there were many things that women shared which men could not understand. The child progressed satisfactorily, according to her mother, throughout infancy.

When Clarissa was 2, Mrs. W. became pregnant again; and again she was troubled—this time by problems in the immediate family. They lived in France where the parents had met, but Mrs. W. was dissatisfied, and longed to live nearer to her mother and siblings. At Mr. W.'s insistence, the family moved to the United States, a decision that Mrs. W. resented bitterly. After their arrival, Mrs. W. was bedridden for 2 months before and following the birth of her son, Noah. Clarissa was cared for by her father who supervised the completion of her toilet training. She seemed to be depressed and inhibited, and she ate little for several months.

It is not clear when Clarissa's symptom of elective mutism

began. Shortly after her arrival in the United States, she joined a play group; although she did not speak English there, Mrs. W. reported that there had been no apparent separation problem. At 3½, Clarissa went through a period of refusing to speak English to her American grandparents, and at age 4, for 2 months, she refused to speak to her father. Just as mysteriously, she resumed speaking to both grandparents and father, although Mrs. W. felt her daughter was rude to them. Both parents reported that Clarissa spoke very little to her father in her mother's presence, preferring to speak about him in the third person to her mother in Hungarian, which he barely understood.

Mrs. W. was a striking woman with large, beautiful green eyes and auburn hair. Her intensity, her vivid manner, and her stylishly bohemian dress conveyed a kind of appealing romantic androgyny. Her articulate, at times almost poetic, style of speech added to the impression that she was a literary creation.

Mrs. W.'s early history was marked by repeated separations from the important people in her life, beginning at age 3 when her parents were divorced and her mother fled Hungary to live in Austria with her lover. Although Mrs. W. joined her mother and her new stepfather in Austria at the age of 5, she was separated again at age 6 to attend boarding school. She recalled her childhood as a time of acute loneliness and unhappiness, living as she was in a foreign country, unable to speak the language, longing to return to Hungary, missing her father whom she was never to see again. In her 20s Mrs. W. moved to France where she met and married Mr. W. The original circumstances of this marriage were not clear, but Mrs. W. later found herself dissatisfied: she considered Mr. W. to be obtuse, rigid, and emotionally unavailable. At the time of the evaluation there had been no sexual relationship for some time and relatively little companionship.

Mrs. W.'s most striking psychological characteristics were her exquisite sensitivity to her daughter, her own acute separation anxiety, and her hopelessness. She complained bitterly of her terrible life, but she felt unable to make any change.

Mr. W. was a tall, slightly stoop-shouldered man. In contrast to his wife's dramatic appearance, Mr. W. was drab and absent-minded. He had an anxious, somewhat obsequious smile as though he was not quite sure he belonged anywhere, but was hopeful one might find a spot for him. The only child of wealthy Americans who had always supported Mr. W. and his family, Mr. W. graduated from college and moved to France. He completed professional training upon his return to the United States, but chose to work part time and in a somewhat casual manner.

Mr. W. felt devoted to his wife. However, although he had ample evidence of her unhappiness in America, he preferred to ignore her complaints and hope she would "adjust" eventually. He was a passive and narcissistic man who tended to deny his many family troubles and to hope vaguely that life would get better.

When his wife was not around, he had a lively, affectionate relationship with Clarissa. Although he was preoccupied and vague, he had periodic flashes of sensitivity toward Clarissa. He was hurt by his daughter's exclusion of him in Mrs. W.'s presence, but accepted it. He had never learned to speak Hungarian, in part because his wife had refused to teach him; the parents conversed in English and French.

TREATMENT MATERIAL

In contrast to her mother, Clarissa was a sturdy, boyishly dressed child, with large, solemn, grey eyes and limp, fine, dirty blond hair. At times, she evoked the sense that she was a waif. When she began analysis, she seemed to be acutely anxious with large staring eyes, rigid body posture, and heavy breathing. Although she was mute during her therapy hours until the fifth week, Clarissa was very communicative through her play, her facial expressions, and a variety of gestures; there was never any doubt about what she intended to convey. As might have been anticipated from her own history, Mrs. W. dealt with Clarissa's separation at the beginning of therapy abruptly and without explanation, but spontaneously acknowledged how anxious Clarissa was. She simply dropped Clarissa off for the third session, having arranged her own schedule so that it was impossible to stay. Clarissa made no protest: she squared her shoulders and marched down the hall to the playroom.

Clarissa's play in the first sessions was dominated by themes of oral aggression, sadistic punishment, and a hunger for contact: there was brutal feeding of many babies who were then angrily thrown away; a biting wolf that wanted to devour everything, especially the therapist; and a little blond girl who both ran away and was thrown away. Very early in treatment, a preoccupation with sexual differences became clear. Clarissa felt that boys could be marvelously exhibitionistic and admired, but that girls could only be "dumb," ugly, and abandoned. Often such phallic themes would be followed by stories in which oral material predominated: stories of greedy children, devouring witches, and two Gobblers, who were always trying to eat people up and were frequently piteously hungry.

During the first months of the analysis, Clarissa's intense preoccupation with the penis and her theories about the cause of her supposed deprivation emerged vividly. Her play suggested that there had once been a golden time when she had been a boy. She seemed to think that this blissful state had been lost through her own greediness, her mother's abandonment of her for her brother, and her mother's oral retaliation for Clarissa's active phallic strivings. Clarissa also imagined that she might have lost her penis through phallic masturbation. There was some evidence that she had tried to turn toward her father in exhibitionistic display but that she had given up her efforts as too dangerous in light of her oral-sadistic attachment to her mother. Clarissa created several specific characters during this period to convey these fantasies.

The most important creation was a little girl named First Class, a phallic girl capable of elaborate gymnastic feats. First Class also had intense oral-sadistic impulses, most frequently turned against her mother and against babies. She seemed to have two mothers—one who was orally gratifying and admiring of her phallic exhibitionism and one who punished her daughter's showing off, preferring her to be "dumb" and ugly. First Class's father, although he enjoyed his daughter's exhibitionism, could not protect her from danger. In the second month, Clarissa picked out the little blond girl doll and named her First Class by sticking a mailing tag on her. Through gestures, Clarissa indicated that this was a fancy girl, very different from Clarissa herself. Clarissa admired the doll's blond hair, then she hugged and kissed her tenderly. First Class turned out to be the boss of the Gobblers; she could make them eat up anyone she didn't like. The only person First Class really liked was Papa. She wanted him all to herself, away from everyone else. Papa loved First Class back. They cuddled and kissed; then they ran away together. Suddenly Mama appeared and angrily went after them. First Class became furious and ordered the Gobblers to eat up all the babies. Clarissa suddenly looked quite worried and began to notice many broken things in the room.

Subsequent sessions suggested that there was a close connection between Clarissa's mutism, her orality, and her attachment to her mother: she got out the Gobblers and pointed to their mouths. She indicated that the Gobblers were friends of First Class and Papa. Then, very playfully, she put Papa inside one of the Gobblers and First Class inside the other. The dolls' feet stuck out, so that they really looked like two huge mouths with feet. I commented that First Class was the boss of the Gobblers, but she also seemed to have very gobbly feelings herself. Clarissa giggled and made the Gobblers walk over and nibble at my fingers affectionately. Suddenly, Clarissa began to hug me, wrapping me and herself up in my shawl. I commented that she wished she could have me all to herself. She hugged me and nodded her head. Speaking for the first time, she said, "No dumb boys!" I said yes, if she were the boss of me and had me all to herself, then I couldn't play with any dumb boys. She giggled and said forcefully, "No dumb boys!" For a long time she sat on my lap, wrapped in my shawl, affectionately touching me, repeating my name softly.

Clarissa's stories began to focus on First Class's delighted exhibitionism as well as her anxiety that there was something wrong with her toes. In the third month, she told a story in which First Class hurt her toes because she wiggled them too much at night. I wondered whether First Class thought it was naughty to wiggle her toes at night, but that she couldn't *not* do it because it felt so good; then during the day she got to worrying that maybe she had hurt her toes at night. Clarissa looked thunderstruck at this, made a bull's-eye motion to my forehead, and exclaimed, "You guessed it!" She then pointed to her baby doll's feet and said, "She loves to wiggle her toes, that's why she never wears shoes"; she giggled. I commented that the doll loved to show off her toes, but Clarissa worried about her toes and wanted to keep them covered. Clarissa solemnly agreed.

In a session a week later, Clarissa told a story in which First Class, wearing my "very fancy watch," went to a birthday party where she danced around delightedly on her father's shoulders. Mysteriously, Mama appeared and took away the watch, saying, "You can't be fancy!" First Class angrily ordered the Gobblers to eat everybody up, but a policeman locked her in jail. Clarissa said, "Now she's all locked up. She can't be angry— she just cries and cries."

A few weeks later, Clarissa had a session in which nearly all these themes were entwined. First Class wanted to play in the water with her friends. Clarissa placed First Class, her girlfriend, Sexy, and some boy dolls in the water and then announced that one boy couldn't play in the water because, "He's a show-off Peepee Boy and First Class doesn't like that. He makes her mad!" Angrily, Clarissa threw the show-off boy across the room. First Class then began to splash around wildly in the water; Clarissa announced, "But she's *not* making pee-pee"! I wondered if First Class might be jealous of those show-off peepee boys, wishing she could do things like that. Clarissa said wistfully, "Oh yes, she *does* want to be fancy like a boy and make peepee with her penis." Clarissa reminded me that in the previous session First Class had had a birthday party and had been given "fancy pearlie shoes." Suddenly, Clarissa said that a monster lived next door to First Class—"all mouth and she just eats people up and won't let them go." First Class became very scared and ran away; the monster pursued her and after a struggle, First Class "killed her dead." Clarissa said, "The monster wants people only to speak French, but First Class fools him—she pretends to speak only French and then he lets her go and then she runs away and speaks ENGLISH!" Clarissa added that this was a very scary story. She remembered the Peepee Boy and said First Class felt very jealous of him. I said that maybe she wished she could show off like that boy. Clarissa said gravely, "Yes she does—she wishes she could be fancy on the outside like a boy and she's not and she gets so *mad* about that!" Then Clarissa noticed a pretty star in the closet. She made First Class clamor for it, saying, "I want that star to wear! Then I can be fancy on the outside too!" I commented that sometimes girls thought boys were special because they were fancy on the outside. Clarissa said solemnly, "Yes girls do get mad—they don't like those fancy boys." She thought about the gobbly monster but reminded me that it was dead. Then leaning against me she said, "You know, a long time ago First Class *was* fancy on the outside and you know what happened? A bad witch-monster came along and this witch *cursed* First Class and made her be a girl and be *cursed* and be *not fancy*—and First Class feels so sad *all the time* and she worries and worries about this. She needs help."

This session conveys the intensity of Clarissa's longing for a penis and how cursed she felt as a result of her supposed lack. She explains anatomical differences as the result of the mother's (the French monster's) oral retaliation for the girl's attempts at separation: an attempt which is active (speaking English) and phallic (wanting to show off). Later in this session, Clarissa suggested that she had been disappointed in her attempts to get love from her father, perhaps in part because of preoccupation with her sadistic attachment to her mother (the witch would curse her and make her a degraded female).

As the third month drew to a close, a more immediate problem arose. Mrs. W. announced that the family planned to visit her childhood summer home in Austria for the next 3 months. As the holiday approached, Clarissa struggled to master her rage and panic at the impending separation from me. Her troubles were compounded by one of her mother's symptoms: Mrs. W. explained that she had been unable to teach her children to say good-bye because she herself had experienced so many good-byes that she found them unbearably painful. She had told Clarissa that she never had to say good-bye to her mother because: "We are always inside each other's thoughts." As the time for separation drew closer, mother and daughter had to be taught how to say good-bye through the introduction of a game of hide-and-seek in the waiting room after each session. At first, they would stand woodenly facing each other while I acted out both roles. Only slowly and with great effort did Clarissa become able to hide, her mother to search for her, and both to find pleasure in their reunion.

Clarissa believed me to be omnipotent, capable of preventing the separation, but unwilling to do so because Clarissa was such a bad girl. She tried to *make* herself bad and disgusting in an effort to preserve my goodness. This mode was often succeeded by a conviction that I was bad. Toward the very end of the month, Clarissa's denial of sexual differences became adamant as she insisted that "both boys and girls are fancy on the outside." This denial apparently enabled her to become more active in coping with what she called "the too many good-byes."

After the holiday, Clarissa struggled to master her overwhelming rage that I had permitted such a terrible separation. The Austrian holiday had proved to be a disaster for both Clarissa and her mother. Various crises in Mrs. W.'s family of origin made it necessary for her to leave her husband and children for extended periods during the summer. She was greatly annoyed by what she perceived as Mr. W.'s childish withdrawal, and she retaliated by abandoning much of the child care to him. Clarissa reacted to the loss of her mother by becoming briefly encopretic.

Clarissa made it clear in the early sessions of the autumn that she was enraged at me for allowing her to go away; for not protecting her from such horrible experiences; for not magically knowing how terrible the summer had been and instead writing her "dumb" cheery letters; she felt acute anxiety because of the intensity of her hostile feelings. In the playroom, she conveyed her experience of helpless terror by hiding in a dark closet and then crying out in a panic-stricken voice, "Mommy, mommy, mommy!" She made it clear that no one could hear her. During one of these episodes of pretended crying, she gouged her forehead with her fingernails so that it bled. In repeated wreckings and messings of the playroom she pretended to be a frightened and helpless child furiously trying to reestablish magical control; I understood this in part as Clarissa's referring to action in the period of encopresis.

Throughout these early weeks, Clarissa was again mute. The sessions became increasingly fragmented, disorganized, and confused, with Clarissa trying to attack me physically and to wreck the playroom. As her fury mounted, she had more difficulty in coming into the playroom; after leaving the waiting room, she would stand immobilized in the hall or dart into a storage closet and refuse to come out; her panic-stricken face and rigid body conveyed her experience of paralyzing anxiety. At the same time she seemed terrified that I would retaliate by making her even more helpless. Clarissa was relieved by an interpretation linking her immobilization with her wish that I use my magic to protect her and her fear that she would, in consequence, be engulfed. I suggested that her feeling of being so frightened that she felt "stuck" was like not being able to speak. Following this interpretation, Clarissa played at being a baby and began to use baby talk. She was never again mute in her analysis.

As she regained the ability to speak, she spun out torture fantasies, shouting angrily, "I'm gonna punish you, the way you punished me!" or "You hurt my feelings and now I'm going to hurt YOU!" She imagined that her feelings of rage were like mud, filling her up and making her disgusting. In contrast, she envied all of my "pretty things" which, if she could only get them, would make her feel better. During one session, Clarissa said that First Class wanted to steal all the pretty things. "She's not pretty," Clarissa added, "She's ugly—she's full of mud." At this she began to torture First Class, attempting to pull off her legs. She began to mutter about "dumb First Class" pointing out that she was "all broken" (the allegation was fast becoming a reality, owing to Clarissa's repeated torture). There followed *sotto voce* remarks about "dumb boys." Suddenly Clarissa started to wreck her magic marker box, saying, "It's mine, so I'm going to wreck it!" This had the quality of her being compelled to assert her prerogative to manage her own possessions, even if this meant ultimate ruination. Her attack on the magic markers and other objects was linked to her insistence that girls were dumb and disgusting, that they felt broken because they didn't have any pretty things. Clarissa announced that she was going to make a beautiful dress for First Class, but just as she began to show some pleasure in how very beautiful it would be, she tore it up savagely, saying, "First Class is ugly. She's full of mud— and she's going to throw up all over everything—mud everywhere!" I said that when First Class was jealous and angry, she felt as though she was full of mud inside and tried to get rid of these disgusting feelings by throwing up. Clarissa became furious, "Shut up! *I* don't have any feelings—you're full of mud, Dr. Mud! You are UGLY and all your pretty things are going to be stolen!" She then attempted to push a tower of blocks over on me.

Clarissa sometimes tried to restore her old feelings of omnipotence by building giant towers, by directing imperious orders at me, and by trying to make me her powerful slave. At other times she shouted in a panic, "You can't know what I'm thinking. You don't know what I'm feeling." All of this suggested a desperate attempt to ward off her annihilating rage, first through projection, and then, when projection failed, by regression to a symbiotic fantasy. Although the latter momentarily restored belief in omnipotent control, it left her vulnerable to the terror that she would become engulfed and helpless.

The dominant theme of the next 2 months was Clarissa's projection of her intense envy of male equipment and prerogatives onto her mother and me. In her view, little girls had indeed been castrated, turned into Nothing at Alls (see below) by wicked, depriving, phallic mothers who preferred boys. Although Clarissa clung to her belief in the phallic mother, she began to relinquish some of her hopes of acquiring a penis herself and to develop a compensatory interest in feminine possessions (e.g., jewelry, curly hair, pocketbooks), which seemed principally valued as assets in winning her father's admiration.

Clarissa was fascinated by the story of Cinderella and her lowly status, sitting by the ashes as ordered by her wicked stepmother. She dreamily imagined how Cinderella would become beautiful and go to the ball. As she neared the end of the tale, however, she shouted dramatically, "No, Cinderella can *never* marry the prince! That isn't allowed! She puts on that wedding dress—it's made of poison—she puts it on and it turns into fire and she'll be burned and burned to *death!*"

A few sessions later, Clarissa created the character of Nothing at All; she said, "Her mama doesn't love Nothing at All because she threw up *two times*—so she has to go off by herself. Her mama *hates* her!" In another story, "Nothing at All lived on a rock in the middle of the ocean all by herself with lots and lots of rats. She was hungry and she tried to get away. She tried to get away to America. But she got to America and the Indians said, 'You don't belong here, little Nothing at All; get out; we HATE you.' So she had to return to the rock in the ocean. That rock is Nothing-at-All Land. And when she got back there, the rats ate her all up. The End."

Clarissa further elaborated on Nothing-at-All Land in a later session:

> This is Nothing-at-All Land, a rock in the middle of the ocean, all bare. But inside is gold stuff and silver and *if you could get it out it would be beautiful.* Here is me, Clarissa. She got sent to Nothing-at-All Land because she's bad and naughty. The terrible thing about Nothing-at-All Land is there's no food there— so Clarissa is VERY hungry. But she doesn't starve because every day she can go to America to be fed. Then Noah gets sent to Nothing-at-All Land because HE was bad—he turned the water tap on two times. He cried and cried because he's so hungry. *He wants his Mama!* And here comes his Mama to rescue him; she takes him home. But she leaves Clarissa there because she hates her forever.

Clarissa became visibly anxious at this point and announced that it was the end of the story. For awhile she played a board game. Then she thought about Hansel and Gretel, saying anxiously, "That witch—she ate them up." I wondered if she was worried that grown-up ladies might have jealous-witchy feelings. Her eyes got very big and she whispered, "Yes!" After a silence she whispered anxiously, "And *do* you have those feelings toward little girls—and you'll take away *my* things—you'll steal my things?" When I asked her what she thought, she said solemnly, "I don't know. Would you?" I said no, I wouldn't, but that she sometimes had such strong jealous feelings she couldn't tell whether they were hers or mine. She relaxed visibly and returned to coloring.

In the next session Clarissa made a plane fly over the ocean to Austria. She said crossly to me, "And you weren't there and you didn't come and the plane might crash in the ocean." I said that she was so disappointed that I had no magic to protect her last summer. Clarissa was so disappointed it felt as though I was no good and all bad. Clarissa grinned broadly and merrily caught my shawl, wrapping the two of us in it; hugging me she said, "And now I have you and you can't get away again!"

Clarissa frequently referred in her stories to Nothing at All and how she had been abandoned for being naughty. Increasingly she began to refer to herself as Nothing at All. She would hungrily grab at pretty things on my desk and then say bitterly, "I'm just nothing! I'm Nothing at All!" Or, drawing a picture, she would ask whether it was pretty; before an answer could be given, she would furiously rip it up, shouting, "It's no good. It's ugly. *It's nothing at all!*" During one session, Clarissa became involved in making a pocketbook; midway through she turned to me and said, "And YOUR pocketbook is yucky!" I commented on her jealous feelings and her belief that little girls couldn't have anything beautiful, that only big ladies could. Clarissa then said her pocketbook was too big. She said, "I want a small one—one that's not too big, something special, just my size." She talked about how pretty curly hair was and how she wished she had curly hair. Suddenly she started to worry that her pocketbook was broken and she said angrily, "You WANT it to be broken!"

She added, "And *you* don't like Noah—you don't like that little boy—that *thing.*" I said that sometimes *Clarissa* felt jealous of that boy for having a special thing—a penis. She grumbled and said, "I don't have those feelings—*you* do!" I wondered if she thought her mother considered boys to be special; that if she had considered girls special, she would have had just Clarissa and not that dumb boy. Clarissa frowned and again began to worry that girls might be somehow broken. She said crossly, "*I* don't have those feelings—other girls might, but I *don't.*" She said something about things being the right size and then told me how her daddy could lift her up in the air.

Suddenly, she darted behind my chair and pulled at my collar saying excitedly, "I want to see your penis! I know it's where your poopy is!" She began to search through the boxes on my desk, saying crossly, "I feel so witchy. I'm going to steal all your things." I said I thought she wanted to steal back what she imagined had been stolen from her. She relaxed and returned to working on her pocketbook, carefully pasting pretty curls on it. When it was time to go she suddenly said the purse was not really hers, "I'm going to give it to Mama." I said that she felt as if she could not keep anything pretty for herself. Clarissa replied, "Well, it's no good anyway—it's just a yucky nothing-at-all thing—throw it away." I said I would not throw it away, that I would keep it until she felt she was able to have it. She smiled and went off cheerily.

As she began to explore her jealousy of her brother and her projection of her witchy feelings onto her mother, Clarissa began to take pride in her own work. This was followed by improved academic performance, a tentative interest in having friends, and the use of speech with some of the children at school. She refused to speak to her beloved teacher, Jane, because of her jealousy of Jane's interest in other children; at one point she said gleefully, "It makes Jane so sad that I won't talk to her; it hurts her feelings!"

There was a renewed interest in exciting boys, especially her brother and her father. In one session she announced that "Doodies are sort of like inside penises," and added excitedly, "That's sexy!" In the next session she repeated this and then said sourly, "Boys have penises and girls have *nothing*." I said, "Boys have penises and girls have *vaginas*." Clarissa looked startled and pleased as though I had given her a gift. "They do? Do you? Do I?" I repeated, "All girls have a special place inside." She drew a picture of a girl who has "sexy feelings," but she was unable to draw the legs or the lower part of the body. I commented that sometimes girls had sexy feelings and liked to touch that special place. Clarissa became silent and completed her drawing. She took up typing. Leaning against me she said softly, "This is sexy." I wondered if she had sexy feelings about me. Angrily she began to push against me. I said sometimes she wished she could be my prince and it made her angry that she couldn't. She said crossly, "Yeah—we're both girls and I can't be a prince." She then said she wanted me to type a story that she would tell:

Once upon a time there was a princess who fell in love with a cat. He was a king cat. The princess and the cat ate a mushroom; it was poison and they died, but they came alive again. They took a walk in the woods and then they got married. They were so happy together—they went dancing, they picked flowers, they took walks together, they read books together. They played music; the princess played the violin and the cat played the guitar. They slept in the same bed together. They were very happy. They slept in the same bed. The end.

In subsequent sessions, Clarissa told stories about her own family, emphasizing that she slept in the same room as Mama and Papa (which was untrue), that Mama and Papa never did things together, except to "ever and ever argue." During the last 3 months of the first year, Clarissa made tentative attempts to work through some of her phallic-oedipal conflicts. She took pleasure in the awareness that I could not know what was on her mind unless she told me and she could "keep secrets." She began to elaborate many fantasies about kings, queens, princes, and princesses. Clarissa said that what distinguished a princess was that she was "a girl who is a boy, too—she's fancy on the outside *and* fancy on the inside!" At times Clarissa imagined that she could be a prince. Sometimes she came to her session dressed in what she called her "fancy pants," adding, "I wear these pants—that makes me a boy." She made a paper ring and, looking at me, said in a voice full of romance, "This is for you. I'm your boyfriend." At other times she said firmly, "Of course I can't be a prince. I'm a girl," but added hopefully, "maybe *you* could be *my* boyfriend."

Her interest in her teacher, Jane, became more openly romantic, with Clarissa saying that she wanted to be Jane's "only one." Remarks like this were frequently followed by a teethgnashing denunciation of Jane's "dumb husband," whom Clarissa would like "to break into little pieces and kill him dead." Toward the end of the ninth month, Clarissa spent a lot of time writing words for her school workbox. She said that she hated Jane and she loved Jane, adding, "Jane doesn't like me because she's always wanting me to do work." Clarissa became extraordinarily bossy toward me. I said that Clarissa wanted to be the only one, the only boss, so that her feelings wouldn't get hurt and she wouldn't feel left out. Clarissa told me that she had seen Jane's husband, adding contemptuously, "He's funny looking." She said furiously, "You know I HATE him; he's so ugly. I'm going to kill him. I'm going to break him into teeny tiny pieces. Now you write that down!" After I wrote it down, she took the paper and ripped it up, saying gleefully, "I'm going to rip him up just like that!" Then she looked romantically at me and lay back, crossing her legs in imitation of me. She said dreamily, "I'd like to eat you up and then I'd have you in my tummy!" I said it sounded as though Clarissa wanted to have *something* in her tummy! She looked startled and then leapt up and asked for First Class, who had been abandoned in her cubby many months before. She searched frantically for the doll and was triumphant when she discovered her, announcing, "Now I'll have First Class forever!" She hid First Class in "a secret place so no one else can find her!"

A few weeks later, Clarissa said that she wanted to dress herself up in beautiful clothes. Having dressed herself and First Class up in beautiful ball gowns, Clarissa happily danced around. At one point she stopped and glowing with pleasure exclaimed, "This is the goodest day of my whole life!" After more dancing she introduced a boy doll to dance with First Class and the three danced together dreamily. When I commented on how everyone looked so beautiful, she said crossly, "No they're *not* pretty." I wondered if she was afraid that the grown-up ladies would get too jealous. She grinned and agreed, adding, "They *are* beautiful, aren't they!" Shortly after this she said with wistful intensity, "The girls always wished when they were little that they could be beautiful and they had wanted to imagine going to fancy dances, but their mother wouldn't even allow them to pretend this. They had to wait until they were grown-up and could get away from their mother." She added righteously, "She was a wicked wicked mother who wouldn't even let them pretend. But now they're grown-up and they're so happy they can be beautiful!"

Relinquishing the powerful preoedipal mother, as well as much of the hostility she had attracted, seemed to free some of Clarissa's libido for sublimation. She became increasingly adventurous, learning to lock my office door behind her and

daring to walk "way far down the hall" all by herself. She created a secret hiding place outside the office and borrowed
many of my "treasures" to hide there. After one of her journeys
down the hall, she urged me to come with her, "Come on. I
have something to show you," she said and took me to the
doctor's scale. With glee, she pointed to the shortest point on
the measuring stick and announced, "That's how little Nothing
at All was. Wasn't she such a tiny girl? But look how big I am!"
and she accurately measured herself. Still standing on the scale,
she surveyed me as an equal and said, "And someday I'll be
even as tall as you are—or taller, because you're really very little
Dr. Dahl—not a tall lady at all [this was, in fact, not true], just
quite little."

Although Clarissa made evident progress during this first
year, she had by no means fully dealt with her conflicts. In spite
of the marked upsurge of interest in learning to read and write
at school, she continued to feel anxious about being active. She
confessed that often she did not really enjoy being a big girl;
during some of her journeys alone down the hall she imagined
that giants or witches might be lurking, and she would turn
back in terror. However, her relinquishment of her preoedipal
attachment to her mother during this opening year of treatment permitted Clarissa to move more firmly into the oedipal
phase. The subsequent 2 years of analysis were spent in exploring and working through fantasies, wishes, and conflicts primarily oedipal in content: the princess who longed to take the
queen's place beside the king; the wicked witch who prevented
the girl from marrying the prince; beautiful girls being courted
by handsome boys; marriage followed by the appearance of
"darling" babies. The particular characteristics of Clarissa's
preoedipal attachment to her mother colored her oedipal fantasies and wishes: the threat of retaliatory engulfment by the
fantasy mother figures remained prominent. Nonetheless, in
both fantasy and "real life," Clarissa was able to triumph. No
longer mute in school, Clarissa developed important friendships with several other little girls. A bright child, she applied
herself enthusiastically to mastering reading and writing, winning her teacher's praise as a committed and imaginative student. Clarissa's father responded to her academic success with

great pleasure, and it appeared that she had succeeded, at last, in engaging his approving attention.

Her relationship with her mother became more problematic; Mrs. W. complained that Clarissa was fast becoming "a little American" and she felt shut out of her daughter's intimate life. During her therapy hours, however, Clarissa gave many indications of blossoming identifications with positive aspects of her mother's femininity—Clarissa took pleasure in dressing attractively, styling her hair in a becoming fashion, and in artistic activity. Therapy was brought to a successful conclusion when Clarissa, age 7½, became happily involved in afterschool activities with her girlfriends. At follow-up when Clarissa was 8½, she was an attractive, sociable child, chatty about her friends and school activities; she was described by her teachers as a leader in her class, an excellent student with a delightful sense of humor and outstanding creative abilities. Mrs. W. continued to complain about the absence of an intimate and exclusive friendship with her daughter, but Clarissa herself seemed unconcerned about her relationship with her mother.

DISCUSSION

Freud (1925) emphasized the critical importance of the discovery of sexual differences to the little girl's hostile renunciation of her mother with the related diminution of phallic strivings; it is only by following this path that she can turn her passive sexual aims toward her father.

Brunswick (1940) elaborated two antithetical pairs which dominate preoedipal and oedipal mental life: (1) active-passive and (2) phallic-castrated. The young child's thrust toward activity is based in part on identification with the active mother. Aggression toward the mother arises when, of necessity, she interferes with this developing activity. Early narcissistic injuries increase the hostility toward the mother which must be repressed. Brunswick comments that "with repressed hostility, a large amount of normal activity must often be forfeited to insure the success of repression" (p. 268). With the emergence of the second pair of psychic antitheses, phallic-castrated, the little girl suffers a further severe narcissistic injury which turns her away from her mother with intense accumulated hostility. The active strivings toward the mother which have become imbued with a phallic character can then be sublimated through activity in the outside world; the passive sexual strivings can be directed toward the father through the wish to be given a baby.

Clarissa illustrates some of these propositions, especially those which pertain to the ambivalence of the preoedipal mother attachment and penis envy. She reminds us that psychological development does not march forward in linear fashion but is best conceived as a series of oscillations between earlier and later points with an underlying progressive momentum. The treatment material demonstrates the intensity of the little girl's struggle to understand the meaning of genital differences and the complex relationship between her fantasies about anatomical differences and her attachment to her mother. Some of what appears to be problematic in the concept of penis envy may lie in the tendency to treat the concept as though it referred to an actual anatomical defect rather than a fantasy configuration created by a small girl in her struggle to solve a central dilemma: why are boys' genitals different from her own? Her solutions in fantasy to this puzzle are limited by her developmental level and will be reworked with increasing complexity as she matures; this may account, in part, for some of the differences between the reconstruction of feminine preoedipal development from the analyses of adult women and the "raw data" from the analysis of a small girl. It is also possible, as Greenacre (1950) suggests, that there may be not only different routes to the resolution of the castration and oedipal complexes, but different types of preoedipal fantasy configurations and "preoedipal phase interorganizations" as well.

Clarissa was born to a mother whose history suggests inadequate resolution of phallic-oedipal strivings and a precarious establishment of feminine genital sexuality; Mrs. W. had to cope with intense conflicts around activity and passivity and a pathological degree of masochism. Clarissa's birth seemed to reawaken her mother's yearning for an undifferentiated, blissful mother-child relationship in which feelings of isolation and loneliness would end; this fantasy is vividly symbolized in Mrs. W.'s insistence on an intimate mother-daughter language from which everyone else was excluded. One is impressed by the likelihood that this narcissistic preoccupation, with its profound intimacy and sensitivity at primitive levels of relationship, drained Mrs. W.'s resources and her availability for supporting Clarissa's efforts to achieve emotional growth and independence at more advanced levels.

Life events brought further narcissistic wounds to this little girl, especially the birth of her brother at a time when her mother was physically and psychologically unavailable. It is probably significant that Clarissa's toilet training occurred at this time and that she was so compliant. It seems likely that she resorted to forceful repression of rage-filled fantasies toward the mother who was the source of the double rejection. Clarissa later became encopretic in her mother's absence when her father was again taking care of her. This situation seemed to replicate the period of toilet training, suggesting that the achievement of bowel control may have been sexualized. Her encopresis may have represented a seductive, oedipal plea to her father couched in anal language, "Take care of me as you once did." Further evidence for this hypothesis lies in the excited, pleasurable quality of her messy explosions in the playroom; her association of being "full of mud" to being "broken"; and her equating "doodies" with "inside penises"—the latter perhaps referring to fantasies of penetration as well. This anal material with its references to internal sensations and fantasies about the inside of the body invites speculation concerning the psychic link between anal and vaginal sensations (Greenacre, 1948); whether this represents a confusion between vagina and rectum, as Freud (1933, p. 118) assumed, or the little girl's attempt to organize vague and unlocalized genital sensations is not clear.

Clarissa's history and material from early in her treatment suggest that her turn toward her father was thwarted by his intermittent psychological unavailability, by his own passivity, and by her mother's furious devaluation of her husband's masculinity. Clarissa probably perceived her turn toward her father as intolerably dangerous because of the sadistic character of her earlier mother attachment; the intensity of this sadism when converted to passivity would invoke unbearable masochistic impulses (Deutsch, 1930, 1932, 1944). Certainly the compliance of her toilet training suggests such a "masochistic surrender." Therefore, Clarissa was forced to settle for her earlier relationship with her mother and to hold under repression the accumulated hostility this relationship entailed. In her efforts to maintain the repression, increasing amounts of activity had to be sacrificed.

Although the focus of this paper is not on Clarissa's elective mutism, this symptom dramatizes the loss of activity to repression. The first clear appearance of her mutism was during her fourth year when she refused to speak to her father and his parents. In Clarissa's inner world, she equated speaking English with the attempt to separate from her mother and an active, phallic turn toward her father; the mother-in-fantasy retaliated for these phallic and autonomous strivings by devouring the child. This fantasy suggests that Clarissa was unsuccessful in her active turn to her father because of the mother's insistence on the exclusiveness of her relationship with her daughter. An additional facet of the symptom was revealed later in the first year of treatment by Clarissa's refusal to speak to her beloved teacher. The treatment material suggests that she experienced her mother's withdrawal at the time of her brother's birth as a punishment. Since this coincided with toilet training, it appears that Clarissa may have felt that she was being punished not only because of her active turn toward her father but for what would have been age-typical exuberant independence as well. Her subsequent surrender left her fearful of reengulfment by her mother to which she responded with heightened rage and hostility. This intolerable hostility was repressed. The elective mutism represented a compromise formation with two levels of meaning: on one, the mutism represented a regression to the exclusive, undifferentiated attachment her mother demanded; at another level, Clarissa could punish her mother (through displacement onto other mother figures) by not speaking as she felt she once had been punished by her mother's not speaking.

In treatment, it appeared that Clarissa could not begin to explore her conflicts around phallic activity until she had recreated a relationship with a "good enough" preoedipal mother who was helpfully omnipotent, but not devouring; in such a relationship sexual differences were as yet without significance. Only within this context could Clarissa begin to recognize and adapt to the narcissistic blow involved in her discovery of the anatomical facts. The analytic material makes clear, however, that Clarissa's struggle with anatomical differences was not a metaphor for the hostile elements in her preoedipal mother attachment. The fantasy configuration concerning the anatomical facts was complex, with many different elements—the equation of the penis with permission to be active; the sense of defect; the wish to penetrate as well as to be penetrated; the fantasy of a "prediscovery" utopia in which there was no genital difference; mother as a phallic woman; theories regarding the cause of the genital difference. Some of these fantasy elements were more closely associated with her relationship to her mother than others. Penis envy and the preoedipal mother attachment are two different fantasy configurations, elements of which intersect and overlap, thereby coloring one another.

Clarissa's intense reaction to the discovery of genital differences points to another major hazzard for the little girl. Active phallic strivings may succumb so completely to the repression aimed at their hostile elements that they are no longer available for sublimation through mastery in the external world. The result may be excessive passivity and crippling masochism.

The emergence of Clarissa's delighted exhibitionism within a dyadic primary relationship suggests the usefulness of the concept of a *preoedipal* phallic-narcissistic phase, which evolves gradually into the first stage of the oedipus complex. Clarissa's fantasies illustrate the long period of oscillation in this phallic-oedipal phase between the mother and the father as the object of phallic strivings. Only very gradually, through the inevitable frustration of her active sexual strivings toward her mother, and supported by positive identification with the mother's own feminine disposition, does the little girl give up her phallic wishes and begin the slow turn toward her father.

BIBLIOGRAPHY

BLUM, H. P., ed. (1976), Female psychology. *J. Amer. Psychoanal. Assn.* 24 Suppl., no. 5.

BRUNSWICK, R. M. (1940), The preoedipal phase of the libido in development. In Fliess (1948), pp. 261–284.

DEUTSCH, H. (1930), The significance of masochism in the mental life of women. In Fliess (1948), pp. 223–236.

—— (1932), On female homosexuality. In Fliess (1948), pp. 237–260.

—— (1944), *The Psychology of Women*. New York: Grune & Stratton.

EDGCUMBE, R. & BURGNER, M. (1975), The phallic-narcissistic phase. *Psychoanal. Study Child*, 20:161–180.

FLIEGEL, Z. O. (1973), Feminine psychosexual development in freudian theory. *Psychoanal. Q.*, 42:385–408.

FLIESS, R., ed. (1948), *The Psychoanalytic Reader*. New York: Int. Univ. Press.

FREUD, S. (1925), Some psychical consequences of the anatomical distinction between the sexes. *S. E.*, 19:243–258.

—— (1931), Female sexuality. *S. E.*, 21:223–243.

—— (1933), Femininity. *S. E.*, 22:112–135.

GREENACRE, P. (1948), Anatomical structure and superego development. In Greenacre (1952), pp. 149–164.

—— (1950), Special problems of early female sexual development. In Greenacre (1952), pp. 237–258.

—— (1952), *Trauma, Growth and Personality*. New York: Int. Univ. Press, 1969.

LAMPL-DE-GROOT, J. (1927), The evolution of the oedipus complex in women. In Fliess (1948), pp. 207–222.

LERNER, H. (1976), Parental mislabeling of female genitals as a determinant of penis envy and learning inhibitions in women. In Blum (1976), pp. 269–283.

NAGERA, H. (1975), *Female Sexuality and the Oedipal Complex*. New York: Aronson.

An Instance of "Displacement from Above Downward" in a Congenitally Blind Child

ANAT FLUG, M.A. AND
JOSEPH SANDLER, Ph.D., M.D.

IN DESCRIBING THE ROLE OF DISPLACEMENT OF SENSATION from the genitals to the lips in the case of Dora, Freud (1905, p. 30) wrote:

> I believe that during the man's passionate embrace she felt not merely his kiss upon her lips but also the pressure of his erect member against her body. This perception was revolting to her; it was dismissed from her memory, repressed, and replaced by the innocent sensation of pressure upon her thorax, which in turn derived an excessive intensity from its repressed source. Once more, therefore, we find a displacement from the lower part of the body to the upper.
>
> [Freud then comments in a footnote:] The occurrence of displacements of this kind has not been assumed for the purpose of this single explanation; the assumption has proved indispensable for the explanation of a large class of symptoms.

A similar displacement from the lower to the upper part of the body has been described by Dorothy Burlingham (1940, p. 268f.) in the case of blind child:

From the Sigmund Freud Center for Study and Research in Psychoanalysis, The Hebrew University of Jerusalem. Anat Flug is a psychologist on the staff of Eitanim Hospital, Jerusalem, and Joseph Sandler is Sigmund Freud Professor of Psychoanalysis at the Hebrew University.

Sylvia rubbed her eyes compulsively, a behavior which the people in her environment considered a very bad habit and for which they had frequently scolded and threatened her in the hope of breaking this habit. . . . The way in which the hand Sylvia uses to rub her eyes is almost completely excluded from performing any other activity and the way in which the environment reacts to the rubbing of the eyes arouse the suspicion that in this case, as in so many blind children, we are dealing with a displacement upwards; that is to say, the rubbing of the eyes is a substitute for masturbation.

In both of the cases cited the displacement occurred from the genitals to an "upper" area, from a primary sexual erotogenic zone to a less "sexual" area. The case which follows illustrates a displacement from a less erotic but highly invested area to a much more erotic one, i.e., from the eyes (or rather the whole visual system as conceived of by a congenitally blind child) to the genitals. Moreover, the case is of special interest in that there is not merely a "symbolic" displacement in which one area of the body comes to stand for another, but a displacement of organized theories and fantasies from one part of the body to another.

The material given below was taken from the psychotherapeutic treatment of Miss F, a blind student of occupational therapy at a college near Jerusalem. The account which follows is strictly limited to the theme of this paper, and the treatment process (including in particular the development of the transference) is mentioned only where relevant.

F was referred to the therapist by the psychologist at the college. In her initial interview she appeared tall and tidily dressed, with no makeup, and with carefully arranged blond hair. Her striking green eyes and mobile facial expression made her appear like a sighted person, and it took the therapist some time to perceive her as someone who was completely blind.

F was 26 years old at the time she was first seen. She had been blind from birth, and had come to Israel with her parents from Bulgaria when she was 16. She posed her problem as being unable to accept her "defect." Although it had always been difficult for her to live with her blindness, she had in recent years become increasingly concerned about her "problem," particularly when she found herself in the company of others. She felt insecure and feared to express her own opinions in case they would be ridiculed. After she had been in treatment for a while, it emerged that her greatest concern was that her blindness stood in the way of her getting married. She said that as she was now 26 this was what was most on her mind. However, she did not like the idea of being married to a blind partner, but wanted someone strong. She was not attracted to blind men, she said. But she feared that sighted men would not be attracted to her, and described how, in her male friendships, the men seemed to "recoil" from the relationship after they had come to know her.

F is the younger of two children, having a brother 2 years older. Her father is a carpenter and her mother has no regular job. She described her parents as simple and sensitive, but although they have always been very concerned for her welfare, she felt that they never really understood her.

According to F, her mother first discovered that F was blind when she was 3 weeks old, noticing that the baby did not look at her while being fed. Her father refused to accept the reality of her blindness until it was confirmed by a specialist when the child was 4 months of age. F's mother was unable to come to terms with her child's blindness, and would not take her out in a baby carriage during her first year.

F was able to attend a regular kindergarten till the age of 6. At about this time F's father experienced a short depressive episode, which, according to F, followed a series of unsuccessful attempts to find a suitable school for her in her native country. He said that he was shocked by the schools he saw, being convinced that they were for blind children who were mentally retarded. As a result, F did not attend school until the age of 9, when she ultimately did enter a day school for the blind. She reported that she had enjoyed being at that school and was well liked.

After the family immigrated to Israel, it was soon confirmed that F suffered from incurable congenital blindness, and she was sent to a boarding school for blind children. She described her first years in Israel as being very difficult. After graduation from school she worked for some years in a nursery school for the blind, and then enrolled in a training course in occupational therapy and rehabilitation.

F agreed to attend weekly psychotherapy, and in her first session expressed her disappointment at being allocated a female therapist. She said that she had hoped for a male therapist. She went on to describe how one of her former teachers had recently died after a prolonged illness, and how she had met this teacher's husband shortly after his wife's death. She expressed feelings of guilt over not having visited her teacher during her illness, and remarked that she had been unable to cry, but tended to find herself laughing instead. She recalled that she had met the husband in a friend's garden where she had been frightened by a rather ferocious dog. She then went on to describe a dream in which she was chased by a dog, and told the therapist that she was afraid of getting dirtied by dogs and of being infected by them. She then said that she was reminded, for a reason she did not understand, of the appearance on television of a mother who had lost her child in a recent terrorist attack. The mother and child had hidden in a small closet, and the mother had tried to prevent the child from crying out, but in doing this had suffocated her. F commented on the contrast between the composure of the woman on the one hand, and the horrifying details of the story on the other.

In a subsequent session F disclosed that the husband of the teacher who had recently died had suggested to her that they should begin seeing each other, and that they could possibly have a sexual relationship. F hesitated about this as she felt in conflict. She told herself that he needed her, and that she did not want to lose his friendship; but he was old enough to be her father, and she did not feel strongly attracted to him.

F began to talk about her sexual history, and commented that her mother had not informed her about menstruation. She remembered the shock of her first period at the age of 10, and how she had entered the living room with cotton and bandages in her hands. Her mother had reacted with anger, and F had left the room feeling upset and confused. Between 12 and 14 she began developing close friendships with boys. Her parents did not know about these, and F enjoyed the secrecy.

After some weeks of therapy, F disclosed that she had been having an "affair" with an older married man since the beginning of therapy. She was attracted to him, both physically and emotionally, and wanted to get close to him. Yet she could not do so because he was married and had children.

In the following session F remarked that, although people would never guess it, she was probably the only one of the therapist's patients who was a virgin at the age of 26. Possibly she was the only such case in Israel! She then described the first time she went to bed with her married friend. They had come close to full intercourse, but, in F's words, he did not "open me up." While she had enjoyed the foreplay, and felt warm toward him, she had had a sudden feeling of "an inner barrier" and became afraid of penetration. She added that she was also repelled by the idea of touching sexual organs which "emitted fluids," and went on to describe her aversion to dirt and bad smells. She told the therapist that, in the end, she was disappointed by the sexual experience, but had liked the cuddling and the warmth of the physical contact. However, she did not want to go any further sexually than she had done so far.

In the next weeks F spoke of her general suspicion of men, saying that all they wanted was sex, that her father degraded women and told dirty jokes. She felt that men's sexual cravings were stronger than women's. Along with such feelings F talked about her own feelings of loneliness and her fear that no one really liked her. She was afraid that her affair would soon end.

F now entered a phase in which she spoke of what she had needed to give up because of her blindness. She recalled that when she was 5 she had wanted to be a nurse who would care for babies in a hospital. She liked to cuddle infants, and wanted to have her own baby. She said that she had the wish to "create" a person, to "shape" him, to "bring him up." She thought that was why she had wanted for so long to become a teacher. She then recalled a doll she had had as a child which she had called "Poppet."

F would feed Poppet through a hole she had made in her mouth. She also gave her injections into her bottom. She had played a game that the doll was ill and that she had to save her. She said, "It was as it had been between me and my mother." She then reported that when she was 6 she had been examined by a neurologist, who had said that her eyes were intact, but that the optic nerve was not passing what she saw from the eyes to the brain. The doctor had raised F's and her parents' hopes by prescribing a series of treatments—vitamins and injections which he said might help. Her skull was X-rayed fairly often, and whenever small changes were detected her father was delighted and bought her a present. She recalled receiving a small sewing machine from her father, and it was of interest that at this point in treatment she developed a special interest in sewing. Following the discussion of the transference implications of this material, F recalled that she had felt guilty as a child when "nothing really changed." She spoke of her doll, Poppet, and of how she had started to dislike the doll, who had begun to smell from all the injections and food that F had pushed into her. She threw the doll away, but remembered dreaming that it had been resurrected.

F then spoke of her fears of marrying a blind person, and her concern that if she did this, her children would be born blind. She referred again to her own anxieties about being damaged, even though she knew she appeared normal on the outside. She said that although as a child she had felt very warm toward babies, she would not now be able to raise children because she was cold and inflexible. She felt the same way in her sexual relationship, and spoke of how she "closed up" when her male friend approached her sexually.

Some sessions later F spoke of her dissatisfaction in regard to therapy. She felt that it was not "deep" enough, had not "opened me up." She wondered whether she should have some other form of treatment, perhaps a course of pills. At this point in the session F heard birds chirping outside the office, and remembered that her parents had kept a number of birdcages in their garden. It was her responsibility to feed the birds, she said, but she had once killed one by accidentally clamping its head in the feeding drawer. After that her parents did not buy any more birds, even though she always wanted her father to do so.

DISCUSSION

There are obvious links, in the material reported by F, between her childhood theories and fantasies about her lack of vision and her current sexual anxieties. As a child she had concluded that although her eyes as such might appear to be normal, there was some kind of "blockage" which stopped her seeing. Because of her early experience of body openings and passages it was probably inevitable that in these circumstances she would conceive of the "blockage" of her eyesight in terms of a blocked or interrupted tube of some sort, and the restoration of her sight as a literal unblocking of a passage. Her strong wish to be normally sighted was certainly reinforced by feelings of shame shared by the whole family about her condition, as well as by her own intense wish to win her father's love. On the other hand, the attempts to restore her sight by means of injections and medication must have been extremely unpleasant and a major source of anxiety, conflict, and guilt. It is possible that the medical interventions were associated in her mind with the creation of further damage, as suggested, for example, by her memories of forcing food into her doll through a hole which she had made, and her resulting disgust when the food began to decay and smell. And there is little doubt that she constantly externalized her own strong aggressive wishes and impulses so that the world was seen as aggressively threatening, with the constant danger that she would be violently penetrated and "bad" things forced into her.[1]

F's present sexual concerns appear to reflect a current un-

1. There are a number of indications that F had carried forward many anal-sadistic interests and preoccupations into subsequent stages of development. Certainly, her later sexual anxieties were colored by fears of infection and contamination, and she viewed her father as sexually "dirty." It also seems likely that her thoughts about her blindness and its possible cure were strongly influenced by fantasies and theories of the anal phase.

conscious theory[2] that she has a blockage in her vagina which
would hinder penetration. If a passage were to be forced by a
penis, this could be violent and damaging, "dirty fluids" would
be deposited in her, and she would be further damaged (there
is a possible connection here with her memories and fantasies
about the onset of menstruation at the age of 10). Her ambivalent feelings toward herself and her mother (who had given
birth to a blinded child) would have lent weight to a conviction
that she would be responsible for violently damaging her
babies, if she were to have any; she certainly thought that they
might suffocate inside her because of her damaged reproductive organs. It is also probable that envy of "normal" babies
played a significant part in all her fears, and her references to
killing the bird she was feeding and to the mother who suffocated her baby are pertinent here. Tragically, for F, penetration was both curative and damaging, and this was very clearly
reflected in her fantasies about and mixed feelings toward
treatment.

In the light of this, it would appear that we have, in the case
of F, an instance of the displacement of theories and fantasies
about the visual apparatus downward to the genitals in a congenitally blind girl, in whose early life the eyes and sight played
a major role. It can be argued, of course, that F's thoughts
about her eyesight were a reflection of more fundamental concerns, during the phallic libidinal phase, over problems of castration and penis envy (Freud, 1908). More convincingly, perhaps, it could be said that F's thoughts and conclusions about her
eyesight developed together with similar theories about her
genitals, and that what she learned, elaborated, or fantasied
about one body opening reinforced her conclusions and speculations about the other. Nevertheless, we have to take into
account the fact that *F's blindness represented, to both her family and*

2. The concept of an unconscious theory is discussed elsewhere (Sandler,
1975). Such a theory reflects *beliefs* about reality which have later been repressed, but which are still acted on as if they were valid and appropriate.
Unconscious theories usually contain many wish-fulfilling fantasy elements,
and have usually been subsumed under the general but less precise heading
of "unconscious fantasy."

herself, a narcissistic wound of major proportions. Her preoccupation with her blindness must have been significantly reinforced by her family's shame about her defect and by her intense wish to gain her father's love and approval by recovering her sight. This wish was nourished and sustained by the hopes of recovery offered to her. As a consequence, the narcissistic investment in her eyesight must have been enormous, and her oedipal fantasies would, it seems very likely, have involved thoughts and ideas about how she could win her father's love if the channels of her eyesight could be "unblocked" and her blindness cured.

In the past we have tended to conceive of special investments in the body in childhood as being derivatives of libidinal strivings linked with specific erotogenic zones. However, equal in importance to any such sexual investment must rank the narcissistic investment of those aspects of the individual's functioning, including parts and systems of the body which are connected with "attractiveness" and power, and with everything which can evoke real or fantasied admiration in others. It is inevitable that such narcissistic investment in "attractiveness" must play an important part in the whole structure of the oedipus complex, particularly in the case of handicapped children. Intense narcissistic cathexis need not be tied to any erotogenic zone, and in F's case it seems clear that her eyesight was, for a significant period of her childhood, the most important and heavily invested part of her body.

It seems certain that F's childhood wishes in regard to her eyes and the recovery of her sight were given new impetus by the overtures made to her by the husband of her dead teacher and by the subsequent sexual relationship with an older man. Her childhood wish to have her eyes penetrated and her vision "opened up," together with all the fears that this entailed, must have been stimulated and reinforced. But such preoccupations and all the associated wishes, fears, and conflicts would not have been acceptable to her adult consciousness; and it seems that the whole area of wishful fantasy and conflict about her sight then found overt expression in the form of a displacement to sexual activity and to a preoccupation with the genitals. In brief, what was originally so heavily involved with her self-esteem, together with all the oedipal and narcissistic wishes, fantasies, fears, conflicts, and hopes connected with her eyesight, can be regarded as having reappeared, later in life, as a displacement from above downward.

BIBLIOGRAPHY

BURLINGHAM, D. (1940), Psychoanalytic observations of blind children. In *Psychoanalytic Studies of the Sighted and the Blind.* New York: Int. Univ. Press, 1972, pp. 227–279.

FREUD, S. (1905), Fragment of an analysis of a case of hysteria. *S. E.,* 7:3–122.

——— (1908), On the sexual theories of children. *S. E.,* 9:205–226.

SANDLER, J. (1975), Sexual fantasies and sexual theories in childhood. In *Studies in Child Psychoanalysis.* New Haven & London: Yale Univ. Press, pp. 149–162.

Determinants of Free Association in Narcissistic Phenomena

ANTON O. KRIS, M.D.

THE GREAT USEFULNESS OF EXPLICIT, ABSTRACT, RELATIVELY experience-distant theoretical formulations for purposes of organizing psychoanalytic observations tends to obscure the disadvantages that may be incurred when these formulations are employed in the clinical situation. One kind of disadvantage is due to differences in conceptual inclinations among analysts: theoretical perspectives of great value to one may represent intrusions for another. So long as theory is available, buffet style, for each to use as the occasion arises, there is little danger of imposing some point of view on an analyst whose way of thinking more readily follows another direction. When theoretical formulations *lead* clinical experience rather than follow it, when theory *defines* rather than organizes, interference in the clinical situation is likely. Another kind of disadvantage stems from competing theoretical influences, either when a new theoretical formulation modifies a previous one or when two parallel, contradictory formulations lead to confusion instead of to the clarity they aim for. The history of the theoretical concept of narcissism—surely one of the most valuable concepts on the psychoanalytic table—is rife with both these sources of disadvantage: the intrusion of excessively influential theories, on the one hand, and competing theoretical formulations, on the other.

Narcissism has been viewed in many perspectives within psychoanalysis (e.g., Freud, 1914; Arlow and Brenner, 1964; Mur-

Training and Supervising Analyst at The Boston Psychoanalytic Society nd Institute.

ray, 1964; Kernberg, 1970, 1975; Kohut, 1971, 1977; Ornstein, 1974; Spruiell, 1975; Rothstein, 1980). At various times it is seen as an entity, as a phase of development, as a perversion, or as a measure of self-love. At times it is a state or condition, especially of well-being. More often it is an indeterminate abstraction, with variable components, conceived to be capable of developmental transformation, of injury, and of pathological disturbance. The term *narcissistic* further compounds the vagueness, for it does not mean merely "of or pertaining to narcissism," as in the case of other adjectives and the nouns they refer to. Narcissistic very frequently implies pathology, especially disorders in regard to self-love, self-esteem, and orientation to power (Spruiell's "three strands of narcissism"). Narcissistic may refer to developmental immaturity in object relations, or to an instability in self-regard that can be manifested throughout a spectrum from depression to megalomania, with defensive forms such as complacency masking dissatisfaction with oneself. Or, again, it may refer to ruthlessness and failure of self-control as episodic or pervasive traits. The indispensable terms, narcissism and narcissistic, unfortunately suffer from such breadth, ambiguity, and imprecision that they sometimes contribute to confusion as they serve their conceptual function.

In this paper I shall present a formulation or, more accurately, a group of closely connected formulations immediately relevant to the free associations of (pathologically) narcissistic patients in analysis. These formulations seem to me to apply in situations in which the narcissistic aspect is relatively minor or transient as well as in those in which it is pronounced and pervasive. That is, I propose to describe what I regard as essential to narcissistic phenomena, no matter where along the spectrum of diagnostic categories the total clinical picture of which they are a part may fall. I shall then make use of these formulations to evaluate some developmental propositions of self psychology concerning narcissistic phenomena.

A CONSIDERATION OF METHOD

The approach I am presenting, a method-based approach to the problem of the *initial* formulation of narcissistic phenomena, focuses on the forms, patterns, and determinants of the free associations seen in the psychoanalytic situation. It is relatively concrete and experience-near. It avoids some of the problems of theoretical formulations centered on a concept of mind or psychic apparatus, but as an initial formulation it can readily articulate with the multifaceted propositions of psycho-analytic theory.

Mutual agreement initiates the method of free association (Kris, 1982), in which the patient attempts to say whatever comes to mind without conscious reservation (the *activity* of free association) and the analyst says only what he believes will facilitate the patient's efforts. No sooner is the process initiated than the limitations of the patient's *freedom of association* confront the participants. I find it convenient to refer to those interferences with freedom of association that the patient is consciously aware of as *reluctances* and to those that the patient is not consciously aware of as *resistances*. (The patient may become aware of the limitation of freedom of association without yet becoming consciously aware of the resistance that produces it.) The determinants of free association include both those that seek and sustain expression and those that oppose it.

In formulating narcissistic phenomena from the vantage point of free association, I must inevitably go beyond a mere transposition of some generally accepted conception into the forms and determinants of the associations. I shall be *defining* narcissistic phenomena in these terms, aware that this definition will not be entirely congruent with any of those previously offered. This definition stands free of any one theory of narcissism, both healthy and pathological, though, I believe, it can be readily correlated with such a conception in terms of mind. I have of course arrived at this formulation in the way that is usual for the clinical method of psychoanalysis. Starting with a variety of published conceptual approaches to narcissistic phenomena, I gradually found the formulation that I present here to be a reliable guide in listening to the free associations and in responding to them.

The formulation I shall present recognizes one pattern of free association, including particular determinants, as the central and most characteristic of the broad spectrum that has generally been regarded as narcissistic. This is the vicious cycle of punitive unconscious self-criticism (unconscious guilt), self-deprivation, and insatiable demand. I want to stress that I am referring to patterns of association of adult patients. I am not outlining a genetic sequence that might lead to narcissistic pathology. The important question of how these patterns and their determinants may develop—how, for example, so relatively late a developmental acquisition as unconscious guilt comes to hold a central position in narcissistic phenomena—will not be addressed here, except in the evaluation of the genetic propositions of self psychology.

THE VICIOUS CYCLE OF UNCONSCIOUS GUILT, SELF-DEPRIVATION, AND INSATIABLE DEMAND

The profound connection between conscious guilt and human sentience has been recognized at least since the *Book of Genesis*. The special link between unconscious guilt, *punitive* unconscious self-criticism, and free association is less widely appreciated.[1] Unconscious guilt tends to restrict freedom of association (resistance) and to interrupt free association (by creating reluctance), because the patient assumes that the analyst holds the same critical attitude. The more urgent the patient's need to express whatever triggers unconscious guilt, the more the patient fears not only punitive criticism from the analyst but rejection by the analyst (Kris, 1982, chap. 6). Formulating narcissistic patterns of free association with an initial focus on unconscious guilt—rather than on self-love, or on a sense of inadequacy, or on exaggerated self-importance and entitlement, or on self-indulgence and self-pity, or on a wish to become perfect, or on envy and hate—draws attention at once to this unusual position of punitive unconscious self-criticism as a re-

1. Unconscious self-criticism does not always have a punitive aim. Self-criticism, both conscious and unconscious, may also aim to limit action or to promote it. This aim can serve an essential, adaptive function, correcting errors, or it may play a pathological role, producing disturbances of function, especially inhibition. I find it useful to distinguish unconscious self-criticism with a punitive aim (unconscious guilt) from unconscious self-criticism with a corrective aim, recognizing that the latter, in excess, can be a source of difficulty.

sistance and as a source of reluctance. The narcissistic patient brings a special vulnerability to the method of free association which must be recognized—preferably early on—if the method is not to be silently derailed. I shall return to the topic of this sort of disturbance of the free association method after outlining further the vicious cycle of unconscious guilt, self-deprivation, and insatiable demand.

The simplest instances of self-deprivation in the analytic situation are those in which the patient fails to say something he wished to say. For example, a patient is very pleased with an achievement and wants to tell me about it. He forgets it and recalls it only late in the session or in the next one. Or a patient wants to show me a drawing or a photograph of his family but decides it would not be "proper" in analysis and then forgets even to mention the wish to do so. Such events link up with a more general inability to feel that the analysis is the patient's, that it belongs to him, and that in analysis the patient has the right to think his own thoughts and to say them. At a still more general level they reflect an inability to allow the satisfaction of wishes to be loved, appreciated, admired, and taken care of. (In terms of drive theory, these are passive libidinal wishes.) Naturally, punitive unconscious self-criticism is not the only influence that can bring about such behavior and attitudes, but, in my experience, it is the most frequent and persistent determinant of such patterns of association.

The frustration produced by self-deprivation contributes to the generally excessive, insatiable demands and self-indulgence that are equally characteristic of narcissistic patients. They must take by force what they cannot allow themselves to accept when it is freely offered. Active wishes are regularly substituted, unsuccessfully, for passive ones (Kris, 1976). One winter afternoon, for example, a patient who deprived himself not only of love but also of some of the ordinary comforts of living became evidently anxious as the room grew dark. I asked if he wanted me to turn the lights on, which meant walking a few steps across the room. He wanted me to do so, but he was sure that that would destroy his analysis, that I was breaking the rules. Analysis, seen in that perspective, was supposed to make him suffer, and, in fact, he maintained for several years that he gained in analysis only when he was most miserable. Yet almost every hour was marked by some attempt to compel my admiration or to pressure me into responding.

Guilt over active wishes, especially in regard to their aggressive component, completes the vicious cycle I have been describing ("Macbeth does murder sleep"). Elsewhere (1976), I have started from that point in analysis when the patient painfully asserts: "I want too much." This self-criticism represents a characteristic step in the therapeutic process for the narcissistic patient, and affords the analyst an important opportunity to help the patient see the vicious cycle of unconscious guilt, self-deprivation, and insatiable demand. It would be vain to suppose, however, that even such a fundamental change in orientation, in which the punitive aim begins to give way to a corrective one and the patient who has previously been unaware of self-criticism acknowledges a sense of guilt, assures the analytic resolution of the vicious cycle. The tenacity of unconscious guilt and of the vicious cycle requires the most extensive working through. Over and over the patient loses sight of the punitive self-criticism and externalizes it onto the analyst. I have found it important at all phases, but especially in the first years of analysis, to distinguish between these externalizations and my own nonjudgmental views. Later on, at times, when I have sought to make such a clarification because I could not tell what the patient was thinking, the reply has often come: "Of course I know you don't hold that view, I'm merely expressing how I feel it." By then the battle has been largely won, but even then surprises have occurred from time to time.

It would be quite incorrect, however, to say that the patient's self-criticism is a wholly unjustified misperception. It may be that the patient overestimates the significance of his destructiveness at times and loses perspective, but hostility, envy, and, at times, hate are always in ample evidence. It is the rule that narcissistic patients have not achieved the ordinary mastery over their aggressive inclinations. Their unconscious guilt is, in that sense, always justified, but as it is directed punitively toward self-deprivation rather than correctively toward modification of these excesses, it exacerbates the problem.

Individual differences and variations in the course of one

patient's analysis create a panorama of alternating pictures, based upon this vicious cycle. The patient may present himself as depressed, or as self-critical and dissatisfied, or as suspicious, ready to take umbrage at a syllable, or as eager to please, but, in fact, refusing secretly to tell the truth, or as determined to prove the analyst and the analysis worthless, and so on. I have found it useful to assume that a variety of aspects are always present at once, though sometimes only one may be in evidence. For example, the patient who feels genuinely understood when her self-critical attitude is clarified worries a moment later that I do not realize how much she hates me and how she has deceived me. Then come her great need for me and fears that I will lose interest in her.

I have described the components of the vicious cycle from the point of view of the patient's current self-criticism, self-deprivation, and insatiable demands. All these aspects occur not only as stable elements of character but also may appear as transference manifestations. Externalized self-criticism joins with criticism attributed to childhood figures; the sense of deprivation and frustration results not only from unconscious guilt but from the unconscious revival of childhood experience; and the insatiable demands repeat earlier ones, never smoothly integrated into an adult personality. The distinction between transference manifestations and other unconsciously determined patterns of association focused on the analyst (Sandler et al., 1975, 1980; Kris, 1982, chap. 9) is most important, and I shall return to it in a later section of this paper.

CONFLICTS OF AMBIVALENCE

The method of free association is intended to re-create to some extent (but not to a traumatic extent) a variety of experiences of conflict. For the narcissistic patient, that is, for the patient significantly limited by the vicious cycle of unconscious guilt, self-deprivation, and insatiable demand, several conflicts arise directly from the *situation* of the free association method, not as a part of the developing *process* of free association. These conflicts can be traced to the characteristic externalization of unconscious guilt, with the consequent expectation of criticism from the analyst and fear of rejection by the analyst. The more the patient wishes to express the associations, free of conscious reservation, the greater the fear of criticism and of loss. It is, for the patient, as though a choice had to be made between a good relationship with the analyst, on the one hand, and the right to associate freely on the other. This is a *conflict of ambivalence,* between two parallel but seemingly incompatible wishes (Kris, 1982, chap. 8). Such conflicts are fundamentally different from *conflicts of defense,* where the determinants are a pair of opposing attitudes or wishes. There, too, fear of the analyst's disapproval may arise, but the more the patient becomes aware of the inner conflict, the more readily the conflict can be resolved. Not so with the conflicts of ambivalence, where increasing awareness of the conflict is accompanied by increasing expectation of inevitable loss, on one side or the other. To gratify one wish, even to express it in the associations, means to forfeit the opposite wish that is in parallel. Often a conscious sense of either-or accompanies such conflicts of ambivalence (Kris, 1977). While it is sufficient, in the case of the conflicts of defense, for the patient to *remember* what has been lost from conscious awareness in order to set the stage for resolution, in the case of the conflicts of ambivalence a painful process akin to *mourning* is required. To put it another way, the vicious cycle is triggered, no matter in which direction the narcissistic patient attempts to express his thoughts, and can only be approached in free association by small alternating steps, each accompanied by a painful tension between conflicting wishes.

For the narcissistic patient, then, the propensity for conflicts of ambivalence contributes to the perpetuation of the vicious cycle in several ways. Unconscious guilt, as I have indicated, can silently derail the free association method because of a conflict between free association and a good relationship with the analyst. Another conflict links guilt over aggressive, competitive action with shame over inadequate performance or passivity and dependence. For example, a narcissistic young man at the beginning of analysis feels himself a failure because he does not dare to assert himself. On the one hand, he has fantasies of enormous success, denigrating others in the process, and is quite unaware of feeling guilty. On the other hand, he wants me to help him, to teach him how to be a man, and fears I will reject him. Then he feels ashamed for what he sees as a homosexual orientation. The latter is not principally a defense against active, aggressive, competitive wishes. It is better understood as the other half of a complex conflict of ambivalence. Inhibition of aggressiveness is caused not only by unconscious self-criticism but also by the expected loss of vital passive wishes if active ones are given free expression. He is critical of both active and passive wishes and cannot gratify either. Even the expression in free association is inhibited and, accordingly, the two sides are at first closely linked in the associations. Dissolution or "analysis" of the linkage comes slowly at best. To conceive of such conflicts of ambivalence as though they were conflicts of defense could lead to a compliant sacrifice of one side for the other rather than to a gradual, painful freeing up of both. Later in analysis, the insistence on a passive orientation may serve as a regressive defense against the dangers attendant on active wishes. The same young man, beset with fears of criticism and rejection, fueled by unconscious castration fears, draws back from active ambition and insists upon a preference for accommodation and a pleasure in being taken care of. The active wishes appear to be temporarily abandoned. The patient does not fear the loss of active wishes in gratifying passive ones. That hallmark of the conflicts of ambivalence is absent. The demonstration of his unconscious fear of active wishes is now sufficient to lead to their further expression and to an understanding of the meaning of the regressive defense against them. This is characteristic of the conflicts of defense, where bringing them into conscious awareness can be counted upon to lead to resolution.

The conflicts of ambivalence that arise from the situation of the free association method link up with conflicts that can be seen throughout life, between old relationships and new ones, between active and passive modes, between a variety of forms of loving, and between love and hate. Most prominent, in my experience, at the beginning of analysis, are conflicts between passive wishes, seen self-critically as infantile or immature, and active wishes, seen as dangerously hostile. It is as though the patient must choose between active genital wishes and passive pregenital ones.

One common example is the view of the young adult patient that he or she should separate more completely from mother or father or from both parents: "I have to give my mother up." Such a statement represents self-criticism for a variety of supposed sins, active and passive, posed as an impossible choice, for no one can or should give up this essential relationship. It is enough to give up, through mourning, the illusion that one can maintain the past in the present and into the future, unmodified.

It is characteristic of the conflicts of ambivalence that the *activity* of free association itself leads to the expectation of loss, as either of the parallel pair of wishes or attitudes is expressed without the other. (This is, again, quite different from the fear of loss that may arise in connection with conflicts of defense. There, it is due to the *content* of the associations, not to the activity of free association. For example, an unconscious hostile attitude seeking expression may lead to a fear of rejection.) While conflicts of ambivalence are ubiquitous, failure to resolve the major conflicts of ambivalence in adolescence is very common if not invariable in narcissistic patients. The conflicts include independence versus dependence, loving versus hating, and the familiar pairs in loving: primary objects and secondary ones, homosexual and heterosexual inclincations, active and passive, genital and pregenital.

A connection between adult narcissistic disorders and the failure to complete the developmental tasks of adolescence in regard to conflicts of ambivalence can be traced through the patterns of association in which a striking persistence of denial in fantasy emerges frequently (Kris, 1979). Just when the patient might be expected to speak of feelings of inadequacy, helplessness, or shame, one hears instead of complacency, competence, and pride. These patterns of association are linked to intolerance of uncertainty and significant problems of self-control. Gradually, in the course of analysis, they can be attributed to a failure in the latency years to develop, with adult assistance, the capacities for tolerance of tension, delay, and uncertainty that are essential for mastering the conflicts of ambivalence in adolescence.

When intolerance of conflict and uncertainty are extreme, denial of one side of a conflict of ambivalence creates the qualities of splitting. I share the view (e.g., of Kernberg, 1975) that splitting of that sort is intimately associated with borderline and psychotic phenomena, of which narcissistic patterns are an invariable part. It is not the usual outcome in the conflicts of ambivalence of narcissistic patients. I do not believe that the denial of guilt, which is a frequent if not invariable component of narcissistic phenomena, has the same diagnostic significance as splitting of conflicts of ambivalence.

THE INTOLERANCE OF GUILT

I have referred to the tenacity of unconscious guilt without spelling out why it is so unyielding. As a rule, the analyst can find no way at first to convey to narcissistic patients their self-critical attitudes without arousing a painful belief that it is the analyst who is critical. Externalization operates, in them, with hair-trigger sensitivity. Beyond that, however, they have the appalling fear of being completely to blame: "It will be all my fault." Again, this fear is always associated with the expectation of rejection and loss. These patients travel through life with the mark of Cain. I attribute the tenacity of unconscious guilt principally to the intense fears with which it is associated and to the consequent denial that interferes with clarification, even in the relative safety of the analytic situation.

Denial of guilt cannot, in my experience, be usefully confronted head on. My own approach has been to delineate as clearly as possible the *consequences* of unconscious guilt: the repeated evidence of self-deprivation ("With friends like you, you don't need enemies") and the expectation that I will be critical ("One of us *is* critical of you"). But this does not mean a one-sided approach to the vicious cycle and to the related conflicts of ambivalence, which would be bound to fail. Eventually, the sources of guilt, especially the insatiable demands and the failures of self-control, must be equally clarified. This always includes problems linked to childhood and adult masturbation, to perversion, or to promiscuity.

THE FAILURE OF REALISTIC APPRAISAL
AND THE NEED FOR CONFIRMATION

Among the characteristic difficulties of narcissistic patients is a particular uncertainty in their appraisal of reality, both external and internal. They have trouble assessing aggression and hostility in relationships, both casual and intense, and in knowing exactly who did what to whom. They are as likely to overestimate as to underestimate responsibility for aggression and hostility, and they doubt their own appraisals. This uncertainty, which directly contributes to the intolerance of guilt, also contributes to a need for confirmation of their opinions by others, especially by their analyst. This need for validation is due, so far as I have been able to determine, to the substitution of punitive unconscious self-criticism for corrective self-criticism that aims at modification and modulation of excesses. The narcissistic patient appears to shut off those affective clues that provide the ordinary guides to such assessment. I have not been able to penetrate this matter further than to say that punitive unconscious self-criticism leads to intolerance of sufficient intimations of guilt and responsibility to permit reliable evaluation by the individual.

I do not of course suggest that unconscious guilt is the only source of the need for validation and confirmation. The specific problem of uncertainty in the appraisal of aggression may have additional determinants and other roots, and other experiences may lead to other kinds of uncertainty and the need for validation. Nor do I mean that this is the only area in which failure to appraise reality correctly may occur. My aim here is to describe patterns of association that reflect the most characteristic features of narcissistic patients.

The patient's need for confirmation presents a problem to the analyst. His main aim is to foster the process of free association by helping the patient understand why he is uncertain in his appraisal of reality. Along the way, I have often found it helpful to assist the patient in marshalling his data to be able to make a correct appraisal—not substituting my judgment for his but helping him to see that his uncertainty derives from inner conflict.

THE NEED TO BE SPECIAL

The feeling of inadequacy and the need to be treated as special are also characteristic of narcissistic patients. Over and over the narcissistic patient, in analysis and outside, seeks to be treated in an exceptional manner. Invariably, there are appeals for something extra from the analyst, especially over time and money, where the analyst's interests intersect with the patient's. Many meanings converge in these requests, demands, and confrontations. From the side of externalized unconscious self-criticism it is a request for reversal of the analyst's criticism; from the side of self-deprivation it is a wish for replacement of love and caring, reflecting inadequately developed self-love. Sometimes unbridled envy, sometimes self-justified hate, sometimes grandiosity are expressed in "narcissistic entitlement" (Murray, 1964). A sense of never having been special, a feeling of having been an unwanted or a least-favored child (often historically as well as experientially accurate) frequently contributes to these demands, both as stable elements of character and as transferences revived in the process of free association.

It seems to me that I have always found it necessary, especially early in analysis, to gratify some of these requests. To refuse to do so often risks much more than may be gained by insisting on the kind of abstinence on which the free association method generally thrives. For example, a patient at the very beginning of analysis seeks one change after another of appointment times and needs to be absent for a variety of reasons. To me it is evident that he is fearful in the analysis and, in addition, that he gains a satisfaction from the control he exerts over me, though there are other, substantial reasons for his requests and actions. Later in analysis I could draw his attention to the several influences, and he would gradually sort them out. At this early phase of analysis any comment would be so overwhelmingly heard as a criticism that I find it better not to interfere with the short-term gratification. The aim of analysis in these situations remains unaltered: to expand freedom of association and to foster the free association process. Achievement of this aim in analysis can lead to such significant changes in modifying the vicious cycle and in resolving the conflicts of ambivalence that an ordinary sense of satisfaction can eventually replace the insatiable need to be special.

The demands made by the narcissistic patient, especially those for interaction with the analyst, run into direct conflict with the requirement of analysis that the patient say whatever comes to mind, for a tendency to withhold further expression of the associations, a reluctance, regularly accompanies such demands. I find it helpful to address this reluctance rather than respond only to the demands themselves. It is often possible to demonstrate it to the patient and to clarify the conflict of ambivalence between the wish to associate freely and the reluctance to do so, with loss expected in either direction. Again, at such a moment the patient's associations are on the point of expressing a wish for a response from the analyst, frequently a need for help with inner tension. This is blocked by unconscious self-criticism and fear of the analyst's criticism, a resistance. The demands express the patient's wish but replace its passive form with an active one, and they substitute dialogue for free association, attempting thereby to prevent the loss that results from reluctance. In the long run, with repeated clarifications of such events, the patient gradually comes to recognize the chronic self-imposed frustration due to unconscious interference with freedom of association (resistance).

ARE "SELF-OBJECT TRANSFERENCES" REALLY TRANSFERENCES AT ALL?

With the aid of the conceptual tools I have presented, I want now to examine one of the most influential but also controversial formulations of the determinants of the associations in narcissistic patients. The *developmental* formulations of self psychology concerning narcissistic phenomena (Kohut, 1971, 1977; Kohut and Wolf, 1978; Ornstein, 1974; Goldberg, 1978) hinge, it seems to me, on the assumption that the characteristic attitudes of the narcissistic patient to the analyst, the "self-object transferences," represent childhood relationships transferred to the analyst. Alternatives to *transference*, not considered in these formulations, include expression of present-day wishes, needs, and fears, externalizations of one aspect of personality or of one side of a conflict of ambivalence, and characteristic, immature modes of behavior (Sandler et al., 1975, 1980; Kris, 1982, chap. 9). The formulations of self psychology appear to ignore the conflicts and consequences attendant upon unconscious guilt. They fail to recognize conflicts of ambivalence. They jump, instead, from the present to the past, regarding the way of relating in analysis as a transference repetition of an early childhood situation in which failure of adult responsiveness led to failure of self-cohesion.

My disagreement with these formulations of self psychology is that they assume that the direct operation of a memory of a past relationship, usually from very early childhood, is the major determinant of the free associations. My own experience demonstrates that a combination of externalizations, wishes, needs, fears, and characteristic modes of relating also are powerful determinants of the associations, with memory producing transference increasingly as the free association process develops.

For example, when things go well at the beginning, the patient experiences a satisfying sense of being understood, which makes the analysis rapidly the central affective experience of his life. Hope, love, and idealization bloom in its warm climate. The patient's sensitivity to self-imposed loss and deprivation leads to the externalized fear that the analyst, who is such an essential part of his absorbing and consuming experience, will fail in one way or another. (It was one of Kohut's significant contributions to demonstrate this sensitivity and the kind of "empathic failure" that readily occurs.) It leads, furthermore, to the attempt to control the analyst and to treat the analyst as though the analyst were not a separate person. Such an intolerance of the other person's individuality also is characteristic of the narcissistic patient's other close relationships, outside analysis. This wish to possess and to control (along with other wishes), however, triggers punitive unconscious self-criticism.

The patient then disapproves of the indulgence of analysis, or feels unworthy, and expects that the analyst, too, will disapprove. The patient may become frantic in the hour or between hours. The hours themselves may become experiences of soothing, fueled by great need.

I am, of course, indicating a number of influences that determine the patient's associations, including his attitudes toward the analyst, none of which depends upon the assumption that a memory of a childhood relationship directly determines the associations in the formation of a self-object *transference*. This is not to suggest that narcissistic patients have not had insufficiently empathic parents. In some instances I have been certain that this was the case, but even in those I have not seen the evidence for the early and exclusive kind of *transference* described in the formulations of self psychology. On the contrary, the transferences have emerged gradually and have characteristically demonstrated conflicts of ambivalence. Most prominent among these have been conflicts between the wish for independence and the fear of losing an essential relationship as a consequence and conflicts between the desire for erotic excitement and the expectation of being rejected and deserted.

There seems to be no place in the formulations of self psychology for the child's conflicts between the wish to stay with mother and the wish to leave her, the wish to be separate and the wish to merge, the wish to be active and the wish to be passive, the pleasure in bodily excitement and the fear of destroying tranquillity, and so on. These conflicts of ambivalence require continual reworking, and there is no doubt that for the child the participation of the adults makes an essential contribution to the outcome. The outcome itself, however, seems to me to follow along paths of conflict resolution—or failure of resolution—in the course of development. Contributions to the formation of the *essential* narcissistic picture are added at successive phases into early adulthood. Accordingly, I believe that the formulations of self psychology, which tend to restrict attention to the empathic attunement of analyst and patient as transference repetitions requiring genetic interpretation, bypass essential components of development and of current conflict that are major determinants of the free associations in narcissistic phenomena.

I do not wish to belabor this discussion of the conception of self-object *transferences* and the related developmental inferences with a point-by-point consideration of self psychology. The valuable emphasis laid by Kohut (1971) on the experience of the self and on the fears of fragmentation of the self in patients with narcissistic personality disorders, however, requires attention here. Kohut *defined* the diagnostic category of narcissistic personality disorder in terms of the characteristic relationships to the analyst, which he regarded as transference. The *experience* of fear of fragmentation was, for him, an immediate consequence of the failure to develop a cohesive self, as a supraordinated configuration, in the context of the original self-object relationship or relationships of childhood. The fear of fragmentation, appearing at times of strain ("failure of empathy") in the adult analytic relationship, was seen by Kohut as a repetition in a transference. That view, however, once again omits consideration of punitive unconscious self-criticism, conflicts of ambivalence, and their consequences at a time of strain in the analytic relationship. The structural conceptualization of an insufficiently cohesive self seems to me far less precise and far less clinically useful than a conceptualization of the failure to establish internalized autonomous capacities to tolerate self-criticism and to resolve conflicts of ambivalence in the course of development through adolescence.

Although it is well recognized that the therapeutic effect of a style of intervention cannot be taken as proof of a particular theoretical formulation, when use of a theoretical formulation improves therapeutic effect it is hard to resist its appeal. Kohut's introduction of a new approach to a group of patients who had very frequently been subject to therapeutic failure brought an electrifying popularity to his conception of self-object transferences and their genetic interpretation. Viewed in the light of the vicious cycle that I have described, the persistent genetic interpretation of empathic failure on the part of the patient's parents can be seen to assist the patient with the problem of punitive unconscious self-criticism and self-deprivation. It could be expected to go far in providing therapeutic effects.

The restriction to genetic interpretation, however, and especially the failure to assist the patient in recognizing inner conflicts of ambivalence and the vicissitudes of unconscious guilt foreclose the analysis of conflicts connected with those phases of development in which increasing individuality and separateness from the parents are essential to the child and adolescent. The difficulty in assessment of aggression and hostility, for example, significantly contributes to the failure of narcissistic patients to find a comfortable balance between competition and relationship. In this light I can account for the radical difference between the description of the oedipal phase in analysis given by Kohut (1977, chap. 5) and my own observations, which follow more generally accepted lines. These considerations also explain why Kohut claimed that there are two sharply distinct groups of disorders, the structural or transference neuroses and the narcissistic personality and behavior disorders, where others find continuum and overlap. This sort of either-or conclusion derives, I believe, from the misapplication of genetic interpretation and from the failure to recognize conflicts of ambivalence. In justifying the formulations of self psychology, Kohut (1977) summarizes the "structural outlook":

> . . . they look upon man's condition as being characterized in essence by the conflict between his pleasure-seeking and destructive tendencies (the drives), on the one hand, and his drive-elaborating and drive-curbing equipment (the functions of the ego and superego), on the other [p. 132].

Recognizing only intersystemic conflicts (conflicts of defense) but not intrasystemic conflicts (conflicts of ambivalence), he fails to acknowledge the full scope of intrapsychic conflict (Rangell, 1963).

Conclusion

In presenting a method-based approach to the *initial* formulation of narcissistic phenomena, I have steered clear of the problem of character versus symptom or reaction pattern. The persistence or entrenchment of narcissistic phenomena cannot alone serve to delineate nosological entities. Other aspects of the patient's personality and condition must be taken into account for that purpose. Similarly, difficulties in the progress of psychoanalytic treatment posed by narcissistic phenomena do not prove reliable as measures of the general severity of the patient's disorder. Close attention to the derailment of the free association method by unconscious guilt and its correlates in these instances can correct such a judgment and reveal the source of interference in the treatment.

I have relied on the adjective narcissistic without coming to grips with that elusive Proteus, narcissism. My aim is to offer formulations immediately relevant to the data of free association in the treatment of narcissistic patients, whether the narcissistic aspect is pervasive or only temporary or limited in scope. Other, more experience-distant and abstract theoretical formulations articulate with the ones that I have presented. Additional ways of formulating the determinants of the free associations at the experience-near level are surely possible and desirable. The ones I have presented are those that serve me in my daily work. Whether they can be of equal use to others remains to be seen.

SUMMARY

The chief determinants of free association in narcissistic phenomena are described. The central defining sequence is a vicious cycle of unconscious guilt (punitive unconscious self-criticism), self-deprivation, and insatiable demand. Unresolved conflicts of ambivalence and failure to develop the requisite capacities to master them are closely linked to the vicious cycle. The intolerance of self-criticism, the connected failure to appraise hostility and aggression in relationships realistically, and the need to be special are considered. These concepts are used to evaluate some developmental formulations of narcissism propounded by self psychology. The assumption that "self-object transferences" are true transferences is challenged. These modes of relationship to the analyst appear to be the product of externalization, wish, need, fear, and characteristic modes of behavior addressed to the analyst, in addition to gradually evolving transferences. The conclusion of self psychology that structural neuroses and narcissistic disorders are sharply distinguished is attributed to the failure to take into account the additional determinants of free association presented.

BIBLIOGRAPHY

ARLOW, J. A. & BRENNER, C. (1964), *Psychoanalytic Concepts and the Structural Theory.* New York: Int. Univ. Press.

FREUD, S. (1914), On narcissism. *S. E.* 14:67–102.

GOLDBERG, A., ed. (1978), *The Psychology of the Self.* New York: Int. Univ. Press.

KERNBERG, O. F. (1970), Factors in the psychoanalytic treatment of narcissistic personalities. *J. Amer. Psychoanal. Assn.,* 18:51–85.

―――― (1975), *Borderline Conditions and Pathological Narcissism.* New York: Aronson.

KOHUT, H. (1971), *The Analysis of the Self.* New York: Int. Univ. Press.

―――― (1977), *The Restoration of the Self.* New York: Int. Univ. Press.

―――― & WOLF, E. S. (1978), The disorders of the self and their treatment. *Int. J. Psychoanal.,* 59:413–425.

KRIS, A. O. (1976), On wanting too much. *Int. J. Psychoanal.,* 57:85–95.

―――― (1977), Either-or dilemmas. *Psychoanal. Study Child,* 32:91–117.

―――― (1979), Persistence of denial in fantasy. *Psychoanal. Study Child,* 34:145–154.

―――― (1982), *Free Association.* New Haven & London: Yale Univ. Press.

MURRAY, J. M. (1964), Narcissism and the ego ideal. *J. Amer. Psychoanal. Assn.,* 12:477–511.

ORNSTEIN, P. (1974), On narcissism. *Annu. Psychoanal.,* 2:127–149.

RANGELL, L. (1963), The scope of intrapsychic conflict. *Psychoanal. Study Child,* 18:75–102.

ROTHSTEIN, A. (1980), *The Narcissistic Pursuit of Perfection.* New York: Int. Univ. Press.

SANDLER, J., KENNEDY, H., & TYSON, R. L. (1975), Discussions on transference. *Psychoanal. Study Child,* 30:409–441.

―――― ―――― ―――― (1980), *The Technique of Child Psychoanalysis.* Cambridge: Harvard Univ. Press.

SPRUIELL, V. (1975), Three strands of narcissism. *Psychoanal. Q.,* 44:577–595.

The Fate of Screen Memories in Psychoanalysis

EUGENE MAHON, M.D. AND
DELIA BATTIN-MAHON, M.S.W.

IN A PRELIMINARY COMMUNICATION (MAHON AND BATTIN, 1981), we described how screen memories can be used as a criterion for the termination of a psychoanalysis. We argued that screen memories are luminous windows on the hidden past that hide, however, more than they reveal. When an analysis nears termination and the hidden past has been transformed into revelations of synthesis and insight, screen memories undergo a clinically measurable metamorphosis. The analysand, in the terminal phase of his analysis, is subjectively aware that his screen memories are no longer the highly cathected, uncanny residues of his past; that is, they have become relatively decathected. This decathexis is a measure of the working-through process and the analysis of the transference neurosis. The patient's subjective sense of this decathexis of his screens is therefore an index of structural change and one indication which can be used, along with others, to alert and guide the clinician in the terminal phase of an analysis.

In this communication, after a brief review of the contributions by Freud and others to screen memories, we shall present the clinical data that led to our formulations and discuss our findings.

Eugene Mahon is a member of the faculty of the Columbia University Center for Psychoanalytic Training and Research in New York. Delia Battin-Mahon is a member of the Psychoanalytic Training Institute of the New York Freudian Society.

An earlier version of this paper was presented at a Scientific Meeting of the New York Freudian Society in December 1981.

REVIEW OF THE LITERATURE

In 1899, Sigmund Freud coined the term "screen memories" for the leftover relics of infantile amnesia. He was fascinated by his discovery that the important elements of the past were omitted from the memory, the trivial retained:

> . . . two psychical forces are concerned in bringing about memories of this sort. One of these forces takes the importance of the experience as a motive for seeking to remember it, while the other—a resistance—tries to prevent any such preference from being shown . . . instead of the mnemic image which would have been justified by the original event, another is produced which has been to some degree associatively *displaced* from the former one. . . . There is a common saying among us about shams, that they are not made of gold themselves but have lain beside something that *is* made of gold. The same simile might well be applied to some of the experiences of childhood which have been retained in the memory [p. 306f.].

Earlier, of course, in the letters to Fliess (October 3, 4; October 15, 1897), Freud had discussed his analysis of his own early memories dealing with impressions of his mother, his nurse, his brother Phillip, and an empty cupboard. It was the analysis of these gaps in his infantile amnesia which led Freud to his momentous discovery of the oedipus complex. Freud returned to the topic in 1900 and again in 1901. The analysis of screen memories plays a highly significant part in his case histories (1909, 1918) and in his study of Goethe (1917) and Leonardo da Vinci (1910). It seems, in fact, that the subject of screen memories was rarely far from his mind. For instance, in a 1920 footnote to *The Three Essays of Sexuality*, he compared a screen memory to a fetish; and in 1937, he tackled the issue again. But it is perhaps in 1914 that he made his most definitive and comprehensive statement on the nature of screen memories: "In some cases I have had an impression that the familiar childhood amnesia, which is theoretically so important to us, is completely counterbalanced by screen memories. Not only *some* but *all* of what is essential from childhood has been retained in these memories. It is simply a question of knowing how to extract it out of them by analysis. They represent the forgotten years of childhood as adequately as the manifest content of a dream represents the dream-thoughts" (p. 148).

Interest in screen memories other than Freud's has been less enthusiastic than one might have imagined. Greenacre (1981) has argued that the interest in ego psychology after Freud's death led to relative neglect of the concepts of reconstruction and screen memories, two concepts which are obviously allied. (Greenacre herself has done much to redress this balance.) A review of the literature before and after Freud's death reveals that this topic was approached from a variety of meta-psychological points of view. Simmel (1925) and Kennedy (1950) focused on the formation of screen memories. Fenichel (1927) provided new information on the economic function of screen memories. Ernst Kris (1956a, 1956b) was interested in the development, in fact, the construction of memory in general, not just its screening function. He argued, convincingly, that analysis is not just a nostalgic proustian attempt to recapture the past and wallow in it, but rather a pursuit of the vicissitudes of "genetics" as they enter the "personal myths" that human beings construct to make some kind of existential sense out of their life histories. Abraham (1913) and Glover (1929) described the screening function of traumatic memories. Helene Deutsch (1932) suggested that hysterical fugues are sometimes reactivated screen memories. The recent tendency to broaden the concept of screening—Lewin's (1950) screen affects, Greenson's (1958) screen identifications, Reider's (1953) screen symptom and screen character—runs the risk, in our opinion, of confusing a useful clinical phenomenon with an overinclusiveness that blurs the distinction of the definition. A useful heuristic phenomenon becomes screened by such ecumenical thinking. It was again Greenacre who brought a developmental point of view to the study of screen memories. Her purpose in a series of papers (1947, 1949, 1979, 1980, 1981), would seem to be twofold: (1) to explain the intensity of the screen memory (what Freud had called its "ultra clear" quality) as a stamp of its genetic origin in the preverbal months of life, when sensory traumas in the visual and auditory spheres are ubiquitous human experiences (Greenacre even suggests that the sharp edges of the screen memory, as contrasted with the vague edges of Lewin's dream screen, can be explained by the latter's less tumultuous sensory birth in the early hours of our oral origins); (2) to highlight the clinical neglect of reconstruction and analysis of screen memories and to renew clinical interest in these areas.

It is interesting, from the viewpoint of development, that there seem to be few studies (none to our knowledge) in which the child's subjective experience of his screen memories becomes available to him. Piaget (1945) did ask children about their understanding of their own dreams, discovering, in his usual genetic epistemological way, that it takes maturity of the mental apparatus to identify the dream as being a product of the mind, very young children experiencing the dream as a foreign body. At what age a human begins to reflect on his screen memories is perhaps an unresearchable topic. But we are inclined to believe that the dissolution of the oedipus complex and the massive repression that ushers in the infantile amnesia leave islands of memory that must erupt into the seas of latency with some chronological regularity that we can only guess at. Freud (1899) himself, describing his own memory, says: "it is not, I believe, until my sixth or seventh year that the stream of my memories becomes continuous" (p. 309). And Piaget suggests that the child does not possess a sense of time as an orderly sequence, past leading to the present, until 7 or 8 (Flavell, 1963). This suggests that by that age the child may have the capacity to reflect a little on his own history, where his memories have gone to, and why only certain pieces of the mosaic of memory remain available to him.

Our interest in screen memories was aroused when a patient, toward the end of his analysis, began to reflect on the working-through process, structural changes that he became subjectively aware of in his own way, and on a new grasp he developed on the meaning of his screen memories. He realized that whereas most of his screen memories had lost their uncanny luminous fascination, one or two others had retained their intensity. The patient felt convinced that the remaining "ultra clear" screens signified unfinished analytic business. As Freud might have said, the complete meaning had not yet been totally extracted from the memories. On the one hand, the patient's subjective sense of the status of his screen memories was an intellectual defense, but it also held a kernel of truth. The analysand's insight suggested an avenue of scientific inquiry to us, which we put to the test in a review of several analyses of children and adults. We had become convinced that attention to the status of a patient's screen memories can guide the analyst in his assessment criteria for termination. The end of an analysis is a complicated, intense series of communications between analyst and analysand, in which a multiplicity of factors have to be judged: like the state of the transference neurosis, the evaluation of the working-through process, assessment of structural changes, to name a few. Full consideration of all termination criteria is clearly beyond the scope of a paper such as this. Our mention of these complexities is in the interest of not appearing simplistic. In other words, we are not suggesting that an analysand can review his memories at the end of an analysis, like a historian, and come to some decision as to the date of his termination. This would indeed be a travesty of treatment and a triumph of narcissistic resistances. However, we are willing to suggest with cautious humility that toward the end of a well-conducted analysis, in the climate of a good-enough working alliance, dual scrutiny of the screen memories can lead to judgments that can be useful in arriving at decisions about readiness for termination.

CLINICAL ILLUSTRATIONS

We turn to the study of screen memories of patients at various stages of their development in order to provide the clinical evidence that allowed us to reach our conclusions.

CASE 1

Two screen memories briefly alluded to earlier and their vicissitudes in the analysis of a middle-aged patient will illustrate our thesis graphically. As previously reported (Mahon and Battin, 1981), the patient became aware that the work of analysis had removed the "uncanny" charge from one memory, but not from another, an insight that had major clinical implications in terms of psychoanalytic work accomplished and work remaining to be done. A narcissistic character armor could not completely conceal residuals of preoedipal pathology and poorly resolved oedipal conflicts. His "success" was often perceived by him as an ambivalent gift to his narcissistic mother or guilt-ridden victory over a castrated father, rather than an achievement of his own growth and development. The screen memories reflected his conflicts and his characteristic approach to them: one memory depicted a childhood scene of separation from the father, but the memory contained a doubt as to whether the father was coming or going. The "confusion" was a defense, of course, against positive and negative oedipal feelings toward the father, but on another level it was a depiction of mistrust that originated in a preoedipal rapprochement crisis with both parents. By focusing on the father, the screen obscured the effective repression of a host of feelings about the mother. The analysis of a poem by the analysand revealed how the screen memory had subtly insinuated itself into the patient's sublimations and into the transference where it could be examined in detail. The poem entitled "Cummings and Goings" was addressed to e. e. cummings and achieved its aesthetic effect through parody, irony, and the obvious play on words (comings in screen memory/cummings in poem). The offer of the poem to the analyst prior to a summer recess was an attempt to undo the "comings and goings" of the therapist with a magical "gift." Analysis of such issues led to an eventual "revision" of memory in which the "coming and going" screen seemed to have lost its emotional impact for the patient, not to mention its "ultra clear" quality.

But another memory had not lost its "illumination," its function as a screen still being under unconscious obligatory control it would seem. This memory depicted a childhood scene in which a practical joke had been played on the patient: a weekend guest of the family sent him to his room to discover, by surprise, a paper replica of a woman in bed. The patient became aware in the analytic process that the inert replication of memory was a screen for an entirely different set of memories that lay hidden in deeper folds of the unconscious: primal scene fantasies of a dangerous seductive mother and an endangered species, namely, his passive father. When the patient brought this differential version of memory to the attention of his analyst, they both realized they had hit on an insight that could gauge the progress of the analytic process. It seemed clear that the preoedipal issues which had found expression in the "coming and going" metaphor had been sufficiently worked through, whereas sexual oedipal components of primal scene fantasy had not.

This understanding of the screen memory allowed the patient to reflect on his inhibition in the sexual transference toward the analyst. If the screen memory was a reflection of the patient's fear that the unavailability and instability of the father could not protect him adequately from his own sexual impulses toward the seductive mother, the patient suddenly became aware that the transference neurosis was a complete recapitulation of his early fears: in a sense, he preferred to think of the analyst as a lifeless paper replica of his mother rather than let the full implication of the reality of his flesh-and-blood contact with the maternal transference emerge. In other words, the analysis of this screen memory allowed the patient to wean himself from a one-dimensional asexual vision of the analyst and the obvious defensiveness of this transference distortion, and engage in a more multidimensional relationship. This insight allowed oedipal sexual memories to rub shoulders with preoedipal tender memories and paved the way to a final undoing of his splitting mechanism—an undoing that was essential to ensure that the analysis would reach a most favorable outcome. It is of significance to report that with the analysis of this aspect of the transference, the corresponding screen memory began to lose its cathexis. As Freud might have remarked, the libidinal residues of the infantile amnesia were extracted.

CASE 2

Robert was 9½ years old and in the fourth month of his analysis when he related his first screen memory. The memory depicted him as 3 years old, in the park, with his father and his newly born baby brother, on a very cold day. He was standing by the baby carriage. His father said, "I'm going to take a picture."

Robert reacted only to the first half of the sentence "I'm going," unable or unwilling to understand that his father was not abandoning him, but was retreating to a relative distance from which he could take a photograph of his two sons. Robert's misunderstanding of this childhood event left him feeling cold and lonely and wishing he could be safe and warm in the baby carriage.

During the fifteenth month of his analysis, Robert became aware of a remarkable trick his memory had played on him. Looking through childhood photographs, he was startled to discover that his screen memory was a direct contradiction of a photographic fact: in the photograph he was *in* the carriage with his baby brother. Not only had his father not abandoned him, as the screen memory suggested; he had actually placed him snuggly and securely in the carriage, before taking the picture. We hope that Robert's need to falsify his memory in this manner will become clearer as we describe the genetic roots of his psychopathology and his symptomatic entry into treatment.[1]

Robert was the firstborn of a depressive mother and an obsessional, argumentative father. While both parents were well-meaning, they were perplexed and confused by an immediate problem that confronted them when Robert was born. The newborn had a large angioma on his neck. Two modes of treatment were suggested to the parents: surgery or parental massage of the skin until the angioma disappeared. The parents chose the latter treatment, which proved highly successful. But the child underwent a 3-month treatment that subjected him to

---

1. This distortion of memory brings to mind Bornstein's case (1953) in which an 8-year-old girl ran away from her father when he shouted "Go away!" to a dog that was close to her and might have harmed her. She completely misinterpreted the remark, so strong was her need to extract punishment for unacceptable oedipal ambitions from even the most protective communication. Bornstein does not take up the issue of screen memories in this paper, but one wonders if the "incident" in its distorted form was not incorporated by the patient and used as a "screen." The patient, as described by Bornstein, was certainly aware of the tricks memory can play. She referred to herself as a "forgettable" child, translating her "active" defensive processes into their passive equivalents in a way that was not uncharacteristic of her.

considerable discomfort and necessitated some neglect of the totality of his oral need.

According to the parents, Robert weathered this initial trauma rather well, and another at 11 months when a cyst on his eyelid required an overnight stay in the hospital for surgical removal. However, the parental reports of his resilience and developmental prowess were belied by his reaction to the birth of a sibling when he was 2½: he threw his pacifier and transitional object (a blanket) into the incinerator, not unlike Goethe who had a childhood memory in which he threw plates out the window, a symbolic ejection of his sibling, according to Freud (1917). In Robert's case, one senses that he was not merely ridding himself of his brother, but he was doing away with his own dependency wishes as well. It seemed clear that he was disavowing dependency while seeking security in his remarkably precocious intellect, but not without significant compromises along the way. After the incineration of his transitional objects, he began to thrust his tongue, for which a corrective brace became necessary. Later, he prided himself in being able to chew his tongue and make it seem as if he was chewing gum. None of these early preschool symptoms attracted too much attention from the environment. But in grade school, when Robert's orality began to explode in symptomatic impulsivity and greedy attention-seeking along with an aggressive argumentative pattern of misbehavior which was clearly a defense against Robert's more passive strivings, psychoanalysis seemed mandatory if his development was to be rescued from permanent maladaptation. This was the opinion of all parties except Robert.

His analysis began, quite expectedly, with belligerent resistance against the very idea of his needing help from an analyst. Every session started and ended with a defiant question, "When can I stop?" as if he had to greet and dismiss the analyst with a slap in the face, to protect himself and his helper from the impact of his needs. (His constant nagging of the analyst also may have reflected the climate of his home where both parents, while remaining married, seemed to need to threaten each other with divorce.) His fear that his insatiable needs could go out of control and overwhelm him and his caretakers forced him to badger the analyst for reassurance that his needs could be controlled: "I don't need you. But if I discover that I do, will there be any end to my greed?" seemed to be the unspoken fantasy.

His screen memory illustrates his defensive posture in the early months of analysis. Compressing the child's account and translating it into adult language, the analyst understood him to be saying: "Since my father is abandoning me, since my brother is the only baby in the carriage, I will stand beside the carriage, develop a personal myth [Kris, 1956b] of myself in which I am deprived but also stoic." A poem that he wrote illustrates the balances of defenses and instincts quite graphically. He called it "Gnore and Bore went to war, etc." Gnore obviously stood for ignore (denial, disavowal, isolation), Bore corresponded to depression, and war represented potential or actual loss of impulse control. Another poem about fog (his favorite) thinly disguised his wish not to see everything so clearly (denial, disavowal with genetic precursors of defense, triggered perhaps by his early eye problem).

The screen memory and the poems were, of course, offered to the analyst in a cautious transference climate in which the patient's trust emerged slowly from the shackles of analyzed resistances, until eventually he was able to rediscover himself not only in the baby carriage of a childhood photograph but also in the newly created psychological baby carriage of the transference neurosis. The memory of the father abandoning the baby carriage was of course a screen that concealed even earlier memories about the angioma and the eye surgery and the cumulative trauma of maternal deprivation.

What we are stressing in this case illustration is the ability of a sophisticated 9½-year-old to review his own falsification of memory, a review that reflected his ability to change his attitude toward his family and his analyst, and, of course, toward himself. We are suggesting that his screen memory was a defensive, self-deceiving internal counterfeit photograph that he could not discard until psychoanalysis made it possible for him to accept a more realistic likeness of himself. We are also suggesting that the revision of his screen memory was of obvious assistance to both analyst and analysand as a chart of the progress of the analytic voyage of discovery.

CASE 3

Alex, a 7-year-old boy with an older sister and divorced parents, began his analysis by saying, "I get angry for no reason." When it was explained to him that there is always a reason for a feeling, even if one cannot remember it, he related a memory in which, as he put it, "at the fourth or third birthday of my sister when I was 2s or 3s [he had a slight lisp], I was wearing blue." He went on to describe how he was the only boy among many girls at his sister's party. He assured his analyst that this memory, in which he seemed to play a very distant second fiddle to his sister, was corroborated by a photograph which confirmed among other details that he indeed had been wearing blue. In subsequent sessions this young analysand was impressed with the analyst's ability to remember the details of the screen memory as it had been told to him. Alex was not always complimentary, however, and when he noticed screwdrivers out of place, he asked how the change had come about. When the analyst confessed that he could not remember how the screwdrivers had arrived in their new habitat, Alex chided him, "How come you can remember what I told you happened to me years ago, but not what happened today?" The analyst was impressed with this piece of wisdom and began to reflect on the countertransference tendency that placed more emphasis on the past than on current events. With this piece of countertransference out of the way, the analyst could see the point of the patient's inquiry. For Alex, the appearance of the playroom was an obvious sign of the analyst's attachment to others; would he (therefore) have to play second fiddle to them and hide his own feelings?

This was a very early moment in the analysis, hardly a time for deep interpretation of all the issues raised by this seemingly innocent question, and yet the analytic situation was vibrating with three dynamic currents: a screen memory, a piece of transference, and an equally important piece of countertransference. In the interest of alerting the patient's insight to the multiple determinants of the transaction, the analyst remarked somewhat humorously, "Other children have been here. You must have feelings about it and you are not even wearing blue." Alex made immediate eye contact with his therapist and

laughed. The analyst was implying that the issues hidden by the
screen memory would be reenacted in the transference and
that the patient might not always have to use defenses to face
them. In a sense, he need not only be blue; all the other colors
of his prismatic development need not be neglected.

A few more details of Alex's life will help us to understand
more clearly the pivotal significance of the memory that strad-
dled a gulf between his understanding of himself and what was
lost to repression. Alex's father left his mother when the child
was one year of age. After the divorce the father would visit,
however, and take Alex's older sister with him, "the baby" left
behind while father and daughter attempted a rapprochement.
"Sister gets everything (including visits with father) while I get
nothing," he must have mused. "An older sibling of the opposite sex, not to mention the even older object of my incestuous desires, for the inside track in the race toward father:
negative oedipal pathways are closed off; with my father out of
the way, positive oedipal pathways are dangerously close to
reality. What a predicament! Let me think of myself permanently as a psychological cripple: all my ambitions can be hidden neatly behind a screen. Every day is sister's birthday, not
mine: I'm an ignored little boy blue. My birthdays don't count.
My depression will extract love, command attention, misery my
weapon against all of them." This dramatization of Alex's adaptation is of course a caricature, but it does represent a condensation of many months of the analytic process. For instance,
Alex developed the habit of collecting stray pens in the office,
pretending to steal them. This was an overdetermined symptomatic act within the context of the analytic process, of course,
but one meaning is worthy of emphasis: Alex would take what
he could not retrieve from primary objects; moreover, this
should not be noticed, prohibited, or interpreted since that
forced many repressed affects out of their hiding places. Alex
was, of course, furious with his father for abandoning him and
favoring another, but he was equally furious with his mother's
remarriage that forced him to deal with a new "father" and
reconsider his relationship with the old. Alex was of course also
furious with an analyst who was unwilling to settle for his
monochromatic estimation of himself. Alex's drawings de-

picted his ambivalence toward working through these issues. Interpretation of his "blue" defenses led to revisions of memory that no doubt reflected rearrangements of defenses as well as structural realignments. Alex informed the analyst that his old memory was only one version of the truth: he could now also remember a birthday party which was a celebration of his own birthday, not his sister's, and he remembered wearing blue on that occasion as well. He would draw both versions and prove his point. Neurosis intervened, however: having drawn the old version (his sister's birthday), he could not draw the new revised version. This is where the story must end since the analysis has not yet proceeded beyond this point. In the future, as the analysis of resistance continues, we hope that Alex will be able to "draw" as many versions of himself as imagination can rescue from screens that would compromise his growth and development.

CASE 4

Prelatency children do not walk into an analyst's office recounting their screen memories. Yet, we know from Piaget (1937) that recognition memory is in existence in the first year of life, evocative memory in the second. We also know that symbolism and rudimentary defenses appear in the second year of life (Jones, 1916; Sarnoff, 1970). This suggests that the screening function might exist from the second year of life on. And yet, clinical data from prelatency children describing their screen memories seem sparse. Is the infantile amnesia that begins at 5 or 6 with the waning of the oedipus complex a prerequisite for the existence of screen memories and their recall? Or could we find precursors of the process even in prelatency? We would like tentatively to suggest the latter.

Willie, a 4-year-old in the full passion of his oedipal romance, was seen in consultation for a sleep disorder, a reaction to the recent divorce of his parents. He described his conflicts in a displaced manner that suggested an incipient screening process. In the second session, he related the following memory: "You know, I had a dog when I was a baby. His name was Silver. He could not be with three people. He bit my daddy who was away a lot: so[2] he did not know him well enough." These were the actual words of the child. The trauma of the parents' separation had occurred one year before the consultation, when Willie was 3; yet, the child created a displacement from the human object to the animal and the concomitant distortion of time as if he needed to soothe himself by saying this did not happen last year, it happened 3 years ago; moreover, it was not me who was angry with my father, it was a dog. This displacement of responsibility in regard to time and object is similar to, if not identical with, the screen memory mechanisms Freud described in 1899. The major difference between this screen memory and its adult counterpart may reside in the amount of insight the patient has into its formation.

This child's parents at first accepted, but later rejected, analytic treatment for their son. Consequently, the vicissitudes of this screen memory received no further documentation.

DISCUSSION

While Freud and others (e.g., Fenichel, Glover, Greenacre) have discussed screen memories from defensive, economic, and developmental points of view, this presentation has focused on the vicissitudes of screen memories in the analytic situation. We argued that the working-through process of analysis allows the analyst objectively and the analysand subjectively to become aware of shifts of emphasis in the reconstruction of the analysand's life history. This awareness of structural change, as seen through the shifting prisms of screen memories, can have prognostic significance.

It is interesting to consider what it is about the nature of screen memories that may afford them a unique role as criteria of termination. Couldn't a similar case be made for symptoms, dreams, parapraxes, character traits, and many other mental phenomena?

Symptom removal was considered the goal of early analysis.

2. The "so" seems to have a double meaning. It can be thought of as a parapraxis or, from an anthropological developmental point of view, as an example of what Freud calls the antithetical meaning of a primal word.

A psychoanalysis that was interested only in symptom removal could obviously use this criterion in its assessment of readiness for termination.

As analysis became relatively less interested in symptoms and more concerned with structures of the mind, character traits, and defense organization, it became clear that symptom removal alone could not be a reliable indicator of readiness for termination. However, the structures of the mind and character traits do not vanish, as symptoms do, after the conflicts and compromises have been understood. They are permanent psychic baggage that cannot be interpreted and then abandoned like unnecessary luggage. They are the essence of human identity itself. They can be modified, they can be understood, they can undergo massive change, but it is unthinkable that they could be totally abandoned. Consequently, it is hard to use their presence or absence as precise criteria for readiness for termination of a psychoanalysis. This is not meant to deny the remarkable changes in character and psychological structure which are the sine qua non of any successful psychoanalysis. We are merely suggesting that these changes are as subtle as they are essential, and that they are extremely difficult for the clinician to measure.

Dreams pose an equally intriguing question. Can we in any way as clinicians use dream content or form as an indicator of readiness for termination? While dreams can obviously reflect not only the primary process elements of condensation, displacement, and symbolism that Freud uncovered in 1899, but also structural elements, most clinicians will surely agree that the royal road to the unconscious is not necessarily a useful road to assess readiness for termination.

What then is so special about screen memories? Are they not creatures of instinct, defense, and compromise formation like most other mental products? Obviously they are made of the same mental stuff as dreams, symptoms, parapraxes, but it is their uniquely contrasting features, not their similarities with these other mental products, that allow them to be prognostic indicators of readiness for termination. What are these unique features?

A man may have a thousand dreams, but he usually has only

a handful of screen memories. From a purely numerical point of view it may be more heuristic to chart the vicissitudes of screen memories than attempt to tackle the labyrinth of a myriad of dreams.

Let us compare and contrast a screen memory and a symptom. Clearly impulse, defense, and compromise are involved in both. But whereas some symptoms seem to rely on somatic compliance for their avenues of expression, the screen memory seems to rely on memory compliance, to coin a phrase. It is as if energies being displaced were not discharged somatically but rather found expression in some rigid, frozen, distortion of memory. This inner distortion, as opposed to the outer distortion of the symptom, if one can be permitted to talk for a moment about the mind in spatial terms, seems to have a heuristic clinical value: whereas symptoms can fade early in the course of an analysis, the inner distortion of memory seems to have an uncanny resistance, as if these deep secrets *corresponded*, as Freud suggested, to the totality of the infantile amnesia. They are deeply buried, tightly sealed forgotten letters of the infantile romance that can be opened only in the utter sensitivity of the therapeutic alliance that characterizes an analysis. It is precisely because these letters cannot be opened at the beginning of a new romance with the analyst that they may have to wait for their final exposition when the transference neurosis—which Loewald (1968) called the recapitulation of the love life of a human being—approaches resolution. Because they can only be fully revealed at the end of the analysis they can be used as criteria for termination.

It is tempting to compare screen memories and dream thoughts. Whereas dream thoughts "can take hold of normal thought, carry the latter away and plunge it into the world of the unconscious" (Mannoni, 1971, p. 54), a screen memory is not plunged into the unconscious, but rather stands at a crossroad between the unconscious history of childhood and all future developmental history, like Janus, one face turned to the past, the other to the future. The screen memory is the point of tension between the two histories, and gets contributions from both sides, or, as Freud (1901) put it, it can be retroactive, displaced forward, contemporary, or contiguous in its chronological relation to what is being screened (p. 44).

The dream thought runs off with the contemporary thought into the unconscious and does not rest until it reaches the end of the mental apparatus in charge of perception and becomes the hallucination, which is the hallmark of dreams. The screen memory, in contrast, runs off with the contemporary thought and most of the infantile amnesia, but, instead of turning up as a hallucination in a dream, it maintains a quasi-hallucinatory image in our waking life.

One might well ask: why does a screen memory maintain such an iconic relationship with what Alvin Frank (1969) calls the unrememberable and unforgettable? Except for recurring dreams, one would be hard pressed to find a mental product that so stubbornly insists on sameness.[3] It is as if the memory behaves like a child insisting that the bedtime story be told exactly the same way each time. In a sense, a screen memory is a caricature of the parent-child relationship in which infantile omnipotence insists that the magical parent will gratify the child on demand and unconditionally. Or, to state it from a historic viewpoint, human beings with complicated histories like to imagine iconic remnants of their past as organizers of their psyches. In a sense, screen memories are to the mind what primitive gods are to the history of culture.

Further comparing and contrasting screen memories and dreams, we immediately realize that while both use similar mechanisms (displacement, symbolism, condensation), there is an essential difference: dreams are forever handling conflict in a cinematic flux of kaleidoscopic images, whereas screen memories are more comparable to one frame of a cinematic sequence in which all the other frames lie hidden in the infantile amnesia.[4] It is this standstill quality of the screen memory that allows one to measure significant increments of change as the

3. A study of the similarity between the persistence of the image in the screen memory and in recurring dreams would help us to understand better the nature of both phenomena.

4. On the other hand, patients may use a film as a screen memory. Schreiber (1974) describes a patient whose memory of the film *The Wizard of Oz* was a screen that shielded her from painful affects caused by separation from her mother as a child. The switch from black and white to technicolor when Dorothy opens the door and first sets eyes on Oz was used by the patient to color over her sense of loss with its opposite, the discovery of a new world.

memory gets revised in the process of working through. It is as if one picture had stolen the pigment from all the surrounding pictures: analysis slowly returns this pigment to the originals and the hyperpigmented fake loses most of its color.

Screen memories may have a special place in reconstructive work. According to Greenacre (1981), "Screen memories are especially helpful, but are often disregarded by students and some analysts who have tried unprofitably to treat them as though they were dreams. Because they are less fluid than dreams and more firmly organized in their enduring defensive function, immediate free association cannot be demanded. Their use depends on the alertness of the analyst for detecting their discrepancies, especially in time and in content. If he is in a good therapeutic alliance with the analyst, the patient becomes interested and begins to question them himself, and later finds ways of checking on the reliability of their content" (p. 42f.).

Greenacre suggests that a patient will not associate to a screen memory. Freud, however, maintained that a patient can associate to an old dream. He essentially says that a patient can free-associate to an old mental product and revive its meaning in a heuristic fashion that can assist the progress of a psycho-analysis. If we compare a screen memory to a fossil dream of childhood, we may ask: why is it that a patient cannot free-associate to this ancient relic and revive its meaning? Surely, what comes between the screen memory and our understanding is the infantile amnesia. If we consider the transference neurosis as a complicated, long-winded association that explains the infantile amnesia, it becomes clear that the screen memory cannot be understood until all its associations which lie hidden in the transference neurosis are revealed. In a sense, all associations throughout an analysis can be thought of as associations to the screen memory. Obviously the screen memory itself is an association to the total metapsychology of childhood experience. This is not meant to be a redundant circular theory in which the transference neurosis reflects the infantile neurosis, the screen memory having a foot in both camps. A simple, more clinical way of saying this would be that the gap that exists between the screen memory and its total elucidation in the transference neurosis is a measure of the repression that exists between childhood psychology and the mental life of adults. In a sense, the transference neurosis is a newly created screen memory that allows screen memories to speak.

The emphasis we are placing on certain unique features of screen memories is not meant to imply that the analysis of memories is more important than the analysis of a symptom, a dream, or a character trait. Obviously, all may be analyzed in contiguity, depending on the free-associative forces.

From the clinical data we have presented, we hope to have demonstrated that analytic work slowly extracts what the infantile amnesia hides by means of screen memories. The extract pours itself into the transference neurosis until finally the vessel of infantile amnesia is relatively empty and the screen memories, which acted like lids, become redundant. This metaphor, while it accurately portrays the gist of our thesis, is surely an inaccurate exaggeration, since no sensible clinician can believe that the creative wells of infantile amnesia could ever be truly emptied. The most we would wish for, as reasonable prospectors of the mind, would be that those underground springs of unconscious processes which directly contribute to human neurosis be traced to their sources, so that their currents can be deflected from symptomatic channels to adaptive ones. If the screen memory is a psychic landmark that not only can lead the prospector toward his destination but also can inform him when certain wells are dry, it is obvious that the prospector can use these signposts to his profit.

BIBLIOGRAPHY

ABRAHAM, K. (1913), A screen memory concerning a childhood event of apparently aetiological significance. In *Clinical Papers and Essays on Psychoanalysis*. New York: Basic Books, 1955, pp. 36–41.

ARLOW, J. A. (1979), Metaphor and the psychoanalytic situation. *Psychoanal. Q.*, 48:363–385.

BORNSTEIN, B. (1953), Fragment of analysis of an obsessional child. *Psychoanal. Study Child,* 8:313–332.

DEUTSCH, H. (1932), *Psychoanalysis of the Neuroses*. London: Hogarth Press.

FENICHEL, O. (1927), The economic function of screen memories. In *Collected Papers*. New York: Norton, 1953, 1:113–116.

478   Eugene Mahon and Delia Battin-Mahon

FLAVELL, J. H. (1963), The Developmental Psychology of Jean Piaget. New York: Van Nostrand Reinhold.
FRANK, A. (1969), The unrememberable and the unforgettable. Psychoanal. Study Child, 24:48–77.
FREUD, S. (1897), Letters 70 and 71. S. E., 1:261–266.
_____ (1899), Screen memories. S. E., 3:301–322.
_____ (1900), The interpretation of dreams. S. E., 4 & 5.
_____ (1901), Childhood memories and screen memories. S. E., 6:43–52.
_____ (1905), Three essays on the theory of sexuality. S. E., 7:125–243.
_____ (1909), Analysis of a phobia in a five-year-old boy. S. E., 10:3–149.
_____ (1910), Leonardo da Vinci and a memory of his childhood. S. E., 11:59–137.
_____ (1914), Remembering, repeating and working-through. S. E., 12:145–156.
_____ (1917), A childhood recollection from Dichtung und Wahrheit. S. E., 17:145–156.
_____ (1918), From the history of an infantile neurosis. S. E., 17:3–122.
_____ (1937), Constructions in analysis. S. E., 23:255–270.
GLOVER, E. (1929), The screening function of traumatic memories. Int. J. Psychoanal., 10:90–93.
GREENACRE, P. (1947), Vision, headache, and halo. In Trauma, Growth and Personality. New York: Int. Univ. Press, 1969, pp. 132–148.
_____ (1949), A contribution to the study of screen memories. Psychoanal. Study Child, 3/4:73–84.
_____ (1979), Reconstruction and the process of individuation. Psychoanal. Study Child, 34:121–144.
_____ (1980), A historical sketch of the use and disuse of reconstruction. Psychoanal. Study Child, 35:35–40.
_____ (1981), Reconstruction. J. Amer. Psychoanal. Assn., 29:27–46.
GREENSON, R. R. (1958), On screen defenses, screen hunger, and screen identity. In Explorations in Psychoanalysis. New York: Int. Univ. Press, 1978, pp. 111–132.
JONES, E. (1916), The theory of symbolism. In Papers on Psycho-Analysis. London: Baillière, Tindall, & Cox, 1948, pp. 87–144.
KENNEDY, H. E. (1950), Cover memories in formation. Psychoanal. Study Child, 5:275–284.
KRIS, E. (1956a), The recovery of childhood memories in psychoanalysis. Psychoanal. Study Child, 11:54–88.
_____ (1956b), The personal myth. J. Amer. Psychoanal. Assn., 4:653–681.
LEWIN, B. D. (1946), Sleep, the mouth, and the dream screen. Psychoanal. Q., 15:419–434.
_____ (1950), The Psychoanalysis of Elation. New York: Norton.
LOEWALD, H. W. (1968), The transference neurosis. In Papers on Psychoanalysis. New Haven & London: Yale Univ. Press, 1980, pp. 302–314.
MAHON, E. & BATTIN, D. (1981), Screen memories and termination. J. Amer. Psychoanal. Assn., 29:939–942.

The Fate of Screen Memories 479

MANNONI, O. (1971), *Freud.* New York: Pantheon.

PIAGET, J. (1937), *The Construction of Reality in the Child.* New York: Basic Books, 1954.

―――― (1945), *Play, Dreams and Imitation in Childhood.* New York: Norton, 1951.

REIDER, N. (1953), Reconstruction and screen function. *J. Amer. Psychoanal. Assn.,* 1:389–405.

SARNOFF, C. A. (1970), Symbols and symptoms. *Psychoanal. Q.,* 39:550–562.

SCHREIBER, S. (1974), A filmed fairy tale as a screen memory. *Psychoanal. Study Child,* 29:389–401.

SIMMEL, E. (1925), A screen memory in statu nascendi. *Int. J. Psychoanal.,* 6:454–467.

Modes of Communication in the Analysis of a Latency Girl

KERRY KELLY NOVICK

PSYCHOANALYSIS IS QUINTESSENTIALLY THE "TALKING cure" (Freud, 1910, p. 13), but there is considerable disagreement about the approximation of child analysis to the ideal of verbal analytic communication with adults. Anna Freud (1965) has sharply contrasted them: "They [children] may communicate verbally, after initial hesitations, but without free associations this does not carry them beyond the confines of the conscious mind. . . . Play with toys, drawing, painting, staging of fantasy games, acting in the transference have been introduced and accepted in place of free association and, *faute de mieux,* child analysts have tried to convince themselves that they are valid substitutes for it. In truth, they are nothing of the kind" (p. 29). Berta Bornstein (1945), not quite so pessimistic, said, "the child is unable and unwilling to produce free associations. The analysis of his play supplies a partial substitute for these free associations" (p. 153). What the child analyst must then work with is a variable mixture of play, action, and speech on the part of the child, while what the analyst offers in return is primarily verbal. The child may not be communicating intentionally, but expressing via physical and verbal modalities impulses and feelings from different levels of consciousness. The therapist, on the other hand, tries to "hear" or "read" all such expressions of the child in the service of (1) understanding the mental life of the patient; (2) integrating the understanding in a secondary process, verbal form; and (3) eventually commu-

Michigan Psychoanalytic Society and Institute, Arbor Clinic, Ann Arbor, Mich.

nicating the understanding back to the patient in the form of verbalizations, explanations, and interpretations. The problem and the excitement of working with children, however, are that this general pattern of therapeutic interaction with the goal of shared verbalizations is difficult to achieve. Words are apprehended according to the developmental level of the child and the specific history of his or her verbal development, and must be used in the analytic process in a way which has meaning for the particular child. In this paper I describe some of the ways a latency girl brought material into her analysis, how I tried to help her put it into forms I could understand, and how we worked together to create a verbal medium of communication in order to bring about interpretation, understanding, and change.

CASE PRESENTATION

BACKGROUND

Louisa H., although born to English-speaking parents, spent most of her early life in the care of au pair girls, nannies, and cleaning women, who spoke a variety of languages. Mrs. H's disinterest in caring for her daughter may have been related to the depression and feeling of uprootedness she described, as the family made frequent moves due to the demands of the father's occupation; a further problem was Louisa's severe congenital strabismus, which the parents claimed not to have noticed. It was only at the insistence of the maternal grandmother that the parents sought medical advice. Surgery was recommended, and Louisa entered the hospital at 10 months. Mr. H. reported that both he and his wife made strenuous efforts to have Mrs. H. stay in the hospital with Louisa, but the doctors did not permit it. The mother remembered only the relief she felt at the prospect of a few weeks' respite from the demands of the infant. Louisa spent 16 days in the hospital, with both eyes covered, restrained in her crib, without a visit from her parents. The mother told me that, on Louisa's return home, she had felt unable to tolerate the change from a passive, dependent infant to a difficult, demanding toddler.

When Louisa was 18 months old, the parents went on a 2-week holiday, leaving Louisa in the care of a familiar Turkish cleaning woman. When they returned, she developed a severe sleeping disturbance: for about a year Louisa often screamed for some 3 to 5 hours a night. During the day Louisa displayed intense clinging or crying whenever mother or father left the room, alternating with aggressive attacks on them. The birth of a sister when Louisa was just over 3 did not affect this behavior, which persisted until the referral at 7½ years of age.

BEGINNING OF ANALYSIS

Louisa brought a torrent of material from the very beginning: she spent each session switching from one topic to another, from talk of the present to the past, from one game to the next, from sadness to glee and back again. Sometimes she was a pale, quiet, "good" girl, compliant and defended; at others, wildly excited, flushed, mischievous, and harder than ever to grasp. All this produced confusion in me and later came to be seen as an important indicator of Louisa's own inner confusion, particularly in relation to affects. The degree of confusion and condensation of thoughts and feelings related to conflicts at all levels may be illustrated by a typical piece of material. Louisa drew a large tongue, in which she put the face of a man. To this man she then added, in sequence, a beard, hair, a bopeep hat, tongue, clothes, a witch hat covering the bopeep hat, brown hair, black hair, and another beard. It took us weeks to begin to disentangle the many threads in this material, but some clues to the defensive nature of Louisa's preoccupation with good and evil witches or ogres came to light around our first separation, one day at half-term.

Louisa was overtly ambivalent about the separation, one day drawing pictures of me as a naughty girl who wouldn't wear my glasses, the next day atoning by drawing me as the good fairy who would bring her twice as much money for her baby teeth as her sister received. I realized later that Louisa conceptualized my understanding her at this point in terms of my looking or listening hard enough; her reproach was that I was not seeing past her anger to her longing for a "fairy godmother." The following week, Louisa brought a story about a friend who was so hungry that she ate a biscuit while sitting on the toilet. She accepted my interpretation that the loss of feces was so unbearable that they must be replaced right away, and followed this with a repetition of the story of "Mrs. Novick who wouldn't wear her glasses." Louisa thus related the feeling of loss to defecation, but used an image directly related to her historical loss in infancy to communicate her reproach that I did not see past the defensive anal preoccupation to her underlying feelings of sadness and rage. Another strand of meaning in this material was her wish that I should need glasses as she did; safety from angry thoughts and wishes appeared to reside in our being similar. It became clear as Louisa's analysis progressed that her wish for us to be the same was accompanied by confusion about our boundaries and perhaps represented a deeper wish for symbiotic fusion of self and object.

As the Christmas holiday approached, Louisa introduced a game of hiding crayons, which we hunted for in turn. She began hiding them more and more often on my person and begged me to do the same with her. She seemed to be wishing for each of us to carry a bit of the other around during the break, to insure against total loss. On the first day back she was very anxious over whether a small split in the sleeve of my dress meant my arm was also hurt.

She played the game of hiding crayons in a compulsive fashion for weeks. When I introduced naming the crayons, Louisa chose for herself the orange crayon which had been lost in the snow on the roof outside our window, and was able to experience consciously and admit to her own lost feeling for the first time. She brought a fantasy about a person searching for someone to take care of her saying, "I'm too cold, I need someone to keep me warm." Louisa added potato chips to the crayons for hiding and began to hide them by eating them; she told me that they were gone for good. A verbalization of her confusion between the chips being incorporated to be saved forever and her chewing destroying them so they were then lost eased Louisa's tension, and she provided a clue to her idea of the reason things get lost by calling the lost orange Louisa crayon "naughty." We could see in this sequence that the material converged around oral aggression, which provided a temporal link to her hospitalization at 10 months.

So far in Louisa's treatment she had played games, drawn pictures, told stories, jumped about the room, been cooperative and friendly, or contrary and sulky at various times. From the form and the content of this mixture of play and talk, I had concluded that she was suffering from conflicts at both oral and anal levels, particularly around aggressive impulses. Her relationships were interfered with by her use of the primitive defenses of denial, generally against feelings of loss, helplessness, and injury; projection, to defend against both aggression and subsequent guilt; and passive into active, which was seen mainly in the transference as a defense against projected aggression and omnipotence. Louisa's difficulties appeared to include a deep sense of the unreliability of other people, with most of her stories and games depicting lonely, lost, pathetic characters.

My understanding was important to me and to the ultimate goals of the treatment, but Louisa resisted what I have described as the third step in the therapeutic interaction: she did not want to hear what I had to say or know what I understood about her. Rather, she wished for unspoken communion between us, with perfect, effortless, mutual understanding. Her terror at the prospect of the fulfillment of this wish in fantasy was also an ingredient in her resistance to my verbal communications. Louisa's main solution to this dilemma was to try to control her surroundings completely; her conflicts were expressed in issues of omnipotent control which she achieved only momentarily in swings between engulfing feelings of helplessness and accesses of overpowering rage. She clung to her mother, refusing to allow her parents privacy at home or a social life outside. Louisa checked the mail and demanded details of telephone conversations. When she could not control my comings and goings at holidays or the ends of sessions, she controlled our means of communication, insisting that we write rather than speak, or write in foreign languages, or backward, etc.

Ferenczi (1913) described stages in the development of the sense of reality which involved a gradual relinquishing of omnipotent manipulation of objects, gestures, and words. Louisa began to progress in first allowing me to verbalize hitherto unnamed feelings of sadness and anger and ultimately taking over that function herself. This paralleled, or perhaps allowed for, an increasing capacity to distinguish between her wishes and reality, her feelings and those of others. We began to see less confusion, and a decrease in projection and reversal of affect. An enhanced reality sense led in turn to the enrichment of her secondary process functioning with the inclusion of more mental content in the autonomous ego.

But Louisa had always functioned adequately in school and outside the home; her secondary process thinking served her fairly well and apparently reliably. How could she function so well when her disturbance dated from such an early phase of development? At one point I thought perhaps some sort of pseudodevelopment had taken place, but Louisa maintained her good functioning even when regressive pulls in treatment were strongest and an "as if" personality might have been expected to break down. What appeared instead was a sort of isolation of her preverbal experience, an impenetrable thicket around which the other trees grew tall, if not quite straight. Anny Katan (1961) distinguishes between verbalization of outside perceptions and that of feelings. Both contribute to ego development, but the verbalization of feelings leads directly to "an increase of the controlling function of the ego over affects and drives" (p. 185). This distinction is relevant in view of what is known about Louisa's parents. Both parents loved Louisa fiercely, if ambivalently, and both were devoted to her upbringing. The father, however, was an extremely inhibited man, particularly constricted in his expression of feelings; and the mother was a chronically depressed woman with flattened emotional expression, except for intermittent temper outbursts which left her guilty and frightened. Louisa's language development would have been idiosyncratic in this family anyway, especially because her major caretakers were non-English-speaking, but, in addition, she suffered two major events which were never integrated into her ego. Her parents could not describe, verbalize, or explain the events and feelings around her hospitalization, or around their holiday from her when Louisa was 18 months old. No one verbalized the feelings for Louisa: she never developed an emotional vocabulary and the effect of this was her skewed ego development, with good functioning in areas related to outside perception, but lacunae in impulse control, reality testing, and secondary process thinking. She could not develop age-adequate object constancy when she had no way to integrate her feelings about loss and separation.

FURTHER COURSE OF ANALYSIS

In this section I shall recount in detail a 6-week period in which we worked on Louisa's wish to be close to her mother and to me in the transference and I shall try to include what I as the analyst said and did and what meaning this had for Louisa. During these weeks two verbal conventions emerged—"saying the opposite" and the use of foreign languages. As we study the uses Louisa and I made of these special locutions, we may further elucidate the nature of the dialogue between patient and analyst, and the meaning verbal interactions took on for Louisa and me in what was becoming a shared goal of verbalization and integration.

On Tuesday of the 17th week of treatment, along with hiding crayons, Louisa initiated a game in which we took turns writing "messages" for each other to guess. The next day we again wrote messages and Louisa made rules for them: they had to be "about your head or my head." To Louisa's message "Your teeth are black," I remarked that she felt the way she did when she hit people. Louisa said, "I was telling you the opposite," but also scribbled wildly over several pages. When her next message consisted of a drawing of my face pulled out into a black blob, I said that she sometimes thought people could come apart and be changed. This again led to scribbling. I wrote over this that it was a secret message from Louisa. She nodded and said it was a letter saying "Boo boo you you moo moo cow cow." I noted that this was the way babies describe things and that she was telling me something she had felt when she was a baby. Louisa then drew another scribble all over the page and said it was my hair in a mess. Some of the wishes apparent in this material are the desire for mutual omniscience and aggressive impulses directed against me (black teeth, blob face, messy hair); she says she is saying the opposite to render the aggressive expression harmless, but this initial statement of the defensive maneuver is ineffective. We also find out that she knows there is a baby wish seeking expression and she is either looking herself for a mode in which to communicate it, or asking me to find one, or, at the end, reproaching me for not understanding "boo boo, etc."

The following day, Louisa came in very excited and started to order me about—it was my turn to write, I must use the red crayon, and so on. I wrote a message about her feeling that she had secrets, to which Louisa responded by writing words in other languages, French, German, Italian, Spanish.[1] She seemed by this both to be agreeing that she had secrets and attempting to disguise them. Louisa went on writing words for a long time until I wrote, in Spanish, "Louisa does not want to talk today." She nodded and smiled, and began to write things in Norwegian, which she knew I could not understand.

We began Friday's session with an exchange of notes; it was my turn first. I wrote, "Does Louisa want to talk today?" She replied, "Does Mrs. Novick want to talk today?" I wrote "Yes" and said that sometimes she was not sure who was who, and who had the secrets. Louisa then wrote in German that she wanted to talk about "book" and "lamp." I wrote, in French, "Louisa is afraid to talk about her secrets," and she said, "Yes." She then turned to a new game of drawing and produced a picture of Cinderella's slipper lost in the snow.[2] Thus in this first week of the central phase of her treatment we evolved the conventions of "saying the opposite" and of using foreign languages, but Louisa circled warily around the edges of the material that was both emerging via these conventions and being defended against by their use.

---

1. Louisa maintained an elementary vocabulary and a repertoire of phrases in several languages, learned from her early caretakers and current au pairs. It was a lucky coincidence that I shared knowledge of the same languages.

2. The links among Louisa's guessing games, hiding games, secrets, and use of foreign languages are visible in this material and could later be connected with her conflicts over control and her wishes and fears about closeness with others.

The following week brought an intensification of Louisa's efforts to defend against emerging oral material; she played games in fits and starts, brought larger than usual amounts of food to sessions, and any attempt on my part to communicate by talking or writing was met with silence or doodling. By Friday, Louisa said she wanted to talk about "writing," which she wrote in Norwegian, but translated for me out loud. I talked about writing being easier for her than talking and the use of other languages as a defense, and she responded with material about the story of the shoemaker and the elves and her feeling that she was magic sometimes and wished I could be too. We drew a series of pictures which showed us in our beds connected by a telephone wire over which we could communicate magically 24 hours a day. Louisa followed this with a picture of me as a witch with a big ferocious mouth full of sharp teeth. I think this material showed Louisa struggling to find ways to share her wish to be together with me and her desperate fear of the possible consequences to us both from her own and her projected aggression. There was a growing awareness on her part that the defensive use of other languages was nonetheless getting us closer to her wishes.

In looking at what I was doing, rather than at Louisa's material or the interaction, we can discern responses at several different levels. First, I simply played whichever game Louisa suggested, and I followed her rules; second, I attempted to link the affect in a particular production to an impulse or fantasy. This premature attempt at interpretation was rebuffed by Louisa when she scribbled in response, but she admitted that the drawings had meaning when I limited my commentary to a descriptive naming, in effect respecting her "secret." She could then let me know it was a secret from infancy. There followed, in the multilingual notes, a phase which I would characterize as one of my providing reassurance that I would respect the defense, while keeping explicit between us that the other languages were being used to avoid something.

The theme of Louisa's material the next week was her wish to be close and her feeling that this was impossible. On Monday she immediately sat down and drew a picture of me in bed with a telephone next to it. I added a picture of her in bed and put a

balloon above her head for "what she was dreaming." Louisa
filled the balloon with a huge telephone, and I interpreted her
wish to communicate everything to me magically. I then drew a
picture of us together in the consulting room and remarked
that we could communicate there. But Louisa rejected this,
crossed out that picture, and drew us again in the beds.

The following day, Louisa drew a picture of me with a balloon
over my head, in which I wrote her name. She changed the
hair color to her own and drew two oblongs, which I guessed
were beds. Louisa said they were the curtains of our room,
but wanted to know more about how they could be beds. I
showed her, and, because the beds were in a circle, associated
them to the beds in the hospital ward where Louisa's mother
had stayed a few months before. Louisa completed the circle of
beds and put people into them, explaining, however, that the
patients couldn't talk to each other because of the central pillar;
besides, they "couldn't really *shout* around the ward." I interpreted her feelings about how hospitalization can keep people from being together and related this to Louisa's frequent
illnesses and the consequent breaks in our communication. She
wrote forcefully under the pictures, "NOT a hospital, a bedroom!" and said it was a big family. I talked about how she said
they couldn't talk to each other easily, and described the closeness of mothers and babies, when there was no need to talk. We
began drawing babies, and Louisa said she could remember far,
far back, even to her parents' wedding and her father's childhood, from pictures. I remarked that that was almost like magic
knowing, as she was not born then.

In those first two days of week 19, I had been pushing Louisa
a bit harder; I tried to say we could talk in the treatment room,
but that was ineffectual, as Louisa's wish was not yet fully conscious. It was necessary that I stay within the image she set up in
our drawings of communicating in bed at night, even when she
tried the compliant maneuver of seeing the bed shapes as the
treatment room curtains. My introduction of the hospital aspect, however, came as a spontaneous product of my own preconscious. No mention had ever been made by either of us of
Louisa's hospitalization in infancy; I was not even sure if she
knew about it consciously. My reference was to her mother's

recent brief hospitalization for tests. The connection between the two hospitalizations was emotional: Louisa was aware of feeling abandoned and cut off when her mother entered the hospital; in her analysis we were moving closer to conflicts over her rage at her early experiences of abandonment and her wish to be close to her mother, all of which was affectively alive in her transference fantasies of 24-hour communication with me. The fruitfulness of my intervention validated it retrospectively, but it is noteworthy that the criteria for my introduction of an apparently extraneous piece of material were intuitive, with roots in the level of transference relationship Louisa was seeking to create.

On Wednesday, Louisa took up the idea of magic, in relation to a picture card of a man using mechanical muscles to lift great loads. I commented on the difference between magical giants who could do such things and men who needed aids with a drawing of a giant. Louisa changed the drawing to that of the man on the card, and I said that her magic feelings frightened her—sometimes she wished she didn't have them. Louisa wrote, "I wish that you . . ." then whispered, "had some m-u-g." I guessed "gum," which sticks things together, and said that she wanted to feed me magically, to get as close as mothers and babies were. Louisa wrote "Jaffa Jaffa."[3] I asked, "Oranges? Are you thinking of our lost orange crayon?" Louisa said yes and blushed. I drew orange halves over the words and interpreted her wish to put them back together again, to get back to the mother-and-baby feeling. I said she was telling me about a feeling from when she was a baby, with a drawing of Louisa as a baby. Louisa then drew two identical women, whom she designated as me and her mother. I noted that she was confused by feeling similar emotions about her mother and me.

Louisa retreated again from this material by staying away from treatment with a cold. She returned on Friday, boasting that she had done only the most difficult math problems in her workbook. I suggested that she felt helpless when she was ill in bed, and was trying to prove to me that she didn't need anything and didn't mind our communication being broken. Half-

3. "Jaffa" is a common brand of citrus fruit.

way through the session, Louisa said that she had really left out
the difficult problems, and I remarked on how she had been
"telling the opposite" to let me know how awful she had felt.
    The material of this week was very important both for under-
standing Louisa's disturbance and for furthering the work of
her analysis, but for the present purpose of elucidating techniques of communicating with children it demonstrates a new
aspect. Techniques aimed at removing resistances are relatively
easy to perceive and describe: at the beginning and end of the
week, the verbalizations of affect and verbal interpretations of
defense were clear. But in the central session, where Louisa
became fully conscious of the intensity of her own infantile
longings, the material had its own momentum; and my role was
more that of facilitation by verbal and nonverbal means, such as
drawing. Each step in the material felt self-evident, that is,
there seemed to be no technical choices to weigh consciously.
    The following Monday Louisa was pale and tense; she drew
telephones and wrote lists of phone numbers. I interpreted her
wish to know my phone number, so that she could really talk to
me at times outside the session, and Louisa turned to writing
words in foreign languages. I asked her to translate them, and
also to translate the "baby talk" phrase of a few weeks before
(boo boo you you, etc.). Louisa said it couldn't be translated, so
I talked about mothers and babies communicating in ways
other than words, and wrote, "Mère, Mutter, m . . . , m . . . ,
m. . . ." Louisa filled in the blanks in the other languages, and I
commented that "mother" is one of the most important words
in all languages—babies learn it early, because their mothers
are so important to them. Louisa responded by writing "daughter" underneath. I drew circles around the pairs of words and
talked about the feeling of being together, and Louisa pulled a
compass out of her pocket and read directions all around the
room. She then produced a "magic eraser" which "could rub
holes in anything—the table and people and everything." I
commented on this rather dangerous magic and described her
own magical feelings as making her feel dangerous and frightening her. Louisa agreed, but stayed home ill the rest of the
week.
    The interesting technical point about this session is Louisa's

need to express the wishes once more in displacement. We could talk about mothers and daughters in general, but she shied away from the previous week's direct experience of her longings for closeness. Her aggression was coming closer to the surface, but again it was only the powerful, omnipotent aspect of her hostile wishes that she would allow me to approach directly. This extra intensity of defensive need seems to me to be typical of latency-age children, who experience the verbalization of affects, with its attribution of disdained feelings, as an intrusive attack. Direct interpretations of drive impulses are likewise perceived as seductions or attacks and often seem to have the impact of permission to indulge in forbidden actions. The words penetrate new and fragile defenses and upset the precarious balance between superego and id. Verbalization in various displacements, talk about "some girls," or writing, or foreign languages, etc., allows the school-age child to begin to feel some confidence in the defenses, that is, it strengthens the ego vis-à-vis the id-superego linkage. Freud (1926) made the general point: "When you have found the right interpretation, another task lies ahead. You must wait for the right moment at which you can communicate your interpretation to the patient with some prospect of success. . . . You will be making a bad mistake if . . . you throw your interpretations at the patient's head as soon as you have found them" (p. 220). This question of timing and analytic tact seems particularly important in work with school-age children, as they retreat quickly into the defensive busyness allowed by the play setting or into acting out.

Week 21 of Louisa's treatment began with my missing Monday's session, and for the rest of the week Louisa was very controlled and defended, with only occasional breakthroughs of the anger she felt about my absence, and hints of further material related to the conflicts we had been working on. All my attempts to bring in the idea that she had been angry at the cancellation were ignored or denied, or Louisa would switch to drawing elaborate irrelevant pictures. She brought the first close derivative of her feelings about her eyes with a vigorous denial of a Japanese schoolmate's unhappiness over having different eyes. By Friday, however, Louisa began the session with a drawing of a "pushmepullyou" (from Dr. Doolittle) which we could use for talking about some things she both enjoyed and felt worried about, like getting into her parents' bed, and fighting with people, and wishes for pleasure, which made her sad because they seemed impossible, like her wish to be close to people. Louisa began talking about the move to our new room, which was imminent, and linked her confusion over moving day to my Monday absence. I again interpreted her anger, which Louisa denied. She turned to the hiding game, in which she managed to give me a stick of gum. I said, "You've given me some m-u-g"; and when she laughed about *my* saying the opposite, I remarked that she only seemed to feed me on days when she really felt angry, but was afraid to express it directly, only doing so by saying the opposite, i.e., giving me something nice. Louisa turned to testing the colors of the crayons; when she made "lemon yellow," I drew a Jaffa lemon in halves. Louisa drew a whole orange, then a split one, and I interpreted her feeling of having been separated and her wish to reunite the halves; I mentioned the lost orange crayon, which had been named Louisa, with a suggestion that the two halves were Louisa and her mother. Louisa then drew "juice" connecting the two halves. In this session the intervention which made the central defense interpretation possible, and which in turn led to an amplification of material related to conflicts and anxieties, was my humorous use of Louisa's form of defense. What I did might be understood as some sort of sharing or participation in the defense, perhaps experienced as reassuring by Louisa in that it made use of the defense permissible but also unnecessary. After this neither of us "said the opposite" again.

The following week brought Louisa's last use of foreign languages. Louisa was defended, but relaxed, at the beginning of the week and began Wednesday's session with a companionable game of table football using crayons. She had brought cupcakes in a bag marked "Princess Cakes" and I drew a picture of her as a princess. She drew herself as a page (her role in a school play) and I added a grumpy-looking Snow Queen. Louisa wrote "mère" on a new page and drew a picture of her mother, to which I added "fille" and a picture of a baby. She then drew an enormous mouth with huge sharp teeth and told me to draw a similar tiny one next to it. I did so and identified them as ferocious mother and baby mouths. Louisa drew the orange halves, and juice between them, and I commented that mother and baby were feeding each other, at which Louisa joined the edges to make a whole orange. A long pause followed, during which I said nothing, and eventually Louisa traced the outlines of the green and yellow crayons. I said quietly that I understood how difficult it was for her to talk about some feelings, and Louisa immediately drew a baby and wrote "fille." I drew a mother with a bottle in her hand and wrote, "Mother feeding her little girl." Louisa covered this up with a figure 8 pattern and said it wasn't anything, and I answered that they were two halves together, like the orange. In the ensuing two sessions, Louisa brought derivatives of this material and linked it with events from her present everyday life for the first time.

The technical vicissitudes of the above sessions again seem difficult to pin down, as the emergence of the material stemmed from Louisa's own growing need to deal with it. It seemed a case of "all roads leading to Rome," as she would have written "mère" no matter what I had drawn. On the other hand, the picture of her as a princess may have been an unconscious narcissistic gift from me to Louisa, which made her feel confident enough to go as far as the fantasy of mutual oral sadism. Once Louisa had joined the edges of the orange, there seemed to be nothing to say; Louisa needed someone to sit with her while she felt sad. From there we could start down the long path of working through these early conflicts and moving on developmentally.

The Easter break marked a focal point in both Louisa's analysis and the life of the family. Just when Louisa had been able to communicate her feelings about separation and change, her father's job necessitated the family's moving yet again. The parents and I agreed that mother and the children should not leave until the summer, while the father went immediately to his new post. Louisa began the new term of treatment with massive defensive denial, but this soon yielded to interpretation, and she began to express her anger through messing, mixing paints, and splashing water. Fantasies of sharks "who must end up made of blood, they eat so much of it," again expressed on the level of oral aggression her feeling of being overwhelmed by her own anger, which had made her totally bad and frightening.

Toward the end of May, Louisa showed increasing insight

into her defenses of denial and undoing against feeling sad and abandoned. She reacted with astonishment to her first real understanding that it was possible to have two feelings about the same thing when she realized that she was both sad about leaving her special swinging tree in the park and excited about all the new ones there would be near her new home. We worked over this theme repeatedly in the following weeks, and Louisa returned from a long weekend very elated. She told me in great detail all about the holiday, which she had never been able to do before. Her own pleasure at this advance was one of the first spontaneous expressions of any consciousness on her part of the previous blanket nature of her defenses. A further absence of two weeks, because of her sister's measles and a school trip, however, produced a setback, and Louisa came back at the end of June restless and depressed, feeling that everyone was scattered in different places, and it was impossible to reach anyone. The following day Louisa told me she felt "sort of mixed inside," and did not, as usual, follow this admission with frantic defensive activity, but spent the session drifting around the room, listlessly fiddling with the paint palette. Her mother reported a dramatic incident that same night. Before going to bed, Louisa and her sister had been playing a mother-and-baby game. In the middle of the night, Mrs. H. heard Louisa sobbing uncontrollably in her sleep, for the first time since the subsidence of her sleep disturbance when she was 3 years old. Mrs. H. rushed in, helped Louisa, still asleep, out of bed and took her on her lap. She held the child and spoke reassuringly for about 15 minutes. Throughout this time, Louisa was still asleep and gave no sign of hearing her mother, interspersing her sobs with cries of "Mummy, mummy, let me, let me, no, no" in a heart-rending voice. According to the mother, Louisa sounded exactly as she had as a baby, even to the pronunciation of the words. When the crying petered out, and Mrs. H. carried Louisa back to bed, asking as she put her down if she had been dreaming, Louisa started and said, "Pardon?" in an awake voice, then settled immediately to sleep. In her session the next day Louisa's subdued mood persisted, and she threw her old paints away, saying "good-bye red, good-bye blue" to the "messy old things," as she described them. This sequence of events lent credence to my sense that in her analysis Louisa had been working through feelings about very early events, and, although she appeared to have no recollection of her night-time experience, it seemed to make it possible for her to relinquish aspects of her anal defenses and move on to integrate affects at a higher level.

By week 35, Louisa not only volunteered information about current events, but described her various feelings as well: she told me that she had been sad when her au pair girl left that week, proud about her ballet recital, happy about her father's visit, etc. This linking of feelings with real present and future events continued; when Louisa had described the skiing lessons at her new school, she began to paint a picture of me with long hair, as I had been at the beginning of her treatment. She crossed it out, then painted me in my clothes that day, standing in shallow "English snow." When a child made a noise outside the room, and Louisa wondered about my seeing other children the next winter when she would be gone, she painted me in a summer dress, standing shoulder-deep in "American snow."[4] This condensed material, in Louisa's usual style, was seen as an expression of her externalized feelings of being cold and lonely, while I was even farther away than England—as far as America. At the same time, I was being punished for leaving her by being made to stand in the snow in a summer dress. Louisa made reparation, however, by painting a warm snowsuit over the dress before the end of the session. The other side of the ambivalence could be seen the following day in Louisa's fantasy of her "very, very, very good friend, who was grown up" and was going to stay overnight with her.

In the last two weeks of Louisa's treatment, we made cardboard models of her house, the subway station, her cousins' house, etc., all of which she planned to take with her when she moved. On the last day we made a telephone. Louisa wrote the office number on it, then changed it to her home number, and we remembered our long-ago drawings of talking on the phone and the good feeling of communicating with each other.

4. Louisa's consciousness of language had early led to her identification of my American accent.

At the end of the year in analysis, it appeared that Louisa had not been able to work through completely her profound feelings of loss, as she still needed the concrete aids provided by our models. Nevertheless, she had made several important advances. Her symptoms had abated, and she was beginning to find pleasure in her relationships with family members and friends. In the realm of affects, Louisa was more able to tolerate some degree of ambivalence; on the ego side, her defenses were more sophisticated and age-adequate, and her self-esteem more realistically based; and, most important, her libidinal development appeared to be proceeding again, with a move into the oedipal phase and the fading away of her anal symptoms. These developments were encouraging, but it was impossible to know if Louisa would be able to retain these advances in the face of the pressure of the family pathology, the move, and the loss of support from treatment. The family accepted my recommendation that they seek further treatment for Louisa. I had a follow-up letter from Mrs. H. 6 months later which confirmed that Louisa was about to start three times weekly therapy and described impressively the way Louisa had held on to the gains from her treatment. Mrs. H. stressed Louisa's independence and pleasure in exploring, talked about her good adjustment to her new school, her improved relationship with her father, and her growing pleasure in doing things with and learning from mother.

CONCLUSION

Early in this paper I referred to the debate over the differences between adult and child analysis; the role of speech and its relation to play constitute the major accepted differences and are perceived as an irremediable gap, due to the developmental realities of childhood. What I would like to suggest, using Louisa's treatment as an example, is that this gulf is not so wide as it appears. Loewenstein (1956) wrote, "What counts in analysis is, not communication by itself, but *what is being communicated* on the part of both patient and analyst, what leads to communication, and what psychic processes and changes occur as a result of this communication as such and of its contents" (p.

467). In describing some of the detail of Louisa's analysis, I have tried to give a sense of the arena in which Louisa and I began to communicate, what helped the process, and how changes then occurred. What I have not yet addressed directly is the building of the arena, which might be described as the interplay of the transference-countertransference relationship and the treatment alliance.

Winnicott (1971) made a suggestion about the treatment situation which aptly described the oscillations in Louisa's analysis: "The thing about playing is always the precariousness of the interplay of personal psychic reality and the experience of control of actual objects. This is the precariousness of magic itself, magic that arises in intimacy, in a relationship that is being found to be reliable" (p. 47). He also said, "resistance arises out of interpretation given outside the area of the overlap of the patient's and the analyst's playing together" (p. 51). Winnicott did not mean "playing" in the concrete sense of games or drawing, but rather referred to a complicated evolution of a capacity for integrated emotional trial action in a "play space" which originated in the mutual trust and satisfaction of mother and child. What was re-created in Louisa's treatment was perhaps something like Winnicott's playground where Louisa could re-experience her wishes and begin to see that fusion with her mother had always been a fantasy, but that love and caring were possible despite her rage. Her mother had indeed been as reliable an object as she could be and was doing her best to change in order to meet Louisa's needs in the present.

Winnicott (1971) further suggests that "we must expect to find playing just as evident in the analysis of adults as it is in the case of our work with children. It manifests itself, for instance, in the choice of words, in the inflections of the voice, and indeed in the sense of humour" (p. 40). Louisa and I constructed our relationship with many different elements, both verbal and nonverbal, but two crucial building blocks were our verbal conventions of saying the opposite and using foreign languages. Our capacity to create a specific form of communication, ours alone, applicable only to Louisa's treatment, exclusive for each of us to our relationship with each other, seems to me to represent the area of overlap of Louisa's and my playing. This is probably an essential element in any analytic relationship, be the patient child or adult. What joins the work of child and adult analyst, then, may be the common experience of creating a treatment-specific idiom which will lead to change through understanding.

SUMMARY

Aspects of the short analysis of Louisa, a multilingual 7-year-old girl, were described in this paper to illustrate different modes of communication between patient and analyst and the ways these contributed to shared verbalizations and interpretations. A detailed description of specific techniques showed how the development of two verbal conventions, "saying the opposite" and using foreign languages, allowed for the creation of a particular form of communication, applicable only to Louisa's treatment, and exclusive for the patient and the therapist to the relationship with each other. The suggestion is made that this creation of a treatment-specific language is an essential element of any analytic relationship and constitutes a common feature of child and adult psychoanalysis.

BIBLIOGRAPHY

BORNSTEIN, B. (1945), Clinical notes on child analysis. *Psychoanal. Study Child,* 1:151–166.
FERENCZI, S. (1913), Stages in the development of the sense of reality. In *First Contributions to Psycho-Analysis.* London: Hogarth Press, 1952, pp. 65–78.
FREUD, A. (1965), Normality and pathology in childhood. *W.,* 6.
FREUD, S. (1910), Five lectures on psycho-analysis. *S. E.,* 11:3–55.
———— (1926), The question of lay analysis. *S. E.,* 20:179–258.
KATAN, A. (1961), Some thoughts about the role of verbalization in early childhood. *Psychoanal. Study Child,* 16:184–188.
LOEWENSTEIN, R. M. (1956), Some remarks on the role of speech in psychoanalytic technique. *Int. J. Psychoanal.,* 37:460–468.
WINNICOTT, D. W. (1971), *Playing and Reality.* London: Tavistock Publications.

Some Meanings of Being a Horsewoman

JOHN E. SCHOWALTER, M.D.

MAN HAS ALWAYS BEEN FASCINATED BY THE CREATURES around him. At first, in the animistic and pantheistic religions, there was a tendency for all life to be seen as a unity, although in the Hebraic creation only Man is made in God's image. The domestication of animals for social reasons is very ancient, and archaeological evidence for the use of dogs as pets is already evidenced by pre-Neolithic, Mesolithic peoples (Zeuner, 1963). At present, over one-half of the families in the United States have pets.

There is an early psychoanalytic literature on the uses and intrapsychic meanings of animals, but then interest waned until recently when there has been an upsurge of medical, psychiatric, and psychoanalytic research on the impact of pets on humans.

In the psychoanalytic literature the two earliest descriptions of the treatment of children, Little Hans (Freud, 1909) and Little Chanticleer (Ferenczi, 1913), both involve youngsters who used animals (horses and fowl) as objects to which they had displaced their sexual interests leading to subsequent phobic fears. In academic psychology, Watson and Raynor (1920) used Little Albert to show how conditioning could cause animal fears. In 1913 Freud commented on the closeness children feel with animals when he stated, "Children have no scruples over allowing animals to rank as their full equals. Uninhibited as

---

Chief of Child Psychiatry and Professor of Pediatrics and Psychiatry, Child Study Center, Yale University, New Haven, Ct.; faculty, Western New England Institute for Psychoanalysis.

they are in the avowal of their bodily needs, they no doubt feel themselves more akin to animals than to their elders, who may well be a puzzle to them" (p. 127). Anna Freud (1936) has noted that "substitution of an animal for a human object is not in itself a neurotic process' (p. 74), but she also comments on and gives examples of how commonly animals are used by children for neurotic symptom formation.

I have reviewed (1983) the sparse child psychiatry literature and through clinical vignettes described the more common ways that interactions with animals influence children's behavior and development. In greater depth, Mahon and Simpson (1977) discuss how 3-year-old nursery school children struggled with their mourning following the death of the class's pet guinea pig. Kupfermann (1977) described in detail the analysis of a 7-year-old boy who imitated a cat, in large part as a defensive denial of his identity as a human being. Most recently, Sherick (1981) detailed the girl's use of various pets during her 3-year analysis and how these changes chronicled gains in her treatment and in her psychosexual maturation.

HORSES

This paper will focus on one type of pet animal, the horse. According to Zeuner (1963), the horse was probably domesticated relatively late in the agricultural phase of man's development, after, for example, sheep, cattle, and pigs. They were domesticated by secondary nomads for transportation and labor. As such, they were the primary responsibility of the males and, for the most part, the horse has been a symbol for strong masculinity. The power and sexuality of the horse symbol was recently portrayed in Peter Shaffer's play, *Equus*. However, compared to the satyr, the centaur was portrayed in myth as sexual, but more reliable and less lustful. The same can be said for that American centaur, the Western Cowboy, whose strong, gallant exploits have been promulgated through generations of novels, short stories, and films (Rappaport, 1968). For a species of animal to become associated with one or the other gender is not unheard of. As long ago as 1904, G. Stanley Hall and C. E. Browne published a survey of almost 3,000 school children which showed that dogs were considered much more "manly" than cats, and nursery school teachers I have queried recently agree that preschool children tend to think of dogs as male and cats as female.

I have been struck by a relatively common but not much studied phenomenon, the "horse-crazy" girl. This too is not only a modern occurrence and indeed was instrumental in the development of Britain's Society for the Prevention of Cruelty to Animals, a forerunner of this country's National Society for the Prevention of Cruelty to Children (Turner, 1964). The SPCA became Royal (RSPCA) because the young Victoria had become interested in protecting horses and an SPCA patron before her accession to the throne. Another woman, Angela (later, Baroness) Burdett-Coutts, was as a young girl devoted to horses and when she later became the richest heiress in England, she in 1870 founded and lavished her wealth and attention on the Ladies Committee of the RSPCA. The latter in 1889 inspired 40,000 essays from school children which extolled the virtues of the horse and other animals and pleaded for their humane treatment.

The modern horse-crazy girl is less exalted but no less committed to her interest. Although I am not suggesting homogeneity, most come from the urban or suburban class. The interest in horses usually begins during latency or early adolescence and is often sparked by a book, a movie, or an opportunity to ride. There may then be a compulsion to do more reading, to collect figures, pictures, or other horse memorabilia, to take horseback riding lessons, and to own a horse. For some girls these interests last for only weeks or months while for others it lasts a lifetime, although a tapering off of interest is common in late adolescence or early adulthood. Riding academy owners state that a similar high level of involvement with horses by boys is relatively rare.

The development of intense interest in horses is by no means necessarily pathological. Indeed, during a study of oedipal-age children's interests in dinosaurs (Schowalter, 1979), I was struck by how many of the same issues of control, fear, and love of a seemingly overwhelming parent were present in the mostly male dinosaur fanatics. Children who are enraptured by dinosaurs, unless it becomes an obsession, usually develop very well, if not precociously. Most girls who are "horse-crazy" also do fine, and in these there is seldom the opportunity to study the meanings of their interest. One young woman's brief period in analysis, however, afforded the opportunity to observe magnified some of what the horse meant for her. While her analysis was not directly focused on this issue, her revelations may well, in exaggerated form, suggest why horses are so important for a subpopulation of young women.

CASE REPORT

C. Z. was a 20-year-old junior at a nearby college when she was referred for analysis at the suggestion of a psychoanalyst who practiced in her hometown. Although she was doing quite well academically, she did not seem to know what to do with her life, was a binge eater, and had recently attempted suicide with a relatively small amount of aspirin.

She was an attractive, tall young woman with auburn hair who tended to wear bluejeans and plaid shirts. She managed to convey both a boyish quality, through her quick, deft movements, and an aura of little-girl confused helplessness. Some days she wore her hair tightly tied and close to her head, at other times flowing long and free.

She was the youngest of four sisters who were considerably older than she. Although she could not help but wonder whether she was a wanted child, her parents had always assured her she was. Both of her parents were successful professionals, and although her mother was careful to spend time with the children, the patient's earliest memories involved fears about being abandoned. She could remember being terrified that her parents would not return when they left to go out in the evening. She also remembered vividly her older sisters leaving home for college and thinking that she herself would never be so self-sufficient. It was in this context that she mentioned that many people mispronounced her name. As a child she was read, and later read herself, the Oz books, and her name was the same as one of the characters. Some of the Oz books featured a sawhorse whose main quality is indefatigability. He could run forever without tiring. In the stories, she said, the horse would be used to carry the children away from impending danger.

She had periods of school avoidance in kindergarten and again in first and third grades. She remembered her mother being gentle but forceful to get her out of the house and to school, but at the time it seemed like cruel coercion. She recalled hoping that her father would save her by giving her a reprieve, but to her great disappointment he remained passive and unavailable. In school she felt unliked by her peers and throughout grade school had few or no friends. During this time, she filled her spare time with reading and music, but she was dissatisfied and believed she would be happier if she were a boy. Toward this end she became interested in sports, asked for tailored clothes, and soon was known in the neighborhood as a tomboy. She had a long-standing interest in horses, but first began riding lessons at age 11, "when some of the other girls began to 'change.'" Riding and then showing horses were described as the most exhilirating experiences of her young life.

She claimed she never thought of herself as a sexual person. Indeed, in the almost a year of once-a-week psychotherapy she had had before seeing me, she contended that sex was never brought up by her or the therapist. When she did think of sexuality, it was in idealized and sanitized terms of "roses and romance." She put her menarche at age 16, when she was a junior in high school, but could not recall breast development until the following year, which was also the time she first began dating. In fact, this memory must have been distorted, since breast formation occurs routinely 2 years prior to menarche. She denied ever having masturbated. Since her senior year in high school, she had had a few short-lived sexual relationships, including orgasms, but denied there had been much of an emotional bond. She dreaded getting close and breaking up.

Although her weight was always within normal limits, her bulimia began about the time of her menarche. She had had no severe gains or drops in weight, but had experienced brief periods of amenorrhea. Her weight was very much tied up with her riding and showing, because she believed that the horses performed better and that she looked better to the judges when her build was slight. She would tend to binge when she felt alone and ignored. Binges often took place in the early morning hours after a day of careful control. She was conscious of "a battle of wills within myself" and hated herself when she gave in to her appetite. To try to offset her lapses of overeating, she would run, lift weights, and row crew (all things she associated as masculine), and occasionally use laxatives and force herself to vomit (things that seemed to her feminine). The former were more ego-syntonic and provided a certain pleasure in "pushing myself through pain." They were experienced as the antithesis of binging, while the purging, although palliative, was linked with the binging as a weakness.

Her thoughts about her parents encompassed strong feelings of both closeness and distance. In the abstract she felt that they were caring and loving, but her predominant affects were terror and anger because they were untrustworthy and inconstant. Her sisters were so much older than she that they remained relatively shadowy creatures, something akin to additional, but even less caring, parents. Often during her childhood she believed her parents hated her, not because of any cruel actions on their part, but because they did not give her the time and attention she craved. Her burgeoning interests in music and sports, she recalled, were efforts to please her mother and father. She had particular problems when her parents went away. Because of this they generally abstained from vacations without her, but she found even short absences terrifying. Both incidents of her taking overdoses of aspirin (neither serious) coincided with her parents' being out of the country on brief holidays while she was in college.

She agreed with her parents that she should enter analysis. She had liked the psychotherapist she had been seeing, but she did not believe anything had been accomplished. She felt her life had little focus, that no one really cared about her, and that she would probably eventually kill herself if these things did not change. What she said she hoped to get out of psychoanalysis were direction and a better sense of who she was.

Following the initial interviews, we agreed to begin a trial analysis 5 times a week. She lay on the couch initially with some misgivings, noting that it made her feel very vulnerable, but she came regularly and on time. The first clear theme and the one that remained most crucial was her belief that no one cared for her. Early memories emerged of her mother telling her she was too old to have another child and did not have the energy to raise her. Very early in life (she dated it to preschool age) she already felt that she was unwanted. Although her parents said they wanted all of their children, she developed the opposite persuasion. As a little girl she decided she would not be a good mother and should not have children herself. While growing up, she had a frequent fantasy of being a nun. An especially appealing part of the fantasy at the time was that nuns sleep alone. As she became older, it occurred to her that being a nun and sleeping alone were tied with her wish not to have children.

It was toward the end of the first month of analysis that her interest in horses came to the fore. She said they were the most important thing in her life and, because of this, she assumed I would believe this involvement was unhealthy. When I asked why, she said she sometimes felt that way herself, but that her interest in horses was what gave stability to her life. At this time vivid memories returned of having no friends in primary school, feeling unwanted by her parents, and longing to love and be loved. Besides the sawhorse in the Oz books, she could at first recall little that was specific about how horses became hypercathected. She did know that she daydreamed about them often and that there were two specific types of fantasies. One fantasy—which later became less important—had to do with a baby horse that was the only baby cared for by a group of horses. The second fantasy involved her caring for a horse that was large, powerful, and "a sort of king" of all the other horses. It was clear that in these two fantasies she could satisfy both her pregenital dependency longings and her phallic and oedipal wishes.

Simultaneously with the discussion of horses in her hours, she began occasionally to be late or miss a session, usually because of a transportation problem associated with her riding lessons. After the second such occasion, I asked about a possible connection. She said it was quite by happenstance, and this was the occasion of her first flare of irritation with me. This irritation did not, however, inhibit her desire to discuss the meaning of horses.

She described her home always having been clean, neat, and

sterile. By contrast, the stables exuded rich smells of sweat, leather, liniments, feed, and manure. While at home emotions were not shown, the people at the stable were passionate and always seemed excited about their relationships with the horses and with each other. The size of the horses was important. The ability to control an animal so much bigger than herself gave her a sense of awe and wonderful power. It was, however, not only gratifying in a physical sense; the caring for, riding, and showing of the horse also represented the mastery of a world that was completely mysterious to the uninitiated. This aspect of being special was reminiscent of the preschool boys for whom knowing better than their parents or teachers the names, sizes, habits, etc., of dinosaurs represented a major impetus for their continuing interest (Schowalter, 1979). For my patient the stable became a separate, "better," and more controllable home.

It soon became apparent that she wanted me to understand her feelings about horses, but the more she told me the more fearful she became that I would be angry or turn against her. When asked about her parents' responses to her interest in horses, she initially said that they had always been supportive. This, indeed, seemed to have been the case, but it became increasingly clear that she believed they would or should be jealous. There was a considerable difference in what she expected each parent's reaction to be. Her main fear was that her mother would suddenly "take them away." At times she thought of her interest as something she secretly shared with her father, but there was the danger that her mother would "force" him to join her in saying that the patient was overinterested and should cut back or stop her riding and showing. It was at the time of this disclosure that she somewhat overdramatically announced she had added another riding lesson per week to her crowded schedule, which I understood as a clear expression of a wish to provoke a maternal transference reaction from me. In response to my interpretation, she described how important the caring for the horse was for her. Although she never owned "a really good" horse and was now renting one, she found the grooming of the horse very satisfying. She would make the horse look "as good as possible." The idea that she was treating the horse as she wished to be treated was close to consciousness. It was also her way, even as a young girl, of having a "child" and probably made it easier for her to say she did not want or need children when she grew up.

By the third month of analysis, the patient's life had settled down remarkably. She was getting along better with the fellow students with whom she lived, her academic work progressed well, and her part-time job which had been marked by frequent disputations with her male superior was going more smoothly. She pondered about this improvement, stated the analysis must be contributory, but complained that, like her father, I was "too distant" to be a truly helpful, caring person. She still had episodes of binge eating, but these became less frequent and less "gross."

She then admitted for the first time that her father had always wanted her to be a boy. This attempt to have a boy, she believed, was an alternative explanation to her birth having been "an accident," coming as it did so long after the births of her sisters. With a gush of feelings, she recounted how badly she had wanted to be a boy. This, she said, had prevailed until her mid-teens when "I changed my bedroom and half of my clothes to pink." To her, in retrospect, this conversion was as inexplicable as it had been sudden. Since then she had undergone two or three other "quick changes" when she precipitously had felt either considerably more like a tomboy or more like a "frills and lace" girl. These shifts seemed to affect her wardrobe more than her behavior, but she did associate these changes with the much more frequent and current alternations between "dieting, being lean, and good with horses" and "pigging out, being soft, and not riding well." Even when she was in the latter phase, a man or "a good time with my horse" could make her feel more stable and more confident about herself.

At about the beginning of the fourth month of treatment, she missed three sessions without warning or notice. When she returned she had a slight limp and said that while jumping, she had fallen off her horse and had fractured three toes. The toes had been attended to medically, but then she had driven into the country to be by herself. She recalled that she had had a relatively bad fall as a senior in high school and following that had run away from home for 5 days. Falling was equated with rejection and abandonment. "It is like the breaking up of a love affair." More importantly, it was like being dismissed by her parents, a fear that haunted her all her life. It was at this time that she described the symbiotic feeling she experienced with the horse. "There is nothing closer than working one-to-one with a horse." She spoke of the "give and take" between rider and horse, the power surging beneath her, and the "flowing sense of oneness" during the jumps. Then, when she fell, she had the dismaying shock of recognition that the oneness was lost. Although some horses were more skillful than others, she believed that a fall was only rarely the horse's fault, but resulted from something the rider did wrong or from the horse being so finely attuned to the rider's mood that it sensed and reacted to the lack of confidence or control. She wondered if the horse sensed a change taking place in her.

My comments during this period were fashioned to help her explore the parallels between what she experienced with the horse and her feelings about her parents and expectations about the analysis and me. I pointed out linkages she had made but not seen: that she (like the sawhorse) always needed to be on the move to escape she knew not what; how important it was for her to control the horse as a substitute for herself, her parents, or her peers; and the fact that immersion in the horse world had proven to be not only an escape but also a detriment to her learning to face her feelings about herself and others.

At times she lashed out at me for either being too distant, trying to rule her life, or both, but she continued to come to her appointments and tried to unravel what was happening. She was considerably sobered for a while after the fall and more silent than usual, but her associations then suddenly turned to a man whom she had met at the stable. She described him as "fantastically" good and intuitive with horses, and said she realized that horses had much sexual meaning for her. She recalled having heard other girls talk about having sexual feelings while riding. She had never personally thought of them as sexual, but knew that being on top and in control of a large horse gave her a sense of power and excitement that was unique. During the next few weeks, she spoke of how sexually exciting she found the somewhat older male rider she was now beginning to date. He had the same first name as I do, was a talented and successful jumper in shows, and was eagerly trying to persuade her to join him on the horse-show circuit, also as a jumper. He was described as a daredevil who "jumped with wild abandon" and who lived an independent life in which he wanted her to join him. Her awe of him caused her to discuss him with an excitement in her voice that I had not heard before. She began to debate out loud whether or not she should leave school, take a summer vacation, or take a whole year off so she could test and perfect her talents as a horsewoman and jumper. I raised the question what these actions would mean in regard to her wish to have a more stable life and whether they were a reaction to what she had been learning about herself. She admitted that she had been uncomfortable about the recent revelations that perhaps she received sexual gratification from grooming and riding. She had thought she was different from the "other girls." However, with her friendship and now burgeoning love affair, she felt less uncomfortable and more convinced that taking time off for the horse-show circuit was sensible.

At this point she had another fall. No bones were broken, but she suffered some "wicked" bruises. She missed two sessions and when she returned she was angrier and more determined than ever before. She now felt the fall was mainly the horse's fault, not her own. She then announced with the quality of a *fait accompli* that she had looked at "the nicest horse in the world." A "magnificent" show horse was up for sale. It was a skilled jumper, and her boyfriend was urging her to buy it; with such a horse she was bound to be a success on the circuit. The horse was expensive, but she had already spoken to her father, who was willing to look at the horse and speak with its present owner.

Once again it seemed as if she was going to use a horse to escape what had become an uncomfortable situation, and in the two weeks that she remained in treatment she acknowledged this intellectually. Emotionally, however, she felt a tremendous enthusiasm and "buoyancy" in anticipation "of being one" with such a perfect steed. While her parents at first counseled her to remain in school and analysis, her father rather quickly agreed to buy the horse and to support her for a year to see what she could do as a horsewoman.[1]

She left the analysis in the high spirits of someone who feels she has narrowly but successfully escaped a serious danger. In contrast to the time when she had been in kindergarten, her father did intervene to extricate her. Although able to admit intellectually that the analytic experience represented repetition rather than progress, she seemed quite genuine in thanking me for all my help.

DISCUSSION

While this young woman's psychopathology, her suitability for analysis, and the technical features of the treatment might be of interest, my discussion will focus on the ways that the horse became important for her. Some of the uses she made of horses are identical to those of other girls and young women I have treated and may have some general applicability.

As would be expected of any abiding interest, the horse came to serve many functions. The horse is ideally suited for gratifying both pregenital and genital needs and for fulfilling aggressive fantasies. It can be an object of identification as well as represent self and object.

In addition to the narcissistic and sublimatory aspect, the horse may also serve defensive functions. Anna Freud (1965, p. 20) noted, "A little girl's *horse-craze* betrays either her primitive autoerotic desires (if her enjoyment is confined to the rhythmic movement on the horse); or her identification with the caretaking mother (if she enjoys above all looking after the horse, grooming it, etc.); or her penis envy (if she identifies with the big, powerful animal and treats it as an addition to her body); or her phallic sublimations (if it is her ambition to master the horse, to perform on it, etc.)." Freud (1926) listed object loss, loss of love, castration, and superego condemnation as

1. The suggestion of a trial of analysis had been made because, among other things, she had a history of trouble finishing things, had only few long-term relationships, and her basic lack of trust and fears of being poorly cared for suggested she might not tolerate the relatively abstemious character of the psychoanalytic situation.

four sources of anxiety. For this patient, the horse served as her protector from these anxieties.

Her intense separation anxieties, whatever their origin, were counteracted by her feeling at one with the horse, the sense of oneness at times representing a primitive fusion.

She believed her parents had never loved her and her peers did not like her. In working with and grooming the horse she felt loved and cared for. As seems true for many other "horse-crazy" girls, she enjoyed feeding the horse special treats. This trait to feed others is, of course, commonly seen in patients suffering from anorexia nervosa and/or bulimia. She could live out the first of her two early horse fantasies by being the cared-for baby. In this she not only identified with the horse, treating it as she wished to be treated, but also demonstrated how she should be cared for by her mother. She had felt that her very being was an aggressive demand on her parents, especially her mother, who admitted to not being up to the task of mothering. By being at the stable rather than at home, the patient consciously believed she spared her mother. Her obvious preference for the stable also, of course, served as a rebuke as well as a neutralization of her aggression.[2]

The horse became a love object par excellence. It would come when called, showed constancy of affection, and was the ticket of admission to a tightly knit and supportive group of afficionados. What has struck me with a number of horse-crazy girls is that although the horse consciously represents primarily a male object, the female instructors and peer group provide important identification figures and a feminine sanction for the experience. This sanction modifies the amount of guilt the girl might otherwise feel for the libidinization of her feelings toward the animal. With this patient's dread of separation, having a regular routine for the horse's care was very stabilizing. It also kept her busy. She had long known that it was important for her to have "things" to do. She did not like free time and racing about indefatigably, like the sawhorse; doing stable connected chores made her feel less alone. In the end, she bought the

2. The preoedipal, especially anal, wishes indulged in and associated with the stable and its sights, smells, and activities were only briefly discussed.

horse of her dreams, the surest way to keep a love object. It is reminiscent of Róheim's (1943) report that as an adult, Arpad, the Little Chanticleer of Ferenczi's paper, bought a poultry farm.

This young woman was brought up believing she should have been a man. She felt castrated and unable to please her father. Even as a young girl she always consciously thought of horses as male, and, in fact, the horses she rode were male. She believed she could acquire a certain amount of maleness through this identification. She feared her large father, but she also loved him. She projected and displaced these feelings onto the horse. She then educated and tamed that wild, powerful force into an obedient servant and at the same time felt more controlled herself. There was much anxiety also, especially because to a young girl the horse seemed so big. Ferenczi (1911) noted that girls' oedipal fears may be enhanced because of their awareness of the relative size of the father's penis in relation to their own small genitals. Therefore, riding well provided the exhilaration of controlling that large beast between her legs ("with just the pressure of my thighs") and of overcoming a great fear. For the patient this was her second girlhood horse fantasy, to be in charge of the "king" horse. In this context it is significant here that the patient dated her riding to when other girls her age had reached menarche. Although her menarche was late physiologically, she realized that riding was linked with a sexual awakening. Indeed, I have known a number of such girls whose menarche was late. Greenacre (1948) emphasizes that horseback riding gives girls a heightened awareness of their genitals. For this girl, riding probably also acted as a substitute for conscious masturbation, which may have been the reason why she became so anxious when the other girls hinted at this meaning. Unfortunately for her, even when most successful astride a horse, she was still a female and never mastered her mixed feelings about her gender. Her ambivalence about being a woman also was expressed in her vacillations between a mannish and feminine wardrobe and between dieting and binging.

Just as she used the horse as a pregenital and a self-love object, it also played a role in her incestuous oedipal wishes and fears. At times she believed her interest in horses was a "secret" she shared with her father, and expected her mother to demand that she "cut back" or "stop" it. While on a defensive intellectual level she polarized the unemotional home from the "passionate" stables, the sanction given for her riding by parents and peers allowed her, for the most part, to feel comfortable about her preoccupation with horses. Indeed, the more she worked with the horse, the more in control she was and the less threatened she felt. That was why following her falls and after the sexual aspects of her interest in horses began to be revealed in the analysis, she needed to "take a year off" and spend it exclusively to learn "how to obtain better control of the beast." Superego condemnation had come to the fore. The fantasy was if she could know and control a horse completely, she would be in control of herself and those around her. Joseph Wood Krutch (1956, p. 136) quotes Thoreau as noting that a hen that is allowed to wander about the house soon looks "too humanized to roast well." Familiarity, it was hoped by the patient, would deaggressivize and desexualize her feelings and protect her from the rising superego condemnation. It was in fact precisely when she revealed her sexual feelings that the analysis became too threatening. She saw me as an impediment to her continued successful use of the horse, in large part because in the transference I was replacing her father as a feared incestuous object. Her turning from me to the horse repeated her earlier turn from father to horse.

She interpreted the falls as signifying rejection and abandonment. In the first she felt the horse sensed her rejection of it and reacted accordingly. With the second fall, she blamed the horse and felt it had turned against her. This time her response was to replace the horse. It was at this point that she concluded that either I or her life with horses, at least as she had known it, must go. The choice was made quickly. It was not, unfortunately, that which Adatto (1958) often found common in late adolescents when the anxiety stirred up in the analysis allows the patient to use the analyst as a bridge from parental to mature love objects. The outcome was more reminiscent of Freud's warnings about the "adhesiveness" of the libido (1916–17, p. 348). As was the case when she had left her parents for horses earlier, she left me as she had felt left. In order to make the decision more understandable and acceptable, she enlisted the aid of her boyfriend and father on the side of the horse. Her sudden and uncharacteristic burst of sexual passion for this young horseman was timed perfectly to defuse the power of and the long-term sexual meanings associated with the horse and the paternal transference that were coming to the fore in the analysis. The boyfriend served as a horseman bridge. The father's agreement to buy her the "nicest horse in the world" and to approve, at least tacitly, of her leaving analysis and college further quelled feelings of guilt and anxiety. Unlike the time when she was in kindergarten, he now supported her wish to regress and not face the age-appropriate tasks confronting her. The original and the peer male love objects joined together in their support of her symbolic male love object. In leaving treatment, she not only felt relieved, she felt triumphant. She was going to be a horsewoman.

It would be an error to suggest that the meanings important for this patient are the same for all girls and young women who love horses. However, it is safe to say that in horseback riding, as in all childhood passions, a greater or a lesser portion of the intensity is due to the fact that it offers ways of fulfilling and working through wishes and fears that are displaced from parents. In this case a follow-up revealed that the patient jumped with her horse for less than a year. She then had a bad fall which resulted in serious injury, broken bones, hospitalization, and prolonged convalescence. She also had a diminished interest in horses, but this is not surprising since more than a year after the fall, she was jobless and still living at home with her parents. The circle was complete. Her horse had done its job. She finally had what she wanted initially—to be cared for by her parents.

BIBLIOGRAPHY

ADATTO, C. P. (1958), Ego reintegration observed in analysis of late adolescents. *Int. J. Psychoanal.*, 39:172–177.
FERENCZI, S. (1911), On obscene words. In *Sex in Psychoanalysis*. New York: Basic Books, 1950, pp. 132–153.

_____ (1913), A little chanticleer. In *Contributions to Psycho-Analysis*. Boston: Richard G. Badger, 1916, pp. 204–213.

FREUD, A. (1936), The ego and the mechanisms of defense. *W.*, 2.

_____ (1965), Normality and pathology in childhood. *W.*, 6.

FREUD, S. (1909), Analysis of a phobia in a five-year-old boy. *S. E.*, 10:5–147.

_____ (1913), Totem and taboo. *S. E.*, 13:1–161.

_____ (1916–17), Introductory lectures on psycho-analysis (Part 3). *S. E.*, 16.

_____ (1926), Inhibitions, symptoms and anxiety. *S. E.*, 20:87–174.

GREENACRE, P. (1948), Anatomical structure and superego development. In *Trauma, Growth and Personality*. New York: Norton, 1952, pp. 149–164.

HALL, G. S. & BROWN, C. E. (1904), The cat and the child. *Pedagogical Seminary*, 11:3–29.

KRUTCH, J. W. (1956), *The Great Chain of Life*. Boston: Houghton, Mifflin.

KUPFERMANN, K. (1977), A latency boy's identity as a cat. *Psychoanal. Study Child*, 32:363–387.

MAHON, E. & SIMPSON, D. (1977), The painted guinea pig. *Psychoanal. Study Child*, 32:283–307.

RAPPAPORT, E. A. (1968), Zoophily and zoerasty. *Psychoanal. Q.*, 37:565–587.

RÓHEIM, G. (1943), *The Origin and Function of Culture*. New York: Nervous and Mental Disease Monographs.

SCHOWALTER, J. E. (1979), When dinosaurs return. *Children Today*, 8:2–5 (May–June).

_____ (1983), The use and abuse of pets. *J. Amer. Acad. Child Psychiat.*, 22:68–72.

SHERICK, I. (1981), The significance of pets for children. *Psychoanal. Study Child*, 36:193–215.

TURNER, E. S. (1964), *All Heaven in a Rage*. London: Michael Joseph.

WATSON, J. B. & RAYNOR, R. (1920), Conditioned emotional reactions. *J. Exper. Psychol.*, 3:1–14.

ZEUNER, F. E. (1963), *A History of Domesticated Animals*. New York: Harper & Row.

A Particular Perspective on Analytic Listening

EVELYNE SCHWABER, M.D.

SEVERAL YEARS AGO AN ARTICLE ENTITLED "MICROPSIA AND Testicular Retractions" (Myers, 1977) caught my interest. Micropsia, descriptively defined as a state in which things appear smaller than usual and more distant, was a symptom that one of my patients had also experienced. Reading the report, I was especially attracted by the author's close attention to clinical detail—the analyst's and the patient's responses—in describing singular moments. Although it was not his stated intent to emphasize the analyst's contribution, that is, the contextual consideration, nonetheless this material was offered—which, in turn, permitted the reader a more reliable opportunity to make his or her own inferences. This kind of presentation of clinical data, even with minimal historical information, I believe is essential for stimulating meaningful, empirically based dialogue.

In the effort to pursue such a dialogue, I shall respond here to those aspects of Myers's report which may bear on his perspective for analytic listening. I shall also consider some issues in the analytic work with my patient, Mrs. G., to try to delineate an alternative perspective and to suggest some gains to be derived from such a shift in the mode of gathering the clinical data.

Myers reports numerous episodes in which his patient experienced micropsia in the analytic situation. The following ex-

Training and Supervisory Analyst, Psychoanalytic Institute of New England, East.

An earlier version of this paper was presented at a meeting at U.C.L.A. in October 1979, and at the Cincinnati Psychoanalytic Society in February 1980.

ample in which we are told what patient *and* analyst said may serve as a prototype of a particular perspective on analytic listening:

> . . . in the last session of the week before the weekend break, he [the patient] was late for an appointment after I had been forced to change the time of the hour.
>
> He expressed intense anger at the time change and spoke of feeling abandoned by me. Obsessions emerged about the presumed differences between the analysis of children and of adults. He speculated about what kind of father I must be and saw me as warm and loving, which seemed unmasculine to him and different from his own father. He then expressed doubts about whether or not to give his current woman friend a gift, something he had never before done with a woman. It seemed obvious that he wished to give her the gift but he was frightened because it seemed adult and masculine. The fear of being a man like me led to his adopting a childlike tone, and he meekly voiced the wish that I might turn off the air conditioner because it was chilly. He said that he could not expect me to do this because he paid me such a low fee. When I pointed out that he was portraying himself as a child, as a defensive response to the fears aroused by exhibiting himself as a man to me, he spoke of experiencing micropsia again.
>
> At this time, he perceived the books on my shelves as appearing smaller, and once again he was reminded of the latency episodes. Those usually occurred . . . when he would contemplate . . . being separated from his mother. He spoke of his present wishes to be little with me, to be my child, and of how "belittled" he had felt by my interpretation, which he took as an injunction to become an adult. . . . [He talked of the injury to his eye] shortly before the onset of the latency micropsia, by the bocce ball thrown by his father [p. 583f.].

Myers then tells us about the link with the patient's testicular movements. He concludes that the "episode was precipitated by anger at the analyst-father arising from an oedipal-level conflict. The rage aroused intense castration (and separation) anxiety" (p. 585).

What are the implications for the listening perspective conveyed here? The patient's symptom was understood as a manifestation of a defensive compromise against the experience of conflictual affect, which was addressed by the interpretation.

That is, the fact that he could no longer maintain his feelings in repression was seen as precipitating the episode, the interpretation serving as the trigger to the patient's ensuing response. The transference—permitted free unfolding—is thus viewed as predetermined by already present instinct and defense derivatives.

The essence of this point of view is one in which the "organization of behavior is the property of the individual" (Sander, 1975, p. 147), the patient's intrapsychic world is the center of its own initiative; his perceptual world is encumbered by distortions (e.g., the analyst as one who "belittles") deriving from his fears and wishes and the defenses against them. As the experiential specificity of the analyst's contribution is not elaborated as intrinsic to the episode, implicitly then the analyst stands "outside," utilizing his own measure of "objective" reality, observing and interpreting the inner reality of the patient.

As an alternative, let us look again at the moment when the symptom appeared, *but in context with* the analyst. When the analyst first commented that the patient was "defensively portraying himself" as a child, the patient responded that he *felt* "belittled" by *this comment.* If we now go back and review the patient's initial remarks, after talking of feeling abandoned, he seemed to have been wondering whether the analyst would be more warmly available to a child, either as doctor or as father, than he was to him. We might consider whether the symptom, communicating the experience of painful affect, would have appeared had the analyst responded to this quest; that is, if the analyst, rather than seeing the patient's childlike behavior as defensive, had commented that it seemed that the patient wished to be responded to with the warmth which he felt the analyst would give to a child. Indeed, when the analyst had at first said nothing, the patient spoke of feeling "chilly." One may conjecture that perhaps that feeling state, as well as the micropsia, arose in the context of a painful perception of the analyst as having "failed" to understand the patient's quest. Thus, to Myers's statement that the episode was precipitated by "anger at the analyst-father arising from an oedipal conflict" I would add: when the analyst *responded* in a way that re-created the patient's perception of the father's earlier response to such a conflict. Listening in this way may offer an added view of the subjective experience of the early interplay between father and child. (Indeed, the father is described in this vignette as neither warm nor loving, and at least inadvertently injuring his son.)

Of course, the analyst cannot necessarily know ahead of time what may be, perhaps uniquely, felt by his patient as injurious. There is no implication that by this mode of attunement he can forestall the occurrence of the symptom, nor even that it is to be his aim to attempt that. Further, even had the analyst recognized and articulated the patient's quest, the patient might still have experienced an injury, feeling that the quest itself had not been met, and the symptom may concomitantly have appeared.

What I am addressing is the effort at systematic elaboration of just *how* the interpretation felt, of *how* the *perceptual* experience became a part of the totality of the ensuing psychic state. The patient's view of the analyst as "belittling," with its historical antecedents, recognized as the expression of his perceptual reality, would become the explicit focus of further exploration.

The shift in perspective to one in which the "organization of behavior," of intrapsychic experience, is seen as the "property of the more inclusive system of which the individual is a part" has considerable impact on the gathering of psychoanalytic data.[1] Listening from within the patient's experience, weaving the perception of the analyst's contribution, silent or stated, into the elucidation of the subsequently emerging material, assigns different meaning to our understanding of transference, resistance, and memory—a relativity continually shifting, though with inherent continuity. Transference, the inner representation of the past amalgamated to the present, is then not viewed as a distortion, for this would imply that there is a reality more "correct" than the patient's psychic view of us, which we as "outside" observer could ascertain. Understood as the prop-

1. Sander (1975) describes his views as an infant researcher and psychoanalyst on some of the new directions in developmental research: "A major difficulty in conceptualizing at the psychological level has arisen from a tendency to view the organization of behavior as the property of the individual rather than as the property of the more inclusive system of which the individual is a part . . . the concept of the 'unity of the organism' relates to an organism functioning in its proper environment" (p. 147). "This represents a major turning point in developmental research" (personal communication).

erty of the system, psychic experience is not separable from its context, the transference is inseparable from the "real." For the effort to distinguish between the "real" relationship and the "transference" implies the perspective of a hierarchy of realities—the one more objective to be distinguished from the other, rather than the recognition of the relativity of each of our realities, our own as well as our patient's. Thus, as reality, for each of us, represents only our own psychic view—even of ourselves—the notion of an attainable certainty of an ultimately knowable reality must be regarded as illusory, a perspective often most difficult to sustain, perhaps because it is disquieting.[2]

In presenting the case of Mrs. G., I shall try to illustrate such an alternate mode of listening. It is characterized by my sustained effort to seek out my place in the patient's experience, as part of the context that is perceived or felt. An essential aspect of my self-reflection is to observe how and when I lost sight of this, when I was listening to her experience as though independent of my participation, even if silent, thereby trying to understand this disparity and to reinstate my original intent. My focus is sharpened on the more experience-near, on the immediate vicissitudes of the patient's state or affect, on shifting defensive patterns, and on her perceptual experience—seen as intrinsic to (rather than distorted by) her emerging wishes, feelings, or defenses. Leaps of inference arising from the domain of the analyst's view of "reality" are thereby taken more systematically into account, facilitating, I believe, more rigorous attunement to the patient's psychic reality.[3]

2. The parallel to Einsteinian physics was cogently stated by the eminent physicist, John Archibald Wheeler, a long-time colleague of Einstein: "What is so hard . . . is to give up thinking of nature as a machine that goes on independent of the observer. What we conceive of as reality is a few iron posts of observation with papier-mâché construction between them that is but the elaborate work of our imagination. . . . For our picture of the world, this is the most revolutionary thing discovered . . . we still have not come to terms with it" (Begley, 1979, p. 62). Referring to this quote, Sander (1979) writes, "The farther scientific investigation goes in these directions, the more it demands that we confront the matter of uncertainty."

3. Clinical material from the analysis of Mrs. G. is also discussed in Schwaber (1981, 1983).

CASE REPORT

Mrs. G. first experienced episodes of micropsia in her analytic hours, when, in the course of our work together, she had become more socially outgoing. In one such hour, she spoke to me of how successful she felt at her job, and compared her work to mine. I said that she was perhaps thinking about surpassing me, and that might stir up what we had seen to be a familiar conflict. The symptom appeared: the walls again seemed further away, the objects in the room smaller. There was a sense of spatial disorientation.

As with Myers's patient, this episode could be formulated as arising in the context of emerging aggressive (oedipal) wishes with concomitant intense anxiety in the transference. Stated in this way, however, this formulation views the analyst's remarks as only triggering the patient's impending response and does not include as intrinsic the intrapsychic specificity of the interaction—the *meaning* of *my* remarks, as an integral part of her re-created past. I then asked: *how* did my comments, interwoven with her experience, bear on this episode? Mrs. G. reflected, "Whenever I shared anything with my mother that I felt good about, she'd say something to take it away, some comment directing me elsewhere—whenever I showed something off to her. What just happened with you is what happened with mother all the time. I was sharing with you my most *adult* self and you talked about a conflict, like suddenly in barges my mother and takes it away."

And so we learned about this historically meaningful dimension of Mrs. G.'s oedipal experience precisely in the effort to elucidate the *experience* of the context in which it was being re-created. The distinction made here is not one which questions the analyst's technical stance, i.e., the intervention about the patient's conflictual wishes; rather, it seeks out the meaning that this intervention has for the patient, thereby lending affectively immediate and genetic specificity to the ensuing response.

Mrs. G. had been told that she was not touched as a baby, with the bottle propped on a rigid 4-hour schedule. In her relationships, she used eye contact to maintain a feeling of connectedness; vulnerable to feeling "disconnected," this state was often experienced in a spatial sense—as she described, "disconnected from the space capsule, distanced, remote." The choice of symptom, micropsia, had meaning richly illuminating patterns arising in the early relationship to her mother, which became interwoven in the conflictual issues of succeeding developmental phases. Viewed in their contextual complexity, it seemed that in the analytic situation one witnessed the re-creation of phenomena that might offer meaningful reconstructive clues about aspects of preverbal experience which otherwise may be bypassed but come into sharpened focus when this mode of attunement is used.

I

Mrs. G. was 35 years old when she first came to see me— tall, thin, with dark-brown Afro-style hair, dressed in darkly colored clothing, somewhat Bohemian in fashion, long-skirted, with no makeup. She had a rather plaintive expression, a kind of wiry, poor-waif look. She appeared somewhat anxious. Articulate and soft-spoken, she seemed rather intelligent. There was something in her appearance and manner that was not engaging.

Mrs. G.'s work centered fully around home and family—wife of a successful lawyer, mother of 3 children ranging in age from 8 to 3. She sought help for what she described as feelings of worthlessness, shyness, inability to study (though she wanted to do graduate work), and anxiety. Sometimes, to her great dismay, she would find herself acting like her own mother toward her children; this thought of "hearing my mother's voice in me makes me weep."

Sketching her history in our early meetings, Mrs. G. told of growing up in a Midwestern city, an only child born to Hungarian immigrant parents. Her parents ran a small business. They lived in a community where to be immigrant was to be alien. There was not much money. In recent years, her father had depressive episodes, occasionally requiring hospitalization. Her mother, who had always taken care of her husband "like he was a baby," was herself quite phobic and continually "nagging." The patient said she did not feel a loving tie to her parents. Her maternal grandparents lived nearby, and she was raised as an only child among four adults. The grandfather died when she was an adolescent, the grandmother soon thereafter. "The best part of my life was that I was *grandfather's child.*" He was a local civic leader who had commanded considerable respect. He disparaged her parents. He was her ally.

From the time of their courtship, some 15 years previously, Mrs. G. and her husband had always had an "intense sexual relationship," spending much of their time together in bed. Though troubled by her husband's Jekyll and Hyde character, his rages and withdrawals, sex was the best and the binding part of the marriage.

The patient had been referred to me by a senior analyst, Dr. A., a much older man of considerable repute, with whom she had wished to go into treatment. She was very troubled by my seeming youth, saying that it stirred up her envy. Besides, as such a junior person, I would have to take whomever I could get; I couldn't pick and choose my patients. If only Dr. A. could have seen her. When I wondered if this wish bore on her feelings about her grandfather, she said, yes, someone more like him in age and status would feel better. Her fear about analysis was that I would come to think that she really belonged to her parents; she did not want to think that about herself. Besides, others had been "bored" by her past; so might I. She spoke of a former therapist, a woman, with whom she had worked some years back; she described her as older, tall, and thin. Mrs. G. had asked her whether she had children, and the therapist answered that she had not. This distressed her. I wondered to myself whether she might have been in search of her "true" parents or wanted somehow to experience a "transference" to the idealized parent of her fantasy. It did seem, I said to her, that the therapist's actual reality was of particular importance to her, and that in asking if she had children, she perhaps wanted to know whether her own feelings as a mother were shared and could be understood. She agreed, "I always felt the need to find someone who had experienced things like me, especially a parental figure. As a child, I always felt myself to be an oddball, different from peers and from parents. Mother had black hair, was short, heavy; she used to think I was an 'odd egg.' She worried about my hair, got me padded bras, orthopedic shoes. I did think perhaps I looked like Grandpa."

After some weeks of struggle around the question of working with me, Mrs. G. decided that, despite her disappointment that I was not the therapist she had in mind, she would stay. She felt that at least I understood this problem.

II

For financial and logistical reasons, we worked together in a vis-à-vis setting, one or two times weekly for about 10 months before beginning the formal analysis. During this period as well, my effort was to maintain the listening perspective of the observer within the experiential world of the observed. I shall try to convey the sense of my own recurrent, groping, often failing attempts to locate my place within that world.

A highlight of our early work together included the focus on the patient's efforts toward, and defenses against, finding and maintaining a mode of attachment and relationship to me. The figures around which the clinical material mainly pivoted, directly and in their transference manifestations, were Mrs. G.'s husband, Alan, and her mother. Father remained a peripheral figure, and grandfather was hardly mentioned. She spoke often with some concern and some satisfaction of her children.

In the initial hours, she told of two dreams, heralding central themes. In one, she had no hands; in their place were bandages, and there was shame about this. In the other, she was traveling with Alan and stopped in a lavish, warm, hotel restaurant for an "intense experience" with a woman therapist, while Alan was staying at a cold, businesslike place. She had the choice of making love with him in his place or having this other experience, which seemed so good, with the woman. Whichever it was to be, she felt that she and Alan must soon leave and drive on. Her associations, experienced with so much shame, led to the untouched child, who fears to touch and fears being unable to touch. She also told of a certain opposition between therapy and Alan, and that therapy could only be a stopover; ultimately, she must choose Alan.

Mrs. G. spoke of her intense dependency on her husband, and of the sense of terrifying aloneness, when she believed she was unsupported by him. "I'm not entirely sure what the fear is, a kind of being disconnected. When he's home, I can't physically separate from him. I need to be in the same room. He can't tolerate this and withdraws further, and then I feel panicky."

Mother emerged as a frightening, alien figure, against whom Mrs. G. was seeking an ally. "Mother envies me, would take from me or spoil what I have. When I became pregnant, I didn't tell her for 6 months, lest she hex me. Mother had difficulty conceiving and had her tubes finally dilated. During her pregnancy with me, she bled and had to remain in bed for much of the time. I don't think she imagined ever being able to have a normal child. I think she was always afraid I was going to die; she told father she'd kill herself if she got pregnant again. She was riddled with anxiety, and could never touch with any comfort." Thus, Mrs. G. could not share her worries or fears, or even "sore throats," with her mother, lest mother's anxiety overwhelm her. Mother's presence was both too much and too little, and seemed best dealt with by disengagement as soon as the child could find someone else; unfortunately, her father was apparently unable to meet this need.

Despite this unfolding history, I often had difficulty in understanding the quality Mrs. G. would try to convey of the present-day injuries inflicted by the mother. When she described mother's words, they did not seem to communicate to me the terrible feelings they evoked in her. For example, when the patient learned to drive, her mother remarked, "Isn't it wonderful, you learned to drive a car!" Mrs. G. felt wounded, "shattered" by this. She said it felt as though mother was again responding to only a part of her, rather than to the *whole* of her, which would have included other feelings, such as the fear and anxiety that go with learning to drive.

There was, then, a discrepancy between the image she portrayed and the one she experienced—at least, I had some difficulty in understanding her experience. I thought about the possibility that the patient may have had defensive reasons for insisting on a negative image; we knew that she sought an ally against mother. But this was an inferential explanation which did not arise specifically from the data offered in the hour by the patient, and which I may have been especially tempted to seek precisely because there was a gap in my capacity to apprehend her experience. Indeed, when there is such difficulty in gaining empathic recognition, our tendency may be to try harder to narrow the gap between our understanding and the patient's experience and to make a broader leap of inference— such as a suggestion of a defensive motive on the patient's part—without data for its experiential immediacy. But awareness of this process in us can be illuminating, and the very fact of the difficulty can be pursued as meaningful in its own right.[4]

Maintaining a sharpened attunement to the affectively charged imagery conveyed, I was led to consider that the degree of mother's felt "injuries" lay in her quality of being, rather than in the words she chose. This may suggest that what is being "telescoped" in these latter-day incidents goes back very early developmentally, perhaps even to preverbal communications. Furthermore, the sense of discrepancy which I experienced in listening to the patient's associations might offer a clue about the difficulty others had in following her, and help us understand the isolation and aloneness she felt in social interactions, particularly with women. It may have a bearing on why experiential similarity between us was so crucial a concern and on the "untouched" quality she had experienced and expressed.

There was another dimension to my difficulty in making sense of the imagery Mrs. G. conveyed. Often I seemed to lose her and had to struggle to find my place in *her* experiential world, while trying to maintain my own self-reflective vigil; for there was a quality of affectlessness about Mrs. G., a kind of lifelessness, with no *manifest* warmth. Unfortunately, often only retrospectively did I become aware of having been impatient, fatigued, or bored—perhaps, in some way, self-protective withdrawals *from* the intense immersion in her experience. The

4. I have (1978) described this difficulty in attaining empathic recognition and the tendency to bridge the gap with broader leaps of inference, in the effort to comprehend the experience of survivors of the holocaust.

clues to such responses on *my* part were frequently signaled by subtle shifts in the patient's communications—a change in tone, sounding more mechanized; or a shift in the style of her stream of associations. In my attempt to maintain sight of the context between us, these clues helped me to more honest reflection, to discover that I had indeed stepped out of her "shoes." As I reread my process notes in preparing this paper, I felt further troubled by seeing things that now seemed so obvious—how could I have missed them at the time? Granted my wish for an answer sparing me narcissistic injury for these errors, I do believe that just as with my difficulty in grasping her meaning from mother's words alone, so, too, Mrs. G.'s words by themselves did not convey the totality of the experience, the quality of disengagement, which made attunement so difficult.

The work with Mrs. G. thus represented a continuing challenge to my capacity for empathic attunement, the refinement of which remained an ongoing process for me to the last moment of our work together. From her perspective, she had a particular quest of me which I was asked to meet in certain, often cryptically defined ways: I must not be vague; I must not be ahead of her; I must be more directive, but not controlling; I must use the first-person pronoun; I must know her meaning, even when she did not spell it out; I must not speak to the mundane, when she was talking of the sublime—all this while she could scarcely tolerate any sustained feelings of being understood, which made her feel too close.

Our task, as the analysis proceeded, was to deepen our understanding of the intensity of her quest for this kind of attunement, as well as the sometimes gross and often subtle ways in which this quest was frustrated and how she responded to these frustrations. It was not that I sought to meet directly the specific aspects of her requests; the effort of our work together remained centered on the systematic search for the multiplicity of their meaning, including variations in the degree of urgency at different moments. Often, she experienced this search itself as a rebuff—her need for my concrete responsiveness was so intense. Nonetheless, she was able to sustain the analytic task without my having to shift my mode of inquiry or response; no parameters were needed.

Instinctual wishes and the defenses against their emergence were viewed within the context of what, at any moment, she was seeking from or re-creating with me. Vigilant focus—as on such nonverbal cues as shifts in affect or state—was maintained on the centrality of how and to what end she was using my interventions. One might otherwise be misled into believing that a deepening analytic experience was taking place when in fact the issue of *apparent* concern lacked affective "reality"—the affectively "real" issue being the way in which she was drawing upon my interpretations to maintain a dialogue or, as we were later to discern more fully, a feeling of connectedness with me.

Further, I maintained the perspective that her quest of me—for my attunement—was itself a sign of hope, representing a core of belief in herself and in me which ultimately was to serve as a source of creative continuity. At times when she seemed to accept without question my "failures" to understand her needs, particularly if she conveyed a sense of "affective" resignation, I became concerned that a feeling of hopelessness might have arisen, a state that then needed to be addressed.

I may note here that this mode of attunement, by elucidating such subtle shifts in affect or state, facilitates illumination of the patient's defensive modes. Focusing upon the defenses at the moment of their experiential and contextual specificity—in contrast to making an inference of affectively unavailable defense against unconscious meaning—offers the patient the opportunity for heightened self-observation and recognition.

III

The transition to the couch, in the second year, was uneventful. The first hour seemed a hopeful one. Mrs. G. spoke for the first time of an artistic interest and skill, describing the beautiful picture she had drawn of her children. She also related several dreams, with associations leading to a time at about age 11 when she had felt much more self-accepting and accepted.

Greeting me, Mrs. G. would now give me a lingering look (perhaps trying to keep my visual image with her, as she was to lie down). In contrast, as she left each session, she seemed to avert my glance, bowing her head low. As may have been anticipated from the initial meetings, a particular quality, intensified by the anxiety of the analytic situation, now presented itself more strikingly and posed somewhat of a challenge to the psychoanalytic method: Mrs. G.'s intense need to know, *in fact,* something about my external reality: "Did you see that movie, read that book? Are you an only child?" Even if on rare occasion I responded directly, relief was only momentary, nor did it seem that anything deepening had been gained.

"I'm thinking of this lovely poem in MS magazine," she said in one early hour when we first came in touch with this issue. "Did you read it? Do you know the poem I mean?" There was a seeming urgency to her questions. I said, "Such a strong wish to have me answer directly—can we look at what that means?" "Yes," she replied, "there is something to that." She paused, then noted, "I—feel—now, a strangeness about myself—alone—different; that's why I don't write; it's not mutual; not mutual makes me feel strange. It's like coming home from school and telling my mother what happened; she'd just sit there and listen, like from another world. Something about asking you if you read that poem is like that. It would have been so nice growing up if mother had said, 'Yes, I had the same experience; I know about that.' My mother never told me things like that; like she grew up in a big fishtank different from mine. If you had said something about the poem, I'd have felt better; otherwise, I get this goldfish-in-the-tank feeling. One looks at it, admires it, feeds it. What I'm saying is I want to get out of the bowl."

Later, she explained, "When I ask you what you've read, what you've seen, it is really, 'Do you experience the same bodily feelings I do?'" It seemed that mother's "failure," originating perhaps in the lack of touch, had somehow to do with an inability to communicate an experiential sameness with the little girl. This then became the essence of how Mrs. G. experienced my "failure"[5] to respond directly.

5. I have in several places put quotes around the word "failure" to indicate that I am addressing such attributes solely as aspects of the subjective reality of the patient. Elsewhere (1981) I said, "A failure in empathy is not synonymous with an error in technique; empathic failure speaks to the subjective experience of the patient and cannot be assessed in any other way" (p. 377).

The patient was continually searching for me to say something to help her maintain focus; "otherwise I get this terrible anxiety, like having asked an inappropriate question, or that I have to produce and there's nothing coming out. I don't look at you, and if I don't hear from you, it's like in my parents' house—once I get in, I can't get out. I get a feeling of 'fogging over,' I feel heavy, rigid, stern, a drawing into myself. As a child I had nightmares, and no sound came out; it was frightening. I equated it with shyness, not being able to talk, as though behind a glass partition; with my mother, I would seek some relief by getting into a fight. Maybe it was a way of separating, maybe a way out of the vagueness . . . such anxiety about me! In childhood I felt safe only as long as every part of me was touching the mattress." And poignantly, "Somehow, I've been told I don't radiate warmth."

As she continued to deepen her awareness of what she was seeking in the transference, she was to learn: "I have come to the recognition that initiative has always been a problem. I see the extent to which I don't even think to do things for myself; someone has to light the match to get me going." She told of how mother, while not comforting or caressing, was constantly "reading" and "attending" to the child's bodily signs well beyond infancy. She was fed until the age of 3, told when to go to the bathroom, and given enemas as cure for illness until about the age of 7—adding to the sense of uncertainty about the integrity of her bodily experiences and sensations. Concomitantly, mother did not seem to validate[6] the *child's* perceptions and affective states, and remained vague and tangential about her own.

The vagueness appeared to be associated with the sense of "disconnection," an experience also represented in her looking away at each hour's end. This feeling at times took the form of her losing a sense of orientation in space. She recalled the film *Destination Moon*, which she saw when she was 9 years old and which had greatly frightened her: "The man walking in space, out of his capsule, without a rope. When I was nursing and

---

6. A term used by Sander (personal communication), referring to the child's developmental need for "validation" of his or her experiences and responses, via recognition and definition by a confirming, approving adult.

Alan walked into the room, it was agony to me that I couldn't get up and go over to him. I feel chronically like a scared only child in a place where I can't reach mother." She had many dreams of this kind of spatial separation from her children— being on a different train or boat. This fear of disconnection also carried with it "the risk of *your* being an ally lest I lose what's outside." At moments of feeling added closeness with me, her thoughts would shift to her husband or children in order to keep the connection to "outside."

The micropsia experience included this sense of spatial uncertainty, "like the hatch opening on an airplane." "Are you too far or are you too close?" was her dilemma, expressed in her character style as well as in the symptom. Our understanding of the *specific* appearance of this symptom evolved only gradually. It seemed at first to occur whenever she felt disconnection between us. Later we learned that it arose when she was sharing with me something of her "mature" or "womanly" side, and I overlooked what pleased her in this experience, maintaining instead the primary focus on what seemed to be distressing her. For example, in one hour she spoke of her involvement in a project at her children's school and turned so quickly to her *fear* of being successful in the interaction with the others that the fear—perhaps of her rivalrous feelings—became our sole focus, with the pleasure being bypassed. (We see here, in the transference as well, that in the emphasis on her conflict about sharing these new steps with me, there was an implicit "failure" to recognize the achievement conveyed in her being able to tell me this at all.)

The appearance of micropsia also evoked an ominous image of mother standing in the doorway to her room at night, sometimes holding an enema bag, sometimes, while she was masturbating—a sense of mother's "hovering, evil presence." She described mother graphically, "like a puffy, white fungus, growing in a dark space, amorphous, asexual; like a food-vending machine, where the one thing you want is empty—the picture of it is there, but it's not there." Mrs. G. began to recall early childhood occurrences of micropsia at about the age of 5 or 6— mother standing in the darkness, seeming so small and far away.

Thus, the micropsia could be understood as a symptomatic expression of a vital aspect of Mrs. G.'s inner state: vague, disconnected, spatially distant, yet with mother still present, looking at but not touching her—too close or too far. As a defensive manifestation, it re-created the disorienting imagery of the darkened room, where it first appeared, the anxiety and bodily confusion evoked by the enemas and expressed in the masturbation experience, and the feeling of spatial disconnectedness from the "intrusive" or "nontouching" mother, who was felt as somehow negating the child's blossoming feminine strivings. The symptom, then, represented a particular phenomenon to be observed and given *meaning* in the presence of the analyst—who was felt to be similarly nonaccepting of the patient's wish to share herself and to have put to question the patient's sense of her very femaleness. The symptom also represented a forward step, a statement of Mrs. G.'s increasing ability to express and experience in the transference her thwarted, competitive, and growth-oriented strivings, albeit still strongly defended against and not yet fully acknowledged.

Memories unfolded about Mrs. G.'s "seemingly endless" masturbation as a child and adolescent. "When I was alone, I used mother's electric foot massager, it was instant orgasm. Erotic tension became a conditioned response when I was home alone. *Masturbating gave me a clearer sense of myself;* it was a way to really feel my own body, but it also made me feel shame and terror. I had the sense like I wasn't completely female; when I got my period, it was like despite the fact that I'm not really a woman; like they were all sitting around waiting for my breasts to develop. If mother discovered an injury, she'd be wildly upset." We could begin to discern the link between the painful, dubious sense of herself as a woman and the earlier sense about her body as being vague or not whole or disconnected.

As she further communicated this dreaded uncertainty about the intactness of her body, particularly in the context of her increasingly emerging feminine and oedipal strivings, Mrs. G. had many frightening dreams and recurrent images of self-induced skin afflictions ("like a leper") or of fragmented body parts (stumps of arms or stumps of breasts). One time, after an injury to her foot, she had a dream which conveyed a particu-

larly despairing and telling self-perception: "I experienced myself as being very bizarre. I was made out of sharp pieces of
wire and cardboard; when I woke up, I felt all elbows and
awkward, a witch feeling, an inhuman feeling that carries with
it the potential for terror; but I was lying next to Alan, and that
made me feel soft. In the dream the sharp parts of me were in
the way. Lovemaking makes me feel good about my whole body
grace."[7]

The urgency of her tie to Alan thus became further elaborated. "He is the only person I can really feel frantic about
losing—his approval overrides everything." She spoke of Alan's
wide mood swings, his "strange behavior," the details of which
she was at first ashamed to share with me: "The fear that I may
have made an awful mistake, giving my life to this man, yet I
overwhelmingly want to stay with him." He was later found to
have a neurological illness, which to some extent was responsive
to medication.

We learned, at this time, only little more about her father—
his own illness, his dependent behavior, which she so abhorred.
"I hated the way mother treated him like a baby, laying out his
pajamas, turning down his covers, protecting him like one does
a defective child. There was a craziness about him; he was like
her propped-up puppet. She never talked about him to me; he
was *her* business. My father so adulated *her* that even her phobias were considered charming; when she and I were in an
argument and she got all steamed up, he'd say, 'Now look what
you did to your mother!' There was something about the way
he looked at me that felt like a terrible reproach. There was a
fear of silence with him, a frantic expression of avoiding eyes; a
feeling, if we *touch*, it would be disastrous, like his frantically
pushing me off. I felt I had no ally, so I ran to grandfather. He
made me feel good; all that ugliness left, and he scolded mother for what she was doing to me, so we each had our champion.

7. Unfortunately my notes do not tell of the effort to elucidate what had
been her experience in the transference that was a part of the evocation of
this dream. Thus it may be that I was listening to her experience independent
of my participation in it. As I have previously indicated, the systematic search
for one's own place in the context of another's psychic experience—even as I
have made an active effort to pursue this—is a task most difficult to sustain.

I felt a fusion at his side; I would just hold on while he went about his meetings."

Some time late in the second analytic year, Mrs. G. started the hour with: "The other day, when I said, 'I'll never know, I can't remember,' you said, 'unless memory returns.' That felt so real, there was so much hope in that, not only for the future, but that there's something in me now. It has the quality of, 'You'll grow up and be a woman'—that someone understands and knows about me. My cousin Vivian would say, patting my backside, 'That's a beautiful ass; some man is really going to like that.' Mother would say, 'Too hippy.' I remember the fear, 'What's wrong with me? Am I a girl?' . . . not feeling whole or intact; to this day, I fear cosmetic prostheses, like false eyelashes, wigs or makeup—anything not real." (Again, "Am I real?" was later translated to "Am I a girl?")

This hour in some way heralded a significant turn in our work. The longing for affirmation—for "touch"—of the positive, womanly side of her had previously been subtly communicated as an underlying thread. Indeed, we came to understand the symptom of micropsia as expressing the complexity of the conflictual dimensions of this quest, including the emergence of homosexual longings; nonetheless, this symptom, even as triggered in regression from oedipal wishes, still had reflected the issue of "connectedness" as a central, if latent, concern. What surfaced now was a more open acknowledgment of hopefulness and a sense of *realness* about this. Though I may have phrased things similarly earlier, Mrs. G. felt, as she subsequently said, that something within *her* now permitted her to hear it. In a certain way, the risk of a fragmenting experience, like the dreaded disconnectedness, had significantly lessened. She felt more autonomously "whole" and so was able to proceed without symptomatic retreat.

One day she recalled a story from childhood, of the "Velveteen Rabbit," a toy so tenderly cared for that it became real.

I thought to myself—how not boring, how much more engaging she had become.

Something more began to emerge, which I was still slow to understand. Mrs. G. came in one hour, looking pleased with herself, and coyly told of a friendly chat with a man who lived nearby, a famous author. She seemed reluctant, however, to reveal this friendship—perhaps flirtation—with this important man. This defensiveness became our central focus. She told of her fear lest the awfulness of her past or parents be exposed, and of her tendency to create an "aura" of sophistication around her, leaving her in continuous fear of exposure. In the succeeding hours she resumed the familiar thread of shame and fear and ignorance. And then, for some time, I did not hear more about this man. Only later, when she again spoke of him, did I come to recognize what had happened. Once more, the emphasis had remained on the conflictual aspects of this relationship without seeking to elucidate her perception of me, which contributed to her fear and shame. Thus, what she felt in the transference was a re-creation of a familiar image of mother, who, whenever Mrs. G. shared something with her that she felt good about, would "say something to take it away, some comment directing me elsewhere—whenever I showed something off to her." Interpreting this to her, I could then add that she had seemed so clearly pleased about this friendship, which she might want to share with me, perhaps in the hope that I, too, would be pleased for her. "Yes," she said, she had always been interested in important people. "If only mother would have said, 'You're very interesting, no wonder that other interesting people take an interest in you.' Instead, mother conveyed a sense of, 'Such an inadequate person as you has such illustrious acquaintances? Tell me all about it.'"

We may note here the oedipal theme, now expressed more overtly. Mrs. G. was seeking to reassure herself about the woman's approval of her interest in an already "taken" man. Again, we could see how the form which this theme—this developmental phase and its attendant conflicts—assumed, was lent particular specificity in her experience of the interaction with her milieu, in what she perceived and what she sought from it. To paraphrase the earlier discussion of Myers's patient: "Mrs. G.'s angry withdrawal from the analyst-mother arising from an oedipal conflict occurred when the analyst responded in a way that stimulated the patient's perception of the mother's earlier response to such a conflict." The transference included the experience of the analyst's intervention as an intrinsic component of this amalgam of the past within the present.

Of course, we had yet to grapple with her defensive posture against the intensity of her own affective states and wishes in relation to me. But as she had attained some resolution of her conflictual feelings about her femaleness, Mrs. G. could express her sexual and competitive strivings with an increasing sense of inner confidence. Her feelings about herself as one woman *to* or *versus* another—with a man in between—thus emerged in the transference at a point when she felt more hopeful. Buried feelings of specialness and grandiosity then unfolded.

As this side of Mrs. G.'s experience continued to emerge, her tone was much more lively. She described a feeling of latent possibilities, like the ugly duckling who turned into a swan. She sang the praises of her children, particularly her middle child, how beautiful she was, much more so than the other children in her class. At times, she walked to my office (about 5 miles), proudly telling of her pleasure in her physical competence, in marked contrast to the constricted immobility that she had felt as a child and had earlier reexperienced on the couch. She said, "I can feel a kind of 'showing off,' and I want you to like me for it." The hours now ended with a direct glance and frequently with a smile.

She had a dream in which she was eating dinner in France at the home of an aristocratic family, the elder gentleman looking like her grandfather. French was spoken in the dream. For Mrs. G., France was a very beloved country—its artistic grandeur, its aristocratic history, and its sensuality adding to its appeal. When she spoke of things "French," there was a subtle enthusiasm in her tone, so different from when she spoke of the "village" background of her parentage. She used to have a childhood fantasy, she said, of being a king's child.

Grandfather was singled out from the others of her family; she believed he was really "upper class." She turned to him (and perhaps also he to her) in her school years. She would sit by his side at meetings, and work with him in writing his memoirs. He filled her mind with heroic stories of his youth. He now emerged as a more central figure in her associations—with an affective connectedness that made him stand out more vividly than he had before. "Grandfather had a 'mind of his own.' I like to think of myself as unconventional—it makes me feel a sense of pride and of being beautiful."

One day Mrs. G. came in wearing a deep green dress, made for her when she lived in France. The dress felt wonderful to her—regal, elegant. The fabric had a softness to it that would invite touch. In front, made of pale yellow cloth, was a rose. After that, for some time, she continued to wear a rose almost regularly. "I love the fact that you notice it, comment on it," she said; "The rose means feminine, off-beat, pretty; it makes me feel more visible."

Her experiential states still vacillated; at times, the old, painful imagery recurred, interwoven with subtle shifts in my own responsiveness. The question of what was "real," what was "legitimate," took on new dimension and import. "As a small child, maybe 2 or 3, I would dance for my parents *or* bob up and down, and they would applaud in either event; I became uncertain about the quality of my performance, and what was real. Sometimes, Mother would call me 'princess,' but she then retracted this with a look of surprise, like it couldn't have been me." Mother, we also learned, had spent some years of her own childhood in Western Europe, which she herself had romanticized.

Thus, another aspect of mother's communications came to view. What seemed to have occurred was that as Mrs. G. felt herself more real, she could accept her own legitimacy as child to her parents and their realness to her—something which, as may be recalled, had been of great initial concern.

The summer after the second analytic year, she spoke for the first time of feelings about the impending interruption. "I think I could even miss you—to miss means to stay connected, even when apart"—a new experience.

The third year was marked by deepening elaborations of her inner experiences and perceptions, further strengthening the feeling of "realness" about herself. She noticed a shift from her childhood style of relating—"What shall I do now, Mommy?"—to one in which she was increasingly able to take the initiative. She observed a change in her relation to Alan; "I had been so exquisitely tuned into his moods; now I can initiate my own. I can see now what is his reality and what is mine. Your not responding directly has made a difference; it has helped me to *know* what comes from me."

Mrs. G. began to pursue more active outside interests and was sending off applications to various local graduate schools for a doctoral program in comparative literature. She made innumerable requests for schedule changes, as she attempted to negotiate school interviews, baby-sitting, and other obligations. Though with some anxiety and some feeling of confusion about her ability to integrate her new experiences, she was clearly more able to assert herself. Even when my response failed to understand or to meet her requests, she did not experience me as hostile, nor did "disconnecting" symptomatology recur. She simply began to object.

She observed a greater capacity for intimacy in her relationships with women, and she continued to feel better about her own womanliness. Retaining the "artsy" style of dressing, her choice of color and fabric was now more varied, often floral, and very soft. Sometimes she wore a hat; other times, a matching scarf in her hair. She even began to wear eye makeup; the fear of cosmetics had abated. Though she spoke at times of things she noticed about what I was wearing, her manner of dress seemed distinctively her own.

An interesting hour occurred when she came in with a cold and said, "It felt so good; it's like I can get sick and not have to hide some terrible affliction."

Mrs. G. began to remember again that good year of her childhood, around the age of 11; "I felt secure in my identity, a favorite of my teacher and a leader of kids." She recalled that it was then that her paternal grandmother had died. Father became devoutly religious and she joined him in that. They sang songs, lit candles, and performed other rituals. "My father saw me as pious and beautiful," she reflected. "When I was very little, 2 or 3, he would sing to me, songs from Hungary; he would hold me, touch me." Thus, it seemed that father, despite his own severe limitations, had offered something sustaining of himself, at least for a brief time in her childhood. Mrs. G. now could relinquish her defensive need to repress this side of her experience and thereby to acknowledge its occurrence.

Letters of acceptance arrived from several graduate schools, and she had her choice of where to go. But the news was marred by Alan's illness. Because of this, she would have to terminate her analysis sometime in the next year. Her own position on this matter was somewhat unclear. Would she herself have chosen at this time to terminate? Perhaps not, she said, because she still wished to learn more about herself. She would come back one day, she thought. But she felt an increasing readiness to continue on her own, give to her family, and pursue an independent career goal.

In this context she reflected on what she had gained. Her view of me had remarkably shifted: "I had a dream in which you made a mistake, and I held your face closer, and it was cute, and we both felt tolerant of your mistake." The dream followed a change I had made in the appointment time. "I've been wondering what you do when you change an hour, a sense of interest in your private life. There was a moment in the dream when I had a realization of how much things were now making more sense; how much I was able to change my view of reality from a confused unknown to one I understand; like the way I changed my view of you—from hostile, mysterious, to uncryptic and comfortable—even when you make a mistake." Another time she said, "Now I can see how I used to pursue anything you commented on, just to stay connected, it wouldn't matter what."

One day Mrs. G. said, "I see now that my old protest against my mother, my saying 'I didn't want my mother,' was a defense against feeling so unconnected. I really only started to get angry with my mother once I started school. Remembering the dream about the guy who floated in space—that's nothing to get angry about; after he gets back into the capsule, then he can get angry with the other guys for having been so foolish."

This statement touches on a critical issue having to do with the place of anger as a primary emotion in the patient's psychic life. It helped us to understand the early absence of experienced anger toward me and toward Alan. She had had to achieve, in the course of the analytic work, the developmental capacity for such a defined emotion, rather than its having been something to be "lifted from repression." (See also Basch, 1976.) She could now begin to get angry with me and, similarly, to broaden the range of other feelings toward me. "Now," she said, "I'm *glad* to see you Mondays . . . like I haven't been disconnected." The capacity to have more defined emotions further lent a stamp of reality to Mrs. G.'s experience.

The patient became increasingly aware of feeling sad to terminate. She had a series of painful dreams which led to a reconsideration of some of the old imagery of her childhood: "always getting abandoned in some way—I will give more to my children." There were dreams of a man coming and stealing her money, with associations that "something has been taken away too soon. Alan, angry with him; he is taking analysis away; but he is sick. I have to do the best I can. I love him. I'm stronger now and not afraid. I feel sad, and that feels so good. I must step back from that so I can get out there and cope. I see how analysis offers the hope for me to continue in this path of really finding myself."

On another day, she said she now wanted to do something for her parents: "I've not felt that before; the connection with analysis—that I feel ready to do something for my parents. I'm beginning to see now that perhaps I didn't give my parents another chance." Mother's own life, her pain and hurt, were reconsidered, as the patient became capable of empathically grasping these feeling states. Mrs. G. went to visit with her parents; her father touched her—it felt warm and good.

The theme of grandfather returned: "That sense of being loved and *special*—his house was countrified, open, simple, animals, plants, quiet; we have a lot of his furniture. I realize now that there's a whole aesthetic part of my life that enjoys beautiful things—not just clothes, also birds, flowers, woods. . . . The rose—I wear it now as it pleases me; there was a time when I felt anxious not to wear it."

One day: "I had said I needed to step back so I can go out there and cope. I see now how I always dismissed things I couldn't have. I see I could have done that here. I see how much my wanting to come each hour makes me want to leave. But now I'm asking you, help me to stay sad, to stay with the feeling of the loss. Yet I see myself wanting to find fault here, so I won't lie in a pool of tears." There was a sense of her recurrent moving closer one hour and then back the next, until finally she was able to modulate the feeling and stay with it.

And in the last hour: "The ending snuck up on me. I've

wanted to give you something. I've been dependent on you for providing the *place*, but I'm ready to go and do more out there; I see that I can move out and be able to hold onto you. I'm feeling something now that I never did experience in this way, good about you and good about myself. I hope you know that I cared and have a continuing sense of that. My caring is something that I would *give* to you, something I haven't had before . . . being *touched* intimately, within my mind. I'll keep that. My parents didn't know me, so I didn't get to know me. I've learned to talk like this from being with you. I'll keep on doing it." Our time was up, we wished each other well, and her eyes filled with tears; we held each other's hands. The moment was deeply moving.

Soon after that, she mailed me her final check. Enclosed was a card. On it was a beautiful picture of a yellow rose, with many buds still to bloom.

IV

I struggled in writing of this termination phase, reviewing it, rewriting it again and again, trying to make things come clearer, to reach a comfortable concluding statement. But was it really a termination phase, or was it rather that her analysis had been interrupted? We never did unravel the full mystery of the rose; we never did establish in genetic depth the "French connection"—her "family romance"; it was not even clear how freely she was choosing her time to leave. Then why did I choose to describe her analysis to illustrate a particular mode of listening, when I did not have a comfortable sense of completion, when other case reports might have lent themselves much more convincingly, I kept wondering to myself? Granted that she had a symptom similar to one described in the literature, offering us a particular opportunity to compare listening perspectives—this explanation did not seem enough. And then I realized that just as I struggled in the writing of this phase of the analysis, I had struggled in the work with her. I repeatedly sought answers to such questions as, "What would *you* now choose if it were not for Alan? How do *you* really feel to leave now?" She had said, "*You* seem to want to know, or want me to know, in some absolute sense; I am quite comfortable with some remaining uncertainty." I thought that statement was an especially meaningful indicator of the strength of her own sense of inner certainty—not to *have* to know. I felt moved by what she had said, and then I thought of my introductory remarks, on the difficulty in relinquishing the illusion of certainty of a knowable reality, and I felt I understood better why it was that I had chosen to present Mrs. G.[8]

APPENDIX

I asked Dr. Sander what he believed might be the consequences for a baby with Mrs. G.'s early developmental history. I indicated only that she had been told that she was minimally touched as an infant, with her bottle propped and on a rigid schedule. I offered no other information about her. He graciously sent a lengthy and scholarly reply, portions of which I briefly excerpt:

> An infant minimally touched or fondled would be lacking in experiences of multimodal, reciprocal tuning. The importance of "multimodal" is in the concurrent integration of posture, touch, olfactory, visual, auditory, motor, etc., modalities in relation to a focus of attention centered upon some aspect of the care-giving partner or upon the infant's own state or perceptual experience during the interactional exchange. The reciprocal tuning of this multimodal exchange places the regulation of the infant within a mutually arrived at feedback context. Such reciprocal tuning leads to the affects of delight and exuberance. Absence of these mutual reciprocal experi-

8. "The polarity to be harmonized in human development is that although our beginnings require the certainty that begets trust, our mature abilities to negotiate life's vicissitudes require the capacity to hold together in the face of uncertainty. There is an unavoidable uncertainty that the analyst is left with and must endure—recognizing and permitting the patient's private and unfound center while facilitating the integrative process necessary for his initiation of new adaptive organization that springs from it and cannot be carried out without it. The recognizing and enduring of this confrontation with uncertainty, paradoxically, is the fruition of the analyst's knowledge and certainty and a facilitation of the maturational process within which the analyst's own development is ongoing" (Sander, 1979).

ences sets the stage not only for lack of trust, that is, being "met" at the moment of need by another tuned to that specific need, but also for the somber affect or seriousness that stems from the failure of spontaneity, delight, and exuberance. There would be a frightening potential of being left with a vast emptiness on taking initiative of her own that the failure of early sensorimotor coordinations and the lack of spontaneous and integrative affective richness would make her heir to. The latter mediate the sense of *reality* which, if one is relying on secondary process and higher level thought, leaves one vulnerable to the feelings of unreality to this kind of human relationship.

Sander stressed the numerous possibilities and cautioned against making predictions of outcome. It was not, however, for its predictive aspect that I sought this communication with the infant researcher. Rather, I feel that the listening mode described here lends itself particularly to pursuing such a dialogue, because it adds an affectively real and immediate dimension to our observable data and offers us a deeper reach to the complexity of early intrapsychic experience and interaction.

BIBLIOGRAPHY

BASCH, M. F. (1976), The concept of affect. *J. Amer. Psychoanal. Assn.*, 24:759–777.

BEGLEY, S. (1979), Probing the universe. *Newsweek Mag.*, March 12, p. 62.

MYERS, W. A. (1977), Micropsia and testicular retraction. *Psychoanal. Q.*, 46:580–604.

SANDER, L. W. (1975), Infant and caretaking environment. In *Explorations in Child Psychiatry*, ed. E. J. Anthony. New York: Plenum, pp. 129–166.

—————— (1979), Polarity, paradox, and the organizing process in development. Read to American College of Psychoanalysts.

SCHWABER, E. (1978), Reflections in response to "A psychoanalytic view on children of survivors," by J. Kestenberg. Read at Symposium on The Holocaust, Brandeis University, Waltham, Mass.

—————— (1981), Empathy. *Psychoanal. Inq.*, 1:357–392.

—————— (1983), Construction, reconstruction, and the mode of clinical attunement. In *The Future of Psychoanalysis*, ed. A. Goldberg. New York: Int. Univ. Press, pp. 273–292.

The Unconscious Still Occupies Us

THEODORE SHAPIRO, M.D.

RECENT DEVELOPMENTS IN PSYCHOANALYSIS BEGINNING with the surge of interest in ego psychology have led us into a number of areas which now account for some of the excitement of our discipline. Studies of narcissism, object relations, borderline conditions, and altered ego states are but a few of the sectors of interest that have encouraged psychoanalysts to extend their scope of inquiry and also have produced significant reformations of theory. Several of these changes have extended our models so that some consider including interpersonalist schools, self psychology, and other variants which the psychoanalytic method itself is said to permit. On the other hand, during the first phase of ego psychology Anna Freud (1936) noted that prior to that time, one considered oneself an analyst *only* insofar as one was a *depth psychologist*. The question raised then also is relevant now. Is depth psychology essential to psychoanalysis? Or stated more boldly: has the proliferation of other "psychologies" led us afield from the initial aims of rendering the unconscious conscious so that the latter is less done than thought of? Has it become an aim that belongs to an antiquarian past?

Some thinkers believe that psychoanalysis became too mechanized following the introduction of the structural theory. Then Hartmann's views (1939) on adaptation became central to what is now generally considered to be the *American school*, and the

Professor of Psychiatry, Professor of Psychiatry in Pediatrics, Director of Child and Adolescent Psychiatry, Cornell University Medical College, Payne Whitney Clinic, New York.

lively discourse around experience-distant theorizing led some
to view ego psychology as dangerous to depth psychology. Indeed, certain European analysts balked strongly; Glover (1961)
even suggested that there was need for an International Association for the Protection of the Id Concept. Extreme forms of
this position were taken by many Kleinians too who are more
prone to direct symbolic interpretative approaches than considerations of level of ego integration in casting their remarks to
patients. The recent upsurge of Lacanian psychoanalysis, an
approach that uses *The Interpretation of Dreams* as the text to be
analyzed, also prescribes greater attention to the unconscious as
a deeply structured, contentful organization, renaming it the
Discourse of the Other.

   While these positions may represent a kind of counterrefor-
mation espousing a radical or radically conservative view of
psychoanalysis, there are many who believe that ego psychology
and some of its variations can very well be melded with the aim
of depth analysis and restated in terms of the central requirements of symbolic transformation. It would be pitiable for the
less flamboyant among us if the central spokesmen for depth
analysis were cast solely in the images of Klein and Lacan. I
think Marianne Kris would have concurred. There is sufficient
solidity in our approach to depth understanding so that we
need not discard all because parts of theory are less tenable now
than earlier. Libido theory may be the stumbling block for
many "moderns." It may, however, be viewed as a theory of
stage- and phase-related fantasies which are anchored in the
development of personality, psychopathology, and even symptom choice. We need not, at this stage, discard it as obsolete
because it is closely tied to energic concepts, which unfortunately blind our way to clarity because of their tenuous theoretical
status. Having supervised with Marianne Kris, I recognized in
her supervisory approach a firm devotion to depth and defense
analysis derived from free association and play. Many *moderns*
seem to forsake free association as the means by which interpretation of dreams and symptoms and traits is achieved
(see, however, Anton Kris, 1982) and have substituted instead
anagogic and analogic paraphrases of observed behavior (see
Stein, 1981; Shapiro, 1982).

The technique that would permit the unfolding of the unconscious was important to Marianne Kris, as it ought to be to those of us working even in the 1980s. This aim also can be accomplished without the fanciful constructions of the Kleinians; interpretation can be brought into close relation to the conscious life of the child and, as experience grows, to include many events. Malcove's (1933) early paper that relates childhood theories of dismemberment to the cutting and mashing of food represents to me the kind of evidential base that is experience-close for human beings. Fantasies derived from such experiences are incorporated into phase-related themes that ought to be reconsidered by analysts and interpreted. How fantasies become guiding forces for life, and the source of childhood theories that lead to misinformation, also ought to concern us more than the pat reinterpretation of experiences as stale derivatives that are the hallmark of wild analysis. On the more conservative side, we dare not ignore unconscious fantasies and substitute warm, caring corrective experiences as *the* therapeutic tool.

T. S. Eliot once wrote that there are three basic experiences in life: birth, copulation, and death. Ernest Jones (1916) added four other basic universal fantasies to these three. But even if these are the base deep structures according to which we order our data, the phenomenology of play sequences, unique life events, and individual family constellations add considerable variability to the way in which these universal fantasies are organized, emerge, and dictate life course.

In this paper I shall recount an experience that is designed to confront the issues mentioned and which reaffirms the central focus of psychoanalysis as a science of symbolic transformation and the discovery of unconscious fantasy by the use of a specific method. In applying it to children we attempt to discover how children respond idiosyncratically and personally to universal themes that are part of growing up as a human because of the need to master life events with both symptoms and character traits. The event that will be recounted is a single meeting with a youngster. Some might view the incident to be told from the standpoint of newer theories and ask if the analyst could not have acted differently in order to help this child. I cannot redo the consultation. However, I believe that I would not have done anything differently today and that may be why I write about it. This most remarkable, poignant meeting firmed my central conviction about what the central aim of psychoanalysis ought to be.

Although Winnicott's (1971) Squiggle game was used as a technical innovation, the essential focus of the meeting was depth psychoanalytic and provided an important clue to understanding a cognitive confusion. Although I claim a depth focus to guide my understanding, the interpretation or, more precisely, the clarification was presented to the child in words directed to the ego. In that sense commonplace childhood problems and symptoms may be said to yield to an essentially linguistic intrusion. I would argue that this procedure is not dissimilar to Freud's interpretative approach as presented in both *The Interpretation of Dreams* (1900) and in the early paper on defense neuropsychosis (1894)—namely, we use words to reveal and render accessible that which until then had been cast in nonlinguistic derivatives of action or symbolic representation. The method holds up but has been neglected in recent writing.

The strength of conviction that I believe accompanies these data derives from what I consider to be the self-evident nature of this child's productions as well as the immediate therapeutic effects of the interpretation. Moreover, the interpenetration of phase-related themes with life events should be noted. I had the opportunity to present the material to Marianne Kris briefly following the excitement of the consultation. The characteristic delight in discovery and the enthusiasm that she demonstrated were lively parts of her teaching style that was so important to the many people she instructed during her long, productive career.

The event to be described concerned a 5-year-old who developed a phase-related sleep disturbance which became more severe in a setting where she was confronted with learning the meaning of death. Her cognitive appreciation of this difficult concept was incorporated into phase-related fantasies that came into full contact with unconscious fantasies and, as Freud suggested, resonated with them just as the day residue grabs hold of a deeper organization. The sleep disturbance was most distressing to her and her parents, but the meaning of the sleep disturbance and the reason for its presence constitute the essential aspects of what had to be analyzed.

THE CASE OF EMILY

BACKGROUND

Recently, at the end of January, Emily's parents consulted me about their 5-year-old daughter. They complained about her sleep disturbance which kept her in a hypervigilant state that made it difficult for her to go to sleep and caused her to wake up frightened in the middle of the night. Once she was awake it was most difficult to help her to relax so that she could again fall off. The family feared that the sleep disturbance had been caused by Emily's learning of the recent death of two cousins, a child of 6 and his mother, in a fire at their country home.

Emily and her family had been away on a Christmas vacation. During the vacation Emily already showed some signs of restlessness and sleeplessness, but not so severe as to warrant concern. They returned to their suburban home just prior to New Year's and were told about the death of Emily's cousins. The disturbance became accentuated after Emily learned of the tragedy.

When Emily awakened she was anxious and trembling, complaining about dinosaurs who would eat her up; she also had fears and worries that the rest of the family would die while she was asleep, and she expressed concern about the possibility that her parents would make a new baby. Emily already had a younger brother, aged 3, who slept in a separate room. The parents were in their late 30s, the father a surgeon. The mother was the firmer of the two parents—more insistent that the child go back to sleep and stay in her room. The father, on the other hand, was somewhat more touched by the child's complaint, more easily cajoled into caring for her and sitting with her until she slept again. Both parents were sincerely disturbed about what had transpired and convinced of the traumatic effect that the cousins' death had on Emily. They could conceive of no other reason why Emily would have a sleep disturbance—despite the fact that the sleep disturbance had begun during the vacation.

The remainder of Emily's developmental and behavioral history was well within normal limits. The family could not bring Emily for consultation until mid-February, on Valentine's day. In the interim, the father wished to give the child mild doses of Benadryl at bedtime in order to see if he could not interrupt some of the desperation of the evening pattern. Just prior to my consultation with the child, he wrote me the following letter:

> Since we spoke with you, Emily's initial hysteria at bedtime has subsided. She has talked some and told me that she is not really afraid of dinosaurs, etc. Emily is afraid of dying; of the family dying. She says whenever she sees her grandmother she is reminded that her grandfather is dead. Emily has always spoken of wanting a baby sister for herself and a baby brother for Ronald. She now says she wants no more babies in the family: she doesn't want daddy's penis in mother's vagina. She spoke about death—I just listened sympathetically; she knows the answer, but does not want to hear that everyone does die. When she spoke about babies, I told her that we were very happy to have her and Ronald and at this time we do not plan to have any more children. She seemed satisfied and reassured with this answer, which is truthful.
>
> Emily now has to sleep with all the lights on and someone to stay with her (since having his own bedroom, Ronald has slept with his room fully lit and last year requested nightly that someone stay with him; once in a while someone did, but usually he was told to wait in bed until we had finished in the kitchen, and he would fall off to sleep by himself—she had never had more than a tiny night light and went right to bed).
>
> I believe her fear and anxiety regarding death and reproduction are genuine. However, although she seems more in control of herself, I do not think it is because she has accepted anything, rather she has chosen not to think about it. Bedtime is a long, drawn-out affair. Emily falls asleep about 9:30 to 10:00 P.M. regularly with one of us in her room, and awakens almost every night at 3:00 A.M. for 15 to 30 minutes.

It was clear that the symptom was under some control even before I saw the child, but that the anxiety persisted and that its meaning was still unknown except in the most general terms. I had scheduled an early morning appointment for Emily. She and her father were waiting outside in the lobby as I arrived to open the front door. My first view of Emily revealed that she was a pretty, slight child, slender, with big dark-brown eyes and long dark-brown hair carefully plaited into a long braid that hung almost to her waist. She was neatly dressed in plaid skirt and tights. She hid behind her father as they entered the waiting room. Although I did not approach her as she undid her coat, she snuggled behind her father pulling at his trousers. She then smiled coyly as I attempted to greet her. She was eating a small sugared breakfast bun which was held neatly in a partially opened napkin. Dots of confectioners sugar showed around her mouth. It was clear to me that at that moment separation from her father would be a terrible tussle and I was not about to venture a consultation with a child assaulted on first meeting by acute separation anxiety. I therefore invited both father and daughter into the office and further invited Emily to help me release a wall-held table and set up the room for our meeting. She immediately disengaged herself her from father and helped quietly. She then made her first spontaneous advance toward me as she turned her face away and held out the bun to offer me a bite. I demurred and began to puzzle about how to approach Emily. I had just been entranced at reading Winnicott's *Therapeutic Consultations with Children* (1971) and thought of the possibilities of the Squiggle game for children who will not or cannot talk. I thought that this technique might be a welcome entry in this circumstance.

As I pulled out a pack of paper and sat down on the floor with her giving Emily her own pencil, I said simply that I would make a scribble. I indicated that she could complete it and make a picture of any sort that she liked. She brightened, took the pencil in hand, looked at her father momentarily, and began. She engaged in the game directly and persistently and was not diverted throughout the entire hour of our meeting. When she finally spoke, she was fluent with speech that was marred by a slightly sibilant "s" slur. She was permitted to elaborate her answers and comments as she pleased, and I did not probe. The increase in fluency and animation was evident in her facial expressions, the music and tonal quality of her voice. In general she was a child who was quite articulate, animated, and affectively spontaneous. Within two minutes of the onset of the consultation simultaneous with the drawing of the second squiggle I casually asked her father whether he would not rather sit in the waiting room. He assented and left as Emily paid almost no attention to his departure.

THE SQUIGGLE GAME

1. I constructed an S-like structure on its side. Emily: A worm—which is all upside down. (Fig. 1.)

2. I then made horizontal and vertical lines as though beginning a square. She completed it. Emily: Pants. (Fig. 2.)

3. I then made another S-like structure. Emily: An 8 for the squiggle. (Fig. 3.)

4. I constructed another S-like figure, she crossed it, placed two zeros and an X on it. Emily: X's for tic-tac-toe board. (Fig. 4.)

5. I made a circle. Emily: A circle—a girl. [What's her name?] Arlene. [Tell me about her?] Her birthday was yesterday, she was 2 years old, she had a Snoopy party and she had a beautiful triangle cake with a standup Snoopy on it. (Fig. 5.)

6. I drew a horizontal line. Emily: A dress. [What about it?] Arlene was wearing a pretty blue dress. (Fig. 6)

7. I constructed an inverted U. Emily: It's a cup—and there were standup cups at the party. (Fig. 7.)

8. I suggested that she do the next one by herself. Emily: It's a boot. There is a zipper on it. [Who has such boots?] Mommy, but Ronald and I have little ones which you can't tell apart, which have fur inside. [Mommy has a big one and you and Ronald have little ones which are just the same!] (Fig. 8.)

9. I drew an inverted V. Emily: It's a clown's hat with a pompom. [Have you ever seen one like it?] We went to the circus and we also saw ballerinas on a horse who went in a circle and stood on top of the horse and danced. [Do you dance?] Yes,

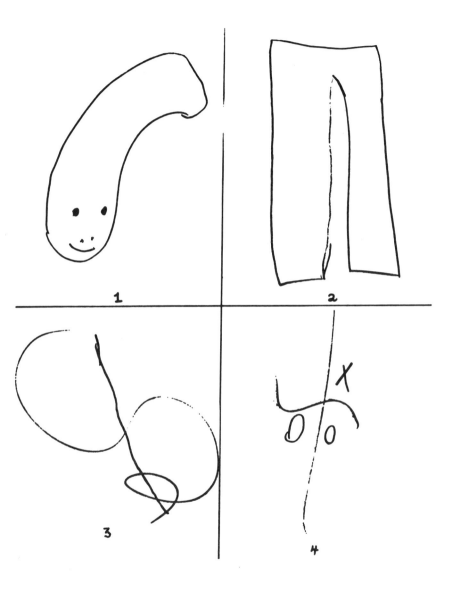

1

2

3

4

Figures 1–4

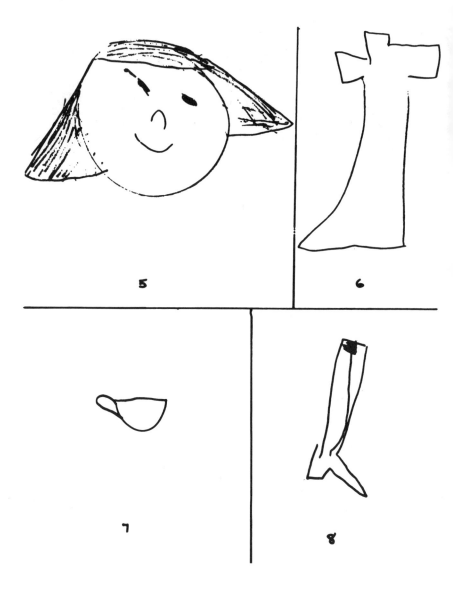

5

6

7

8

Figures 5–8

I go to dancing school, but I am going to be a *nurse* and work with my daddy in a hospital. Do you know that he takes care of little children? And does surgery on them, and puts children to sleep with sleepy air? [Why does he put them to sleep?] So that he can take out their hernias and appendixes! [What are those?] Those are little bumps that people have. (Fig. 9.)

10. I made another S figure. Emily: A tree. [Tell me about it.] It is going to develop apples! [Oh?] We have an uncle who lives on a farm in Massachusetts, and an aunt, and there are two cousins in the house. I forgot the older one's name. Do you know they have a dog who let me pour raisins on his back when I was 2 years old [giggles]. [Such good things happen to 2-year-olds!] I'll be able to do it again. (Fig. 10.)

11. She now drew a house on her own. Emily: That's a house—Aunt L. and Uncle B. have a house that looks like that, and it's made of bricks, I mean wood. [Is that good or bad?] Well, it has bricks on the outside and wood on the inside. [And that's what makes it good?] Because bricks and wood are good for houses. Wood is not as good as brick, because it can chip, splinter, . . . and rust. [And what else can it do?] It can break. (Fig. 11.)

12. I made another deeper S-like structure. Emily: A cat [Fig. 12]—my friend has a guinea pig and a cat, and I am going to get one for my birthday. [When is it?] In the spring. Ronald had a Snoopy party in November when he was 3, and a Fireman party when he was 4. [I know you like a Snoopy party, but how do you like a Fireman party?] It's okay . . . firemen are good for putting out fires [noticeable sadness in her voice]. [I heard that there was a sad fire recently in your faimly.] Yes, I felt sad that they died; you know a sister did get out. . . . I look at my daddy's surgery book and see pictures of them doing dog surgery. My mother and Amy had their appendixes out. [Your mother and Amy?] Well, they only have it out if it is infected, and you cut a hole in a blanket when they are asleep—I saw my mother's scar. [Maybe you would like to draw it.] What if it comes out like a child? [Do it as you like to. She draws and says,] The oval part of the scar is what I'm going to show, and she has a pony tail. [You have one too! Disdainfully she says,] I have a braid. My hair is as long, no longer than my mother's. (Fig. 13.)

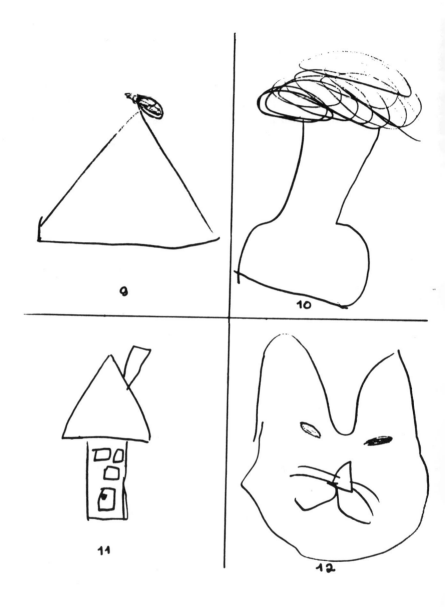

9

10

11

12

Figures 9–12

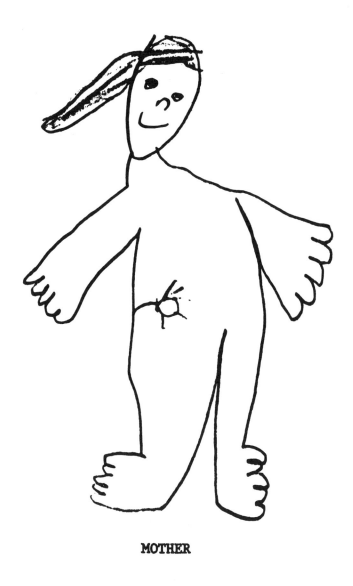

MOTHER

Figure 13

At this moment, our time was drawing to a close, and the aims of the Squiggle game had been achieved. Winnicott believes that as preconscious ideas become available to verbalization and reveal the willingness of the child to explore some of the feelings associated, enough work has been done and one need not press the child further. Moreover, the ego defenses should also be reconstituted to help master the traumatic constellations. I considered that I would have the opportunity to see her again. But I also had witnessed the emergence of defensive structures that seemed to me to be adequate to effect the linkages between death and surgery as well as the regressive pull toward the oedipal attachment to her father. I therefore shifted ground and asked if she would like to draw a person. She responded, "Clothes on or off?" When I said, "Whichever way you like," she drew a female first, and then made a male (see fig. 14).

She spontaneously began to describe the drawings as if there was pressure to reveal more and said, "The girl is 8 years old. It's supposed to be pink and yellow in her dress, but I couldn't draw it. She is going to a party with her dress on and she is very happy." (Why?) "Because she is going to dance and she likes to do that." She then turned to the boy and said that the boy was going fishing. First he is going to go inside and get his fishing pole, and then go down to the creek and fish. And then he's got to find some worms. She made a sour face. (Oh, you don't like worms?) "They are squiggly and icky and yucky." She became animated and suggested that her brother and she once found a toad and made it jump on her mother, which made her jump, and then they made a special place behind their house, out of chicken wire to keep the toad. They supplied the toad with ample moss on the bottom, and they made a *toad bed* out of moss and *put it to sleep* one night. In the morning they found that it was so sleepy that it couldn't get up. Her father was asked to examine it, only to declare: *"The toad is dead!"*

I suggested to her that it was a hard thing for children to tell the *difference between sleeping and dying,* and that makes going to sleep very worrisome. I then added that even though children sometimes get confused, grownups know the difference very well. She exited from the meeting, smiling, attached herself to her father, and coyly reengaged him as she left.

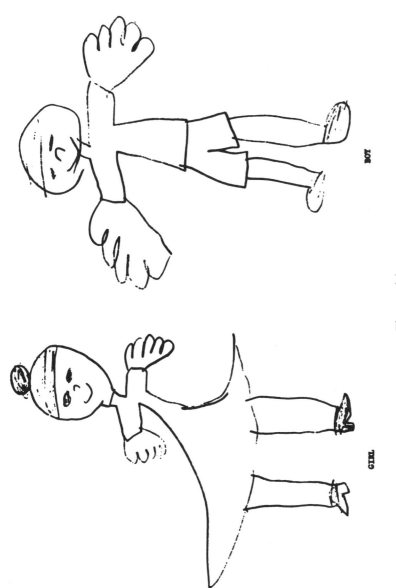

BOY

GIRL

Figure 14

The second session, one week later, saw a happy, bright, and interested child. In the interim, she had sent an affectionately decorated Valentine's card. This time she was very interested in my toy closet and the materials in it; she focused most acutely on folders of other children, wishing to make her own and thereby to establish a place with me.

The subsequent meeting with the parents designed to round out the consultation revealed that Emily was sleeping well, that she was no longer as anxious, and that there was a major diminution of disturbing behavior. Since the meeting had been initiated around a single symptom, I did not feel justified in suggesting treatment, and indicated to the family that they were welcome to call as they needed. They were not eager to continue either.

DISCUSSION

I have presented this case verbally to many psychoanalysts, and have been asked: Why did you not insist on carrying the analysis further? Why did you not approach the child's narcissistic injury at having an unempathic mother? Why did you not interpret the clearly defined oedipal constellation and castration anxiety? Why did you not approach the preoedipal ambivalence toward the mother? Why did you not do parent counseling?

These queries are legitimate and relate well to the central issue of how one practices; that is, how can our grasp of depth psychology lead to better understanding and then help us to make our interventions at the appropriate level without stirring up more sediment than is necessary, and also permit development to proceed? Moreover, when should we stop even when we understand more? The answers are determined by our theory of change and how that theory interacts with our ideas about normative development and the growth of meaning. Technique should follow directly from how we understand theory and how we use our knowledge of unconscious functioning.

This case is an apt example of how a common symptom of sleep disturbance (Hertzig and Beltramini, 1983) can become a violent assault on a family and a most distressing and uncomfortable symptom to a child. The confusion of meaning between death and sleep is quite natural given the child's wish for death to be reversible, and sleep signifying loss of conscious control of the known world. Indeed, even our cultural tendency to refer to death in terms of sleep must add to childhood confusion and anxiety. The often-repeated bedtime prayer that admits to "if I die before I wake" is probably so ritualized that most children hardly appreciate the significance of the words; otherwise Emily's symptom might be more widespread.

The appreciation of death as irreversible and an end to which we all must come has provoked a vast literature on the stages in the appreciation of death and the capacity for mourning. While these themes are not central to my presentation, this case and other clinical experiences suggest that the understanding of death may be a discreet event in time rather than a gradual acquisition. Appreciation of its significance may occur as early as 3 and as late as the senium. The degree of cultural and personal defense that accrues is not so much existential *but,* as Freud (1926) suggested, a recasting of developmental anxieties ranging from separation to castration. Emily's case presents elements of both.

Emily wished to be in control. Her light must be on, her eyes open. She wanted a parent in her room. Her father gratified her wishes. Separation themes surely abound. Yet, her loving protector also was a "castrator" of women and children who lie helpless when they sleep. He cut holes in blankets and surgically removed bumps—her mother and Amy were living examples with their appendectomy scars. However, and fortunately, their long ponytails or big boots with fur remained testimony to the wished-for equality between brothers and sisters and mothers and daughters. Indeed, what better altruistic surrender and defense against anxiety than to become father's helper, a nurse, and participate actively in symbolic castrations while awake rather than risk sleep, passivity, and mutilation. The fire, in turn, was a trigger that caused the bitter realization that death is indeed possible for the young as well as the old and that it is not reversible. Thus sleep also leads to mortal danger.

It is almost a pity to belabor the obvious in this case. Emily's words are far more poetically rich as her story unfolded than a dry rehash. However, the multiple layers of this *translation* will, I think, better help us to find the appropriate level of interpretation if we spell out the trends.

If nurse Emily is to succeed, then father surgeon dare not join mother to make babies, however that is done. The regressive suggestion of oral ingestion by a dinosaur or an assault while asleep is frightening enough to wish for times when the world was happy as a warm puppy (a Snoopy party with raisins and standup everything)—a regressive paradise when knowledge of death need not even be considered.

All the foregoing is not very fanciful even to a behaviorist given the data of our Squiggle game, but it is familiar because we have had 90 years of psychoanalysis—the derivatives and dynamics leap out at us. What might have been more remarkable in 1910 or 1930 was: why did Emily not have more than a sleep disturbance? The answer comes from within our science; psychodynamics is not psychopathology! Marianne Kris (1957) wrote in her paper on prediction in a longitudinal study, "in general we have been more accurate in predicting areas of conflict, difficulty and pathology than we have been in predicting conflict-free functioning and the use of normal defenses. This may be due to a general tendency in many of us to look for the 'defect'" (p. 186); or, as Anna Freud (1965) would put it, regressions in developmental lines. These views are useful for a modern consideration of Emily's problem. Except for her sleep problem she was made of good stuff. Her ego functions were well in place, and she had an encapsulated anxiety that made sense psychologically.

The central theme of this presentation rests on the idea that it made sense psychologically because we could visualize the depth features of the symptom as the child permitted us to see the layered fantasies that supported the surface manifestation. The logic of the symptom was made understandable by finding the depth fantasy. This is the age-old claim of psychoanalysis. It is also the hallmark of any structuralist model since linguistics was born. The technique of listening without excess intrusion permitted the fantasies to emerge, and the pressure of the peremptoriness of the fantasies suggests their close relation to significant drives. Were the latter not so, we would not so easily have been permitted to construct a story that makes sense. With another story, another method, another theory, our ideas might emerge differently—but I think not as self-evidently. The recent hermeneutic approach to psychoanalysis suggests that any story told to a patient might be equally therapeutic. I doubt this because only the fit to the facts of the child's life permits conviction. Indeed, I believe that the patient's conviction does not emerge from fluff or "any story"; rather, his or her own story is a derivative of a universal grammar of stories that constitute the store of base human fantasies; these result from our ontogenesis and our prewired central nervous system that has weathered Darwinian survival.

I return to Emily and the question why I did not belabor her oedipus complex and its regressive components once I had uncovered them. The answer lies in the description of the process and in Winnicott's claim (1971) for the Squiggle game: "The child may of course feel to have been more understood than in fact he or she was understood, but the effect will have been to have given the child some hope of being understood and perhaps even helped" (p. 5).

The description of the play reveals that the child's fantasies were emergent and preconscious. According to Ernst Kris (1956), their interpretation is then timely. Winnicott's claim is that the feeling of being understood participates in the strength of the interpretative force. I chose to limit my comments to the cognitive confusion because of both factors stated.

I had not contracted with family or child to engage in further work. I did not wish to risk the effect of a grander intervention by its too rapid association with a more far-fetched notion. The risk of defensive denial, the question of love for and ambivalence to parents with whom the child still resides and on whom she depends are significant here. Besides, the rules of symbolic transformation (Werner and Kaplan, 1963) would suggest that Emily's dim awareness of the source of her anxiety was sufficient for this time in her young development.

1. The fantasies were universal in form and phase-adequate, although idiosyncratic to her unique life.

2. The emergent representation in a symptom was time- and ego-bound. No other functions were encroached on.

3. Her relationships suffered only around the anxious focus.
4. Her development was proceeding.

These factors seem sufficient to have dictated the narrowness of what I told her in words.

However, some will see in this a direct counter to the purpose of this presentation, i.e., my claim that the unconscious still does and still should occupy us. I do not think so, for it seems evident that my circumscribed treatment of Emily's dilemma was dictated by the very notion that the unconscious fantasies were most relevant and that my restraint in telling all was part of our general psychoanalytic knowledge that telling all is wild analysis and that ego factors must be considered to determine the limits of what we may convey in words.

The richness of psychoanalytic theory would suggest that every surface derivative could lead to an associative path to complete self-knowledge. Yet we cannot formularize that except in a few base forms or universal fantasies. The latter, however, are indeed empty without significant sensitivity to experiential and ego anchors. This is even more so during the current Freudian era where the excitement of the unconscious has become banal. This banalization of the unconscious is a result of common usage and popularization. For this reason special attention must be paid to interpreting derivatives within the patient's *personal* idiom. On the other hand, there is no reason for us to give up approaches centering on the interpretation of unconscious content for new theories or to suggest new models of analysis that completely overturn Freud's basic discovery.

We have come full circle to discover that the unconscious does occupy us, *but* what may be different now is the care with which we interpret it—rather than discard it. I submit that my language suggests a new reification of the unconscious. I refer to an "it." I do not intend to do so. I am using "it" as a convenient, though regressive metaphor for latent fantasies that comprise the base grammar of conscious behavior and thought. This "it" or "id" should not be neglected if we are to provide patients who are children (the ambiguity is deliberate) with a feeling that they are understood—or, to paraphrase Winnicott, that there is "some hope of being understood and perhaps even helped."

BIBLIOGRAPHY

FREUD, A. (1936), The ego and the mechanisms of defense. *W.*, 2.
——— (1965), Normality and pathology in childhood. *W.*, 6.
FREUD, S. (1894), The neuro-psychoses of defence. *S. E.*, 3:45–61.
——— (1900), The interpretation of dreams. *S. E.*, 4 & 5.
——— (1926), Inhibitions, symptoms and anxiety. *S. E.*, 20:77–175.
——— (1937), Constructions in analysis. *S. E.*, 23:257–269.
GLOVER, E. (1961), Some recent trends in psychoanalytic theory. *Psychoanal. Q.*, 30:86–107.
HARTMANN, H. (1939), *Ego Psychology and the Problem of Adaptation*. New York: Int. Univ. Press.
HERTZIG, M. & BELTRAMINI, A. (1983), Individual differences in the longitudinal course of sleep and bedtime behavior in preschool children. *J. Amer. Acad. Child Psychiat.* (in press).
JONES, E. (1916), The theory of symbolism. In *Papers on Psycho-Analysis*. London: Baillière, Tindall & Cox, 1948, pp. 87–144.
KRIS, A. O. (1982), *Free Association*. New Haven & London: Yale Univ. Press.
KRIS, E. (1956), The recovery of childhood memories in psychoanalysis. *Psychoanal. Study Child*, 11:54–88.
KRIS, M. (1957), The use of prediction in a longitudinal study. *Psychoanal. Study Child*, 12:175–189.
KUBIE, L. S. (1953), The distortion of the symbolic process in neurosis and psychosis. *J. Amer. Psychoanal. Assn.*, 1:59–85.
MALCOVE, L. (1933), Bodily mutilation and learning to eat. *Psychoanal. Q.*, 2:557–561.
SHAPIRO, T. (1982), Empathy. *Psychoanal. Inquiry*, 1:423–448.
STEIN, M. H. (1981), The unobjectionable part of the transference. *J. Amer. Psychoanal. Assn.*, 29:869–892.
WERNER, H. & KAPLAN, B. (1963), *Symbol Formation*. New York: Wiley.
WINNICOTT, D. W. (1971), *Therapeutic Consultations in Child Psychiatry*. New York: Basic Books.

On Anxiety and Terror

ISIDOR SILBERMANN, M.D., F.A.C.P.

IN A PREVIOUS PAPER (1981), I HAVE SUGGESTED THAT ANX-
iety is the ego's response to its perception of a disturbance to its
equilibrium. Anxiety is the alarm which the ego sounds in its
attempt to mobilize its defenses and discharge mechanisms to
reestablish balance (Freud, 1926). The intensity of anxiety depends on the degree of imbalance. Thus, anxiety can "whisper
or roar" and, in extreme cases, swell to an overwhelming cre-
scendo of terror.

Features common to anxiety are: feelings of impending danger, failure, etc., or of threat to life, to security, to sanity, and to
control over aggressive and libidinal impulses. Due to these
feelings of threatening dangers or loss, anxieties are rarely, if
ever, free of depressive features, just as depressions rarely lack
anxiety. The deep withdrawal of depressed patients is therefore frequently, if not always, loaded with anxiety. The cata-
tonic stupor of schizophrenics is another illustration.

Balance is always temporary, precarious, and unstable. Once
established, it is often jarred, disturbed, and reestablished. In
addition to minor shifts of equilibrium, however, there are always changes with greater impact on the ego, and deeper reactions in it. Those minor shifts in mind and body, wavelike and
incessant, in their daily course are regulated, within limits,
without stormy upheavals. They are for the most part mute and
their mental representations are subliminal. There are, however, functional shifts which force a *total* alteration of equipoise.
These shifts via their mental representations are experienced
by the ego as consciously disturbing emotions, as "feelings of

Faculty, New York Psychoanalytic Institute.

anxiety." These latter may be called "threshold anxieties." Finally, there are high waves of disturbance which keep the ego's balance in long-lasting or even constant turmoil; these we call "pathological anxieties."

In other papers I have described anxiety as the experience of disequilibrium: in disturbances of the vegetative centers (1929), in cases with disbalance of the ego due to its regression before and during menstruation (1950), in climacterium (1961), and during maturation and development (1979). Now I return to a major and severe balance disturbance and its resulting stormy emotion, terror, the abysmal escalation of anxiety. I refer here to patients with dramatic pathological changes of blood sugar levels.

A woman returned after many years of successful analysis and requested further therapy. She had developed sudden overwhelming attacks of anxiety which appeared out of the blue, at home and at work. I requested an examination by an internist who, after confirming a suspected diabetes, ended her hypoglycemic attacks and with them her terrifying fits of anxiety.

In 1940 I reported observations and conclusions which I had made in a mental hospital in Hatton, England, on patients undergoing insulin-coma treatment (under Dr. D. N. Parfitt). The hypoglycemia produced a grave balance disturbance in the ego, experienced as a pathological anxiety in the form of a terror of death. My report concluded with the statement that one of the essential features of the hypoglycemic coma is the intense fear of death with the subsequent experience of rebirth and the associated euphoria.

On their descent into the strange realm of unconsciousness, these patients' egos showed progressive "fragmentation at its worst" and severe disequilibrium; and as their hold on reality vanished, they experienced mounting terror. On the return to consciousness there was a reversal of the phenomena. With the ego's now "modified" reintegration and resynthesis, feelings of hopefulness and happiness followed.

Another observation proved of value. Some patients could not shake off the heavy weight of their disequilibrium and regained consciousness only with great difficulty. This happened when, during their restitution, they encountered unfriendly and demanding attitudes on the part of nurses. When this observation was shared with the nursing personnel, more caring approaches facilitated quicker recovery from the coma. All the observations and conclusions of 1940 found confirmation in the dramatic experience of a patient in psychoanalytic therapy, during which his diabetes was discovered. He had frequent attacks of hypoglycemia with high-pitched anxiety; but on two occasions his equilibrium was so severely disturbed that he sank into a state bordering unconsciousness, which he recalled as a deep sleep with peculiar dreamlike experiences:

I am suddenly aware of a red blanket of a peculiar texture, of an unusual weave. It feels strange. I feel that I am moving into another world, that I am between two worlds, and I experience growing and tormenting panic. I tell myself that I must come back before it's too late. The question whether I will be able to come through that gate holds terror and danger; the question whether I will be in control at that moment is petrifying. I can't find the words to describe that nightmarish dream. I become progressively sleepier and I would like to sleep, sleep, and sleep. I must have fallen into a very deep sleep.

Then slowly I cross a bridge to a wonderful place. Although I still have some fear that I might have missed that bridge and remained in the land of agonizing terror, I feel reprieved. Soon I find myself in a vast space surrounded by a great light. There are exquisite paintings covering the walls and ceiling, with shades of light grays and pearly pinks. But they do not remain still; they move, change shapes, break apart, and come together again in a fantastic ever-changing dance.

Although everything is puzzling, there is a feeling of increasing peace. I feel excited that I have created all this beauty and that I am becoming my own self. Then I feel no fear anymore. I am enchanted. Although the fabulous light holds the whole dream together and there is a whisper of music around me, I feel that I have been in another world, a strange land, and that I have taken a very long journey through it. I am aware that my wife and you [the analyst] are here; but it seems that you are not participants but only silent onlookers. I feel that I am getting my own self together again, and that I am elated to be alive again. But I cannot get my bearings yet; the environment moves slowly into focus, and objects only leisurely assume their distinct forms. I want to speak; but I cannot. I hear myself mumble; but I am unable to put my dreams into words. Although I feel that I have crossed the bridge from unreality to reality, I also feel that I am still too weak to grasp and to hold on to things. I feel dizzy and suspended.

His wife, aware of his condition, encouraged him to drink orange juice. But he refused, turned away, and closed his lips tightly. He described those moments:

> Her voice sounded far too loud, too demanding, too threatening; her movements too forceful and aggressive. I felt that if I wanted to remain secure in my regained life, I must resist her attacks. But the terror slowly subsided, her words lost their sharpness, things lost their haziness, and I lost my fear. Finally I felt assured by her compassion and solicitude. I felt that she had helped me to hold on to reality and face the tasks ahead. My feelings of beauty and enchantment and my lack of fear stayed with me for quite a while.

We find in that rather poetic description of his nightmarish state many features similar to my formulation in the previously mentioned paper (1940): the terrifying sinking into the dark abyss of the unconscious, the progressive loss of reality on the way into the strange world of nothingness; and then, on his return to the world of real life, the slow reconstruction of his self and his environment. He also saw colors in a variety of bright lights. He perceived strange acoustic phenomena, forms disintegrating and reintegrating in a fantastic, ever-changing dance. Although there was fear at the beginning, when he crossed the bridge, he returned from the foreign land of death. He was also bewildered by his inability to speak. He could not formulate words, syllables became mixed up; at first only sounds crossed his lips. Then he mumbled incoherently until he finally regained his ability to express himself freely. He also felt threatened by his wife's too aggressive attempts; and he rejected her help. His still very weak ego had not yet gained proper differentiation and judgment.

In 1940 I decided to utilize the elevated mood following the deep regression of these hospital patients after insulin-induced hypoglycemia for exploratory purposes and for supportive psychotherapy. Many patients seemed to respond favorably; many who were previously able to communicate could speak more freely and express their emotions without great distress. Many became more sociable and participated in various work or play activities.

Now, with my diabetic patient who underwent psychoanalytic therapy because of anxiety (feelings of inefficiency and incompetence), the question forced itself on me whether the *temporary* changes following his coma could possibly be connected with the dramatic assaults on his ego, and with his regression and his ego's reconstruction. Not wanting to confuse post hoc with propter hoc, I shall limit myself to a description of my observations. Although they were not made in connection with an artificially produced state, they nonetheless involved a genuine pathological one. While my patient's experience of terror was induced by *physical* factors, it subsequently led to dramatic *psychological* changes.

The sessions following his spontaneous hypoglycemic shocks showed noteworthy changes. For a time after his attacks, he described himself as more alive, more self-assured, less restrained, and freer in all respects. His associations flowed with greater ease; he was more alert; and his often negative, doubting attitudes had given way to a more positive cooperation. His transference became more tractable, his speech more fluent and better modulated, and his language showed more color and variety. His mood was better and his life seemed to move on smoother tracks. He expressed his feelings by saying, "Now I can do all I have to." A feature came to the fore which previously had been kept in repression. He was now able on his own to discover the subtle links so essential for psychoanalytic therapy. He found connections which until then seemed to have been beyond his reach; dreams were described with greater facility; and his artistic personality seemed to unfold with greater freedom. His resynthesized and reintegrated ego had seemingly gained new strength and solidity. It did not flutter and scatter as easily as before. The treatment moved along as if a breeze had swelled the analytic sails.

Somehow it had dawned on him that the concept of a forest

as a collection of trees is too narrow and too concrete; that words are not empty but possess substance, shades, and facets; that the interstices between lines are filled with meaning and suspended feeling; and that silences and pauses carry melodious sounds and speak an expressive language of their own; that symbols and metaphors are like the colors of the rainbow condensed into light. They are concentrated and supercharged; and if their veils are lifted, they depict, with a paucity of strokes, many panoramic views.

The closeness to death apparently cleared the road to greater insight. It helped him to see that life does not move on one simple plane; that it has not one but many facets and aspects; and that light and shades as well as the harmony of colors create beauty.

Balance between body and mind, between past and present, between one's self and others, between the unconscious and the conscious, between reality and fantasy—in short, *equilibrium plus the absence of anxiety resulting from equipoise*—has always been man's deep-seated goal.

BIBLIOGRAPHY

FREUD, S. (1926), Inhibitions, symptoms and anxiety. *S. E.*, 20:77–125.

SILBERMANN, I. (1929), Über eine eigenartige Störung der vegetativen Zentren. *Z. ges. Neurol. & Psychiat.*, 118:752–772.

———— (1940), The psychical experiences during shocks in shock therapy. *Int. J. Psychoanal.*, 21:179–200.

———— (1950), A contribution to the psychology of menstruation. *Int. J. Psychoanal.*, 31:258–267.

———— (1961), Synthesis and fragmentation. *Psychoanal. Study Child*, 16:90–117.

———— (1979), Mental transitional spheres. *Psychoanal. Q.*, 48:85–106.

———— (1981), Balance and anxiety. *Psychoanal. Study Child*, 36:365–378.

APPLICATIONS OF
PSYCHOANALYSIS

The Contribution of Psychoanalysis to the Psychotherapy of Adolescents

PETER BLOS, Ph.D.

SELECTED PRINCIPLES OF ADOLESCENT PSYCHOTHERAPY

PSYCHOANALYSIS IS A THEORY OF THE HUMAN MIND AND A method of healing its ills. As a theory of the mind psychoanalysis has a bearing—either as a technique or an explication—on all kinds of systematic endeavor to influence and change human behavior within the limit of the individual's wish to do so. True enough, this wish is not always present as our ready ally, and it becomes our job to induce a desire for change. What we always can rely on is the patient's wish to be relieved of an unpleasant mental state. Only too often the deliverance from mental pain is expected to come about by that legendary recovery of a repressed childhood memory which has become the popular mystique of psychotherapy in many of its varieties. The romantic concept of therapy, so widespread today, is simply being "made to feel good." Contemporary language uses the word therapy with this kind of connotation in mind. People speak of going skiing, talking to a friend, or listening to music

Faculty, New York Psychoanalytic Institute, Columbia University, Center for Psychoanalytic Training and Research, The New York Freudian Society.

A shortened version of this paper was presented at the first Institute of the Association for Child Psychoanalysis on "Child Therapy from an Analytic Perspective," San Diego, California, March 1981; and at the congress of the International Association for Child and Adolescent Psychiatry and Allied Professions, Dublin, Ireland, July 1982.

as "therapeutic," equating the experiences of pleasure and relief from distress as the essence of the therapeutic process. Such expectations brush aside the fact that therapy not only resolves old conflicts but introduces by its very nature new conflicts which—by their continual resolution—lift psychic functioning onto a higher, more complex level. This level, which we call maturity, can never be maintained easily and effortlessly. It is, assuredly, a life task.

The specific therapeutic endeavor of which I speak here is psychoanalytic psychotherapy of the adolescent. Its method, generally speaking, aims at restoring or advancing optimal psychic functioning in harmony with the self and the social world in which the patient lives. Contrary to the popular conception of psychotherapy, I think of optimal psychic functioning as encompassing the capacity to tolerate a modicum of anxiety and depression (Zetzel, 1964), since both these disquieting affects are irreducible attributes of the human condition. Insight, in and by itself, does nothing; its therapeutic effectiveness always remains contingent on the use which the ego makes of it toward the expansion of its realm in mental life. The actuality of this expansion is reflected and observable within the contemplative and expressive interplay which ceaselessly flows between the self and the object world.

We are initially confronted in therapy with two basic variables: one refers to the manifestation of a psychological disturbance (be it a neurosis, a phobia, a delinquency, a social inadequacy, etc.); the other variable is reflected in the patient's thoughts or fantasies about therapy and the therapeutic situation. We have learned from psychoanalysis that resistance to change not only represents an impediment in the course of therapy but also denotes a healthy capacity of the psychic organism to protect an established and familiar way of functioning against outside interference. With the slow emergence of the therapeutic alliance the patient yields—ever so cautiously—to a restructuring of his personality organization. The conservation of the psychic status quo is reflected in specific self-preservative mental activities to which we refer as defenses. Both resistance and defense denote capabilities of the psychic apparatus which are basic and indispensable in human life; they protect the psychic organism against the infliction of injury or the incapacitation of functioning.

In order to ascertain where the elusive line of demarcation lies which divides normal from abnormal resistance and defense (in therapy and in life), psychoanalytic theory serves as a useful guide. To triangulate the line of demarcation, we must focus our attention simultaneously from three points of view. First, we investigate the patient's present condition; to this we refer as diagnosis or, less rigidly and more dynamically conceived, as assessment. Second, we explore the life history of the patient in order to discover enlightening clues for a more discriminating, i.e., genetic understanding of his present condition. Third, we hold both these investigative efforts up against an age-specific model or norm in order to determine the degree of deviation. In short, what I suggest here is a developmental approach to adolescent psychotherapy in order better to coordinate assessment and therapy. As is well known, it remains a most difficult task in working with adolescents to tease out in the clinical picture what is a normal disturbance due to the developmental upheaval of the age and what constitutes a truly psychopathological condition. One of the inherent tasks of adolescent psychotherapy is to expose the adolescent to the painful recognition of inner conflict and of the illusions which a wished-for self tries to maintain. This transaction requires from the therapist the most genuine empathy, the most delicate tact, and the firmest and most consistent attitude. In making this remark I hear the echo of an older adolescent's irate response to my reminding him that, even though he wishes fervently to be a writer, the unalterable fact remains that he has never written more than a line—if that much. He shouted with a pleading desperation in his voice: "What is this? I thought you are supposed to make your patient feel good about himself." What motivated this adolescent to enter therapy was his desire to attain the narcissistic self-image of fame through the magic of therapy. The source of his failure in actively pursuing any goal lay camouflaged behind self-deceiving illusions. Confrontation with these irrationalities in his life represented the opening move in the emotional struggle called psychotherapy.

The note I struck in telling this incident leads me to a basic theme of adolescence. I have often been asked what in my opinion is the most difficult developmental task with which the adolescent has to cope. My answer has not always been the same, but years of experience have convinced me that the most painful task which faces the adolescent is the deidealization of self and object. With this statement I wish to convey the developmental fact that many of the narcissistic supplies which the young child receives from the "holding environment" (Winnicott, 1965) are drying up with the advent of puberty. At this stage of the life cycle, biological and social demands are voiced relentlessly by the maturational process and urge the individual to renounce the infantile sources of emotional security. Similarly, the external sources of identity constancy and self-esteem regulation are gradually to be replaced by internal sources and by object relations of a different order. The new and extrafamilial object ties of the adolescent are not just replacements or displacements of infantile attachments; on the contrary, they are new creations, even though they contain elements of familiar object qualities. By the same token, they also reflect the exclusion or rejection of qualities which the familiar objects of childhood possessed. The adolescent does not simply replicate his past by either repeating it in fact or in disguise; rather, he actively employs his expanding mental and social resources to shape for himself a wider, more inclusive and exclusive surround by breaking through the bounds of the familiar patterns of his childhood. From a changed and changing body and surround the adolescent receives and elicits an array of novel and untested sensations and stimulations via a widening and more complex interaction system between the self and the object world. This process, if vigorously sustained by the individual and his surround, furnishes those developmental activators necessary for keeping the adolescent's forward thrust toward adulthood in motion. I must leave the itinerary of this developmental journey unexplored on this occasion because issues more urgent to the topic of this paper require our attention.

We know from the work of Mahler et al. (1975) that the young child passes through a phase of psychic structure formation designated as individuation. Briefly, this process encompasses the period when the toddler—from early to late toddlerhood—internalizes the caretaking person or persons, usually the mother, and thus acquires object representations which possess an internally available object presence. Obviously, this acquisition of psychic structure memorializes the virtues as well as the flaws of the object world as it was originally experienced. We must not ignore the fact that these early internalizations remain under ceaseless scrutiny by the ego, whose work is governed progressively by the growing influence of the reality principle. To the extent that this process is successful, the autonomy of the ego gains in scope and, by the same token, the ego's dependency on the environment diminishes. Concomitantly, the line of demarcation between fantasy and reality becomes drawn not only more sharply but also more indelibly.

Mental and sexual maturation require an overhauling of internalizations, identifications, and object relations. These changes are effected or practiced via social ritualizations; among these we refer to social role assignments as powerful agents in the adolescent's life. I have formulated these internal changes, designated as the structural reorganization of the adolescent personality, in dynamic terms as the second individuation process of adolescence (Blos, 1967). The first individuation facilitated the young child's existence as a demarcated psychological entity through the internalization of the caretaking persons and the impinging surround. Thus, psychic structure formation takes its origin. We can discern the consolidation of nuclei of the self around which experience becomes organized. These are the steps in psychic differentiation which afford the young child a forward move toward physical independence; the internalized objects have become the guardians of the self or the protectors against abandonment anxiety.

In contrast to the infantile individuation process just outlined, the second individuation process represents the adolescent task of achieving independence from the internalized objects and their early formative influence on ego and superego. These internal changes not only effect the normative adolescent personality transformations but also account for much of the proverbial emotional turbulence of this age. The second individuation process proceeds either noisily and agitatedly or calmly and silently vis-à-vis the surrounding world and the self-observing ego. In any case, we witness often enough affective states and forms of behavior which are abnormal or bizarre. Adolescent abnormalities, emotional and behavioral, can best be assessed as to their transient or irreversible nature by viewing the disturbance in the light of adolescent psychic restructuring. The unavailability of the accustomed and dependable internal stabilizers of childhood seems to be responsible for many of the typical and transient personality characteristics of this age. Since every therapist is well acquainted with them, I refer to them only briefly by mentioning the swing from avid object hunger to bleak object avoidance and emotional withdrawal; from motoric impulsivity and action craving to lassitude and limp indifference; from the idealization of ideas or heroes to cold egotistical cynicism; from narcissistic self-sufficiency, imperviousness, and arrogance to the depressive and dejected state of shame and guilt. We always find one or the other of these characteristics in the clinical picture of adolescent psychopathology, regardless of whether it is definitive, namely, irreversible by development, or accompanies development and is therefore transient in nature and self-liquidating in time. The unrelenting malfunction of the adolescent personality is the sign of a miscarriage of the adolescent process, namely, the failure to yield adaptively to the challenges of the second individuation process.

Paradoxically, progressive development during adolescence requires the capacity to regress in order to rework those infantile tasks which had been too taxing to master at the tender age of early childhood. At the advanced age of adolescence they have to be dealt with anew by an ego that has acquired in the intervening years a resourcefulness commensurate to the task of the second individuation process. Internal conflicts, manifest in adolescent mental disturbances, lie within a defensive spectrum which extends from the irresistible urgency to regress to the frantic forward thrust into adultomorphic behavior, thus sidestepping a developmental progression that requires *time* to lend firmness and durability to psychic restructuring. Transient regressive movements are characteristic of this task and are at no period of life as obligatory as during the adolescent process. I have designated this regression "regression in the service of development" (Blos, 1967). Clinical observation renders the differentiation between normal regression and pathological regression at adolescence a knotty and puzzling problem. I have found that a discriminating review of the individual life history will throw light on the diagnostic and prognostic understanding of the case at hand. Let us admit that we are often reluctant to say that an adolescent does not require therapeutic attention when his or her behavior gives cause of concern to parents, teachers, and the community; we are equally hesitant and cautious not to err in the opposite direction. At such critical junctures we turn for clarification to the dynamic conceptualizations of development which psychoanalytic psychology offers us.

At this point I shall shift my presentation from a theoretical to a clinical focus. The case I shall present not only exemplifies my antecedent remarks but also opens up new territory in which to advance the exploration of the topic. I have chosen this case because it demonstrates the clinical usefulness of psychoanalytic theory in the field of psychotherapeutic work regardless of its official designation, which might be psychotherapy, casework, or child guidance. In the context of this discussion I pay attention to the application of psychoanalytic principles in the treatment of the adolescent outside the treatment modality of psychoanalysis proper.

I have selected a case of psychoanalytic psychotherapy because the vast majority of disturbed adolescents is treated—if treated at all—by this treatment modality. I also wish to demonstrate my conviction that a psychoanalytically grounded comprehension of a case influences more decisively and favorably the conduct and outcome of therapy than does the frequency of weekly sessions. The intensiveness of therapy is by no means proportionate to the frequency of therapeutic contacts. Which treatment modality is finally chosen as the treatment of choice is ideally determined by the assessment of the presenting disturbance, but in clinical practice extraneous factors affect the decision, such as the ability to pay, the patient's psychological accessibility, or the therapist's geographical accessibility. This consideration does not deny the indisputable fact that a certain kind of emotional illness requires a specific treatment modality in order to effect cure. Even though we wish to render a perfect match between type of illness and treatment modality, we must admit that reality factors often taint the purity of our principled judgment. Every clinician has discovered to his surprise that a judicious recourse to what, pejoratively, is called a compromise of treatment choice might bring about a remarkable amelioration of the presenting disturbance. It has been my experience that this kind of rewarding outcome can occur most often when treatment is undertaken during the stages of primary development, namely, during the years of pre-adult life (Blos, 1970).

THE CASE OF MARY

The patient I shall report was seen over a period of 5 months in individual sessions once a week.

Mary, a 15-year-old girl, was brought to my attention by her parents. She was an only child. From the description the parents gave me of their daughter's troubles emerged the typical clinical picture of an agoraphobia in an adolescent girl. This condition had for some time exerted a seriously confining influence on her life. She was unable to leave her home and walk on the street without being accompanied by her mother or a girlfriend. The companion had to be female. She felt uncomfortable or actually anxious in the presence of males if they were older than herself. Being in the company of her father made her apprehensive and uneasy. She had confided to her mother the fear of men which possessed her and over which she had no control.

Mary attended a parochial girls' school with only women teachers. Once inside the school building she felt safe, was anxiety-free, and enjoyed the time with her many friends. However, after school Mary's life was restricted to her home. She never visited a friend unless picked up by a companion; she never visited her beloved grandfather in the country where she had spent many happy times when she was younger. In fact, for several years she had shunned his company. The parents had observed over the last year a drop in her academic work and also a detached, morose, and worried moodiness. Mary was particularly nasty and impertinent to her mother on whom she depended not only for traveling to and from school but for all her movements outside her home. She accused her parents of hating her, of wanting to get rid of her, and of wishing her out of the house. While she hurled such accusations at her parents, she never believed a word of them to be true. The mother was a hardworking, caring, and proper woman, who was closely attached to her daughter; the father was a responsible provider, even though he displayed at times a flighty, impulsive, and self-indulging disposition. During the prephobic period Mary looked neither right nor left when walking alone to school but kept staring at a static object like a building, a billboard, or the pavement, always sensing around herself a presence of men, whether they actually were there or not. It is reasonable to assume that men were constantly on her mind without being associated with any conscious mental content. In fact, Mary was a reserved and shy girl who behaved in public with extraordinary decorum.

I shall now report a secret which Mary had told her mother 1½ years earlier with the explicit request never to tell her father. This secret—so I later discovered—was to be of crucial importance for the understanding of the case. The secret which the mother reported to me in the initial—and only—interview I had with the parents was a memory that had troubled the girl for a long time, but more persistently during the last several years. When she was about 4 years old, so she remembered, she was in her parents' bed as was the family custom on Sunday mornings. That particular morning the mother was up already, dressed, and ready to go out. Mary and her father were fooling around in bed, when she suddenly heard her mother say in a stern voice: "You do that only with your wife." This phrase struck like a bolt of thunder and stayed silently in her mind until she repeated it to her mother some 10 years later.

Mary entered psychotherapy with the determination to get well. Should her mother be unable to bring her to my office, she would arrange to travel with one of her girlfriends. Mary unburdened herself eagerly of her thoughts, experiences, and memories which had lain buried alive in her mind since early childhood. She told me that for the last 2 years she had avoided to be in the presence of her father. "Even though I love him," she said, "I don't like to be in his company or near him; often I hate him." She talked freely about her romantic, childish daydreams or about the troubled times of her childhood. Lately she often cried when alone in her room listening to sentimental music, or she sat brooding over her parents' unhappy marriage. She described quite graphically her father's drunken binges, his coming home late at night with the help of an unfamiliar woman, shouting, cursing, and toppling over furniture. She remembered well the sights, the sounds, and her hate of the other woman who—so she thought—had degraded her father.

In the course of talking about herself Mary told me "the secret" which she had confided to her mother. She began her narrative with saying that on Sunday mornings "I used to cuddle with my parents in their bed. That day I asked my dad to put his arm around me, when I heard my mother say—she was just ready to leave the room and go out—'You do that only with your husband!'" After a pause Mary continued, "Not until I was 10 years old did the meaning of that remark become clear to me; I knew then it had something to do with sex, love, and necking."

As soon as Mary had finished telling me her secret, I realized that her version was different from the one reported to me by her mother. Let me point out the discrepancy between the two stories. In one, as told to me by Mary's mother, the girl had heard her childhood mother say, "You do that only with your wife." In the version Mary told me she had heard her childhood mother say, "You do that only with your husband." In the first comment the father stands accused; and in the second, Mary is the guilty one. In both statements the child heard herself addressed in the forbidden role of a presumptive marriage partner. Both role arrogations represented for Mary a psychic reality of traumatic consequences. What the girl had heard was the mother's accusation that the father loves his little girl as he loves his wife or, in other words, that he desires forbidden sexual relations with his little daughter. The enigmatic sentence, etched indelibly in her memory, had acquired elaborate and formidable meanings with the advancing years of puberty.

The self-accusatory and guilty state, both implicit in Mary's version, was confirmed by her through a dream in which she kisses a man who is a distant relative. Mary explained, "I hardly know him and I really do not like him," adding quickly that she was related to him "by marriage only and not by blood." To my astonishment she was acutely surprised by the fact that in the dream it was she (not the man) who made the sexual advance by kissing him. Via this nonincestuous and nonattractive man in the dream she came to acknowledge the sexual wishes and fantasies which—so we had good reason to assume—lay hidden behind the phobic symptom.

Her reaction to the dawning awareness of her sexual memories, fantasies, and wishes which she had shared with me was a surprising one. For the next session Mary arrived "dressed to kill." From under a shock of blond hair, fluffed up into a spectacular aura, there peeked out a child's face, painted clumsily with rouge, lipstick, and mascara. Tight white sailor pants completed her shapely appearance, which amounted to a caricature of a juvenile make-believe streetwalker. I shall return to the patient's sexual acting out in the transference when I arrive at the discussion of the case.

Let me state at this point that the discrepancy between the two versions of the "secret"—we will never know for certain which is the true one[1]—made me form the hunch that the different versions represented the opposing sides of the mental conflict which had become manifest in the phobia. I therefore decided to bring the version, told to me by the mother, to Mary's attention,[2] thus making her aware of the fact that two versions of the secret existed simultaneously, but in a dissoci-

1. I was prepared to discover that both versions were auditory projections of guilt with a delusional realness that remained attached to the memory.
2. The reader must have noticed that I committed an indiscretion when I quoted to Mary from my interview with her parents. It must have been obvious to her that her mother had reported the secret to me in front of her father, thus having broken the promise of silence the mother had given her daughter who requested it. In spite of all these considerations, I did not hesitate to use the therapeutic potential of the double-faced secret and run the risk of complicating and perhaps aborting the good work with the patient by involving the parents at this point in her treatment. I was confident that the therapeutic alliance was strong enough to ride out safely any emotional storm in case Mary should take me or her mother to task. As it turned out, none of these complications came to pass. The girl was too profoundly occupied with past traumatic events to bother with their faint reverberations in the present.

ated state, in her mind. I expected from this intervention that her realization of the bewildering disparity would activate the synthesizing faculty of the ego. This psychic effort, so I reasoned, might bring about an active striving toward the resolution of a conflict which had been kept in mental limbo by the irreconcilable content of a memory whose double-faced nature was the cause of a pathological accommodation, namely, symptom formation. As was to be expected, Mary felt gradually less anxious and socially less constrained.

At this point the summer vacation intervened. I saw Mary again after an interval of 2 months. She had stayed at home during the beginning of her vacation until she realized that her mother had "too much of a need for my company." It was then that she decided to accept an invitation to her grandfather's house in the country where she had not visited for 2 years. She stayed with him for 3 weeks. With joy and pleasure she summed up her stay by saying, "I had a real good time." She experienced no anxiety when outdoors alone. She made friends, boys and girls, and became romantically attached to a boy from the village neighborhood. Ever since she returned home and after she had started school, Mary was free of her phobic symptom. She was no longer in need of a companion on the street. On some days she preferred her girlfriend to pick her up rather than meet her at an appointed place. On weekends she played golf with her father.

Mary seemingly had lost her symptom as smoothly and completely as a snake slithers out of its skin. Emotional transformations do not occur in this fashion. Simultaneously with the symptomatic improvement Mary's demands on her mother became more exacting and frenzied, leading to passionate love and hate arguments. The mother reacted with resentment and hurt to Mary's bullying and demandingness; to this the girl responded with wild accusations of the mother's unkindness and lack of love. She burst into teary complaints about the cold indifference she received from her mother for the many pleasures Mary provided for her, such as cleaning the house in order to cheer her up upon her return from work. Obviously, Mary's accounts of her dutiful household chores were wild distortions and exaggerations within the typical emotional struggle between an adolescent girl and her mother. In resentful anger Mary told me that she would not ask her mother anymore to accompany her to school "even if it kills me."

With the decline of the phobic symptom I saw the discord between mother and daughter mount and move into the center of Mary's emotional life. She was now engaged in a conflict with her mother, finding herself unable to face the intensity of her ambivalence at this stage of her postphobic psychic restructuring. I was therefore not surprised when she told me of her wish to terminate treatment. I decided to put no obstacle in the way of her decision, even though the mother was pleading for a continuation of therapy. A talk with the mother had convinced me that Mary's growing independence had aroused in her an anxious feeling of loneliness and estrangement. In the wish that Mary continue therapy I suspected her intention to use Mary's therapy as a way for preserving the close bond of emotional attachment between mother and child unaltered. This dimension added weight to my decision to let her terminate treatment at this juncture.

DISCUSSION

The discussion of this case has the express purpose of extracting from it certain psychoanalytic principles which have an applicability far beyond the treatment of Mary. My first comment dwells on the human faculty of listening. It is common knowledge that the psychoanalyst's most time-consuming interaction with the patient is listening. In using the word "interaction" I attribute to the therapist's listening an active, not merely a receptive, quality. This kind of listening provides the therapist with information which is unintentionally conveyed by the patient and lies beyond what is literally communicated. The trained faculty of hearing what is communicated by the patient without his conscious awareness lifts the act of listening onto a special plane quite remote from the receptivity of a natural good listener. Under the tutelage of a psychoanalytic orientation, listening is done by an educated ear. Theodore Reik (1948) has felicitously called it "listening with the third ear." This kind of listening proceeds in a state of suspended judg-

ment to which we refer as free-floating attention. Content and
sequence of the patient's communications are constantly viewed
against the backdrop of psychoanalytic theory or, in other
words, they are perceived in association with multiple references, be they of a dynamic, genetic, adaptive, or developmental nature. While listening, the clinician elaborates hypothetical
formulations in his mind, letting the clinical evidence that follows render the verdict whether the tentative construct was
accurate or not. The therapist should be pleased with whatever
the verdict might be, because it brings the truth closer within
his reach. In addition, the therapist listens simultaneously to his
own inner promptings which never fail to be elicited by the
help-seeking individual as a patient and as a person. These
promptings receive their buoyancy from the therapist's personal associative sensitivities, thus evoking in him a state of empathy. The voice of empathy is listened to with the same discriminating ear as is the voice of the patient, thus making audible—
by a kind of mutual enforcement—what is often too faint a
sound to be perceived in the patient's direct communications.
From the multitude of these perceptions in the field of listening
and observing, there emerges insight into the patient's psychological state; based on this information we formulate guidelines
for our therapeutic work. The point just outlined is illustrated
in Mary's case by the elucidation of the secret as the vortex of a
conflictual turbulence which was pathologically brought under
control by her symptom. The insight into the content and dynamics of the secret pressed upon me various options of the
therapeutic lines from which to choose.

During the entire course of therapy we constantly grope for
reliable guidelines, particularly at certain way stations which
challenge our clinical sagacity. At such times we project before
our mental eye the whole therapeutic encounter in order to
determine the direction into which treatment should move.
This process scrutinizes not only how therapy has progressed
so far, but also what to expect from its continuation and where
its limitations might lie. For an illustration of this point I refer
to my assention to Mary's decision to terminate treatment. Why
did I do this? I did it after I had carefully juxtaposed the
relative reasons for or against continuation of therapy. What

weighed heavily in this act of decision-making were the considerations which prompted me initially to take this girl in psychotherapy. After a brief acquaintance I could see that Mary was a deeply troubled girl, anxious rather than depressed or emotionally withdrawn. Her reaching out for help was genuine, and her therapeutic cooperation could be engaged. Furthermore, I formed the opinion that her phobia was a symptom in formation, partially still operating on the level of acting out a fantasy. In other words, the conflict was not yet fully internalized; it had not yet progressed to the state of a neurotic condition, but was still on the way toward consolidation into a structured symptom. Her emotional illness was still enmeshed in the adolescent process and accessible to psychotherapy. It seemed to me that the testing of this preliminary assessment was an effort worth undertaking.

It is noteworthy that in the treatment of Mary a phase of "working through" was not discernible, even though this phase supposedly brings treatment to its successful and natural conclusion. Two comments are in order at this point. Whenever treatment is undertaken while development is still in potential progress, it remains the aim of psychotherapy to bring impeded development into flux and redirect it into the mainstream of adaptive growth. Furthermore, I wish to emphasize the incongruous fact that during adolescence therapeutic achievement becomes manifest not only by a symptomatic improvement and a more satisfactory performance in life generally, but also by the appearance of a new wave of disturbances; these, however, are now of a developmentally more phase-adequate nature. In Mary's case, this turn was signaled by her forward thrust into an active social and academic participatory life and by the appearance of an acute daughter-mother conflict. These adaptations usually are compromise formations which will serve the adolescent well enough to move toward a reasonably satisfactory closure of adolescence. In cases where this goal remains out of reach, we must conclude that another therapeutic modality is indicated.

Pursuing the lines of thought I have just outlined, I wish to make a further remark about Mary's recovery. When the phobic symptom was abating, I observed that the focus of her disturbance had shifted to a regressive acting out of a typical mother-daughter ambivalence struggle. This reengagement in preoedipal dependency and attachment issues represents a normal and transient stage in female adolescence. In Mary's case it was kept in abeyance by the fixation on the oedipal level. We must, however, not overlook that the passionate turn to the oedipal father provided simultaneously a bullwark against the regressive pull to the mother of early childhood, the preoedipal mother. This typical, i.e., normative regressive pull in female adolescence usually gives rise to all kinds of attachment and dependency needs as well as to rebellious and distancing behavior. Seeing the developmental picture in this light, one might have been inclined to offer Mary's liberated emotions an opportunity to find their adolescent-adequate balance with the help of continued psychotherapy. However, as my therapeutic stance indicates, I elected in this adolescent case to suspend treatment after a reasonable resumption of a developmental flux or reengagement had been attained. This I did with the thought in mind that treatment might be resumed if another insurmountable impasse were to arise in the course of her growing up. We could well speak here of an age-appropriate therapy delivered in installments. The risk of leaving the therapeutic work incomplete has to be gauged against the benefits of an autonomous developmental advance; this in turn furnishes that confidence and trust in therapeutic work which are necessary for its resumption whenever a decisive need for it should arise.

Some readers may have wondered why I had neglected—if neglect it was—to deal with the girl's acting out in the therapy situation or—to be more precise—in the transference. I refer here to the session in which Mary appeared "dressed to kill." Her exhibitionistic and seductive behavior was obviously for my benefit. In order to explain my nonintervention I must mention the fact that my work with adolescent girls has taught me the paradoxical lesson that the interpretation of sexual acting out in the transference, done with the purpose of rendering sexual fantasies or wishes conscious and consequently subject to ego control and insight, quite to the contrary stimulates sexual excitation, which in turn provokes other forms of acting out such as, for instance, absenteeism or breaking off treatment. A complication of this nature becomes particularly virulent if the therapist is a man.

Acting out in the transference, as demonstrated by Mary's behavior when she appeared for her session "dressed to kill," presents a most delicate situation which has to be approached with utmost tact, sensitivity, and circumspection. A forthright interpretation should be given only if a breakdown of therapy is imminent due to a persevering and unmodulated, i.e., direct sexual transference. This cautiousness is suggested by the fact that the adolescent girl who develops a rapid and massive sexual transference to a male therapist equates his talking about transferential sexual feelings, wishes, and fantasies with his seductive intentions—indeed, with his desire for sexual intimacy with his female patient. The projective component of this reaction is obvious. While we are familiar with the ease and casualness with which most contemporary adolescents discuss matters of sex, it is noteworthy that the taboo—encompassing guilt, embarrassment, and shame—of incestuous emotions, when they come to life in the transference, has not lost any of its original stringency. Indeed, the adolescent state of sexual freedom has not affected at all this infantile realm.

Returning once more to Mary's transference behavior, I wish to emphasize that in forgoing an interpretation of her acting out in the transference, I gave expression to my opinion that the resolution of her symptom would be feasible by pursuing her pathogenetic past without exposing to the light of awareness the sexual arousal in the transference. I attempted therefore to affect Mary's sexual acting out in the transference by helping her to rework, namely, resolve the emotional conflict she had once experienced in the parental bed. My knowledge of the secret had laid out the path into this festering region of her mind. At any rate, by this incongruous therapeutic twist, the usual direction of analytic technique was reversed. It succeeded in bringing the repressed component of her infantile conflict to her attention by using a lost memory that was recovered by outside information. I was persuaded to take this course because the concrete treatment situation had reestablished the original triadic constellation with both Mary and therapist alone in the consulting room and the mother in the nearby waiting room as an absentee participant. This treatment approach was further strengthened by the fact that Mary possessed an unusually clear memory of her childhood and was in vivid touch with her pathogenetic past. It should be noted here that the particular kind of acting out in the transference which I described was never repeated.

In this connection I want to comment on the puzzling fact that Mary entered treatment—and indeed a productive one—with a man. Her phobia presented no hindrance to her therapeutic engagement; quite the contrary, it rather seemed to help it along. As hinted at above, on a psychological level, Mary was never alone with me during her visits to my office; the presence of her mother in the waiting room completed the triadic constellation in which her pathology was embedded. The *dramatis personae* were all in their proper places: they replicated the traumatic experience and set the stage for the fateful drama of early life to unfold in therapy. What might have eased this psychological transfiguration with a male therapist was perhaps his advanced age; it blended, so to speak, oedipal passions with a more benign grandfather transference.[3]

There remains one more observation to be made: the symptom was never dealt with directly as a focal entity. The obvious and painful pathological condition, the phobia, was treated with a kind of attentional neglect. This therapeutic attitude is based on psychoanalytic theory and practice which have taught us that a neurotic symptom exists only as long as an unresolved conflict requires its presence; the function of the symptom can be seen in protecting the sense of self, and in averting catastrophic anxiety from flooding the psychic organism. By laying open the discrepancy in the two versions of Mary's secret, I exposed her divided self in front of her mental eye. By confrontation rather than by offering an interpretation of the phobic symptom—the dynamics of which were well understood—I

---

3. Mary's first move away from her parental home was a prolonged vacation visit at her beloved grandfather's house which she had avoided for several years. It should be mentioned that the grandfather was a single man, a widower.

made the dissociated drive components (embodied in the two versions of "I want you" versus "you want me") available to the synthetic work of the ego. I expected from this effort that the patient would structure a conflictual organization of a different order than the pathological one—the phobia—which was built on repression, displacement, and projection. The endeavor just outlined was followed by an abatement of the phobia. Concomitantly, the conflictual focus shifted into the realm of the dyadic, preoedipal phase. With this shift Mary had attained a second chance to complete some of the unfinished business of her early childhood. Should she be equal to this adolescent task, I expected that she would move into adult life less impeded and burdened by her past.

FOLLOW-UP

The case of Mary would be left incomplete if there were no follow-up attached to it. Too many questions were raised, too many prognostic and alternative hunches were advanced for silence to descend at this point on Mary's posttherapeutic development. Our curiosity is justifiably directed to the specific ways in which therapy had affected her life.

Before Mary left my office at the end of our last session, we agreed that she would get in touch with me in the near future "just to let me know how she was getting along." I never heard from her. Half a year had passed when I got a call from her saying that she wanted to see me. When we met it was as if no time had elapsed. She was obviously happy to see me again. She admitted readily that she had avoided me because she was afraid that being in my office or in my presence would bring to life all the memories she had shared with me and wanted to forget. She told me that she had not been able to manage her life as well as she had expected and would like to resume therapy.

In the following report I shall summarize Mary's life since I had seen her last and as told by her in the initial interview after her return. I shall focus upon the use of this information in assessing whether or not a second installment of treatment was indicated.

Mary reported that she had experienced pleasant changes on three fronts of her life: (1) she and her mother had come closer together ("We can talk about everything and we enjoy each other's company. My mother has become my best friend"); (2) she had been out on several dates; and (3) she had improved remarkably in school. The gentle climate of family closeness recently was blown away by a tornado of family fights which always culminated in Mary's accusation of her mother: "You don't love me!" The emotional intensity of these fights evoked Mary's decision to see me. Although I was not able to elicit the cause or provocation of these fights, it was clear that the fighting made Mary dejected and miserable to the point that she felt compelled to make peace with her mother at any price. Mary reported that she was now on reasonably good terms with her father but felt "uncomfortable and uneasy" when greeted by him "with hugs and kisses" upon his return from work.

Mary expressed great dislike of her tendency to daydream and had made efforts to counteract it by doing something or being in her mother's company. She used her room less as a refuge from the world or as a place to cry, sulk, and pity herself. However, she reported spells of moodiness; she said, "They just come and go without any rhyme or reason. But I feel much happier now than before I came to see you." She voiced the wish to be more like the girls of her age and "have fun," while decidedly disapproving of their preoccupation—in thought and deed—with sex. "My generation moves too fast" she said, and, "I'm really afraid of guys." Within her rather proper social conduct the fact that 2 weeks prior to her revisiting me she had gotten drunk at her girlfriend's birthday party stood out like an unaccountable apparition from the unknown.

While the street phobia was no source of trouble any longer, Mary still moved outdoors with a certain restraint; for example, she would not pass the corner filling station on her street because the men there could be counted on to whistle at her. She added, "I am quite prudish." However, she now could walk by herself to and from school as well as go downtown to do her shopping.

At this point we have to ask ourselves how the life history data, covering the last 6 months, can be translated into an assessment of Mary's present psychological status and be used for the purpose of defining changes in her functioning which would speak clearly for or against the resumption of treatment. What struck me in Mary's account was the keen alertness of her self-observing ego. In contrast to her previous grasp of causality, namely, her pathological use of projection, she was now able to realize that the origin of her various emotional discomforts was internal. Furthermore, her wish to return to therapy signified that her first acquaintance with treatment had been a positive experience; in other words, she had invested the therapeutic process with a sense of trust and confidence. She could now keep separate her relatedness to the therapist and his function to help her from the therapist as a sexual being, a man. In other words, her response and attitude to the father figure (imago) and its reexperience in the outer world had become more discriminating and complex.

In an effort to strengthen her ego autonomy she had abstained actively from the self-indulgence in daydreams and self-pity. Her florid fantasy life had become ego-alien. She had become determined "to do things," one of which was academic work, with the result that she had received praise and was considered a success by teachers and parents alike. Thus, she had created for herself a source of legitimate narcissistic pleasure. She literally beamed as an answer when I asked her, "Do you enjoy the A's on your report card?" In an effort to gain ego control over situations which she had previously avoided due to anxiety arousal, she had faced them head-on: she had accepted dates and gone out. These friendships were short-lived in most instances because she became frightened by the erotic physical contact which the boys demanded. As a result she stayed away from them. This defeat on her first forays into heterosexual sociability had thrown Mary back into closeness to her mother. She was now caught in the double pull of returning to the safety of her home and of entering the enviable world in which her peers moved. At one point in the interview I asked her what, in her opinion, was her present trouble? She answered without hesitation, "My insecurity." At the first stage of treatment the answer would have been a description of her phobia.

I shall now define Mary's answer "My insecurity" in dynamic

terms. It is evident from the clinical picture that the girl's ego
proved incompetent to deal with the emotional tasks of adolescence. The gratification of any sexual urge from holding hands
to kissing (such was the extent of her love life) had to be renounced entirely (so to say: *en bloc*) due to the unreliability of
her ego as a protector of her moral and physical integrity. This
conflict was subjectively experienced by Mary as "insecurity."
Her mental state was of the neurotic modality. In essence,
Mary's illness was due to the tension between opposing wishes
or needs, irreconcilable in their nature. I call attention to the
juxtaposition of her getting drunk and being her mother's
good little girl. This impasse or bind had by now congealed into
an emotional and behavioral pattern which can best be described as an oscillating state between regressive and progressive trends and movements. This was the condition in which
Mary reentered therapy. Due to the first stage of treatment an
advance in the internalization of conflict was noted; this change
rendered Mary a promising candidate for the resumption of
psychotherapy. (However, the tale of that enterprise will be
told on another occasion.)

Before I leave the follow-up of Mary I wish to make some
general comments on this subject. I consider a follow-up of
particular significance and urgency in all treatment reports
concerning children or adolescents. This opinion is based on
the fact that child and adolescent therapy, when undertaken
while childhood development is still in progress, operates within given delimitations. These delimitations are conceived of as
integral aspects of child development itself and lie beyond the
particular effectiveness of a given therapeutic enterprise and its
unique partnership. Therapy during childhood and adolescence can neutralize[4] the noxiousness of pathogenetic nuclei,
formed in early life, only up to the developmental level or,
more exactly, up to its potential normative presence (i.e., age)
which the patient has attained at the time of treatment. Under
the most fortunate circumstances the child emerges from therapy with a restored ego competence which proves equal to the

4. Within the framework of the structural theory we refer to this process in
terms of stages in conflict resolution.

developmental challenges that lie ahead. But we can never be certain whether new developmental tasks will not be found too taxing, in which case symptom formation—not necessarily symptom repetition—may be resumed.[5] In other words, we can never be certain whether a new developmental thrust will not activate pathogenetic remnants or residues that have survived the earlier therapeutic work.[6] The so-called and misnamed failures of child therapy are rarely predictable, especially after a satisfactory completion of therapy during preadult life.

It is an empirical fact that a large number of children who were successfully treated during childhood or adolescence resume therapy again later in their lives. Follow-up studies promise to be of invaluable help for comprehending more clearly the delimitations inherent in child psychotherapy and child psychoanalysis. Even if follow-up studies cannot be pursued systematically, I suggest that they be undertaken randomly (as in the case of Mary), because they add a worthwhile edge of discriminating foresight and humility to any clinician's skill.

This brings my presentation to an end. The nature of the case chosen for illustration determined the selective attention to certain clinical issues drawn from the vast borderland that lies between psychoanalysis and psychoanalytically oriented psychotherapy. I am certain that many a reader wished I had given more attention to one or the other theoretical or technical problem. But even though I could not fully attend to the topical richness of the subject under discussion, I nevertheless hope I conveyed and strengthened the conviction that the judicious use of psychoanalytic knowledge enhances significantly the scope and effectiveness of our psychotherapeutic work with adolescents.

5. In such an instance the normative developmental task is comparable to a trauma inflicted on the psychic organism. In these instances, the trauma coalesces with dormant pathogenetic residues.
6. I am fully aware of the fact that development is not restricted to the period of childhood but is an ongoing process during the life cycle. But I submit that, within this broad spectrum, the developmental stages of preadult life are of an order that differs distinctly in terms of the internalization of prototypical experiences and their effect on psychic structure formation, from that of the stages following later in life.

BIBLIOGRAPHY

BLOS, P. (1967), The second individuation process of adolescence. *Psychoanal. Study Child,* 22:162–186.
—— (1970), *The Young Adolescent.* New York: Free Press.
MAHLER, M. S., PINE, F., & BERGMAN, A. (1975), *The Psychological Birth of the Human Infant.* New York: Basic Books.
REIK, T. (1948), *Listening with the Third Ear.* New York: Farrar, Straus.
WINNICOTT, D. W. (1965), *Maturational Processes and the Facilitating Environment.* New York: Int. Univ. Press.
ZETZEL, E. R. (1964), Symptom formation and character formation. *Int. J. Psychoanal.,* 45:151–157.

On Ventriloquism

EDGAR L. LIPTON, M.D.

A PSYCHOLOGICAL STUDY OF THE ART OF VENTRILOQUISM seems not to have been attempted in either the psychoanalytic or other scientific literature available to me. The reason for this may be that ventriloquism is so frequently regarded as a lesser art form, associated with music halls and charlatans. It has a slightly disreputable aura. There are very few professional practitioners. The main national professional organization of ventriloquists in this country has about 800 members, most of whom perform infrequently, usually for church groups but also for children's parties, nightclubs, and television.

In contrast, a strikingly large number of latency-aged children and adolescents answer advertisements in pulp magazines for booklets promising to teach them the art. Moreover, plays and motion pictures featuring a ventriloquist, although few in number, are repetitive occurrences. The practice of ventriloquism is known in many cultures and is a very old profession.

The present study has modest aims. After a brief review of how ventriloquism was viewed historically, I shall present the case history of a ventriloquist to demonstrate how he used this minor art form as an aid in the resolution of some of his anxieties and personal conflicts.

PHENOMENOLOGY AND HISTORY

The word ventriloquism derives from *venter*, the belly, and *loqui*, to speak. It is the art or practice of speaking in such a

Associate Clinical Professor Psychiatry, Cornell University School of Medicine; examiner in child psychoanalysis, New York Psychoanalytic Institute.

manner that the voice appears to come from some source other than the vocal organs of the speaker.

Since voice cannot be produced in the stomach or anywhere other than in the larynx, the commonly accepted idea of a ventriloquist as one who throws his voice is based on acceptance of an illusion. It is physically impossible to throw a voice in the ventriloquial sense. In fact, the exact location or even the direction from which sounds originate is not very clearly recognized by our ears, so that it is usually very easy to infer from a visual suggestion (as the sight of the moving mouth of a dummy) that the voice is coming from the dummy. Modern practitioners, as Edgar Bergen and Paul Winchell, achieved their effects by using dummies or large dolls; but hand puppets, finger puppets, shadow graphs, and cardboard dummies also have frequently been employed. These are examples of near ventriloquism. Textbooks on the subject stress the importance of creating believable characters with specific ages, sex, and personalities. The illusion is maintained by a flow of conversation in which the ventriloquist uses one or more voices sounding different from his "own," plus a certain amount of action on the part of the dummy.

A variant of "near" ventriloquism is called the "muffled voice" or "telephone voice." It employs techniques creating the illusion of a person in a nearby closet, closed box, or at the far end of a telephone conversation. "Distant" ventriloquism relies on the illusion of voices coming from large objects·such as idols or from distant spaces.[1]

In the public's eye, ventriloquism is allied to the practice of magic—the belief that demons or secret forces directly affect nature and humans for good or evil. This is distinct from religion, in which there are appeals to divine powers by sacrifice and prayer (Middleton, 1967). Magic is viewed by scholars as historically older than the belief in gods (Budge, 1901; Frazer, 1905, 1911; Leuba, 1912). Magic in ancient times could be good or bad magic, but ventriloquism is invariably characterized as

1. I would like to express my gratitude to my teachers, the master magicians and ventriloquists Clinton Detweiler, Dan Ritchard, George Schindler, and Todd Stockman for their help and generosity in sharing their secrets.

evil or black magic. For example, Philo Judaeus of Alexandria, known as the mediator between Hellenistic and Jewish-Christian thought, speaks of good and bad magic. He cites ventriloquists as an example of the "vulgar impostors" or bad magicians—sorcerers, enchanters, and jugglers.

The Old Testament concept of monotheism forcefully negates the existence of magic and in several places makes it clear that, since there is no power above God or in competition with Him, God's hand cannot be forced by divinations. Further, in the Old Testament, the dead have nothing to offer the living (Psalms 115:17–18). Thus, if the dead cannot tell us anything and divination is totally out of the question, then necromancy and divination are mere superstitions, or at the worst ways of resorting to forbidden idolatry. The ban on necromancy is mentioned in several places in the Torah.

Leviticus (19:31) says: "Do not inquire of ghosts [*obot*] or familiar spirits [*Yidoneem*] to be defiled by them." According to Rashi, the foremost commentator on the Bible and Talmud, this passage is directed against the practice of necromancy and divination. He explains the Hebrew terms *obot* and *Yidoneem* in the following way. *Obot* is a *pitom Hamaidaber* (the classical word for ventriloquist) who speaks out of his armpit. In his commentary on the Babylonian Talmud (Tractate Sanhedrin, p. 65-B), Rashi explains that this *ba' al ha -obot* is a charmer who puts a corpse under his armpit and creates the impression that the corpse is speaking. A *Yidonee* is defined as a person who puts a bone from an animal into his mouth and the bone talks.[2]

The warning is repeated again in Isaiah (29:4) and in Deuteronomy (18:10–11). This time, according to Rashi, it is a warning not to be tricked by these wizards and charmers. Another reference to this form of necromancy is in Samuel (1:28), where the desperate King Saul, violating the Biblical injunction against consulting such persons, goes to the Witch of Endor to

2. It would seem impossible to talk with something like a bone in the mouth. However, if one visualizes this as held in the edge of the mouth, as a cigarette is held between the lips, it is not at all impossible. Indeed, some modern ventriloquists do this cigarette stunt to demonstrate their skills in lip control.

query her about a forthcoming battle. She divines up the ghost of the dead prophet Samuel to give Saul answers. Scholars of ventriloquism believe this to have been an example of a ventriloquial trick.

"Far" or "distant" ventriloquism also is mentioned in early Greek and Roman writings. Ventriloquists believe that the miracles of early oracles such as that of Delphi were probably utterances of priests referring ventriloquial sounds to statues.

Belief in magic and open fears connected with ventriloquism as a subdivision of bad magic have receded as science and rational thought have gained ascendancy in modern times. As the secrets of how ventriloquism is performed have become known, the attitude of the public to it has changed markedly. Indeed, a recent survey (*Newsy Vents*) of professional practitioners revealed that by far the widest use of the skill is in the field of religious education! Nowadays ventriloquial shows are performed in Sunday Schools, as they would be at children's parties or on TV advertising, as entertainment in the service of presenting educational material in an attention-arresting manner.

On the other hand, a brief review of the trade journals as well as of plays, novels, and motion pictures that contain ventriloquists shows striking recurrent fictional themes of horror. In spite of the modern pragmatic entertainment-oriented function of ventriloquism, a strong current of the ancient emotional connotation of ventriloquism as frightening black magic remains. The main fictional elements include a blurred comparison between dummy and operator, so that the audience is held in a state of suspense as to who is the live and who the dead or inanimate. Each of these tales expresses a theme with the explicit assumption of evil magic and perhaps insanity. The issues of confused identity, magic, death, and the uncanny recur again and again. And the illusion on which the acceptance of the act is based has its counterpart in the performer's concern with issues of identity, sincerity, and "magically" fooling people, as my patient taught me.[3] They are perhaps representative

3. While these issues clearly appeal to the audiences, I know of no cases of ventriloquists getting confused about their identities and the dummies', of going insane in this manner, or of using the dummies for evil purposes.

of childhood fears of the unknown, loss of control, strange agressors, and the breakdown of the distinction between animate and inanimate, the revival of which evokes a feeling of uncanniness. In this context Freud's (1919) words are appropriate:

> Let us take the uncanny associated with the omnipotence of thoughts, with the prompt fulfilment of wishes, with secret injurious powers and with the return of the dead. The condition under which the feeling of uncanniness arises is here unmistakable. We—or our primitive forefathers—once believed that these possibilities were realities and were convinced that they actually happened. Nowadays we no longer believe in them, we have *surmounted* these modes of thought; but we do not feel quite sure of our new beliefs, and the old ones still exist within us ready to seize upon any confirmation. As soon as something *actually happens* in our lives which seems to confirm the old, discarded beliefs we get a feeling of the uncanny [p. 247f.].

The audience's enjoyment of the ventriloquist's performance may be based on the arousal of a sense of the uncanny in connection with old, but mastered infantile conflicts. The issues and conflicts in the ventriloquist may not be all that different, but perhaps more intense.

CASE REPORT

Although I did not work psychoanalytically with Mr. V.—I saw him twice a week for some 2 years—the material he presented is useful and valid because of the availability of his history and the insights gained during his work with me and in a previous lengthy analysis. Intelligent and introspective, he was highly motivated for treatment. He consulted me at the age of 37 because of a depression and feelings of inadequacy. A few months prior to this consultation he and his wife had participated in natural childbirth training and he had been present at the delivery of their first child. When the baby appeared, he experienced a feeling of great amazement and had the conscious thought, "I can't do that with the dummy." Shortly thereafter he became depressed and feared he would die.

Edgar L. Lipton

Several years before seeing me he had terminated a long analysis with an older, very authoritarian female analyst in another city. His reasons for entering that analysis centered on feelings that he had no penis and no personality of his own. He had been hypochondriacally anxious and chronically depressed and saw himself as very passive, capable only of imitating other men, and afraid of adult women. He had suffered from compulsions to look at and touch little girls, accompanied by great feelings of shame and guilt.

I shall present the salient points of this man's development as they could be reconstructed at the end of the treatment. Mr. V. was told repeatedly by his mother that he was a "miracle" child. He was an only child born after several years of attempts at conception. His mother was informed by her doctor that she would be unable to have any other children. Birth and pregnancy were said to have been uncomplicated. The mother delighted in telling many ghost stories in a playful way, but she often included the idea that if she had died in childbirth, he might not have lived. He was given many enemas until his fourth birthday. At 4½ years he was moved out of his crib into a bed of his own and was said to have regressed for a few months to a short period of bed wetting. He was bathed by his mother in a small tub in the bedroom until he was 11 or 12 years old. He saw his entire childhood as lonely and isolated from peers. His mother catered to him in many ways and treated him like a prince, but tried to stay very close to him and afforded him very little privacy.

When the patient was 4 years old, his father was fired from a job as a night watchman on a construction site, probably for sleeping. For the next 5 years he then held a number of unskilled jobs until, at the urging of his wife, he stopped his work and tried to operate a small business to which he commuted some distance, coming home only on weekends. The patient, with his bed, was moved back into the parental bedroom which he had left only a year previously. After a few months the business failed, the father returned home and began the work he continued for the rest of his life on the night shifts as a machine shop worker. The patient continued sleeping in the parental bedroom, and left it only at age 16, when he insisted on moving into the living room.

Mr. V.'s mother went to the toilet, dressed, bathed, and changed her menstrual pads regularly within his sight.[4] Even after Mr. V. moved out of the bedroom, she continued to be immodest before him, but by that time he was more successful in evading her.

This difficult picture was further complicated when the patient's mother, in order to augment the family income, boarded a disturbed foster child 2 years older than the patient. This boy stayed only for a few months because he became unmanageable. The patient, then 7 years old, was at first very excited to have an older brother, but his feelings changed quickly when this boy regularly terrorized and bullied him.

Shortly after the removal of the foster child, the patient became ill with mumps and had to stay home from school for several weeks. Previously he had stayed home occasionally because of colds or stomachaches, but from that time on his absences became much more frequent and were encouraged by his mother. She wrote dishonest excuses to the school on every occasion in order to keep him home with her. This pattern of school truancy persisted for many years.

Another series of incidents in which my patient remembers being terrorized occurred soon after he became a truant. A neighbor boy, somewhat older than he, pursued and hit him for many months. It was during this period that the patient began performing magic shows for friends and family, but especially for his mother. He recalled fantasizing that he was more powerful than this boy and that through his magic he could control all bullies.

At that time he saw a motion picture starring the singer Al Jolson. He came home and began imitating his voice and soon

---

4. Clinical experience has alerted us to the effects of such exposures. Greenacre (1968) in particular stressed the defective body image of such patients. Mr. V.'s untutored self-description as having no penis of his own aptly confirms these findings.

thereafter the voices of other people. Later, after watching the very popular television ventriloquist Paul Winchell, he tried to copy him. In this he was aided by his mastery of voice mimicry, generally considered to be the hardest and most important part of the ventriloquial act. His self-taught ventriloquism pleased his mother even more than the magic acts. She encouraged him to enter a contest for young ventriloquists, a nationwide competition for children sponsored by Paul Winchell, and purchased a commercially manufactured dummy for him.[5] He did not win any prizes, but his mother told neighbors and relatives that he had won the dummy as a prize for his performance. He did not contradict her in this deception, just as he made no effort to resist collaborating with her in the school truancy deceptions.

When V. was 10 years old, his father was involved in an accident and stayed in bed for several months in order to build up the legal aspects of several court suits, which eventually he lost. The patient perceived these law suits and his parents' behavior as shameful family secrets. This period of dishonesty augmented his old feelings of shame connected with his truancy, the father's business failures, and memories of his own enuresis when he was 4 years old.

Mr. V.'s mother always had had one or two cats as house pets, but when her husband's business failed she began to acquire more and more pet cats. The patient recalled counting 22 cats in residence in their 3-room apartment. When he was 16, he and the family were mortified when the superintendent asked them to move from their basement apartment because of the neighbors' complaints of the nuisance created by the sights and smells of the cats.

At age 18, in spite of his mother's pleading that he stay, he moved out of the house into an apartment of his own. By that time she had deteriorated further; she had become a "bag lady" who, looking bizarre, walked the city streets talking to herself and collecting garbage and old clothes in paper bags.

During these years he saw very little of his father, who had

5. Winchell's book (1954) mentions, probably in exaggeration, that nearly 15,000 entered this contest.

adapted to the peculiarities of an aggressive and odd wife by absenting himself for most of the time from the house. Once the patient moved out of the home, he emulated his father in seeing his mother as little as possible. He was deeply ashamed of her and on several occasions when he was in his 20s and saw her on city streets, he avoided meeting her. He had only sporadic contact with her except for a few dutiful telephone calls from the age of 18 until 30, when he visited her at the hospital where she lay dying of an inoperable cancer.

The father also died of cancer when the patient was 26. Mr. V. visited the dying father in the hospital, but had seen very little of him for several years prior to these last visits. There was very little mourning for either parent before treatment.

His eleventh year had been a particularly traumatic one for him in terms of the loss of several older male figures. An especially important person was his paternal grandfather, who died of cancer after a long illness. Earlier during that year he had taken one of his mother's cats to a veterinarian to be altered and it had died at the kennel after the operation. He did not mourn deeply for either the cat or his grandfather, but was saddened. These were his first meaningful exposures to death. After the grandfather's death his fears of the dark, which had existed for about a year, changed to fears that he would die of cancer.

From age 20 to 23 he worked in a funeral parlor with no more than an initial squeamishness when he began to assist in the embalming procedures. Simultaneously, he attended college at night, studying business administration and accounting. He was an excellent student, and after graduation he was able to leave the funeral parlor for employment in his professional field.

In this large firm, he saw himself as the protégé of an admired older man, but became troubled by his shyness in approaching women. Depressed and feeling very unmanly, he sought psychoanalysis. He described his first analyst as a very authoritarian person who told him in many ways how to run his life, and apparently entered quite actively into his fantasy that he was only a little boy. Nevertheless, in the 12 years of this analysis a great deal was accomplished. He ceased being chronically depressed; got a firmer sense of himself as having substance and ideas of his own; fell in love and married a loving, strong woman with whom he achieved a very satisfactory relationship in all respects. He advanced steadily in his company and changed from a shy, unassuming, and rather withdrawn man to one who, while still feeling shy, was a well-liked leader in both his job and his local community center.

One of the major conflictual themes in Mr. V.'s life was that of separating from his mother and becoming an individually functioning person. The difficulties in separation and in asserting himself were aggravated by his mother's intrusiveness, on the one hand, and by her encouraging interests of his on the other. In many respects she forced him into a shared world, not only keeping him home with her physically but also involving him in the duplicity of her various schemes. With regard to his interest in ventriloquism, his mother indeed treated him like the stereotyped mother of a child actor who pushes her child from audition to audition. She repeatedly told him that he would be her savior and that his successes as a ventriloquial performer would surely solve all of their financial difficulties. It is of interest that his first ventriloquial act consisted of the ventriloquist constantly scolding and correcting a little boy who made many stupid errors. This act was a thinly disguised repetition, albeit in a humorous vein, of his day-to-day life with his mother.

An important change in his life occurred at 14 or 15 when he began to attend a local community center and became attached to a religious leader who treated him in a fatherly way. Thus by 16 he became able to separate emotionally as well as physically from his mother. It is of special interest that at that time he also put away his ventriloquial dummies. It seemed that once he detached himself from his domineering mother, he no longer needed "to speak in two voices." He left the dummies in a closet for most of his adolescence. Although he gave a few performances, he did not practice or work out any new routines until much later when he was asked to give some performances for pay at his local community center or volunteered to perform for church groups and Sunday school classes. On these occasions he primarily enacted parent and child characters or Bible stories. He basked in the adulation and praise bestowed on him as a lovable actor and avoided giving the impression of a feared and powerful magician.

While many aspects of this man's psychopathology are of interest, I shall confine myself to those that have a direct bearing on his interest in magic and ventriloquism.

Mr. V. grew up dreading constantly that his truancies would be discovered. He had only marginal relations with his peers because he was timid and afraid of exposing his family secrets and revealing himself or his parents as liars. The ventriloquism allowed him to meet the world outside of his family in an active yet separate way. Prior to his interest in ventriloquism, his mother had dominated his life and allowed him virtually no privacy. The ventriloquial play not only allowed him to gain love and admiration from his mother, but also provided an acceptable vehicle for establishing some independence. He could use the dummy to express aggressive feelings without much fear of retribution. In addition, the male dummy permitted him to express positive feelings for a male figure without incurring the wrath of a mother who derided her husband and men in general. The hobby helped him to obtain an entrée with peers and others, as well as an identity as someone special.

Wangh's (1962) ideas on the evocation of a proxy illuminate some of the functions of ventriloquism in Mr. V. Wangh described patients who mobilize another person to function as an "alter ego." The anxiety the patient arouses in the proxy stirs the proxy to do what the patient himself dare not carry out or feel. The proxy's actions reinforce the patient's ego control, maintain his reality testing, and ward off threatened loss of object relationships by temporarily allowing a partial fusion with the proxy as an object. The ventriloquist can be thought of as using the dummy as a kind of proxy in Wangh's sense. The dummy does and says what the ventriloquist would not allow himself to do or say in his own identity. The dummy can also be compared to the children who act out their parents' unconscious but warded-off wishes (Johnson and Szurek, 1952). The main difference is that while in Wangh's proxy and in the children described by Johnson and Szurek other people are used to act out or voice the warded-off feelings and thoughts, the ventriloquist plays both roles himself, merely splitting his voices and projecting the unacceptable ideas onto the dummy. For this reason it might be more appropriate to compare the dummy to an imaginary companion, the child's own creation with whom he interacts. Indeed, Mr. V. as well as several of the performers I interviewed told me that they in fact often spoke in private to their dummies.[6]

In the patient's previous analysis, as far as I could determine, his ventriloquism was interpreted as an extension of himself, the dummy being symbolic of his penis, as though in compensation for his feelings of not having a penis. The ventriloquial performance was interpreted as an act in which the patient was both the powerful manipulator behind the scenes and a weak little boy who could not speak for himself. In short, the ventriloquist stood for the mother and the dummy for himself. This scene was indeed played out in the 12-year analysis in which the transference was characterized by awe and feelings of being a puppet in the hands of a powerful woman.

The predominant transference fantasies in his treatment with me were similar, especially his fears of being discovered as an inadequately functioning professional person (rather than sexual man). Much of our work centered on his fears of aggressive strivings directed against men and the symptomatic and characterological sequelae of the emotional and physical absence of his father who was berated as a failure, as weak and a poor provider, but who in fact was a physically strong man.

The patient was obsessionally preoccupied with questions of whether or not he had betrayed or would betray professional secrets in his work and thus bring about some disaster to others and himself. His excessive concern with secrets and with "giving them away" was intimately tied to the dishonesty of both

6. After a ventriloquial performance members of the audience often ask the performer: "Do you talk to your dummy?" The standard answer to this is, "No, of course I don't. We stopped talking after our argument two years ago."

parents and the familial secrets to which he had been privy—
the school truancies, the insurance fraud, and other lies. In his
childhood he was ashamed and mortified, feelings he partly
released in his ventriloquist acts by letting the dummy express
them. In addition, however, he was also demonstrating to his
parents how they *should* behave. Yet, speaking with two voices,
each expressing opposing aspects of his conflict, he himself felt
dishonest or at least sensed that there was something fraudulent in his ventriloquist act—that he, like his parents, was getting away with fooling and tricking people into believing something which he knew was not so.[7] Thus, in a certain sense, the
ventriloquist performance itself contributed to his fear of
"being found out" or the fear-wish to be exposed and expose
others.

Focus on this problem led to an interesting sequence in the
treatment. The patient talked about his having witnessed a girl
playmate's nude genital at ages 8 and 10 and feeling that he
had observed her "secret." He then described his lifelong ob-
sessive impulses to rip off the wigs and/or beards of adult men.
His associations led to memories of his father who was prematurely bald and often complained of arthritic back pains
which caused him to walk with a limp. Following an interpretation of a possible connection between his father's physical defects, the sights of the female genital, and his wishes and fears
of aggressively revealing secrets in order to expose a genital
secret, the symptoms of wishing to rip off disguises disappeared. Working through the reality factors of an absent but
not so weak father, and the implications of a mother who herself seemed to have had major separation and other problems,
led to a resolution of his own current phobic states, depressive
moods, and ambivalences.

A recurrent preoccupation that started when he was 8 was
related to his interests in magic and ventriloquism. He had
frequent daydreams of having superman powers. Through
these superman fantasies he could compensate for his helpless

7. It is significant that in his adult life he performed only for superego-
approved purposes. This was true even in the case of his superior (see below)
who had "tricked" Mr. V. and who therefore "deserved" to be exposed.

feelings in response to bullies as well as to his domineering mother. They constituted a variation of the family romance fantasy, enabling him to achieve an oedipal triumph by winning the admiration of women. They also gratified wishes for a powerful father in that in fantasy he gained the admiration of men for his prowess. Similar daydreams recurred during his treatment with me. He reported that when he was anxious, he walked the streets and daydreamed that he was Superman scaling the heights of tall buildings on the way to my office. Fearing nothing and being invisible, he could discover my "secrets." This Superman fantasy expressed his wishes to be powerful and aggressive and to compete successfully with a feared authority figure in the transference.

At one point in his treatment with me, Mr. V. worried about being ill at ease with his infant son. He felt he did not know how to play with him. He started to play regularly with the little boy via the ventriloquial dummy. The child responded with smiles, which greatly relieved Mr. V. When the child was about 18 months, he began to want to play with the dummy himself. Mr. V. became extremely anxious. He expressed fears that the dummy would be broken; but there was an undercurrent of jealousy, as though he feared that his proxy, the dummy, was more interesting to the child than he was. He was greatly concerned with not letting the baby play with the dummy lest this fragile instrument be damaged, but it became clear that the dummy could not be so easily broken. The injury anxiety screened the patient's actual competitiveness with the doll. Earlier he had shown similar competitive strivings in relation to his wife when he witnessed the birth of his son. His depression at that time thus was determined by a revival of murderous fantasies connected with the wish to be the only child.

As was true in his childhood, ventriloquism permitted Mr. V. to express aggressive feelings without retribution fears. This was illustrated by his description of a ventriloquial performance he gave for the managers of his accounting firm. His direct superior, an alcoholic, had been overbearing toward him and had been taking advantage of Mr. V. by using his reports without giving him credit for the work. Mr. V. structured his act by saying to his dummy that they would be going on an underwater exploration. At one point in this tableau he pointed to his superior in the audience and asked the dummy whether he saw the wreck out there. The dummy replied, "Careful, V., Mr. Green [he used the actual name of the superior] can sue you for that." The audience loved it.

SUMMARY

Magic acts, the performance of tricks, and ventriloquism normally attract the interest of many latency-aged children and adolescents. The interest in ventriloquism, like the choice of other hobbies or professions, is multidetermined and serves both conflict-free and conflictual ends. In the case I presented, the child's interest in ventriloquism was actually encouraged and promoted by the mother, though for her own ends. He used his ventriloquial skills in the service of emancipation from his stifling attachment to her, as an aid in improving his marginal relationships with peers, as a means of coping with his conflicts over his aggressive strivings and murderous and competitive fantasies. His ventriloquial performances also were based on an identification with his parents. On the one hand, he caricatured their insincerity and dishonesty; on the other, he himself fooled people and spoke with several voices. The issues of being found out and exposed were central in his life experiences and entered into his choice of ventriloquism.

In latency when he took up magic tricks and ventriloquism, he was unable to leave his mother, was timid, was afraid of the dark, and terrified by bullies. After his first exposure to human death, some of these anxieties coalesced into a common final pathway of a fear of death. Later in his 20s his occupational choice of the mortuary industry was certainly multidetermined, but probably had a counterphobic element as one determinant. Attempts to deal with the fear of death have throughout the ages been channeled into rituals and religious practices. It is interesting to note that ventriloquism, as it was used in ancient magical rituals and religions, functioned as a means of simulating communication with the dead. If the dead can speak, death does not exist and we need fear neither object loss nor our own death wishes. In denying death, ventriloquism performs the ultimate magic.

BIBLIOGRAPHY

BERGEN, E. (1938), *How To Be a Ventriloquist*. New York: Gross & Dunlap.
BUDGE, E. A. W. (1901), *Egyptian Magic*. New York: Dover, 1971.
FRAZER, J. G. (1905), The beginnings of religion. *Fortnightly Rev.*, 48:162–172.
———— (1911), *Folklore in the Old Testament*, 2 vols. London: Macmillan.
FREUD, S. (1919), The uncanny. *S. E.*, 17:219–256.
GREENACRE, P. (1968), Perversions. *Psychoanal. Study Child*, 23:47–62.
HERTZ, J. H. (1979), *The Pentateuch and Haftorah*. London: Soncino Press.
INTERNATIONAL BROTHERHOOD OF VENTRILOQUISTS (1950–60), *The Oracle* (official publication).
JOHNSON, A. M. & SZUREK, S. A. (1952), The genesis of antisocial acting out in children and adults. *Psychoanal. Q.*, 21:323–343.
LEUBA, J. H. (1912), *A Psychological Study of Religion*. New York: Macmillan.
MIDDLETON, J. (1967), *Magic, Witchcraft, and Curing*. Austin: Univ. Texas Press.
RASMUSSEN, K. (1965), A shaman's journey to the sea spirit. In *Readings in Comparative Religion*, ed. W. A. Lessa & E. Z. Vogt. New York: Harper & Row, 2nd ed., pp. 460–464.
RUSSELL, F. (1898), *Ventriloquism and Kindred Arts*. London: Keith, Prowse.
SCHINDLER, G. (1979), *Ventriloquism*. New York: David McKay.
THORNDIKE, L. (1923–58), *A History of Magic and Experimental Science*, 8 vols. New York: Columbia Univ. Press.
WANGH, M. (1962), The evocation of a proxy. *Psychoanal. Study Child*, 17:451–469.
WINCHELL, P. (1954), *Ventriloquism for Fun and Profit*. Baltimore: I. & M. Ottenheimer.

Hans Christian Andersen and Children

PHYLLIS GREENACRE, M.D.

AS HANS CHRISTIAN ANDERSEN IS KNOWN AS ONE OF THE world's most famous writers of fairy tales for children, he is naturally thought of as a great lover of children. This, however, is not quite true. His relation to children was complex, full of contradictory feelings with ambivalence that bred ambiguity. This could be said of many other aspects of his life and is only noteworthy here because it is by the fairy tales that he won, almost against his will, great and lasting fame. Only those who have studied his life know of his six novels, which in their day won some acclaim. In addition, he wrote a number of very popular travel books, several plays, as well as books of poetry and several autobiographies.

His first ambition was to be a singer. He had an excellent voice as a boy soprano, but had to give up this ambition when his voice broke in late adolescence. Subsequently he aimed to be a ballet dancer, and after 2 years of lessons, had to renounce this too, as he was so awkward and ungainly that he was once referred to as looking like an orangutan. He sketched tolerably well and had developed an extraordinary ability to make elaborate paper cutouts that often embodied figures that had some significance in his inner life and early memories. But there were few children and no babies in them. The early cutouts resembled doodling as he often did them while he was listening to someone else.

The fairy tales actually contain very few fairies, though an-

Member, New York Psychoanalytic Institute; Professor of Clinical Psychiatry, Emeritus, Cornell University, New York.

gels are mentioned as being at hand and magic is not unknown. Perhaps the greatest fairy tale of all was the *Fairy Tale of My Life*, his last autobiography. Its first chapter starts with:

> My life is a lovely story, happy and full of incident. If, when I was a boy and went forth into the world poor and friendless, a good fairy had met me and said "Choose now thy own course in life, and the objects for which thou will strive, and then through development of thy mind, and as reason requires, I will guide and defend thee to its attainment," my fate could not, even then have been directed more happily, more prudently or better. The history of my life will say to the world what it says to me—"There is a loving God, who directs all things for the best."

We see then that the good fairy is God's helper, even as the angels are in some of his stories.

He then gives an account of his birth: "On April 2, 1805, in the town of Odense,—the only child of a young couple who were extremely attached to each other. The father, a young man of 22, though only a shoemaker, was richly gifted and of truly poetical mind. His wife, a few years older,[1] was ignorant of the world and of life, but possessed a heart full of love." With many details he describes the trim little one-room home where he was born and spent the first decade of his life. They were so poor that his father had made a bed out of a trestle which had recently borne the coffin of Count Trampe.

Very little of this was strictly true. Obviously his good fairy had been at work to make a suitable birthplace for him. The time but not the place of his birth was registered. The parents did not occupy this home until some time toward the end of the first year or during the second year. Both parents came from very impoverished and unstable backgrounds. Andersen probably had some knowledge of this for he sometimes referred to himself as a swamp plant. The marriage was apparently a reluctant one, achieved only 2 months before he was born. While it was true that Hans Christian was the only child of these two parents, the mother had already an illegitimate child, Karen Marie, who was 6 years older than Hans Christian. He never

_____

1. Actually she was 11 years older.

knew her and had seen her only once to the best of his memory, though he may have seen her during the first, the unrecorded year. His father had some ambitions to be a student, but had become instead a discouraged and unsuccessful shoemaker.

The one-room home was close to the Grey Friars Hospital, a group of buildings caring for the mentally sick and the aged, with the gaol adjacent. Andersen's paternal grandfather was probably a manic-depressive patient, periodically housed in the asylum, while his paternal grandmother worked around the grounds. His maternal grandmother and his maternal great-grandmother were known to have served short gaol terms as they were so unlucky as to have had third illegitimate children, and the law only permitted two without punishment. This grandmother does not appear in person in Andersen's autobiography, and it is possible that she had agreed not to intrude on her daughter's family after the marriage actually took place. Since Karen Marie and her grandmother lived in the same town with the young Hans, it is probable that he heard something about them and that this knowledge was soon repressed. He spoke rarely of Karen Marie, and then referred to her as "my mother's daughter."

With no younger siblings or neighborhood playmates he may have had little contact with or special interest in human babies. He had no animal pets and was quite afraid of dogs. There was, however, a fanciful interest in storks and other large egg-layers, and in his later stories, these clearly substituted metaphorically for humans. He could, in a way, bypass direct knowledge of human birth. He had very little formal schooling until he was about 16.[2] As a young child he often saw carnivals and the guild parades, and at 7 he was taken to the theater. This remained always a strong influence and preoccupation. It is reported that at one time he was so taken up with acting that he actually believed that he was a character in the play. This alarmed his mother who feared that he was becoming mad like his (paternal) grandfather. It may have been at this time that his father

---

2. He had three short periods in school, terminated by his mother who considered him too delicate for the usual discipline. She also may have feared that he would hear something derogatory about herself.

built a little theater for Hans, and the mad grandfather contributed strange carved animals and people for it.

As a precocious reader, he was preoccupied with his own daydreams and meant in a few years to write plays that would compare with those of Shakespeare or be novels like Scott's. His interests also turned inward, and for a time he was concerned with the functioning of the human body. Always ready to be on stage, he soon began to share his knowledge with the old ladies whom he visited in the spinning room of the hospital. He lectured to them on human anatomy and drew pictures to illustrate his talk. He presumably dealt with the vital organs: heart, lungs, and alimentary system. The ladies were interested and thought him too bright a child. There was no reference, however, to anatomical differences between the sexes, or to babies. The genitals seem to have been ignored.

This period of relative solitude and active daydreaming ended decisively at 14, 3 years after his father's death, when he left Odense to seek fame and fortune in Copenhagen. Here he found a patron and surrogate father in Jonas Collin, a member of the board of directors of the Royal Theater. This began a staunch relationship in which Andersen became an "almost member" of the Collin family and developed a strong, lasting, and mutually ambivalent friendship with Edvard Collin, oldest son of Jonas. Andersen wrote innumerable letters to and about the various members of the Collin family. These and his autobiographies contain little or no references to two younger brothers, who must have been quite young when Andersen joined the family. There is, however, a later letter from Edvard in reply to one from Andersen (then 41) reminding Andersen of how in much earlier years Theodore, one of the brothers, used to tease Andersen by sitting on the floor and tickling Hans Christian's legs to distract him when he was drinking his afternoon coffee (Bøøk, 1962, p. 188).

The death of a young child and the anguish of the mother were recurrent themes throughout Andersen's young adulthood. While a student at the Slagelse Grammar School, he wrote a poem "The Dying Child," which was ultimately published. It became quite popular, although the headmaster attempted to suppress it, saying that writing it had interfered with serious studies. Andersen seemed to be expressing through it his anguish lest his own poetic creative ability might be destroyed. He continued to be preoccupied with thoughts of the grief and sometimes guilt at the loss of a child. Aspects of this theme appeared in one guise or another in his fairy tales, notably "The Angel," "Story of a Mother," "Anne Lisbeth," and "The Dead Child."

Andersen in fact never liked to have children touch him. It was characteristic of him to demand a listening audience for anything he wrote before he offered it for publication. This is a common enough need and practice among writers generally, but with him the situation was essential and highly charged. Yet he did not want any corrective criticism, only affirmations and praise. This need for applause led to many difficulties because he felt any suggestion for change as an attack. To others he seemed irritable and vain. He liked children who were old enough to read and would sit quietly at a little distance, and just *listen.* He referred mostly to boys. It is not clear how these audiences were recruited or how often they were assembled. He seemed to need confirmation not only of what he wrote but of his own physical presence and appearance. He did not just report what had happened in the story, he told it as though it was happening right then, and was vitally experienced. To a lesser degree this was true in his travel books. He made the reader a fellow traveler.

He was uneasy if children sat next to him or leaned against him, or physically touched him in any way. Some friends thought that he could be at ease only with children whom he knew personally, but this was not generally true. There is a good deal of presumptive evidence that he felt that he had inadequate genital equipment and was inordinately sensitive on this score. As a boy of 14, he had suffered humiliation at the hands of fellow workers in a cloth factory. He had sung, recited bits of Shakespeare, and imagined that he was pleasing them, when two of them seized him and pulled down his pants to determine whether he might be a girl. This surely contributed to his sensitivity about his body, but did not cause it.

Most of all he dreaded physical contact in a crowd of any kind, and the idea of children milling around him was torture.

As he approached 70, admirers in his own country planned to
honor him by having his statue placed in the Kongens Have, a
park in Copenhagen. On his birthday, April 2, 1875, he was
told that the money was collected, and late in May the sculptor,
August Saabye, brought him a sketch which showed him seated
in a chair reading, surrounded by a crowd of eager children.
The very sight of this threw him into such a rage that he refused to pose. He objected especially to the idea of a tall boy
who seemed to be lying right up against his crotch.

Even on a second visit from Saabye he had not cooled down.
He soon wrote an emphatic letter to Jonas Collin, grandson of
the older Jonas Collin,

> My blood was boiling, and I spoke clearly and unambiguously,
> saying, "None of the sculptors knew me, nothing in their at-
> tempts indicated that they had seen or realized the characteris-
> tic thing about me,—that I could never read aloud if anyone
> was sitting behind me or leaning towards me, and even less if I
> had children sitting on my lap or on my back, or young
> Copenhagen boys leaning up against me, and that it was only a
> manner of speaking when I was referred to as 'the children's
> writer'—my aim being for all ages; and so children could not
> represent me. Naïveté was only part of the fairy tale, humour,
> on the other hand was the salt, and my written language was
> based on the folk language, that was my Danishness
> [Bredsdorff, 1975, p. 271f.].

The statue that was finally placed in Kongens Have has no
children in it. Andersen is sitting with a book in his hand evidently reading aloud to an invisible audience. This statue is
somewhat similar to one in New York's Central Park, though
the latter has a little duckling looking up expectantly. It is clear
from his protest to Jonas Collin that he still carried, or had
relapsed into, an extreme neurotic body shyness that had been
most apparent in his young manhood. This state of mind is
vividly presented in the character of Otto Thostrup in the novel
O.T., published when Andersen was 31 years old. At 70 he still
felt embarrassed and reluctant to be honored so exclusively for
his stories for children. He would have preferred to be thought
of only as a great creative artist, proficient in many fields, a
digter.

Some of his first fairy tales were refurbished folk tales, written to earn money, and when published they were marked "For Children." Later he felt better when he had found a way in which to write a story so that the patent action would be enjoyed by the children while the deeper significance would reach adults. He was pleased and relieved when the announcements of new groups of stories did not carry the phrase "For Children." Some of his later tales were witty, even commentaries on human foibles, social customs, and pretentions (e.g., "The Collar," "The Happy Family," "The Professor and the Flea," "Great Grandfather").

Andersen twice found himself literally surrounded by children, and appointed without any warning to play a part in the detested story of the Pied Piper. On his first visit to England in 1847, Mary Howitt, who had translated much of his work, very soon invited him to a country party, where he found himself welcomed and surprised by a bevy of children gathered to greet him. He clearly was expected to respond by telling them stories. The trip had been hot and fatiguing, and he spoke English so poorly that he was unable to respond. After an attempt, he gave up and tried to entertain the hoard by making small flower arrangements, at which he was very skillful. In the end it was quite a fiasco; the children drifted away to their own games, while he retreated to find refuge in a cooler spot. Mrs. Howitt, who sometimes seemed more energetic than sensitive, was disappointed and attributed his withdrawal to his jealousy of an American writer, Henry Clarke Wright, who was also a guest and came to the rescue, substituting for Andersen in amusing the children with his stories (Bain, 1895, p. 272ff.).

Fourteen years later he again unexpectedly found himself selected to participate in a play about the Pied Piper. It was on a smaller scale, and he did not have to play the Piper himself. On a visit to Rome together with young Jonas Collin (Edvard's son) he met and was invited to the home of an American sculptor, William Wetmore Story, where an impromptu party was going on. Elizabeth and Robert Browning were there with their 12-year-old son, as well as a number of others with younger children. Andersen amused some of the children with his paper cutouts and attempted to read "The Ugly Duckling," but his

English was so halting that he gave it up. Browning struck up with the *Pied Piper,* and organized a grand march in which he played the leading part, with Story playing a flute. Andersen's further contribution is not clear, but anyway a little girl crowned him with a wreath of laurel and gave him some lovely roses. He recorded this very scantily in his autobiography (p. 462), did not mention it at all in his letters to friends at this time, and gave it slight attention in his diary. Forty years later a much more detailed and fulsome account was given by Henry James (1903), in a book he wrote about his visit, having been one of the notables who took part in the merriment. One gets the impression that Andersen was uncomfortable in the crowd of children and wished to forget it, whereas James may have embellished it in this much later account. It may be that on this occasion Andersen felt reassured by the very nature of the participants in the Pied Piper parade. If so, his fears were allayed but by no means gone, and surfaced again in a full-fledged panic and rage at the age of 70 at the thought of his own image being cast in stone, a solitary man surrounded forever by a crowd of children.

One cannot know with complete assurance from what his terrible fear arose. It would seem, from the very nature of his symptom, that he had been—or thought he had been—threatened by a sexual attack by an older boy. But this can only be a reasonable assumption. It is clear from the accounts of his childhood that he had so vivid an imagination that at times he did not distinguish objective thought, dream, or fantasy from fact.

His very situation in the snug little one-room home, which he idealized so much in his autobiography, clearly predisposed him to early and constant participation in whatever sexual or other activities went on between his parents. This situation might have colored and distorted his development of sexual interest and promoted as well a fear of hostile aggression in himself and in others. There was also a more than ordinary feminine quality in his appearance and behavior that caused him at one time in his later school days to refer to himself as being somewhat *airy-fairy*.

Andersen's unease with boys was mostly with those who came to listen to his stories. He wanted them to keep at a (physical) distance, to sit and *listen*. There is no mention of little girls at these readings, but our information is limited. He could be both cordial and friendly to children, both boys and girls who wrote to him *after having read* his stories. He carried on a prolonged correspondence with Annemarie Livingston, the daughter of Dr. Livingston, the famous African traveler. They exchanged 13 letters between 1869 and 1874, when she wrote him about her father's death and the funeral in Westminster Abbey (Bredsdorff, p. 255f.). She was to lose this good friend very soon, for Andersen died in August 1875.

That he might have a warm heart for special little ones too young to come to his listening sessions and so disturb him is illustrated by his correspondence with William, the nephew of Mrs. Melchior, who with her husband had filled the benevolent family role after Jonas Collin's death. On July 31, 1874, Andersen wrote to Mrs. Melchior, "Please tell William that a little while ago a fly came to rest in my ear; it told me that it had seen William writing a letter to me. The fly wanted to know what he had been writing, but he chased it away. Is that true?" Mrs. Melchior replied on August 5, "Little William, who was here yesterday, found your story about the fly amusing, but said he did not chase it away at all." Andersen replied 2 days later, "Please tell my friend William from me that he did in fact chase away the fly, who was supposed to have brought him greetings; the fly assures me this is so and tells me that it can swear that his hand was dirty; she quite clearly noticed a splotch on his hand when he chased her away. Who shall I believe, the fly or William? By the way, please tell him that the fly is a flying princess; her father is alive and reigns over all human noses." Five days later he again wrote to Mrs. Melchior, "Please tell William that I have sent off a sparrow with greetings; it will fly past him in the garden three times which means 'Hello, William!'" (Bredsdorff, p. 256). This certainly was just the sort of provocative banter that a 5-year-old would cherish, when he is poised between babyhood and being a school boy.

In the last 5 to 6 years of his life, Andersen did not travel as much as he had in the past, nor find it as invigorating.[3] He was

3. The last journey was 2½ months in Germany and Switzerland (1873).

somewhat slowed down and may not have had as ready a response to fellow travelers, or eagerness to find himself praised and recognized. With his diminishing strength his neurotic vagaries became more troublesome. In this situation he became more responsive to the children of friends in Copenhagen whom he visited frequently. Edvard Collin, writing some time after Andersen's death, remarked that Andersen had then told spur-of-the-moment stories to children of friends. These became so vivid that they soon were serial stories that continued from visit to visit. Rigmore Stampe, the granddaughter of Ingeborg Drewson (thus the great-granddaughter of Jonas Collin) in a book about Andersen wrote that she had always felt at ease with him, that he was always good and kind; he brought presents from abroad and after telling fairy tales sometimes later sent small printed editions as they were published.

Paper cutouts were important at this time. It was a talent that Andersen developed early and brought to great refinement. Sir Henry Dickens who was only 8 and not particularly responsive to Andersen at Gad's Hill, in 1857, was entranced by the paper cuttings that produced "lovely little figures of sprites and elves, gnomes, fairies and animals of all kinds—delightful in their refinement and delicacy," while Rigmore Stampe described them as "little fairy tales, not illustrations for written fairy tales, but expressions of the same imagination.—He was essentially concerned with a limited series of motifs which he went on repeating, especially in his paper cut-outs. There were castles, swans, goblins, angels, cupids and other imaginary characters, many hearts, a dead man hanging on a gallows, a 'chamberlain with his key hanging on his back,' a windmill in the shape of a man—the wings being his arms and legs—and many others" (Bredsdorff, p. 303).

Kjeld Heltoft, a contemporary Danish painter, in 1969 wrote an amazing and beautiful book on *Hans Christian Andersen as an Artist*. It contains reproductions of Andersen's pencil drawings of his puppets, pen-and-ink drawings recording his travels; and finally a section with bold pictures of his colored paper cutouts, which refer—one way and another—chiefly to the fairy tales, and so were basically meant for children.

Heltoft emphasizes that the extraordinary acuteness of Andersen's vision was more important than words in producing a sense of animation especially when he read his fairy tales.

> Andersen could *use* his eyes. He remembered a detail with amazing accuracy and had a feeling for figures and landscapes that brought to his writing something immediate and enduring. The colloquial tone became his specialty in literature, but where his art is at its best, the thought is supremely integrated with day-to-day speech; a pronounced visual element is always present as well. Indeed, it can be argued that a visually artistic approach, converted into literature, is the essential reason for the ease with which his writings have succeeded, despite often inadequate translations, in crossing national borders. People may not have appreciated fully the stylistic or philosophical subtlety, but the actual *picture* sank in. Can there be any other author, including Shakespeare and Dickens, who has so many *figures* permanently in daily international speech and awareness!" [p. 8].

When one reads Andersen's notes about his fairy tales, one becomes aware that some actual visual experience often had set off a whole story in which inanimate objects become alive and assert themselves to produce a story, telling a tale of poignant relationships among adults. After all, is this not a revival of a young child's view around him, when vision is the primal initiator of communication before words are adequately achieved and reliable? Vision was of great importance to Andersen and a bit of primitive magic in eye-to-eye contact lasted into his adulthood.

There was a significant incident soon after his arrival in Copenhagen in his mid-teens. Seeking to soften the hard heart of a landlady whose rental fee he could not meet, in her absence he wept, and gathering the tears on his fingers, he smeared them on the eyes of a portrait of her deceased husband. He hoped in this way to arouse the dead man's sympathy which in turn would somehow soften the landlady. In fact it seemed to work for when she returned she was willing to accept a lesser rental. Throughout his life, he responded to *any* strong emotion with tears.

Andersen's fairy tales never begin with "Once upon a time" reporting of past events; the reader is at once introduced into a live emotional situation often through the antics of inanimate objects that have come alive in representing their owners.

In Heltoft's appraisal of the paper cutouts, one misses any recognition that many of them represent disturbing events in Andersen's life which were etched into his memory and reproduced in sharp distorted forms. These represent real experiences as well as screen memories, and sometimes are grotesque and macabre, with nightmarish qualities. He sees these as coming from Andersen's private mythology played out in his childhood with his puppet theater, and others as coming from folk legends and classical myths. One theme that is often repeated in the paper cutouts presents a gallows tree sometimes with one, but more often two human figures dangling from the cross-bar, while at the foot of the gallows there may be one or two hearts. Sometimes a tiny heart is seen resting on the top of one of the bigger hearts.

Heltoft interprets these cutout pictures as referring to death and life. I believe that there was also a specific personal origin, in a horrifying experience that Andersen had in his teens when he was a student in the Slagelse Grammar School. The senior students were given a free afternoon in order that they might view an execution of three people convicted of murder. A girl of 17 had persuaded her lover, by whom she was pregnant, to murder her father who wanted to prevent the marriage. The plan had been that the mother of the girl would marry the assistant murderer. The whole situation haunted Andersen interminably, though most of the audience seemed more concerned with the question of who would get the clothing of the dead convicts (Bredsdorff, p. 53). There had been a much earlier impressive experience when, at the age of 3, he had seen a Spanish soldier being dragged away to be executed for having killed a French soldier. He did not see the actual execution, but a vivid memory of incidental details of the setting remained always with him, in the fashion of a screen memory.

Among many paper cutouts, one male figure recurs prominently in different settings. This is a man whose body is peculiarly angular, as though there were hinges at every joint. He plunges forward as though in a hurry. His posture conveys both pretentiousness and subservience. In one cutout, he carries a tray held over his head, like a waiter hurrying to serve an impatient master. On the tray are small objects that refer to Andersen's fairy tales—a windmill, a swan, a church steeple, and a country house. The figure is almost a replica of a cartoon of Andersen himself as a toady too eager to please, on a visit to Sweden in 1849. At that time, and earlier, he had been ridiculed as a social climber, finding his way not only into the manor houses of the local aristocracy, but into the courts of the nobility and even the royal castles in other countries (Bredsdorff, p. 223).

There are other strange, sometimes androgynous figures. A particularly bizarre cutout presents a broad male (or female?) figure whose body is a windmill with four sails that represent the arms and legs. Two large hearts are where the breasts might be. The mouth is a dark, irregular oblong. In the lower part of the body there is a large open door approachable by a ladderlike structure rooted in the genital area. The legs are widely spread. Each foot is attended by a little girl holding a parasol, while a tiny ballerina hangs upside down, with one foot held in the hand of the monstrous windmill man. It is hard to say at first whether this creature has two arms and four legs, or four arms and two legs, and whether it represents a single creature, or a male and female in coitus. When one scrutinizes this cutout picture more fully, it is evident that if the picture is folded horizontally at the level of the bottom of the monster's body, whoever or whatever was on the ladder would be catapulted into the space of the wide open door. Thus the cutout picture is given a third dimension and coitus is achieved.

It is possible that, since not even a phantom is on the ladder, the ladder itself stands for the implied rhythmic movement necessary in mounting it, and so represents masturbation with a fantasy of the ballerina whom he admired so much and perhaps envied in his late adolescence. In the cutout she is dangling upside down from the hand of the monster. There was some evidence that Andersen was at times a frequent masturbater. This is indicated in some way in his diary, but is not mentioned directly. In other cutouts the ballerina appears in graceful and joyous poses. That the ballerina in this cutout is important is indicated in the title: "Miller with a dancing girl

and Ole Lukøje (the Sandman, also known as old Shut Eye)."
Further pursuing the choice of a windmill to represent the
human being, one can ask: may this not portray how much
human destiny may be determined by the uncontrollable winds
of fate?

From any description such as I have just given, one might
readily think that this cutout was the product of a psychotic
patient. With further thought it seemed to me that this particular cutout might be a composite of many early, never adequately understood impressions and questions about the nature
and actual functioning of the human body. Clearly, the genitals
are the most mysterious and dramatic of all body parts, and yet
were the most unmentionable in Andersen's childlike life. This
cutout is made up of unassimilated primal scenes and other
scoptophilic experiences. These are brought together in an extraordinarily precise and economical way such as may occur in
some dreams. It is clear that in his childhood both at home and
in the adjacent Grey Friars Hospital, he was exposed to many
situations that he could not understand. He made an attempt to
organize his information about the human body in his lectures
to the old ladies in the spinning room, but kept safely away
from questions about genital activity and function.

The windmill man cutout may be regarded as a concise and
condensed accumulation of free associations, such as are connected and verbally expressed in the work of analysis of dreams
in psychoanalytic therapy. Perhaps the relation to dreams is
implicitly recognized in attributing the cutout to the Sandman
who puts children to sleep. Somewhere lurking around, too,
there were memories of his mad grandfather who was subject
to joyous outbursts in the spring when he bedecked himself
with flowers and danced on the highways, while at other times
he furnished his young grandson with strange carved figures of
humans and animals. These could be used in young Hans's play
theater.

Andersen's visual acuity and responsiveness were almost uncanny. In making cutouts of faces, he was able with a few simple
snips of the scissors to give an impression of the character or
state of mind back of the face. It is an indication of the strength
of his integrative and synthetic functions involving all senses
working together, combined with extraordinary manual dex-

terity to produce a "simple" and vital impression of his subject. This multiple linkage was phenomenal. While vision seemed his leading function, Andersen's own eyes would not have been well thought of; they were small, deeply set, and rather pale in color. He referred to them as looking like green peas. But they certainly *worked.*

During the last decade of his life, Andersen felt less vigorous and gradually became aware that old Chronos was there as a constant companion looking over his shoulder and disturbing him at night. Traveling no longer stimulated him. In 1867, the prediction of the wise woman of his childhood came true. His native city of Odense was ablaze with light and festivities in his honor. Severe toothache and general fatigability made the occasion one of endurance rather than exhilaration. In 1869, he attempted to attend a series of lectures on fairy and folk tales and was dismayed to find that the lectures were about himself. He felt he was dead, to be so lectured about in a university (Bredsdorff, p. 253). He kept a small apartment in Copenhagen but spent much time in the country homes of the Melchiors and the Henriques. He was on good terms with Edvard and Henriette Collin, but saw them only occasionally.

In this period his paper cutouts flourished, with a growing tolerance of and then friendliness with children. Many of the cutouts then were decorative strips of dancing children, especially little girls. Alone with himself he experimented with new forms of paper pictures and produced a number of collages.

In summary, this paper attempts to describe and define Andersen's strangely varied behavior toward children. For a deeper understanding, however, one needs not only a more thorough study of his life than the condensed sketch given here, but a consideration of his writing, especially of his six novels. It has been said, with some justice, that he never wrote about anything but himself. This gave him a reputation for being vain and stubbornly self-important. The vanity and the preoccupation with himself were secondary, however—the products of an ever present anxiety which spawned innumerable neurotic symptoms. Ambivalence attended all and permeated many aspects of his life.

There was also a deep and stubborn conviction of his own

worth, an intimation of genius, which he accepted as a gift from God. This sustained him in the long stretch of his life, even when he was most tormented by self-doubt and the criticisms of his colleagues. He always tended to feel an outsider. He had a superb sense of humor and wit, which was usually reserved for his closest friends, though it crept into some of his fairy tales as well. He was never able to marry, and I suspect that basically he envied little boys and was afraid of the anger that envy and jealousy could generate in himself.

We may consider briefly Andersen's plight in life: (1) "Who was really my father?"; (2) his relation to his mother, especially in infancy; (3) his bisexual identification; and (4) his problem with rage. I believe that Andersen knew—in the way that children often do know the secrets that the parents think they are keeping from them—that his mother had been a prostitute, at least a practicing if not an established one; and it is probable too that he knew something of the delayed marriage and the "swamp plant" period. This unspoken knowledge carried with it the realization that a child conceived in a brothel could never know who was really his father, or who might be a half-brother or a half-sister, as Karen Marie was. Doubt opened the door to a variety of fantasies about his own identity and increased his tendency to family romance expectations. All in all it contributed to a feeling of not being a whole person by his own birthright, and one of his less happy fantasies was of having been born in the gaol.

Andersen's mother, Anne Marie, was proud of her baby, her pleasure undoubtedly increased by the facts that he was legitimate and that his father accepted the responsibility of supporting them, in contrast to her experience with Rosenvinge, who had fathered Karen Marie and given her his name but failed in every other way. She could feel superior too to her sister Christiane who had gone to Copenhagen and prospered, but had no children.[4] There is no doubt that in her own proprietary and narcissistic way his mother loved her baby very much and was determined that he should become famous. But she came from

4. Some years later when Andersen went to Copenhagen, he found Christiane, the madame in a brothel. She had no children of her own, but two adopted daughters helped her in her profession.

the most meager background, was illiterate, superstitious, and shallow. She may have given him the best she had. She tied him too much to herself, especially as his father tended to be taciturn and morose, without ebullience or merriment. The intensity of her attachment increased his feminine identification, especially as he had little contact with boys or men. He undoubtedly got his love of books from his father, while his mother's blind insistence on his future greatness contributed to his courage and confidence. This situation furnished the background for further ambivalence and increased his doubts of his ability as an ordinary husband and father. His father deserted him and soon died just as Hans approached puberty, and a few years later he deserted his mother (who had remarried), and struck out for himself.

This brings me to consider the fourth major difficulty in the development of his character and personality, namely, his lifelong struggle with *rage*. This may surprise many who have idealized him in a rather simple way, seeing him as one who met repeated adversity with courage and ingenuity—to become world famous by his love for children and his extraordinary ability to tell fairy tales. It is amazing how many twentieth-century writers have tidied up his life story—or perhaps never investigated it—and have given him a childhood and a character that were quite inaccurate. Of course, he did this for himself to a very considerable degree, and wrote autobiographies in his own honor, in a period when biographies were not meant to be too truthful, but to do honor to the deceased one. In the present day we may go rather far in the opposite direction. At any rate, Andersen's struggle with rage was, in my estimation, a major problem and a fact in his life. It made him miserable and often reduced him to tears, for which he was famous among his contemporaries.

The rage began, I believe, in his infancy, perhaps even in the lost unaccounted-for period, before his father had become the legalized father and was at hand, the "swamp" period. In his account of his own life, he commented on how much, according to reports, he cried like a cat—when he was born, when he was baptized, and when he was taken to a party in the gaol! All this crying was supposed to indicate that he would be a great singer.

Chiefly from clinical observations and from material gained

in psychoanalytic practice, I have come to think that adult individuals who have sudden violent attacks of rage, on slight, inadequate provocation, suffered in infancy from particularly severe distress that could not be alleviated. This distress might be from physical pain such as is associated with operations, from abuse, or from chronic discomfort that was not attended by care and attention. Andersen did have attacks of some kind in childhood which have been accepted by some biographers as epileptic, but seem possibly to have been severe tantrums such that his mother was reluctant to allow him to go to school.

His rage came to a head in a violent outburst at Edvard Collin whom he had taken as an alter ego and the closest of friends, when he felt that he was not accepted fully by Edvard and the Collin family. At another time, feeling hurt and rebuffed by his colleagues in the criticism of his work, he wrote a sizzling letter to his friend Henriette Wulff damning the whole Danish nation and praying for its mass extermination. In each situation there was justification for his feeling hurt, but his response was an explosive wish to kill. In his old age, there was the time when he was so angry that he could hardly speak to the sculptor who conceived of him as surrounded by children. More often his anger was repressed, but left him oversensitive, depressed, irritable, and habitually tearful with thoughts of suicide and fear of madness. His novels are extraordinarily autobiographical in thinly disguised ways. Through writing them he may have gotten some periodic relief. It was through his fairy tales (that might better be called his wonder stories) that he could reluctantly claim his fame, being at first fearful that he would be considered childish because he wrote them for children.

BIBLIOGRAPHY

ANDERSEN, H. C. (1855), *The Fairy Tale of My Life*. New York: Paddington Press, 1975.

———— *The Complete Fairy Tales and Stories*, tr. E. C. Haugaard. Garden City, N.Y.: Doubleday, 1974.

BAIN, T. N. (1895), *Hans Christian Andersen*. New York: Dodd, Mead; London: Lawrence & Bullen.

BØØK, F. (1962), *Hans Christian Andersen*, tr. G. C. Schoolfield. Norman: Univ. Oklahoma Press.

BREDSDORFF, E. (1975), *Hans Christian Andersen*. New York: Scribner's.
HELTOFT, K. (1969), *Hans Christian Andersen as an Artist*, tr. R. Spink. Copenhagen: Royal Danish Ministry of Foreign Affairs Press and Cultural Relations Department; Andelsbogtrykkeriet Odense, 1977.
JAMES, H. (1903), *William Wetmore Story and His Friends*. Boston: Houghton, Mifflin.

A 70-Year Follow-up of a Childhood Learning Disability

The Case of Fanny Burney

KATHRYN KRIS, M.D.

SHAME AND IMPAIRED SELF-ESTEEM ARE WELL-KNOWN
consequences of childhood learning disabilities. There is wide
agreement on the need to maintain and restore self-esteem by
means of relationships until developmental lags remit or until
alternate modes of cognition or other avenues for success develop (Bender, 1958; de Hirsch, 1975; Eisenberg, 1975; Klein,
1978; Silver, 1974; Weil, 1977). Among the many excellent case
reports of children and young adults (Berger and Kennedy,
1975; Blanchard, 1946; Bryant, 1964; Buxbaum, 1964; Critchley, 1964; Hellman, 1954; Mahler, 1942; Newman et al., 1973;
Pearson, 1952; Rosen, 1955; Thompson, 1966; Walsh, 1966;
Watson et al., 1982), I could find none that extended throughout a lifetime. Therefore I was specially interested in Fanny
Burney's description of her own, severe childhood dyslexia,
written when she was 74. In her autobiographical account,
Frances Burney (later Madame d'Arblay), the first important
English woman novelist, vividly portrays the way in which a

Psychiatrist, Harvard University Health Service (Medical Area); Associate
in Psychiatry, Brigham and Women's Hospital and Beth Israel Hospital,
Boston, Mass.

The idea for this paper was originally presented at the Workshop on Literary Adolescence of The Boston Psychoanalytic Society and Institute, chaired
by Professor Patricia Spacks and Dr. Jo Ann B. Fineman. I am indebted to
Professor Spacks for her encouragement and for her critical reading of an
earlier draft.

childhood disability may be associated with a lifelong propensity for shame and cognitive disorganization. She shows also how relationships and her writing helped her master this problem. I will draw on autobiographical material from her adolescence, young adulthood, and old age to show these interactions.

FAMILY HISTORY

Fanny Burney was born in England in 1752, the third child in a family of six living siblings. Her parents were middle-class professionals. Her father was Dr. Charles Burney, the famous musician and historian of music. Her mother shared her husband's literary interests and was a writer of ability herself. She died in her 30s when Fanny was 10. When Fanny was 15 her father remarried and two half-siblings were born. Two of Fanny's siblings became prominent. James, the older brother, became an Admiral, and Charles, several years younger, a Greek scholar. Fanny was the most renowned, exceeding even her father. At 25, after writing in secret, she published anonymously her first novel, *Evelina* (Burney, 1778), which was to become a best seller. At first, only members of her family knew the author's identity. Later, her fame and talent gained her a place in the Queen's household. At 41 she married an impecunious French nobleman, and had one son. She lived to the ripe age of 87. For most of this time she wrote novels and plays to support her family, maintained an abundant correspondence, and kept voluminous diaries as a way of life.

CHILDHOOD

Although Fanny Burney's diaries are filled with examples of her trepidation at public notice, whether as a writer or as a person of note, it is only at age 74, writing her father's memoirs and stirred by Sir Walter Scott's interest in her early writing, that she reveals publicly something of the childhood roots for this trepidation. To fulfill her obligation to her father, and to honor him, she had sorted his multitude of letters and papers for 12 years after his death in search of material for his literary biography: the *Memoirs of Doctor Burney* (Arblay, 1832). During these 12 years, her two brothers, Charles and James, and her husband General d'Arblay, had died. Her closest remaining family were Hetty, her older sister, and her grown, unmarried son, Alex. At this time Sir Walter Scott, himself the anonymous author of The Waverly Novels, visited Fanny Burney and inquired about the secret atmosphere in which she had written and published *Evelina*.

Once the impetus for personal reminiscences and reconstruction was set in motion by this visit, 25 pages of personal history poured out, interpolated into her father's biography. The turgid, heavy prose that she employs elsewhere in the *Memoirs* to eulogize her father is relieved by a partial return to her more spontaneous style as she recaptures her past. She begins with her childhood backwardness and leads up to the history of the publication of *Evelina*, a time when she was particularly close to and shared the limelight with her father (Hemlow, 1958, p. 465). Fanny Burney describes her intellectual difficulty:

> FRANCES . . . was during her childhood the most backward of all his family in the faculty of receiving instruction. At eight years of age she was ignorant of the letters of the alphabet; though at ten, she began scribbling, almost incessantly, little works of invention; but always in private; and in scrawling characters, illegible, save to herself [2:123].

Her father, in an autobiographical note that Fanny Burney includes in the *Memoirs* (2:168), is more specific about her difficulty. Dr. Burney contrasts her slowness in reading and writing with her inventiveness. Her parodies of the actors when they went to see Garrick on the stage were composed and recited by heart before she could read. Today such visual perceptual difficulty, in sharp contrast to auditory fluency, would be recognized as a form of dyslexia.

Fanny goes on to tell us how her relationship to her mother protected her from the worst loss of self-esteem during her early childhood. She recalls hearing

> . . . a neighbouring lady recommend to Mrs. Burney, her mother, to quicken the indolence, or stupidity, whichever it might be, of the little dunce, by the chastening ordinances of

Solomon. The alarm, however, of that little dunce, at a suggestion so wide from the maternal measures that had been
practised in her childhood, was instantly superseded by a joy of
gratitude and surprise that still rests upon her recollection,
when she heard gently murmured in reply, 'No, no,—I am not
uneasy about her!'

But, alas! the soft music of those encouraging accents had
already ceased to vibrate on human ears [referring to her
mother's death when she was 10], before these scrambling pot-
hooks had begun their operation of converting into Elegies,
Odes, Plays, Songs, Stories, Farces,—nay, Tragedies & Epic
Poems, every scrap of white paper that could be seized upon
without question or notice; for she grew up, probably through
the vanity-annihilating circumstances of this conscious intellectual disgrace, with so affrighted a persuasion that what she
scribbled, if seen, would but expose her to ridicule, that her
pen, though her greatest, was only her clandestine delight
[2:123f.].

Seven years before writing this autobiographical portion of
the *Memoirs,* in a letter to her older sister, Hetty, Fanny Burney
refers to her mother's literary guidance (Arblay, 1904–05):

. . . she very early indeed began to form your taste for reading,
and delighted to find time, amidst all her cares, to guide you to
the best authors, and to read them with you, commenting and
pointing out passages worthy to be learned by heart. I perfectly recollect, child as I was, and never of the party, this part
of your education. At that very juvenile period, the difference
even of months makes a marked distinction in bestowing and
receiving instruction. I, also, was so peculiarly backward, that
even our Susan [2 years, 7 months younger] stood before me;
she could read when I knew not my letters. But though so
sluggish to learn, I was always observant: do you remember
Mr. Seaton's denominating me, at fifteen, the silent, observant
Miss Fanny? Well I recollect your reading with our dear mother all Pope's Works and Pitt's *Aeneid.* I recollect, also, your
spouting passages from Pope, that I learned from hearing you
recite them before—many years before I read them myself
[6:401].

In the *Memoirs,* Dr. Burney, in a letter to a close friend,
describes his wife's last wish, on her deathbed:

She told poor Hetty how sweet it would be if she could see her constantly from whence she was going, and begged she would invariably suppose that that would be the case. What a lesson to leave a daughter!—She exhorted her to remember how much her example might influence the poor younger ones; and bid her write little letters, and fancies, to her in the other world, to say how they all went on; adding, that she felt as if she should surely know something of them [1:143f.].

This suggestion reinforced Fanny's developing capacity to read and write, as a means of maintaining the relationship with her mother.

In addition to the strong support from her mother and identification with her, Fanny identified with her father's example. During her preadolescent years, while four of her brothers and sisters were away, she and the baby, born a year before her mother's death, remained at home with her father. Busy with teaching music, he began to study and travel, preparing himself for his own writing career which was to culminate in his *A General History of Music,* published when Fanny was 23 (Hemlow, 1958, p. 59). Though he was away often, his example was there, with his library and his friends, particularly the elderly bachelor, Mr. Crisp, who took an interest in Fanny's education and development, promoting her letter writing by his evident pleasure and friendly advice.

In his recollection of her childhood learning difficulty, Fanny's father describes an anecdote with her much-loved and admired 2-year-older brother, James, which provides a clue to one of the relationships in which her lifelong embarrassment and confusion may have originated (Arblay, 1832):

She was wholly unnoticed in the nursery for any talents, or quickness of study: indeed, at eight years old she did not know her letters; and her brother, the tar, who in his boyhood had a natural genius for hoaxing, used to pretend to teach her to read; and gave her a book topsy-turvy, which he said she never found out! [2:168].

Perhaps not, but she could hardly have failed to sense his mood. She seems to return to this childhood relationship in the experience of "vanity-annihilating circumstances of this conscious intellectual disgrace" whenever a man takes interest in her writing. The fine sense of parody, particularly of masculine self-importance and self-aggrandizement, that runs so boldly through her writings may also reflect such painful experiences with James. Her pleasure in the confusions and evasions with her father in her adolescence, and later with Mr. Crisp over the authorship of *Evelina,* reverses this helpless childhood situation.

ADOLESCENCE

Fanny's adolescence comes to light spontaneously, and with humor, pleasure, and feeling, in her adolescent diary (Burney, 1768–78). Hers was a prolonged adolescence, necessary if she was to develop her literary talent and differentiate herself from her sisters and stepsisters who married early. Her intense relationship with her father was *very* slowly attenuated and modified through identification with his literary ambitions and skills, through humor and satire to diminish her awesome love for and dread of him, and through intellectually provocative relationships with young men in which she interested them and successfully competed with her older sister. Her appreciation of her father's responsiveness to her and her full responsiveness in return are touching and unwavering, and were characteristic of her throughout her long life of loving and being loved.

Family dramas related to her writing appear, time and again, in her adolescent diary. When she was 15, her father remarried, and at this time Fanny burned all her writings, including a precursor to *Evelina,* based on a romance of Evelina's parents. Dr. Burney's marriage was kept secret from his new mother-in-law, who objected to him as a suitor for her daughter because his income was too modest. When Fanny's stepmother became pregnant and moved into the Burney home and the secret was out, Fanny began her diary. On one occasion she is overcome with trepidation when her parents find her diary on her father's piano, but on she goes. Undaunted by her father's teasing and despite a gentle caution from an old family friend, Dolly Young, about the dangers of such personal, private musings, she insists stubbornly on continuing.

A charming vignette from her diary illustrates how she involves her father in her writing. At 17, Fanny sent a poem in a letter to her father at Oxford when he received his doctorate in music. Full of love, humor, and satiric references to his lack of doctorly corpulence, the poem follows a family tradition of responding to separation by creative writing.

And here is her reaction to her father's response (Burney, 1768–78):

> Charles appeared curious, I was horridly ashamed. "What do you think," continued papa, "do you know this abominable girl calls me Dr. Last?"—Charles and Hetty both laughed, and papa took up the letter, and holding it out to me said—"Come, do me the favour of reading this!"—I would fain have torn it, but papa drew it back, and was going to read it—I beg'd him not—but *in vain,* and so I ran out of the room. But, to own the truth, my curiosity prevailed so far that I could not forbear running downstairs again with more speed than I ran up, and into the next room, where I found . . . by papa's voice and manner that he did not appear displeased—though he half affected to be so—he read it loud—. . . . "I assure you" said papa, "'tis very good stuff! I read it to Mrs. Playdel, and she was much pleased—particularly with the last stanza—and to one or two of my new Oxford friends at breakfast, and we had a very hearty laugh—"
>
> This was enough—I ran once more upstairs and lighter than a feather felt my heart!
>
> ....
>
> O—but one thing has very much vexed me—my papa has read my nonsense to Mrs. Skinner, an intimate acquaintance and a very clever woman, and she insisted on having a copy which papa desired me to write—I was horrid mad, and beg'd most earnestly to be excused, for such trash, however it may serve to read at the moment, must be shocking a second time; but papa would take no denial—"It's very sufficient," said he, "for the occasion, and for your age." However, I am as much mortified at doing this, as if my first fear had been verified, for I cannot at all relish being thus exposed to a deliberate examination. . . .
>
> Once more I take up a pen to write to my Journal, which I thought I never again should do [1:60f.].

Here is the same horrid shame as in her childhood, now

associated with an inhibition of reading her work aloud, followed by relief and a heart as light as a feather. Her curiosity
about her father's response wins out, but mortification recurs
when her poem is shown to Mrs. Skinner, "an intimate acquaintance and a very clever woman." Temporarily she interrupts
her diary writing. Her adolescent need to separate from her
father alternates with the pain of feeling replaced and betrayed
by his interest in another woman at the time of his remarriage.
The experience becomes a "deliberate examination," perhaps
reinforced by her recent Confirmation (Hemlow, 1958, p. 28).
Years later, at the time of her son's Confirmation, she would
write her brother, Charles (Hemlow, 1958):

> I remember well that, when I was preparing . . . I had such an
> idea I should undergo an examination, & I was so fearful of
> some *wry* question that might discountenance me, That I learnt
> nearly the whole common prayer Book by heart!— Besides
> reading the Bible *quite through* 3 times! I was so indefatigable, I
> rose to nothing else; & never went to rest while I could procure
> light for my labours. Alex would not be much led to imitate
> me, if he knew that, after all this hard work—the fat clumsy
> stumpy worthy Bishop of Norwich clapt his hand upon my
> head, & off it, as fast as he possibly could, & never made a
> single interrogatory, nor uttered a single doubt or demur upon
> my fitness or unfitness for this blessing [p. 29].

The "deliberate examination" suggests a link to her experience
with James and other intellectual failures, and, predictably, the
Bishop is portrayed as a fool.

Young Adulthood

Fanny Burney says she was busy composing in her imagination
the scenes of *Evelina* from the time she burned its predecessors
until she actually began writing it in her early 20s. She loved the
imaginative effort, but it was hard to find the time and privacy
for the actual writing. She made it a rule never to "indulge" in
reading or writing early in the day. She did her needlework in
the mornings to avoid her stepmother's criticism and thereby
held her "Hobby Horse" in limits. Unfortunately, her step-

mother, Elizabeth, became increasingly jealous and suspicious of all the children's activities, so Fanny kept her writing to herself. Furthermore, Elizabeth was faced with the first Mrs. Burney's translation of Maupertuis's Astronomy Letter accompanying Dr. Burney's publication of an *Abridged History of Comets*.[1] For Fanny to write a novel at this time would have overburdened her stepmother, already taxed by sharing Dr. Burney. But, when it did appear, *Evelina* included a satiric rejection of her stepmother's coarseness and wildness.

So Fanny wrote her novel in secret and published it with the help of Charles and Susan, her younger sister. She had her father's approval, though he had not seen it and believed that nothing would come from her "sport." In the *Memoirs* she gives center stage to two experiences at this point. In the first, *Evelina* is read aloud by Hetty to a gathering at Mr. Crisp's home (Arblay, 1832):

> With flying colours, therefore, the book went off, not only with the easy social circle, but with Mr. Crisp himself; and without the most remote suspicion that the author was in the midst of the audience; a circumstance that made the whole perusal seem to that author the most pleasant of comedies, from the innumerable whimsical incidents to which it gave rise, alike in panegyrics and in criticisms, which alternately, and most innocently, were often addressed to herself; and accompanied with demands of her opinions, that forced her to perplexing evasions, productive of the most ludicrous confusion, though of the highest inward diversion [2:138f.].

Fanny turned first, as always, to Mr. Crisp as an intermediary between her family and the public, for an opinion about her novel. But how carefully modulated it was, to turn a childhood passive and painful experience into an active source of pleasure, with no one badly hurt by the hoax. Where earlier she sought to hide her shame for her intellectual deficits, now she revels in keeping a secret. Fanny is the playful trickster, Mr. Crisp the unsuspecting victim. But Hetty must read, not Fanny, who could never read her own works aloud (Arblay, 1904–05):

1. With obvious pleasure, in the *Memoirs*, Fanny describes her father "appearing before the public by the side of his Esther" (1:216).

> I dared not trust my voice with the little introductory ode [to her father], for as *that* is no romance, but the sincere effusion of my heart, I could as soon read aloud my own letters, written in my own name and character: I therefore skipped it. . . . Indeed, I have since heartily repented that I read *any* of the book to him [Mr. Crisp] for I found it a much more awkward thing than I had expected: my voice quite faltered when I began it which, however, I passed off for the effect of remaining weakness of the lungs; and in short, from an invincible embarrassment, which I could not for a page together repress, the book, by my reading, lost all manner of spirit [1:29f.].

The *Memoirs* continue with a report of her first meeting with her father, after he read her novel. She had already heard, in a letter from her sister, Susan, that he was greatly pleased with it (Burney, 1768–1778, Vol. 2, p. 222). Her dread focuses on the novel's ode of dedication to him, in which she claims her incapacity to extol sufficiently her father's numerous virtues and worth (Arblay, 1832):

> Yet, earnestly as she coveted his sight, she felt almost afraid, and quite ashamed, to be alone with him, from her doubts how he might accept her versified dedication.
> She held back, therefore, from any *tête-à-tête* till he sent for her. . . . But there, when he had shut the door, with a significant smile, that told her what was coming, and gave a glow to her very forehead from anxious confusion, he gently said, 'I have read your book, Fanny!—but you need not blush at it—it is full of merit—it is, really,—extraordinary!'
> She fell upon his neck with heart-throbbing emotion; and he folded her in his arms so tenderly, that she sobbed upon his shoulder; so moved was she by his precious approbation. But she soon recovered to a gayer pleasure—a pleasure more like his own; . . . She had written the little book, like innumerable of its predecessors that she had burnt, simply for her private recreation. She had printed it for a frolic, to see how a production of her own would figure in that author-like form [2:144f.].

Fanny becomes startled and frightened, once again, at her father's request to tell Dr. Johnson's Mrs. Thrale of his daughter's authorship. She is reassured only and "ashamed to demur" because of his promise not to reveal the secret unless Mrs. Thrale is pleased with the book.

DISCUSSION

Though Fanny was always shy and inhibited in public, her passion for anonymity and her dread, embarrassment, and confusion appear specially intense in triangular relationships. She seems to be greatly influenced by persistent oedipal fantasies and conflicts. Her ecstasy over her father's love and approval of her writing is tempered by concern for restrictions and envious criticism, especially from her stepmother, from whom the secret of *Evelina*'s authorship is kept much longer. Secrets, and the excitement they entail, abound in the Burney family and throughout Fanny's writings. The atmosphere of the household no doubt contributed to Fanny Burney's love of secrets, with all their meanings.

It is always difficult to know and to state precisely how a learning disability may interact with oedipal and preoedipal conflicts in relationships. It seems, however, that for Fanny Burney the failure in learning and the humiliation that followed from it linked up with the sense of oedipal failure and inadequacy. At the same time, especially after the death of her mother, Fanny found her father to be the safest port in a stormy sea. Not unusually, this combination led to inner conflicts and complex identifications, largely associated with writing and with authorship.

Remarkable woman that she was, Fanny Burney managed not only to adjust to her difficulties; she mastered them creatively. The extraordinary support from her mother and then from her father enabled her to follow the pace and style she needed. With her father's support she rejected all the well-intentioned advice (including the recommendations of her beloved Mr. Crisp) for early marriage. With the publication of *Evelina* and her ultimate acknowledgment of authorship she became a celebrity and remained so. Subsequently, as a member of the Queen's household, she literally walked and talked with kings. Relatively late she married and became a mother, continuing as a writer throughout her life. With success on all these fronts, she remained, however, susceptible in some degree to the earlier conflicts and their associated fantasies and images. An incident from her later life reflects these enduring characteristics.

The visit from Sir Walter Scott at 55 to the 74-year-old widowed Madame d'Arblay, which led her to write the section of the *Memoirs of Doctor Burney* that chronicles her literary development from dyslexic childhood to celebrated authorship, itself follows the pattern of a lifetime. Here is Fanny Burney's account of the visit from the *Memoirs:*

> . . . she is tempted to disclose, in self-defence—a proud self-defence!—of this personal obtrusion, the LIVING names of Sir Walter Scott and Mr. Rogers, who, in a visit with which they favoured her in the year 1826, repeated some of the fabrications to which this mystery of her early life still gave rise; and condescended to solicit a recital of the real history of Evelina's *Entrance into the World.*
>
> This she instantly communicated; though so incoherently, from the embarrassment of the subject, and its long absence from her thoughts, that, having since collected documents to refresh her memory, she ventures, in gratefully dedicating the little incident to these Illustrious Inquisitors, to insert its details in these memoirs—to which, parentally, it in fact belongs.†

---

†The first volume of this work was nearly printed, when the Editor had the grief of hearing that Sir Walter Scott was no more. In the general sorrow that his loss has spread throughout the British Empire, she presumes not to speak of her own: but she cannot persuade herself to annul the little tribute, by which she had meant to demonstrate to him her sense of the vivacity with which he had sought out her dwelling; invited her to the hospitality of his daughters at Abbotsford; and courteously, nay, eagerly, offered to do the honours of Scotland to her himself, from that celebrated abode.

In a subsequent visit with which he honoured and delighted her in the following year, she produced to him the scraps of documents and fragments which she had collected from ancient diaries and letters, in consequence of his inquiries. Pleased he looked; but told her that what already she had related, already—to use his own word—he had "noted;" adding, "And most particularly, I have not forgotten your mulberry tree!"

This little history, however, was so appropriately his own, and was written so expressly with a view to its dedication, that still, with veneration—though with sadness instead of gladness—she leaves the brief exordium of her intended homage in its original state [2:121ff.].

This little paragraph and its sad explanatory footnote reveal the persistent echoes of the old sequence: admiration, excitement, embarrassment, dread, confusion, the sense of incompetence and sadistic examination, and subsequent mastery through writing. She had felt Scott's vivacity and generosity, to which she wished to respond with a "little tribute" in the form of a collection of scraps and fragments to document the "real" history of *Evelina*. In between came a startle reaction, a feeling of ignorance, embarrassment, and a sense of incoherence. She makes a joking reference to Scott and Rogers as "Inquisitors." Scott apparently was not aware of incoherence or embarrassment to judge from what he "noted." Here is Sir Walter Scott's description from his diaries of the visit to Fanny Burney (Lockhart, 1838):

November 1826—Was introduced by Rogers to Mad. D'Arblay, the celebrated authoress of Evelina and Cecilia,—an elderly lady, with no remains of personal beauty, but with a simple and gentle manner, a pleasing expression of countenance, and apparently quick feelings. She told me she had wished to see two persons—myself, of course, being one, the other George Canning. This was really a compliment to be pleased with—a nice little handsome pat of butter made up by a neat-handed Phillis of a dairy-maid, instead of the grease, fit only for cartwheels, which one is dosed with by the pound.

Mad. D'Arblay told us that the common story of Dr. Burney, her father, having brought home her own first work, and recommended it to her perusal, was erroneous. Her father was in the secret of Evelina being printed. But the following circumstances may have given rise to the story:—Dr. Burney was at Streatham soon after the publication, where he found Mrs. Thrale recovering from her confinement, low at the moment, and out of spirits. While they were talking together, Johnson, who sat beside in a kind of reverie, suddenly broke out—"You should read this new work, Madam—you should read Evelina; every one says it is excellent, and they are right." The delighted father obtained a commission from Mrs. Thrale to purchase his daughter's work, and retired the happiest of men. Mad. D'Arblay said she was wild with joy at this decisive evidence of her literary success, and that she could only give vent to her rapture by dancing and skipping round a mulberry-tree in the garden. She was very young at this time. I trust I shall see this lady again [6:274f.].

CONCLUSION

The extraordinary circumstances that brought together childhood dyslexia, a strongly supportive environment, and enormous literary talent in Fanny Burney provide a serendipitous
opportunity for a personal account of the lifelong vicissitudes
of her reading disability. The early experience of shame and
intellectual disgrace and the passion to write are interwoven
with conflicts over loving and public display. The persistent
anticipation of failure appears, in Fanny Burney's case, tied to
the love of men and the wish to be found interesting by them. It
seems to date to her oedipal relationships and, especially, to her
relationship with her much-admired older brother, James.

It is both obvious and curious that Fanny Burney's great
pleasure, satisfaction, and public achievement in writing do not
erase the early failure to read and write. Success, whether in the
area of earlier failure or in some other area, may enormously
strengthen self-esteem and may contribute indirectly to mastery of conflicts. For Fanny Burney writing served, among
other purposes, as a means of communication, as a means of
identification, as a means of overcoming inhibitions in seeking
admiration, and as a means of expression closely connected to
mourning and to subsequent reorganization. The early experiences of inadequacy and the associated affective reactions remained lifelong, however, and though much muted still played
their part when Scott brought *Evelina* and the secrets back.

In traversing the path from shame, guilt, and defectiveness
in reading and writing to pleasure in open acknowledgment of
her writing, Fanny Burney shows the persistent characteristics
of a keen observer, an outsider, not "personally guided" by
mother or father. She wrote in secret. Could these characteristics reflect an early or innate propensity to observe, listen, and
learn at a distance, as well as a response to the dangers of
regression in ego functions when overexcited? It is not possible
to distinguish how much the tendency to regression is a liability
from the early anlage of her dyslexia and how much is the
traumatic residue from the dyslexia. It is also not possible to
determine whether her exceptional auditory memory originated with endowment and early parental stimulation or whether

it developed in compensation for the failure to be able to read. The writings of Fanny Burney do, however, permit us to see the interplay of cognitive capacities and object relationships in successive developmental phases of her life.[2]

BIBLIOGRAPHY

ARBLAY, F. B. D' (1832), *Memoirs of Doctor Burney*, 3 vols. London: Edward Moxon.
_____ (1904–05), *Diary and Letters of Madame D'Arblay* (1778–1840), 6 vols., ed. A. Dobson. London: Macmillan.
BENDER, L. (1958), Problems in conceptualization and communication in children with developmental dyslexia. In *Psychopathology of Communication*, ed. P. H. Hoch & J. Zubin. New York: Grune & Stratton, pp. 155–176.
BERGER, M. & KENNEDY, H. (1975), Pseudobackwardness in children. *Psychoanal. Study Child*, 30:279–306.
BLANCHARD, P. (1946), Psychoanalytic contributions to the problems of reading disabilities. *Psychoanal. Study Child*, 2:163–187.
BRYANT, K. N. (1964), Some clinical notes on reading disability. *Bull. Menninger Clin.*, 28:323–338.
BURNEY, F. (1768–78), *The Early Diary of Frances Burney 1768–1778*, 2 vols., ed. A. R. Ellis. Freeport, N.Y.: Books for Libraries Press, 1971.
_____ (1778), *Evelina*. London: Oxford Univ. Press, 1968.
BUXBAUM, E. (1964), The parents' role in the etiology of learning disabilities. *Psychoanal. Study Child*, 19:421–447.
CRITCHLEY, M. (1964), *Developmental Dyslexia*. London: Heinemann, pp. 81–89.
DE HIRSCH, K. (1975), Language deficits in children with development lags. *Psychoanal. Study Child*, 30:95–126.
EISENBERG, L. (1975), Psychiatric aspects of language disability. In *Reading, Perception and Language*, ed. D. Duane & M. Rawson. Baltimore: York Press, pp. 215–229.
HELLMAN, I. (1954), Some observations on mothers of children with intellectual inhibitions. *Psychoanal. Study Child*, 9:259–273.
HEMLOW, J. (1958), *The History of Fanny Burney*. Oxford: Clarendon Press.
KLEIN, C. L. (1978), Developmental dyslexia in adolescents. *Bull. Orton Soc.*, 28:160–174.
LOCKHART, J. G. (1838), *Memoirs of the Life of Sir Walter Scott, Bart.*, 7 vols. Philadelphia: Carey, Lea, & Blanchard.

2. As I became familiar with Fanny Burney by reading her diaries, I was impressed by the similarity between her and Marianne Kris whom this volume honors. Both overcame childhood intellectual difficulties, developing characters of unusual integrity, personal responsiveness, and independent initiative, enabling them to become pioneers with their respective talents.

MAHLER, M. S. (1942), Pseudoimbecility. *Psychoanal. Q.*, 11:149–164.

NEWMAN, C. J., DEMBER, C. F., & KRUG, O. (1973), "He can but he won't." *Psychoanal. Study Child*, 28:83–129.

PEARSON, G. H. J. (1952), A survey of learning difficulties in children. *Psychoanal. Study Child*, 7:322–386.

ROSEN, V. H. (1955), Strephosymbolia. *Psychoanal. Study Child*, 10:83–99.

SILVER, L. (1974), Emotional and social problems of children with developmental disabilities. In *Handbook on Learning Disabilities*, ed. R. E. Weber. Englewood Cliffs, N.J.: Prentice-Hall, pp. 97–120.

THOMPSON, L. (1966), *Reading Disability*. Springfield, Ill.: Thomas, pp. 112–137.

WALSH, M. N. (1966), Strephosymbolia reconsidered. *Int. J. Psychoanal.*, 48:584–595.

WATSON, B. U., WATSON, C. S., & FREDD, R. (1982), Follow-up studies of specific reading disability. *J. Amer. Acad. Child Psychiat.*, 21:376–382.

WEIL, A. P. (1977), Learning disturbances with special consideration of dyslexia. In *Issues in Child Mental Health*, 5:52–66.

Bibliographical Note

S. E.   *The Standard Edition of the Complete Psychological Works of Sigmund Freud,* 24 volumes, translated and edited by James Strachey. London: Hogarth Press and the Institute of Psycho-Analysis, 1953–1974.

W.   *The Writings of Anna Freud,* 8 volumes. New York: International Universities Press, 1968–1981.

Index

Anger
absence of, 542
see also Aggression, Rage
Animal, 288, 392, 432, 471–72, 501–16,
619
Anna O., 62, 71, 79, 90
Anniversary reactions, 301
Anorexia, 294, 513
Anthony, E. J., 163, 191, 306, 378–79,
546
Anticipation, 175–77, 186, 237, 284,
313, 375
of danger, 211, 218–19, 225–30
Anxiety, 54, 120–21, 174, 524–25, 528,
532–35, 631
attack, 323, 392
concerning death, 214, 295, 407,
552–66
8-month, 129; *see also* Stranger anxiety
and equilibrium disturbances, 569–74
in infant, 243–54
in mute child, 409–17
sexual, 429–38, 514–16, 532–33
signal, 211, 214–15, 388
situation, 325, 327, 512–13
tolerance, 578
see also Danger, Fear, Phobia
Apathy, 248, 254
Apfel-Savitz, R., 217, 231
Arblay, F. B., *see* Burney, F.
Arend, R., 183, 190
Aristotle, 18, 20, 22–23
Arlow, J. A., 305–06, 383, 387–89, 400,
402, 439, 458, 477
Arnold, M. B., 183, 187–88
Arnold, W., 189
Arousal, 170–72, 258
Asher, H., 79, 107
Assessment, 134
developmental, *see* Developmental
testing
diagnostic, 579, 583–84, 591, 596–97
Assimilation, 174
Asthma, 223
Attachment, 183, 202, 226, 236, 249,
261, 271, 283, 332, 335, 343, 385,
387, 401, 527, 589, 592
preoedipal, to mother, 405–27
Attack, sexual, 621, 624
Attention, 170–71, 198, 242, 270
free-floating, 590
Autism, 201
Autistic phase, 197
Autoerotism, 399, 512
Automatisms, 98
Avoidance, 253, 329, 582, 585, 597, 609

of physical contact, 236–46, 621–22
see also Object, Touching
Axelrad, S., 197–98, 206

Bach, S., 275
Bachrach, A., 136
Bain, T. N., 623, 634
Balint, M., 302, 306
Bandler, L. S., 224, 226 27, 231
Bank, S. P., 293, 304, 306
Banks, J. H., 175, 187
Barber, V., 354, 378
Barlow, D., 78–79, 108
Barlow, G., 190
Barnes, M. J., 300, 306
Basch, M. F., 179, 187, 542, 546
Basch, S. H., 298, 306
Battin-Mahon, D., 459–79
Beating fantasy, 287–88
Bed wetting, 606–08
Begley, S., 523, 546
Behavior
exploratory, 218–21, 225–26, 259
impulsive, 209–30
organization of, 521–22
regressive, 343
social, 238–53, 262–68
stimulus-seeking, 201–05
Bell, S., 171, 186
Bellak, L., 198
Beltramini, A., 562, 567
Bender, L., 637, 651
Benedek, T., 163, 354, 378–79
Benjamin, J. D., 193, 195–98, 203, 205
Bergen, E., 602, 616
Berger, M., 399, 401–02, 637, 651
Bergin, A., 109
Bergman, A., 132–33, 138, 167–68,
174, 183, 190, 272, 277, 302, 308,
372, 377, 379, 580, 600
Bergman, P., 195, 201, 206
Bergmann, T., 298, 306
Berman, L. E. A., 301, 306
Bertalanffy, L. von, 170, 187
Bettelheim, B., 55, 58
Bibring, G. L., 354–55, 377–78
Biller, H. B., 259, 275
Binger, C. M., 298, 306
Biological principles, 165, 169–73, 179, 186
Biology, 20, 23, 34, 124, 160, 169–73,
186, 194, 258–59, 270
see also Neurobiology
Birth, 605, 614, 618
of hero, 149
psychological, 132
see also Pregnancy, Siblings

preoccupation with, 214, 295, 407,
552–66
reaction to, 10–13, 551–63, 603–05
of sibling, 11, 225, 287, 300–02
Death instinct, 212, 214
Death wishes, 286–88, 386
Decarié, T. G., 170, 187
Defense, 97, 121, 127, 129, 563–64
and adoption, 142–44
and affective disturbance, 520–46
and aggression, 227, 236–37
anal, 497
conflict, 446–48, 456
confusion as, 464
development, 123, 253, 384
interpretation, 85, 531, 538–39, 548
in latency child, 483–98
against passivity, 467
and resistance, 578–79
and screen memory, 466–77
and sibling rivalry, 317, 320–21,
325–26, 329
and stimulus barrier, 195–97, 202–05
see also specific defense mechanisms
Deficiency disorders, 129, 133
de Hirsch, K., 637, 651
Delinquency, 578
Delusion, 587
Dember, C. F., 637, 652
Dement, W., 200, 207
Demos, V., 219
Denial, 144, 152, 235, 298, 384, 414,
449, 468, 485, 493, 495–96, 502,
504–05, 565, 615
Dependence, 391, 448–49, 467, 507,
516, 528, 581, 592
to self-reliance, 134, 388, 391
Depletion, 225–26, 230
Depression, 11–12, 130, 151, 154–55,
212, 230, 268, 301, 431, 445, 468,
569, 582, 591
in child, 243–45, 248, 254–55, 368,
407, 470, 496
chronic, 605–06, 609–10, 613–14,
619, 634
in father, 525
in mother, 243–45, 249, 368, 395,
466, 482, 486
tolerance, 591
Deprivation, 97, 170, 281, 323
maternal, 233–55, 468
Despair, 248, 254
Determinism, 19
Deutsch, H., 143, 148, 163, 426, 428,
461, 477

Development
arrest in, 391–94, 400–01
autonomous, 124, 132
biological principles, 169–73, 179–80,
186
concept of, and technique, 113–36
continuity, 165, 178–80
decline in, 239–55
delayed, 385
deviations, 391–94, 579
discontinuity, 116, 126
disharmony, 385, 387–89, 394–98
fetal, 199–200
impact of siblings on, 325–51
normal, 281, 311–13, 385–86
organizers, 129, 177, 271
phase dominance, 320, 339
phases: 115–22, 126–28, 130–32,
136; interdependence of, 384–85;
and pathogenesis, 383–88; *see also*
specific phases
polarities, 173–86
primary functional phase, 391
principles, 173–79, 186
role of parent-child relation in, 130–32
self-righting tendencies, 170
transformations, 115–17, 126–27,
170, 179
undifferentiated phase, 121–23, 129
uneven, 116, 129, 245, 253–55,
387–88
see also Maturation
Developmental defects, 387, 391–94
Developmental dissolution, 401
Developmental disturbance, 390–402
Developmental lines
of anxiety, 327–29
of body management, 216–17, 388,
395–98
concept, 133–34
egocentricity to companionship, 394
of object relations, 134, 391–94
regression on, 564
Developmental point of view, 114–15,
117, 461, 579
Developmental psychology, 165–92,
233–34
Developmental testing, 236–52, 260,
262, 266
Diabetes, 570–73
Differentiation, 114, 123–24, 126–28,
131–32, 328, 334, 581
external and internal, 328, 384
object and self, 127, 131, 134,
174–76, 406

168, 215, 297, 316, 387–88, 398, 502
defective, 227
and development, 126–29, 204–05, 213, 239–42, 248–49, 255, 570
sexual, 581; *see also* Puberty
Maury, L. F. A., 27
Mayman, M., 109
Mead, G. H., 174–75, 190
Medea complex, 295
Meissner, W. W., 114, 139, 228, 231
Meltzoff, A. N., 178, 190
Memory, 12–13, 176–78, 186, 253, 392, 429, 446, 522, 537
    childhood, 445, 453–54, 460–62, 467, 469–70, 504–07, 534–35, 541, 585–87, 613, 617, 630
    compliance, 474
    distortion, 466–68, 474, 586–87
    fallibility, 63, 75, 87, 93–94
    preoedipal, 464–65
    recognition vs. evocative, 471
    recovery, 71, 74–75, 89
    and transference, 453–54
    see also Screen memory
Menning, B., 146, 163
Menninger, K. A., 212, 230
Menopause, 11–12, 570
Menstruation, 432–33, 436, 505, 514, 570
Metaphor, 575
    Freud's use of, 17–58
    universal, 287
Metcalf, D. R., 203, 206
Micropsia, 519–25, 534–35, 537
Middleton, J., 602, 616
Mill, J. S., 107
Mind, theory of, 18, 30, 37–58, 441
Mintz, J., 79, 90, 101, 109
Mintz, N., 224, 226–27, 231
Mirroring, 334
    parental, 178–79
Money, J., 168, 190
Money, withholding of, 152, 154
Mood, 641
    basic, 133
Moodiness, 584, 596
Moore, M. K., 178, 190
Moran, G., 389
Morris, 269, 276
Mother
    and daughter, relation, 154–58, 405–27, 524–46, 584–89, 596
    depletion state in, 225–26
    dishonest, 606–15
    disidentification with, 271

emotional availability, 183–86
facilitating, 127, 130
failing to protect child, 218, 225–26
good enough, 214–15, 264, 426
intrusive, 606–15
as pathogenic agent, 383, 385–86
phobic, 525
preoedipal, 592
relinquishing nurturing, 270
revival of sibling experience in, 353–71
sadistic impulses of, 236–49
seductive, 464–65
unable to separate, 610, 613
unempathic, 385–86, 562
wish for boy, 235
see also Death, Depression, Parent
Mother-child relation
    disturbed, 234–55, 358–69, 399–401
    early, 170–73, 175–79, 214–15, 225–26, 259, 383–84, 524–25, 532, 535–37, 545–46
    and sibling relations, 286–87, 292–93, 313–14, 317, 325–27, 330, 332, 338–48
    unity, 134, 197, 384, 388
Mothering, deficits in, 235–55
Motor development, 127, 171, 176, 260–66, 273
    disturbed, 235–52
    precocious, 218, 225–26
Mourning, 9–13, 287, 446–48, 502, 563, 609, 621, 650
Mouth-hand contact, 237–39
    aggressive, 240
Murphy, G., 114, 136, 138
Murphy, L. B., 251, 255
Murray, J. A., 439–40, 451, 458
Musatti, C. L., 301, 308
Mutism, elective, 407–26
Muybridge, E., 31
Muzio, J., 200, 207
Myelinization, 203
Myers, W. A., 519–21, 524, 538, 546
Myth, of descent, 149–50

Nagera, H., 295, 308, 406, 428
Narcissism, 211, 298, 384, 439–41, 457, 514–15, 547, 582
    familial, 147–62
    see also Personality, narcissistic
Narcissistic injury, 143, 148–52, 154, 162, 406, 423–27, 436, 440, 530, 562
Narcissistic phenomena, and free association, 439–57